Infective Endocarditis

INFECTIOUS DISEASE AND THERAPY

Series Editor

Burke A. Cunha

Winthrop-University Hospital
Mineola, and
State University of New York School of Medicine
Stony Brook, New York

Infective Endocarditis

Management in the Era of Intravascular Devices

edited by

John L. Brusch
Cambridge Health Alliance
Cambridge, Massachusetts, U.S.A.

informa
healthcare

New York   London

Informa Healthcare USA, Inc.
270 Madison Avenue
New York, NY 10016

© 2007 by Informa Healthcare USA, Inc.
Informa Healthcare is an Informa business

No claim to original U.S. Government works
Printed in the United States of America on acid-free paper
10 9 8 7 6 5 4 3 2 1

International Standard Book Number-10: 0-8493-7097-3 (Hardcover)
International Standard Book Number-13: 978-0-8493-7097-7 (Hardcover)

Library of Congress Cataloging-in-Publication Data

Brusch, John L.
    Infective endocarditis : management in the era of intravascular devices / John L. Brusch.
        p. ; cm. -- (Infectious disease and therapy ; v. 41)
    Includes bibliographical references and index.
    ISBN-13: 978-0-8493-7097-7 (hardcover : alk. paper)
    ISBN-10: 0-8493-7097-3 (hardcover : alk. paper)
    1. Infective endocarditis--Treatment. 2. Cardiovascular instruments, Implanted. I. Title. II. Series.
    [DNLM: 1. Endocarditis, Bacterial. 2. Defibrillators, Implantable--adverse effects. 3. Heart Catheterization--adverse effects. 4. Heart Valve Prosthesis--adverse effects. W1 IN406HMN v.41 2007 / WG 285 B912i 2007]

RC685.E5B78 2007
616.1'106--dc22   2006101797

Visit the Informa Web site at
www.informa.com

and the Informa Healthcare Web site at
www.informahealthcare.com

This book is dedicated to my beloved wife,
Patricia Brusch, whose support makes
all things possible. She is my heart and soul.

To my children Amy Claire, Meaghan, and
Patrick, who have accomplished so much
at an early age.

A special acknowledgment of my gratitude
for the prodigious efforts of my friend,
Fred Centanni, who ensured that the layout of the book and
the tables and figures are of the highest quality.
He has become a virtual author.

Preface

My experience with infective endocarditis extends back to my third year in medical school when I was assigned to present a case on endocarditis on teaching rounds to Dr. Louis Weinstein the next day. To prepare, I read Dr. Weinstein's three-part *New England Journal of Medicine* article, "Infective Endocarditis in the Antibiotic Era." Because of the lateness of the hour and the encyclopedic nature of Dr. Weinstein's review, the only thing I was able to comprehend was that I, a third-year medical student, was presenting to a world's expert on the subject. This unnerved me to the point that when I opened my mouth really nothing came out. Dr. Weinstein calmed me down and I managed to get through the presentation. Despite this less than auspicious beginning, I persevered in learning as much as I could about endocarditis. I became one of Dr. Weinstein's fellows. In the early 1990s, he asked me to co-author a text on infective endocarditis. It was a wonderful opportunity. I had access to his case files, library, and his unique experience. His generation was the one that saw the disease before and after the advent of antibiotics. Our book (*Infective Endocarditis*, Oxford University Press, 1996) presented the disease from its first recognition through the onset of AIDS.

This new volume covers the recent profile of this disease. Classic subacute valvular infections still exist. However, *Staphylococcus aureus* and coagulase-negative staphylococci have become the prominent pathogens. They have assumed this prominence not simply because of their increasing resistance to antimicrobial agents. The major reason for the increasing involvement of the staphylococci in valvular infections is the proliferation of intravascular devices.

This realization inspired the title, *Management of Infective Endocarditis in the Era of Intravascular Devices*. Subacute disease is thoroughly presented. However, the dominant theme throughout this book is the ability of the staphylococci and other bacteria to infect prosthetic material. I have attempted to cover this topic from the perspective of the pathogenic properties of the organisms as well as of the defects in the defenses of the hosts who require these intravascular devices.

Because of the specialized nature of many of the areas to be covered, I called upon Drs. Cunha, Picard, Jassal, and Kradin to contribute their extensive knowledge and experience to the book. I am deeply grateful for their efforts.

John L. Brusch

Acknowledgment

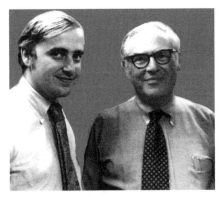

John L. Brusch, MD, and Louis Weinstein, MD

In grateful acknowledgment of the many contributions to the study of infective endocarditis made by the late Louis Weinstein, M.D.

Contents

Contributors

John L. Brusch Harvard Medical School and Department of Medicine and Infectious Disease Service, Cambridge Health Alliance, Cambridge, Massachusetts, U.S.A.

Burke A. Cunha Winthrop University Hospital, Mineola, New York, U.S.A.

Davinder S. Jassal Cardiac Ultrasound Laboratory, Division of Cardiology, Massachusetts General Hospital and Harvard Medical School, Boston, Massachusetts, U.S.A., and Bergen Cardiac Care Center, Division of Cardiology, St. Boniface General Hospital, Winnipeg, Manitoba, Canada

Richard L. Kradin Departments of Pathology and Medicine, Massachusetts General Hospital, Boston, Massachusetts, U.S.A.

Michael H. Picard Cardiac Ultrasound Laboratory, Division of Cardiology, Massachusetts General Hospital and Harvard Medical School, Boston, Massachusetts, U.S.A.

1 Epidemiology

John L. Brusch

Harvard Medical School and Department of Medicine and Infectious Disease Service, Cambridge Health Alliance, Cambridge, Massachusetts, U.S.A.

INCIDENCE

Infective endocarditis (IE) is an infection of the endocardium of one or more valves. Rarely, it may involve the mural endocardium. It currently is classified into one of the four major types: native valve endocarditis (NVE), prosthetic valve endocarditis (PVE), intravenous drug abuser IE (IVDA IE), and healthcare-associated IE (HCIE). Classically, this infection has been categorized as either acute or subacute. The clinical courses were quite different with the pathogens that were highly associated with one type or another. Acute IE was, and still is, a rapidly progressive disease that can be fatal in a few days. Without treatment, subacute IE may smolder for months or even longer than a year (Chapter 6). Until the 1980s, the vast majority of cases were subacute, caused by viridans streptococci. In this era of IE of intravascular devices (Table 1), there has been a dramatic reversal of this pattern. At times, the differences between these two may be blurred by indiscriminately prescribed antibiotic therapy. Infective endocarditis, caused by *Staphylococcus aureus*, may assume an indolent course when exposed to inadequate dosage regimens of antibiotics that are given on the basis of faulty diagnoses. This situation could be labeled as "muted endocarditis." Nonetheless, the clinical classification of acute and subacute disease remains useful, as it still retains a good amount of clinical predictive value.

An accurate rate of new cases of IE is difficult to determine. This is attributed partly to the intermittent courses of antibiotics given because of failure to make the correct diagnosis. The recognition of IE often may be very challenging, especially when its signs and symptoms are noncardiac. Five to 10 percent of the cases of IE have negative blood cultures. In the past, only postmortem examination reliably differentiated uncomplicated bacteremia from that caused by cardiac infection. The declining rate of autopsies has only worsened this situation. In 1981, von Reyn et al. published strict case definitions for diagnosing IE (1). The Duke Endocarditis Service combined echocardiographic findings with various clinical measures to improve the accuracy of diagnosis (2). These criteria have positive and negative predictive values of at least 92%. The International Collaboration on Endocarditis is an initiative to establish a global database of IE patients who have been studied with standard methodology (3).

Based on the studies conducted within the last 25 years, the incidence of IE throughout the world varies from 1.5/100,000 to 6/100,000 per population per year (4–7). There are marked variations in the incidence of IE among nations and even within a given country. This probably is related to the proportion of urban versus rural populations (8,9), and their differences in socioeconomic class and intravenous drug abuse.

In 1940, Hedley estimated that there were approximately 5000 cases of IE in the United States, at a rate of 4.2/100,000 per population per year (10). Overall, the

TABLE 1   The Eras of Infective Endocarditis

The preantibiotic era (1725–1943):
1885—William Osler presented the first comprehensive account in English of infective endocarditis
The antibiotic era (1943–1980s):
1966—Louis Weinstein presented an in-depth review of the pathophysiology, clinical presentation, diagnosis, and treatment of infective endocarditis
1980s—Infective endocarditis in the era of intravascular devices

availability of antibiotics does not appear to have made a significant decrease in the incidence of this disease (10,11). There might have been a transient decrease during the early days of antimicrobial therapy (12). This could be attributed to several factors, including (*i*) widespread use of antibiotics that decrease the rate of sustained bacteremia, originating from many types of extracardiac infections; (*ii*) antibiotic prophylaxis in patients with significant underlying heart disease; and (*iii*) admission of patients with endocardial infection to referral hospitals. The increase in the resistance of bacteria to various types of antibiotics and the increase in cardio-vascular surgery and intravascular devices have blunted this advantage. These same factors have changed the clinical profile of IE from a predominantly subacute disease to an acute one. Newsom reported that the incidence of IE had changed little since the 1930s (3.8/100,000 per population per year between 1950 and 1981) (13). Currently, there are approximately 2000 to 15,000 new cases of IE yearly in the United States (14).

The incidence and type of IE in any given hospital is dependent on the types of patients it serves (15,16). Institutions that have a large population of IVDA, congenital heart disease or patients with prosthetic valves, have a higher rate of IE than a community hospital. The IE owing to *S. aureus* occurs more often than those admitted to a community hospital, whereas enterococcal disease is cared for more frequently in tertiary-care hospitals (1).

AGE AND SEX

The age distribution of IE has changed considerably since the 1940s. This was formerly a disease of young adults. In 1920s, the patients were usually <34 years of age (17). The mean age of those with subacute IE has increased from 36 (1923) to 32 (1930s and 1940s) to 46 (1950s), and to 56 years (1960s) (18–20). The current median age is 58.0 (3). Gladstone and Rocco observed that the elderly are more susceptible to IE. Older patients present with more subtle clinical manifestations than younger ones to the degree that the correct diagnosis was missed in two-thirds of them early in the course of disease. They postulated that their vulnerability is related to a decrease in the activity of their immune system and to the dysfunction of the heart and other organs that marks the aging process (21). Other proposed causes of this "graying trend" include (22): (*i*) a heightened susceptibility of the endocardium to infection during a transient bacteremia because of an increase in calcific valvular disease; (*ii*) a marked increase in cardiac surgery and intravascular devices among the elderly; (*iii*) 67% of those with nosocomially acquired staphylo-coccal bacteremia are elderly compared with the 30% of those with community-acquired staphylococcal infections (23); (*iv*) almost complete disappearance of rheumatic fever and rheumatic heart disease (RHD) in the United States (24); (*v*) individuals with congenital heart disease live longer and often require valvular replacement; and (*vi*) people, in general, are living longer (25). In adults, the major exception to this aging pattern is IVDA IE. The median age of these patients is approximately 30 (26).

Pediatric IE is quite uncommon. Infective endocarditis accounts for 0.55 per 100,000 admissions to tertiary-care pediatric hospitals (27). As would be expected, most cardiac infections are attributed to congenital abnormalities in children more than two years of age. In the very young, pediatric IE more commonly occurs in the setting of normal cardiac structures, and is usually secondary to a catheter-related bloodstream infection (BSI) (28).

Infective endocarditis occurs at least twice as often in men as in women (11,26). This ratio increases to 9:1 in patients 50 to 60 years of age and to 6.5:1 in individuals 61 to 70 years of age. This sexual distribution generally is not dependent on the specific infecting organism. However, women <35 years of age are disproportionately involved in cases of enterococcal endocarditis (29).

PREDISPOSING CARDIAC LESIONS

Approximately 40% of cases of IE affect the mitral valve alone, and 5% to 36% affect the aortic valve alone. Infection of both of these valves occurs less often (30). The pulmonic valve is seldom infected. Cases of right-sided endocarditis occur primarily in IVDA and HCIE owing to intravascular lines.

Almost any structural lesion of the heart may give rise to IE as long as it can result in the formation of a sterile platelet/fibrin thrombus, the indispensable precursor of all types of IE (Chapter 5). The specific type of cardiac abnormality underlying a given case of IE is closely associated with certain characteristics of the patient (age, history of drug abuse, or immunosuppression) and the nature of the infecting organism. Bacteria, such as *Streptococcus viridans*, with a low invasive potential, opportunistically infects abnormal valves. *Staphylococcus aureus* has the ability to infect normal valvular structures. Cabell and Abutyn commented that "there are studies available to quantify the risk of developing IE for patients with specific cardiac conditions. It is more clear which conditions, when associated with active IE, are more likely to be associated with complications and death" (31). For certain cardiac conditions, the risk of developing IE is better established. In the case of mitral valve prolapse (MVP) with significant regurgitation, it is increased 10- to 100-fold (32), whereas for prosthetic valves and for patients with prior IE, the risk for valvular infection may be increased >100-fold (33,34).

Durack and Petersdorf (22) have concluded that the advent of antibiotics has made no change in the contribution of congenital heart disease to the development of IE. Overall, congenital heart disease is the underlying factor in 5% of adult IE. Bicuspid aortic valves may account for up to 20% of the cases of IE in individuals older than 60 years. Among congenital heart diseases, the tetralogy of Fallot exhibits the greatest incidence of IE. Even when surgically corrected, it remains a significant factor for the development of endocardial infection. Approximately 25% of tetral- ogy patients, who undergo an anastomotic correction develop infection at the surgical site. This is attributed to the turbulent blood flow at the point where the vessels are joined. Lesser, but still significant, risk factors for IE include coarctation of aorta, ventriculoseptal defect and bicuspid aortic valve. Secundum atrial septal defect and congenital pulmonic stenosis pose negligible risks for IE, probably because of the minimal pressure gradient across these lesions (35,36). The risk of congenital aortic stenosis becoming infected is directly proportional to the pressure gradient across the valve (37).

Although RHD has become a negligible predisposing factor for IE (38,39) in the developed world, it remains the largest cardiac risk factor for IE in the developing countries (50% of cases). The lifetime risk for patients with RHD to develop endocardial infection is 6% (39). The majority of cases of RHD IE occur in females (67% of cases), and involve the mitral valve (85% of cases).

Mitral valve prolapse accounts for up to 30% of cases of NVE. It has supplanted RHD as the chief underlying condition for the IE of younger patients (32,40,41). Mitral valve prolapse is found in approximately 5% of the population. It is inherited in an autosomal dominant fashion. It may be a part of a syndrome (von Willebrand's disease, ophthalmoplegia, and distinctive female habitus) that is associated with an abnormality of chromosome 16p (42). Cases of MVP that do not exhibit any significant regurgitation are at little increased risk of IE (43). Thickened anterior mitral leaflets and male sex >45 years of age are additive risk factors for the development of IE in MVP (40,44). On the whole, the cases of IE of MVP have relatively lower rates of morbidity and mortality (45) than do other types of valvular infection.

The term degenerative cardiac lesions represents a wide range of entities, including degenerative valvular disease (DVD), calcified mitral annulus, and atherosclerotic calcifications of the endocardium. They all have in common a roughened endocardium that enhances thrombus formation. Often there is no significant pressure gradient across these valves (40,46–48). If a murmur is present, it usually is classified as innocent. Thirty-three to fifty percent of people >60 years of age have evidence of wear-and-tear aortic valve disease. Degenerative valvular disease accounts for approximately 50% of IE in elderly patients (25). It coexists with a number of other significant medical conditions in >50% of patients. These include diabetes mellitus, renal failure, current artery disease and chronic lung disease. Their presence accounts for the increased fatality rates in these patients.

An underappreciated predisposing cardiac lesion for IE is asymmetric septal hypertrophy. The risk of developing IE is directly related to the level of obstruction—the higher the peak pressure, the greater the chance of infection (49,50). The lifetime risk of developing IE in these patients is 5%. Most cases involve the mitral valve, and rarely the aortic valve. This distribution is attributed either to displacement of the anterior leaflet of the mitral valve by the abnormal contractions of the septum or by the jet stream affecting the aortic leaflets distal to the obstruction. *Streptococcus viridans* is the causative organism in 75% of cases. The outcomes of valvular infection are worse among the one-third of patients who clinically develop a new murmur.

Infective endocarditis occurs in approximately 5% to 10% of prosthetic valves (51). The greatest risk of infection occurs within two months of implantation (early PVE). Initially, mechanical prosthetic valves were most vulnerable. With time, the rate of infection of bioprosthetic valves equals or exceeds that of mechanical ones. After the first year, the rate of infection averages about 0.3%. Over time, the process of endothelialization partially protects prosthetic valves from being infected by transient bacteremias. However, it is important to emphasize that no matter how old the valve is, it will always be at some risk (52). Prosthetic valve endocarditis accounts for 7% of the total cases of IE (8,14). Similar in nature to PVE is IE of pacemakers and other intracardiac devices (53). Most become infected within a few months of implantation.

EXTRACARDIAC PREDISPOSING FACTORS

The incidence of IE in IVDA ranges from 1% to 5% per year (54). Those who inject cocaine are at the highest risk of developing valvular infection (55). Intravenous drug abuser IE might be decreasing in certain populations because of the increased use of sterile needles and syringes in an effort to decrease HIV transmission (56). Intravenous drug abuser IE is a disease of urban areas with few cases seen in rural ones. The male to female ratio is 9:1 (57). In certain areas of the country, up to 90% of patients with IVDA IE are HIV-positive (58). Those suffering from advanced AIDS do significantly worse with their valvular infections (59). Pure right-sided IVDA IE occurs in >50% of cases, usually involving the tricuspid valve. The aortic valve is involved in 25%, with the mitral valve in 20%. Polymicrobial IE is seen most frequently in IVDA. Of all the types of IE, the chance of recurrence is highest among IVDA. Most likely, this is the result of the persistence in the use of injectable drugs by those who have already had an attack of IE (20–40% of cases).

The shift from the use of the term nosocomial IE to HCIE reflects the fact that healthcare is increasingly delivered outside the walls of the hospital. In the 1970s, von Reyn (1) was one of the first to recognize that hospitalization itself could be a major risk factor for acquiring IE. In his study, 20% of the patients acquired IE on being hospitalized for some other condition. HCIE is defined as a valvular infection that occurs within four weeks of an invasive procedure or the development of signs and symptoms of IE 48 hours or longer, following admission to a healthcare facility (1).

Finland and Barnes (60) associated the rise in the cases of IE, caused by *S. aureus*, enterococcal sp., *S. epidermidis*, and gram-negative bacilli with the institutalization of the patient. Friedland et al. characterized patients with HCIE as being older, with a higher rate of valvular disease, and whose bacteremias are related to various intravascular procedures (61). The mortality rate of HCIE is approximately 50%.

The cases of HCIE appear to be on the rise, accounting for approximately 30% of the cases in many hospitals (61). It correlates with the escalating employment of intravascular devices, such as hyperalimentation lines, dialysis catheters and pacemakers. Much of this is related to the increase in staphylococcal bacteremia, associated with the infection of intravascular catheters and other devices (62–66). Staphylococci followed by enterococcal species, are the predominant organisms. They usually originate from the skin or urinary tract. There appears to be a close association between particular healthcare procedures and the risk of IE. A particularly strong connection exists between bacteremias associated with hemodialysis and the development of *S. aureus* IE (66). Thirteen percent of staphylococcal bacteremias acquired in the hospital result in HCIE.

There are two varieties of HCIE (67). Type 1 is attributed to various traumatic types of injury to the endocardium of the right ventricle produced by various types of intravascular lines. Type 2 is produced by bacteremias that infect the left ventricular structures. At least 50% of the cases of either type occur in the setting of normal valves. This most likely reflects the predominant role of *S. aureus* and its potential to invade healthy cardiac structures. Friedland pointed out the importance of recognizing the risk factors for developing HCIE (68). He stated "nosocomial endocarditis occurs in a definable subpopulation of hospitalized patients and is potentially preventable."

TABLE 2   Changing Patterns of Infective Endocarditis Since 1966

Marked increase in the incidence of acute IE
Rise of nosocomial, IVDA, and prosthetic valve IE
  (a) Change in the underlying valvular pathology: rheumatic heart disease, <20% of cases
  (b) Mitral valve prolapse, 30% of cases
  (c) Prosthetic valve endocarditis, 10–20% of cases
  (d) 50% of elderly patients have calcific aortic stenosis
These changes are attributed to:
  (a) The "graying" of patients (excluding cases of IVDA IE, 55% of patients >60 years of age)
  (b) The increased numbers of vascular procedures

Abbreviations: IE, infective endocarditis; IVDA, intravenous drug abuser.

The definable sets of hospitalized patients are those that are at risk of developing bacteremias, especially those caused by *S. aureus*.

Dental procedures have been inextricably linked to the development of endocarditis in the susceptible patient. Recently, several human studies have failed to support this connection (69,70). The risk may be as low as 1 in 115,000 patients with predisposing cardiac lesions (71). The risk is much greater for patients with prosthetic valves in place (1–2%) (72).

Various types of immunodeficient states have been identified as risk factors for the development of IE (73). These include diabetes mellitus renal failure, liver disease, pregnancy, many types of neoplasms and organ transplants (Chapter 11) (74).

Table 2 summarizes the current major underlying abnormalities for the development of valvular infection.

MICROBIOLOGY

The organisms that are involved in NVE differ somewhat from those that produce PVE or IVDA IE. Gram-positive cocci predominate in all types of IE. *Staphylococcus aureus* accounts for 30% of cases overall—coagulase-negative staphylococci (CoNS) 16% and *S. viridans* 16%. The frequency of *S. viridans* IE has lessened by 35%, whereas that of *S. aureus* has increased by 50%.

Non-*S. viridans* streptococci, such as nutritionally variant streptococci (currently classified as Abiotophia), have also become more common. They also have become increasingly more resistant to penicillin-culture-negative endocarditis, and currently account for approximately 5% of cases. Tables 3, 4, and 5 summarize the microbiological and clinical correlates of IE.

TABLE 3   Microbiology of Infective Endocarditis in Different Risk Groups

Microorganism recovered (% of cases)	Native valve endocarditis	Intravenous drug users	Prosthetic valve endocarditis	
			Early	Late
Viridans-group streptococci	50	20	7	30
Staphylococcus aureus	19	67	17	12
Coagulase-negative staphylococci	4	9	33	26
Enterococci	8	7	2	6
Miscellaneous	19	7	44	26

TABLE 4   Epidemiological Characteristics of the Four Major Types of Infective Endocarditis

	NVE	PVE	IVDA IE	HCIE
Mean age	50 (15% >70)	50 (15% >70)	30–40	50 (15% >70)
Underlying abnormalities	Congenital heart disease 13% RHD 6% MVP 30% Degenerative valvular disease 21% (especially calcific aortic stenosis) Hypertrophic cardiomyopathy 5%	Prosthetic valve	75% have no underlying pathology	45% involve prosthetic valves
Total cases of IE (%)	>40	10	15	30

Abbreviations: HCIE, healthcare-associated IE; IVDA IE, intravenous drug abuser infective endocarditis; MVP, mitral valve prolapse; NVE, native valve endocarditis; PVE, prosthetic valve endocarditis; RHD, rheumatic heart disease.

TABLE 5   Clinical Characteristics of Organisms Commonly Involved in Infective Endocarditis

Organism	Comments
Staphylococcus aureus	The most common cause of acute IE, including PVE, IVDA, and IE related to intravascular infections. Approximately 35% of cases of *S. aureus* bacteremia are complicated by IE.
Streptococcus viridans (*S. mitior*, *S. sanguis*, *S. mutans*, *S. salivarius*)	70% of cases of subacute IE. Signs and symptoms are immunologically mediated with a very low rate of suppurative complications. Penicillin resistance is a growing problem, especially in patients receiving chemotherapy or bone marrow transplants.
S. milleri group (*S. anginosus*, *S. intermedius*, *S. constellatus*)	Up to 20% of streptococcal IE. Unlike other streptococci, they can invade tissue and produce suppurative complications.
Nutritionally variant streptococci (NVS)	5% of subacute IE. Isolates require active forms of vitamin B6 for their growth. Characteristically, they produce large valvular vegetations with a high rate of embolization and relapse.
Enterococci	Third most common cause of IE. They may produce alpha, beta, or gamma hemolysis. Source is GI or GU tracts, associated with a high rate of relapse. Growing problem of antimicrobial resistance. Most cases are subacute.
Nonenteroccocal group D streptoccoci (*S. bovis*)	50% of group D IE; associated with lesions of large bowel.
Coagulase-negative *S. aureus*	30% of PVE; <5% of IE of native valves; subacute course that is more indolent than that of *S. viridans*.
Pseudomonas aeruginosa	Most commonly acutely seen in IVDA IE (right-sided disease is subacute) and in PVE.
HACEK organisms (*Hemophilus aphrophilus*, *Actinobacillus actinomycetocomitans*, *Cardiobacterium hominis*, *Eikenella corrodens*, *Kingella kingae*)	Most common gram-negative organisms in IE (5% of all cases of IE); presents as subacute, culture-negative IE. Part of normal flora of the GI tract. Intravenous drug abuser is a major risk factor. Complications are arterial macroemboii and congestive heart failure. Cases usually require the combination of ampicillin and gentamicin, with or without surgery, for cure.

(Continued)

TABLE 5   Clinical Characteristics of Organisms Commonly Involved in Infective Endocarditis (*Continued*)

Organism	Comments
Bartonella species (*Bartonella quintana, Bartonella henselae, Bartonella elizabethae*)	*B. quintana* is the most common isolate. Culture-negative, subacute IE in a homeless male should suggest the diagnosis. Usually treated with a combination of a beta-lactam antibiotic and an aminoglycoside.
Fungal IE	An increasing problem in the ICU and among IVDA. *Candida albicans* is the most common example (especially in PVE) as compared with IVDA IE, in which *Candida parapsilosis* or *Candida tropicalis* predominate. *Aspergillus* species recovered in 33% of fungal IE. Most cases of fungal IE follow a subacute course.
Polymicrobial IE	Most common organisms are *Pseudomonas* and enterococci. It occurs frequently in IVDA and cardiac surgery. It may present acutely or subacutely. Mortality is greater than that of single-agent IE.

Abbreviations: GI, gastrointestinal; GU, genitourinary tract; ICU, intensive care unit; IE, infective endocarditis; IVDA, intravenous drug abuser; PVE, prosthetic valve endocarditis.

REFERENCES

1. von Reyn CF, Levy BS, Arbeit RD, et al. Infective endocarditis—an analysis based on strict case definitions. Ann Intern Med 1981; 94(Part 1):505–518.
2. Durack DT, Lukes BS, Bright DK. Dukes endocarditis service. New criteria for the diagnosis of infective endocarditis: utilization of specific echocardiographic findings. Am J Med 1994; 96:200–209.
3. Cabell CH, Abrutyn E. Progress toward a global understanding of infective endocarditis. Lessons from the International Collaboration of Endocarditis. Cardiol Clin 2003; 21:147–158.
4. Delahaye F, Goulet V, Lacassin F, et al. Characteristics of infective endocarditis in France in 1991: a 1- year survey. Eur Heart J 1995; 16:394–401.
5. Bouza E, Menasalvas A, Munoz P, et al. Infective endocarditis—a prospective study at the end of the twentieth century. Medicine 2001; 80:298–307.
6. Griffin MR, Wilson WR, Edwards WD, et al. Infective endocarditis, Olmstead County, Minnesota 1950–1981. JAMA 1985; 254:1199–1202.
7. Durack DT, Petersdorf RG. Changes in the epidemiology of endocarditis. In: Kaplan EL, Taranta AV, eds. Infective Endocarditis: An American Heart Association Symposium. Dallas: American Heart Association, 1977:3.
8. Berlin JA, Abrutyn E, Strom, et al. Incidence of infective endocarditis in Delaware Valley, 1988–1990. Am J Cardiol 1995; 76:933–936.
9. Hogevik H, Olaison Andersson R, et al. Epidemiologic aspects of infective endocarditis in an urban population. Medicine (Baltimore) 1995; 74:324–339.
10. Hedley OF. Rheumatic heart disease in Philadelphia hospitals. III. Fatal rheumatic heart disease and subacute bacterial endocarditis. Pub Health Rep 1940; 55:1707.
11. Lerner PI, Weinstein L. Infective endocarditis in the antibiotic era. N Engl J Med 66, 274, 199.
12. Wilson al M. Etiology of bacterial endocarditis: before and since the introduction of antibiotics. Ann Intern Med 1963; 58:946.
13. Newsom SWB. The treatment of endocarditis by vancomycin. J Antimicrob Chemother 1994; 14:79.
14. Bayer AS. Infective endocarditis. Clin Infect Dis 1993; 17:313.
15. King J, Nguyen L, Conrad. Results of a prospective statewide reporting system for infective endocarditis. Am J Med Sci 1982; 31:517.

16. Kim E, Ching D, Plen F. Bacterial endocarditis at a small community hospital. Am J Med Sci 1990; 299:487.
17. Thayer WS. Studies on bacterial (infective) endocarditis. Johns Hopkins Hosp Rep 1926; 22:1.
18. Robbins N, DeMaria A, Miller MH. Infective endocarditis in the elderly. South Med J 1980; 73:1335.
19. Kaye D. Changing patterns of infective endocarditis. Am J Med 1985; 78(suppl 6b): 157–162.
20. Cabell CH, Jollis JG, Peterson GE, et al. Changing patient characteristics and the effect on mortality on endocarditis. Arch Int Med 2002; 162:90–95.
21. Gladstone JL, Rocco R. Host factors in infectious disease in the elderly. Med Clin NA 1976; 60:1225.
22. Durack DT, Petersdorf RT. Changes in the epidemiology of endocarditis. Infective endocarditis. Am Heart Assoc Mono 1977; 52:3.
23. Terpenning M, Buggy B, Kauffman C. Infective endocarditis: clinical features in young and elderly patients. Am J Med 1987; 83:6, 26.
24. Land M, Bisno A. Acute rheumatic fever: a vanishing disease in suburbia. JAMA 1983; 249:89.
25. Cantrell M, Yoshikawa TT. Aging and infective endocarditis. J Am Geriatr Soc 1983; 31:216–222.
26. Watanakunakor C, Burkert T. Infective endocarditis in a large community teaching hospital, 1988–1990: a review of 210 episodes. Medicine (Baltimore) 1993; 72:90–102.
27. Coutlee F, Carceller A, Deschamps, et al. The evolving pattern of pediatric endocarditis from 1960–1985. Can J Cardiol 1990; 6:169.
28. Baltimore RS. Infective endocarditis in children. Pediatr Infect Dis J 1992; 907.
29. Weinstein L, Rubin RH. Infective endocarditis in 1973. Prog Cardiovasc Dis 1973; 16:239.
30. Nager F. Changing clinical spectrum of infective endocarditis. In: Horstkotte D, Bodnar E, eds. Infective Endocarditis. London: ICR Publishers, 1991:25.
31. Cabell CH, Abrutyn E. Progress toward a global understanding of infective endocarditis. In: Durack D, ed. Infective Endocarditis in Infect. Dis Clin NA 2002; 16:255–272.
32. Zuppiroli A, Rinaldi M, Kramer-Fox R, et al. Natural history of mitral valve prolapse. Am J Cardiol 1995; 75:1028–1032.
33. Sidhu P, O'Kane H, Ali N, et al. Mechanical or bioprosthetic valves in the elderly: a 20-year comparison. Ann Thorac Surg 2001; 71(suppl):257–260.
34. Steckelberg JM, Wilson WR. Risk factors for infective endocarditis. Infect Dis Clin N A 1993; 7:9–19.
35. Normand J, Bozio A, Ettiene J, et al. Changing patterns and prognosis of infective endocarditis in childhood. Eur Heart J 1995; 16(suppl B):28–31.
36. Morris DC, Reller MD, Menashe VD. Thirty-year incidence of infective endocarditis after surgery for congenital heart defect. JAMA 1998; 79:599–603.
37. Gersony WM, Hayes CJ, Driscoll DJ, et al. Bacterial endocarditis in patients with aortic stenosis, pulmonary stenosis or ventricular septal defect. Circulation 1993; 1121.
38. Johnson CH, Rosenthal A, Nadas AS. A forty-year review of bacterial endocarditis in infancy and childhood. Circulation 1975; 51:581–588.
39. Kaye D. Changing pattern of infective endocarditis. Am J Med 1985; 78:157.
40. McKinsey DS, Ratts TE, Bisno JL. Underlying cardiac lesions in adults with infective endocarditis. Am J Med 1987; 82:681–688.
41. Weinberger I, Rotenberg Z, Zacharovitch D, et al. Native valve infective endocarditis in the 1970s versus the 1980s: underlying cardiac lesions and infecting organisms. Clin Cardiol 1990; 13:94.
42. Disse S, Abergel E, Berrebi A, et al. Mapping of a first locus for autosomal dominant myxomatous mitral-valve prolapse to chromosome 16p11.2-p12.1. Am J Hum Genet 1999; 65:1242–1251.
43. Clemens JD, Horwitz RI, Jaffe CC, et al. A controlled evaluation of the risk of bacterial endocarditis in persons with mitral-valve prolapse. N Eng J Med 1982; 307:776.
44. Devereaux RB, Kramer-Fox R, Kligfield P. Mitral valve prolapse: causes, clinical manifestations and management. Ann Intern Med 1989; 111:305–317.

45. Nolan CM, Kane JJ, Grunow WA. Infective endocarditis in mitral prolapse: a comparison with other types of endocarditis. Arch Intern Med 1981; 141:447.
46. Weinstein L. Infective endocarditis. In: Braunwald E, ed. Heart Disease, a Textbook of Cardiovascular Medicine. 3rd ed. Philadelphia: Saunders, 1988:1098.
47. Mansur A, Grinberg M, Bellotti G. Infective endocarditis in the 1980s: experience back at a heart hospital. Clin Cardiol 1990; 13:623.
48. Venezio F, Westenfelder, Cook F. Infective endocarditis in a community hospital. Arch Intern Med 1982; 142:789.
49. Chagnac A, Lobel H, Rudnicki C. Endocarditis in idiopathic hypertrophic subaortic stenosis: report of three cases and review of the literature chest. 1982; 81:346.
50. Weinstein L. "Modern" infective endocarditis. JAMA 1975; 233:260.
51. Toronos P, Almirante B, Olona M, et al. Clinical outcome and long-term prognosis of late prosthetic valve endocarditis: a 20-year experience. Clin Infect Dis 1997; 24:381–386.
52. Calderwood SB, Swinski LA, Waternaux CM, et al. Risk factors for the development of prosthetic valve endocarditis. Circulation 1985; 72:31–37.
53. Eggimann P, Waldvoge FA. Pacemaker and defibrillator infections. In: Waldvogel FA, Bisno AL, eds. Infections associated with indwelling medical devices. Washington D.C.: American Society for Microbiology Press, 2000:247–264.
54. Haverkos HW, Lange WR. Serious infections other than human immunodeficiency virus among intravenous drug abusers. J Infect Dis 1990; 161:894–902.
55. Chambers HF, Morris DL, Tauber MG, et al. Cocaine use and the risk of endocarditis in intravenous drug abusers. Ann Intern Med 1987; 106:833–836.
56. Currie PF, Sutherland GR, Jacob AJ, et al. A review of endocarditis in Acquired Immune Deficiency Syndrome and human immunodeficiency virus infection. Eur Heart J 1995; 16(suppl B):15–18.
57. Matthew J, Adai T, Anand A, et al. Clinical features, site of involvement, bacteriologic findings and outcome of infective endocarditis in intravenous drug abusers. Arch Intern Med 1995; 55:1640–1648.
58. Levine DP, Crane LR, Zervos MJ. Bacteremia in narcotic addicts at the Detroit Medical Center II infectious endocarditis: a prospective comparative study. Rev Infect Dis 1986; 8(3):74–83, 96.
59. Pulverenti JJ, Kerns E, Bentson C, et al. Infective endocarditis in injection drug users: importance of human immunodeficiency virus serostatus and degree of immuno-suppression. Clin Infect Dis 1996; 22:40–45.
60. Finland M, Barnes MW. Changing etiology of bacterial endocarditis in the antibacterial era: experiences at Boston City Hospital 1933–1955. Ann Intern Med 1970; 72:341.
61. Pellitier LL, Petersdorf RG. Infective endocarditis: a review of 125 cases from the University of Washington Hospitals 1963–1972. Medicine (Baltimore) 1977; 56:287.
62. Gaynes R. Healthcare-associated bloodstream infections: a change in taking. Editorial Ann Intern Med 2003; 137:850–851.
63. Fowler VG Jr., Sanders LL, Kong LK. Infective endocarditis due to Staphylococcus aureus: 59 prospectively identified cases with follow-up. Clin Infect Dis 1999; 28:106–114.
64. Safar N, Kluger D, Maki D. A review of risk factors for catheter related bloodstream infections caused by percutaneously inserted noncuffed central venous catheters. Medicine 2002; 81:466–474.
65. Gouello JP, Asfar P, Brenet O, et al. Nosocomial endocarditis in intensive care unit: an analysis of 22 cases. Crit Care Med 2000; 28:377–382.
66. Fernandez-Guerrero ML, Verdejo C, Azofra J, et al. Hospital-acquired infectious endo-carditis not associated with cardiac surgery: an emerging problem. Clin Infect Dis 1995; 20:16–23.
67. Lacassin F, Hoen B, Leport C, et al. Procedures associated with infective endocarditis in adults. Eur Heart J 1995; 16:1968–1974.
68. Friedland G, von Reyn CF, Leavy BS, et al. Nosocomial endocarditis. Infect Control 1984; 5:284–288.
69. Strom BL, Abrutyn E, Berlin JA, et al. Dental and cardiac risk factors for infective endocarditis. A population-based, case-control study. Ann Intern Med 1998; 129:761–769.

70. Pogrel MA, Welsby DD. The dentist and prevention of infective endocarditis. Br Dent J 1975; 139:12–16.
71. Horstkotte D, Rosin H, Friedreichs W, et al. Contribution by choosing the optimal prophylaxis of bacterial endocarditis. Eur Heart J 1987; 8:379–381.
72. Garvey GJ, Neu HC. Infective endocarditis—an evolving disease. Medicine (Baltimore) 1978; 57:105–127.
73. Brusch JL. Cardiac infections in the immunosuppressed patient. In: Cunha BA, ed. Infections in the Compromised Host. Infectious Disease Clinics of North America Philadelphia: WB Saunders, 2001:613–638.
74. Weinstein L, Brusch JL. Microbiology of infective endocarditis and clinical correlates: gram-positive organisms. In: Weinstein L, Brusch JL, eds. Infective Endocarditis. New York: Oxford University Press, 1995:35–72.

2 Microbiology of Infective Endocarditis and Clinical Correlates: Gram-Positive Organisms

John L. Brusch
Harvard Medical School and Department of Medicine and Infectious Disease Service, Cambridge Health Alliance, Cambridge, Massachusetts, U.S.A.

INTRODUCTION

This chapter, along with the following one, presents the distinctive properties of the principal organisms that are involved in infective endocarditis (IE) in the era of intravascular devices. In the last 10 years, there has been a significant increase in our knowledge of the pathogenesis of IE. Much has been learned of the manner in which pathogens infect both native tissues and prosthetic devices of all types. Much remains to be discovered. Hopefully, this expanded knowledge base will provide targets for antimicrobial therapy that were not even dreamed of about a decade ago. Later chapters examine the interaction of specific pathogens and the host that results in varied presentations of native and prosthetic valve endocarditis.

Gram-positive cocci have remained the premier pathogens of IE. The advent of intravascular devices, cardiac surgery, antibiotics, potent immunosuppressive agents, and the increase in intravenous drug abuse have led to the decline of *Streptococcus viridans* and to the ascendency of both coagulase-positive and negative staphylococci in IE (Chapter 1). Although the target of these organisms is the same—native or prosthetic materials, the manifestations of each can be markedly different. *Staphylococcus aureus* typically produces an acute type of valvular infection, whereas *S. viridans* and coagulase-negative staphylococci (CoNS) an indolent/subacute one. Unusually, the course of *S. aureus* IE may be subacute. This reversal of clinical course is often attributed to the administration of suboptimal doses of antibiotic (1). Much less frequently, *S. viridans* results in acute disease. These organisms differ greatly among themselves as to their pathogenic factors. What they have in common is the ability to resist decolorization by alcohol during the process of Gram staining. This is attributed to their thick peptidoglycan layer with extensive teichoic acid cross-linkages (2) compared with the far thinner peptidoglycan structure of the gram negatives that completely lack teichoic acid. Exposure to antibiotics may lessen the ability of gram positives to retain the crystal violet stain. Some cells will appear pink and others purple. This state is classified as Gram variable. Characterization by their gram-staining properties and morphology of organisms, isolated in blood cultures, remains clinically useful. It is usually the first "hard" information that the clinician receives regarding the nature of the suspected case of IE. There is no diagnostic technique on the horizon that usurps this role of the Gram stain. Figure 1 presents an algorithm for the identification of gram-positive organisms.

THE STAPHYLOCOCCI

Staphylococci are members of the Micrococcaceae family. The genus *Staphylococcus* consists of 31 species. They are gram-positive cocci that cluster irregularly.

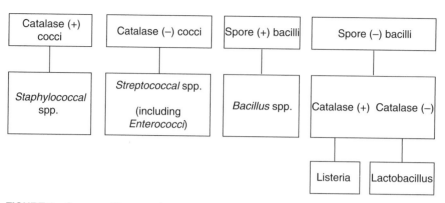

FIGURE 1 Gram-positive organisms.

All examples are anaerobic/facultatively anaerobic and catalase positive. Only *S. aureus* is coagulase positive.

Staphylococcus aureus

Finland and Barnes observed that *S. aureus* caused approximately 6% of IE in the decade prior to the widespread use of penicillin (3). From 1944 to 1966, the frequency of IE, caused by this organism, increased to 16% (4). Currently *S. aureus* produces greater than 30% of cases of IE. In the past, most cases of staphylococcal IE originated in the community; 4% of these at present are cases of healthcare-associated IE (HCIE) (5,6). As early as 1982, it was recognized that staphylococcal IE is "… part of what is to be called a staph pandemic which was presumably reflected in large hospitals and all the highly developed countries" (7).

S. aureus is uniquely qualified to take advantage of the aforementioned advances in medical care, especially when used in the treatment of the elderly and immunosuppressed. This section will examine the properties that facilitate *S. aureus* distinctive ability to produce IE. *S. aureus* exhibits three classes of virulence agents (8). The first are those that govern the organism's attachment to a variety of cells and extracellular material. As an initial step, staphylococci must be able to bind to the integument or mucosa of the host to establish a "beach head" from which to invade the bloodstream. Teichoic acid is a phosphate-containing polymer that has been implicated in the ability of the bacteria to attach to the nasal mucosa (9). Mucosal binding is also facilitated by upper respiratory viral infections, intravenous drug abuse, hemodialysis, and diabetes. More recent work indicates that *S. aureus* employs several bacterial surface proteins that interact with the host's extracellular matrix proteins to promote colonization and invasion (10). These are termed "microbial surface components recognizing adhesive matrix molecules" (MSCRAMMs) (11). These molecules are covalently attached to the peptidoglycan layer by a common core of six amino acids, LPXTGX. The LPXTGX has to be cleaved by sortase, which then transfers and attaches the MSCRAMMs to the peptidogycan layer. The expression of these factors is governed by several gene regulators—most important of these is the accessory gene regulator (*agr*) and the staphylococcal accessory regulator (*sag*) (12,13). Attachment factors are expressed only during the exponential phase of bacterial growth (14). Table 1 lists the most significant MSCRAMMs. Of these, those with the best-established role in the pathogenesis of

TABLE 1 Attachment Virulence Factors of *Staphylococcus aureus*

MSCRAMM	Demonstrated pathogenic role in IE
Clumping factor A	Yes
Clumping factor B	No
Coagulase	No
Fibronectin A and B	Yes
Collagen-binding protein	No

Abbreviations: IE, infective endocarditis; MSCRAMM, microbial surface components recognizing adhesive matrix molecules.

IE are clumping factor A and fibronectin-binding protein A and B (15,16). *S. aureus* surface proteins G and H appear to to be highly associated with the the organism's potential for tissue invasion (11).

In addition, *S. aureus* may attach to a prosthetic device by means of its production of a biofilm (17). This extracellular matrix probably is less significant for infection of medical devices by coagulase-positive staphylococci than for CoNS.

At any given time, 10% to 40% of healthy adults are nasal carriers of *S. aureus* (18). From the nares, microorganisms spread to the skin (19). A minor cut, an abrasion, injury to the mucosa or intravascular line placement can serve as an entry point to the vascular system for *S. aureus*. Once the dermal or mucosal barriers are breached, the staphylococci must avoid or overcome the host's defenses. These constitute the second class of virulence factors (Table 2). The pathogen has at its disposal many resources to do so. At the early stages of tissue invasion, the patient's primary defense is the polymorphonuclear leukocyte (PMNL). These cells are summoned to the point of infection by a complex series of events (chemotaxis) (20). Concurrently, the pathogens are opsonized in order to prepare them for phagocytosis by the PMNLs. The process of opsonization involves primarily activated C3 of the classic pathway of complement and immunoglobulin (Ig) G. Occasionally, the alternative pathway and antibodies directly reacting against the peptidoglycan component of the cell wall are involved. The polysaccharide capsule of *S. aureus* interferes with opsonization to a variable degree per given isolate. Antibodies against the *O*-acetyl group of the polysaccharide component are the primary means of opsonizing encapsulated *S. aureus* (21). Paradoxically, Baddour et al. documented that unencapsulated strains were more efficient in producing IE in an experimental model (22).

The other principal means by which *S. aureus* evades opsonization is by its expression of protein A, which takes place primarily during the exponential growth

TABLE 2 Host Defense Evasion Virulence Factors of *Staphylococcus aureus*

Factor	Demonstrated pathogenic role in IE
Protein A	Yes
Lipase	?
V8 protease	?
FAME[a]	?
Leukocidins	No
Antibiotic resistance	Yes

[a]See text.
Abbreviations: FAME, fatty acid-metabolizing enzyme; IE, infective endocarditis.

of the organism. The role of this protein appears to be more important in the beginning stages of infection when there are low concentrations of organisms. By its ability to bind with the the Fc portion of IgG, protein A interferes with successful phagocytosis of the pathogen in three ways. Extracellular protein A may bind with the Fc end of IgG. The resulting aggregates consume complement that is required for phagocytosis. Extracellular protein A also may attach to the Fc portion of antistaphylococcal antibodies that are already attached to the bacteria. This blocks the Fc receptor of the PMNLs. Protein A that remains bound to the staphylococcus may attach to the Fc portion of any IgG molecule, and hence functionally inactivates them (23).

Complement appears to be the most important component of opsonization. There is an increase in staphylococcal infections of all types in individuals deficient in complement. However, there is probably no such extra risk for those with a significant decrease in their immunoglobulins (24,25). It is challenging to separate the intrinsic risk of gammaglobulin deficiencies from the exposure to staphylococci in the nosocomial environment.

Defects in cellular immunity do not appear by themselves to increase the rate of staphylococcal infection. The actual rate of staphylococcal infections in patients with T-cell deficiencies depends on the particular situation. In AIDS patients, *S. aureus* infections probably occur significantly more often than in comparable individuals without AIDS. This augmented rate probably reflects the multiple immunodeficiency components of HIV infection. These include an increased rate of nasopharyngeal colonization and complicating bacteremia with *S. aureus* (26); the frequency of eczema that makes this population susceptible to bloodstream invasion by *S. aureus* (27); the common usage of intravascular lines; and the increased incidence of both neutropenia and decreased phagocytosis in AIDS patients (28) (Chapter 11).

Five percent of *S. aureus* remain viable for at least 30 minutes within normally functioning PMNLs. A few bacteria completely escape intracellular killing. This seems to be strain dependent, and may be associated with a particular coagulase genotype (29). Additionally, strains of *S. aureus* may differ in their susceptibility to being killed by the intracellular oxidants of PMNLs. It is possible that the isolates exposed to sublethal concentrations of H_2O_2 may develop tolerance to this important molecule (30). In comparison, 100% of CoNS are killed within minutes after being phagocytized. Circulating white cells lower the concentration of *S. aureus* that has been injected into the bloodstream of experimental animals, by more than a 1000-fold within 20 minutes. However, the small percentage of staphylococci, which resist intracellular killing, can be released back into the bloodstream upon the death of the PMNL. Their intracellular survival sustains the initial bacteremia and increases the risk of developing IE. The greater the numbers of *S. aureus* in the bloodstream, the greater the chance of developing a sustained bacteremia (31).

Other staphylococcal compounds that interfere with the host's defenses include gamma toxin and Panton–Valentine leukocidin. These are synergistically toxic for PMNLs, macrophages, and monocytes. They probably play little, if any, role, in the development of IE (32) that are associated with a type of catastrophic, necrotizing pneumonia in children and young adults. Lipase and fatty acid metabolizing enzyme (FAME) are able to break down the host's fatty acids that can damage the staphylococcal membrane by their surfactant action (33).

S. aureus produces several extracellular proteases. The most studied of these is the serine protease, V8 protease. This substance can inactivate IgG and the neutrophilic antimicrobial peptides (defensins) and platelet microbicidal proteins (8).

The resistance of *S. aureus* to a growing list of antibiotics has to be considered an essential part of its ability to escape the host defenses. A dramatically increasing therapeutic challenge is the proliferation of methicillin-resistant *S. aureus* (MRSA) infections, acquired both in the community and in healthcare facilities (34). A recent meta-analysis indicates that the mortality associated with MRSA IE was significantly greater than that associated with methicillin-sensitive *S. aureus* (35).

A particular isolate of *S. aureus* may exhibit intolerance to a number of antibiotics. When an organism expresses tolerance, it requires much higher concentration of the antibiotic to kill rather than suppressing its growth. The minimal inhibitory concentration (MIC) and minimal bactericidal concentration (MBC) of penicillin cephalosporin for nontolerance strain are essentially the same, whereas in the intolerance ones, the MBC may be 128 times higher than the MIC. The clinical importance of tolerance still has not been clarified (Chapter 14) (36).

In addition to the loss of dermal and mucosal integrity, other common sources of staphylococcal bacteremia include prostatitis and pneumonia. In these latter situations, the organism usually enters the vascular space by way of lymphatics that drain into the small venules (37,38). *S. aureus* infects the endothelium of the microcirculation (endotheliosis) in a manner similar to that by which *S. aureus* infects normal endocardial cells. Fibronectin both anchors *S. aureus* to the venular endothelium and promotes bacterial aggregation. Clumps of *S. aureus* are then ingested by the endothelial cells. When the capacity of these endothelial cells is reached, a prolonged bacteremia can occur (Chapter 5) (39).

For a bacteremia to develop into IE, it is essential that the circulating pathogens be able to affix to the intact endothelial cell or to the platelet/fibrin thrombus (40). This process is facilitated by the same adhesions, MSCRAMMs, as described earlier (8,11). The complete description of the way *S. aureus* produces IE in both previously normal endocardium and have normal endocardium is described in detail in a later chapter (Chapter 5).

Once *S. aureus* has attached itself to the valve, it must survive long enough to reach the point where it is capable of successfully invading the tissue. It appears that the growth of the platelet fibrin thrombus is vital. On reaching maturity, this complex serves to protect the invading organisms from host defense mechanisms and antibiotic effect. Production of tissue factor (TF) and the aggregation of platelets are key to this. Tissue factor is a membrane glycoprotein which when combined with activated factor VII activates factor X. This latter factor converts prothrombin to thrombin which eventually leads to the production of fibrin. *S. aureus* can induce TF activity (TFA) from a variety of cells. Monocytes are its chief target in early vegetation formation. Eventually, the endothelial cell becomes the chief producer of *S. aureus*-induced TFA (41) and a variety of cytokines. These componds promote both coagulation and local inflammation, thus allowing the fibrin/platelet thrombus to grow.

The platelet has a dual role in the pathogenesis of IE. The ability of *S. aureus* to directly aggregate platelets by utilizing fibrinogen as a bridging molecule is essential to the infectivity of the organism in the immature thrombus (42). Strains of *S. aureus* that lack this ability are up to 100 times less infective than those that possess it. The platelet also may play a role in the defense of the host. Once they are exposed to thrombin, they release a variety of platelet microbicidal proteins (PMPs) that reside in the alpha granules of the intact platelet (43). The PMPs appear to break down the bacterial cell wall, and may work synergistically with certain antibiotics.

TABLE 3 Tissue Invasion Virulence Factors of *Staphylococcus aureus*

Factor	Demonstrated pathogenic role in infective endocarditis
Alpha toxin	Yes
Beta hemolysin	?
Hyaluronidase	?
Metalloprotease	?
Stimulation of tissue factor activity	Yes
Platelet aggregation effect	Yes

When the staphylococci are adequately sheltered by the growing vegetation, they may then start producing the third type of virulence factors (Table 3). Chief among these cytotoxic agents are the hemolysins (43). Although they may injure the membrane of many types of cells, their clinical importance in IE has not been established. The role of other enzymes, such as hyaluronidase and the metalloproteases is even less understood (44).

Persistence of *S. aureus* within the endocardial vegetation may be attributed to small-colony variants (SCV) (45). These isolates have a slower growth rate with lessened hemolytic and coagulase activity that is caused by a decrease in bacterial ATP (46). The SCV of *S. aureus* also produce less alpha toxin. This downregulation promotes the organism's survival within the host cells. Presumably, reversion of the SCV phenotype would be a mechanism for relapsing infection. This topic is further discussed in relationship to CoNS (see later).

Coagulase-Negative Staphylococci

Over the last 25 years, CoNS have become an increasingly prominent cause of IE. Formerly, only about 5% of all types of valvular infection were attributed to CoNS. In the past, only 6% of blood cultures, positive for CoNS, were considered to represent true infection. No longer can we assume that the presence of CoNS in a blood culture signifies contamination. Currently 6.6% of cases of native valve endocarditis (NVE) are produced by this group (47). Coagulase-negative staphylococci are also the most frequent cause of prosthetic valve endocarditis (PVE) occurring within one year of valve implantation (48). It is also the most commonly found organism in healthcare-associated bloodstream infections (HCBSI) (49). This change in the profile of CoNS infections is understandable in the light of the increased use of intravascular catheters. Fifty percent of hospitalized patients receive some type of intravascular catheter (50). Up to 18% of these devices are associated with a primary BSI and 31% with CoNS (51).

There are at least 15 species of CoNS that are part of the resident flora of humans. Fifty to seventy percent of these belong to the *Staphylococcus epidermidis* group (*Staphylococcus epidermidis*, *Staphylococcus hemolyticus*, *Staphylococcus hominis*, and *Staphylococcus capitis*) (52,53). As compared with particular areas of skin and mucus membranes inhibited by other species of CoNS, *S. epidermidis* is widely distributed throughout the body. Because of this, it is important to identify particular strains of *S. epidermidis* both in order to verify the presence of a true bacteremia and to rule out common sources of nosocomial transmission. Several commercial kits are available to identify subspecies. Biotyping system and the use of antibiogram of an isolate is the most commonly employed approach to accurately characterize an organism retrieved in blood culture (54).

However, it appears that the predominant role played by *S. epidermidis* goes beyond its dominance of the flora of the human skin. This species appears to have intrinsic pathogenic mechanisms. In an experimental model, IE was produced in all animals infected with *S. epidermidis*, but only in 12.5% of those given *S. hominis* (55). Coagulase-negative staphylococci possess several virulence factors that are analogous to those of *S. aureus*. They often show variation in their colony morphology. This has been described in cases of both NVE and PVE (56). These observations have given rise to the possibility that this phenotypic variation may contribute to the pathogenesis of CoNS infections (57). The small cell variation (SCV) of *S. epidermidis* were found within the endothelial cells of rats after the establishment of experimental IE. However, the small colony type is less able to initiate infection than the usual type. The significance of these findings is not clearly known. Extrapolating from the situation of the SCV of *S. aureus*, one can speculate that this is a type of survival mechanism. The phenotypic conversion permits the organism to enter and persist within the endothelial cell. There they are safe from phagocytosis by PMNLs (58). Most SCV have defects in hemin or menaquinone synthesis (59) that are attributed to a disrupted electron transport chain. Downregulation of the electron transport system leads to overall decreased metabolic activity.

The primary virulence factor of CoNS is its distinctive ability to attach and adhere to a variety of prosthetic materials, and then use the medical device as a part of a multifactorial shield against the defenses of the host and most antibiotics (60).

The infection of prosthetic material by CoNS is a two-step process. The first phase is an initial rapid attachment, brought about by electrostatic forces (61) and a capsular polysaccharide adhesion, PS/A (62). Some CoNS isolates possess a fibrinogen-binding protein (Fbe) that promotes the adherence of the organism in a manner similar to that of *S. aureus* (63). Fbe may explain in part the ability of some CoNS to infect native valve tissue. The second step is intercellular adhesion of the individual CoNS bacteria to one another. This is the result of several cellular antigens. Probably, the most important of these is polysaccharide intercellular adhesion (PIA) factor. It is a very complex *N*-acetyl glucosaminoglycan polysaccharide that imbeds the bacterial cells in a thick matrix of slime (biofilm) (64). It appears that PIA and PS/A share many similar antigenic components, and may be identical (65). Norepinephrine and certain types of antibiotics (suprainhibitory levels of vancomycin) increase the production of slime. Subinhibitory concentrations of vancomycin and cefazolin decrease its formation (66). In general, slime producing CoNS have a higher MBC to most antibiotics than nonslime-producing examples. The MIC is not affected.

Biofilm formation is the major virulence factor of CoNS, because it both enables the infection of prosthetic material and protects the bacteria from the host's defenses and many types of antibiotics. Slime interferes with the migration of PMNLs, opsonization, and T-cell activation (67). Isolates of CoNS, which are imbedded in the biofilm, are more resistant to antibiotic action than the same strain tested outside this envelope (68). This resistance is not intrinsic but reflects the fact that bacteria in slime multiply much more slowly (69). This decreased reproduction rate reflects the cellular adherence phenomena and not deficiencies of nutrition.

Within the biofilm, CoNS downregulates genes that control the production of adhesion factors and aerobic metabolism (70). Poly-D,L-glutamic acid (PGA) is secreted by CoNS. It aids in the resistance of the bacteria at high salt concentrations (71). Currently, it appears that PGA is an extremely important part of the infectious process. Conversely, CoNS upregulates genes that control osmoprotection and an antibiotic resistance determinant (Drp 35). This upregulation process may indicate that the bacteria perceive the slime cocoon as hostile.

Hemagglutinins of CoNS may play a role in infecting prosthetic material in humans (72). DNAse, fibrinolysins, hemolysins, and proteases have been named as potential virulence factors of CoNS (73). Eighty percent of CoNS, which are retrieved from nosocomial infections, are resistant to the beta-lactam antibiotics (74). Their methicillin-resistant gene (mecA) is the same as that found in *S. aureus*. Because of the high rate of heterotypy among CoNS, methicillin resistance was not clinically evident until the patient was given antibiotics either for therapeutic or prophylactic reasons (75). More than 50% of these isolates are resistant to multiple antibiotics, including macrolides, trimethoprim/sulfamethoxazole, and gentamicin. This may well be attributed to the high rate of resistance plasmids among CoNS. Studies that show that the carriage of these plasmids by the hands of nurses gave rise to the spread of multiple antibiotic resistance in a cardiac thoracic intensive care unit (76).

It would be appropriate now to discuss *Staphylococcus lugdunensis*, as it produces an extremely aggressive type of IE, similar to that of *S. aureus*. It has only been recently identified as a cause of human IE (77,78). However, this figure may be a significant underestimation. A recent study, both a prospective and retrospective review of the world's literature, profiled 69 cases of *S. lugdunensis* IE. This organism is capable of producing infection of native (77%) and prosthetic valves (13%) along with pacemaker IE (10%). The mitral valve is the most commonly infected native valve. Prosthetic valve endocarditis primarily involves the aortic valve. Both types are associated with a high rate of abscess formation, embolization, and heart failure. Pacemaker IE has a better prognosis with a death rate of 25%. Mortality was 42% in the former type and 78% in PVE. Surgery was performed in >2% of cases. Because they are coagulase negative, they may be erroneously identified as a species of CoNS in a clinical laboratory using routine commercial identification approaches (79). Many cases of CoNS NVE might have been caused by this organism. Their yellow pigmentation and alpha hemolysis may cause the isolates to be classified as *S. aureus*. As compared with other CoNS, they usually are sensitive to all of the beta-lactam antibiotics. No definitive virulence factors have been yet identified.

THE STREPTOCOCCI

Streptococci are gram-positive cocci that arrange themselves in pairs or in chains. They are frequent colonies of the respiratory, gastrointestinal (GI), and genitourinary tracts. Most are facultative anaerobes and all are catalase negative. The genus Streptococcus is composed of streptococci and enterococci. Members of this genus can be identified by the type of hemolysis that they produce; by their antigenic and serologic properties; by biochemical tests; and by molecular testing (80). The nomenclature of the subdivisions of streptococci has become extremely confusing as the classic well-known classification systems do not necessarily correspond to those that are based on genetic taxonomic techniques. Because the older terminology is a well-established one, it will be used when appropriate, and the newer term placed in parentheses.

Streptococcus viridans

Currently, the members of the viridans group of the streptococci group are responsible for less than 25% of cases of IE as compared with >75% before the availability

TABLE 4   Clinically Important Viridans Streptococci Groups

Streptococcus mitis group
  S. mitis
  Streptococcus sanguis (biotypes 1, 2, 3)
Streptococcus mutans group
  S. mutans
Streptococcus salivarius group
  S. salvarius
Streptococcus bovis group
Streptococcus anginosus group (also known as *Streptococcus*
  milleri group)
  S. anginosus
  Streptococcus intermedius
  Streptococcus constellatus

---

of antibiotics (81,82). *Streptococcus viridans* remains the most common cause of mitral valve prolapse associated IE (83). The term viridans (Latin, for green) was applied to the original recognized members of this group because of their characteristic alpha hemolysis (green hemolysis) on blood agar. Many, however, are gamma hemolytic (nonhemolytic). Their cell walls are composed of peptidoglycans, teichoic acids, and lipoteichoic acids. As compared with the pyogenic streptococci (groups A, B, C, and G), there is no relationship between their particular Lancefield serogroup and the pattern of biochemical reactions used to classify them. Currently, we focus not on an in-depth discussion of the biochemical and enzymatic assays used to identify the various types of *S. viridans*, but present their most clinically relevant properties (Table 4).

In the current classification of viridans streptococci, *Streptococcus mitior* has been classified as a subtype of *Streptococcus mitis* (84). Streptococcus morbillorum is now classified as Gemella morbillorium. Long considered as part of the *S. mitis* group, nutritionially variant streptococci have been reclassified as Abiotrophia (85). The species of viridans streptococci most commonly involved in IE are *Streptococcus sanguis*, *Streptococcus mutans*, and *Streptococcus mitior/mitis* (86). There has been an increasing involvement of microaerophilic streptococci in IE. Most prominent of these is *S. mutans*. It is quite fastidious and difficult to grow from the blood. Sixty-six percent of *S. mutans* hydrolyze bile-esculin XL, which could be confused with enterococci.

Viridans streptococci are part of the normal microflora of the mouth, upper respiratory tract, and upper intestinal tract. *Streptococcus mitior/mitis*, *S. sanguis*, *Streptococcus milleri*, *Streptococcus salivarius*, and *S. mutans* constitute up to 60% of the microflora of the mouth. *S. mutans*, *S. mitis*, and *S. sanguis* (formerly known as Streptococcus SBE) reside most commonly on the surface of the teeth. *S. mitis* is also found in the oropharynx. *Streptococcus salivarius* resides on the tongue, pharynx, and hard palate (87). This propensity to adhere to dental enamel provides insight into how these bacteria produce IE.

Most viridans streptococci lack classical virulence factors. They, as a rule, do not produce toxins, hemolysins, or cytotoxins. As we shall discuss, it is their ability to adhere, to infect, and to promote the growth of the fibrin/platelet thrombus, which makes the viridans streptococci the classic organism of subacute IE. Unlike the situation with *S. aureus*, this group requires a preformed fibrin/platelet thrombus that is the result of previously damaged endothelial cell production of extracellular matrix proteins that trigger its formation. From this point on, the process is very similar to that of vegetation formation by *S. aureus* (15,88). The production of extracellular dextran (glucan) is positively associated with both attachment of the bacteria to the dental enamel and to the fibrin platelet thrombus. Those strains that adhere best to dental enamel have the highest rate of IE complicating bacteremia. *Streptococcus sanguis* I and II produce 16.4% of streptococcal IE. In an experimental model, dextran production has been shown to shield viridans streptococci from the effects of penicillin (89). The production of dextran is not an absolute requirement for the development of endocarditis. However, nondextran-producing *S. mitior* (*mitis*) also are involved significantly in subacute IE, whereas 7.3% of all cases of IE was produced by dextran-producing *S. mitior* (*mitis*). These figures represent data collected in the 1970s. Clearly because of the decrease in subacute IE and the rise in acute disease, the percentage of all cases of IE caused by *S. mitior* would be less (86). More recent data indicates that dextran production is found in equal frequency in the isolates of *S. viridans* that were obtained from the oral cavities of individuals with and without IE (90).

Fibronectin is produced by the endothelium, fibroblasts, and platelets in response to vascular injuries. Although fibronectin constitutes a small percentage of the platelet/fibrin thrombus, the IE-associated strains of *S. viridans* bind more avidly to this substance than do those not so involved in valvular infections (91,92).

Fim A and homologous adhesions enable viridans streptococci to adhere to fibrin and the extracellular matrix. Platelet adhesions of *S. sanguis* appear to promote the growth of the infected vegetation (93). The binding of these streptococci to fibronectin and other extracellular matrix components is probably quite heterogeneous involving multiple adhesion components (94).

Table 5 presents the MSCRAMMs of the viridans streptococci for which there is significant experimental evidence supporting their role in the pathogenesis of IE. In short, there are strains of viridans streptococci that are associated with IE and others that are not. This division of pathogenic potential occurs for a variety of reasons, many probably not yet defined.

There is evidence that certain types of *S. viridans* can invade and kill endothelial cells. *Streptococcus gordonii* were demonstrated to be cytotoxic to monolayers of human umbilical vein endothelial cells. Several surface proteins were vital for cellular invasion. Death of the endothelial cells was felt to be to the result of peroxidogenesis by the streptococcus (95). The relevance of this endotheliosis to clinical IE is yet to be determined.

The *Streptococcus anginosus* group, formerly known as the *S. milleri* group, is composed of three species—*S. anginosus, Streptococcus intermedius,* and *Streptococcus constellatus* (96). They have varying abilities to produce IE. *Streptococcus anginosus* isolates do so frequently; *S. intermedius* the least (97). They are microaerophilic with

TABLE 5 Streptococcal MSCRAMMs–Ligand Systems Relative to the Pathogenesis of Infective Endocarditis

MSCRAMM	Ligand
Dextrans of *Streptococcus sanguis* and *Streptococcus mutans*	Fibrin/platelet thrombus
Tn917 of *S. sanguis*	Fibronectin
Extracellular matrix molecules	Fim A proteins
Phase I, II of *S. sanguis*	Platelets

Abbreviation: MSCRAMM, microbial surface components recognizing adhesive matrix molecule.

characteristic small cavities and a distinctive caramel-like odor when grown on agar. They may exhibit alpha, beta, or gamma hemolysis on blood agar plates. They were initially called *minute hemolytic streptococci,* and are most frequently serotyped as Lancefield group F.

Their most important characteristic is their ability to invade and produce abscesses in a variety of tissues, including myocardium and valvular structures (98). They produce adhesin factors similar to those of other viridans streptococci. The majority of isolates involved in bacteremia adhere strongly to fibronectin, laminin, and fibrinogen. These are substances found deposited on an exposed basement membrane (99). In addition, several distinctive properties have been reported to contribute to their virulence. Anginosus streptococci are able to grow in the acidic and anaerobic environment of an abscess (100). It appears that concurrent infection with fastidious anaerobes actually accelerates the replicative ability of this group (101). This symbiosis may have significant therapeutic implications (102). Various cytolysins (hemolysis) and hydrolytic enzymes are produced by these streptococci (103,104). The presence of a polysaccharide capsule appears to interfere with phagocytosis (105). By unidentified means, particular species are able to generate disproportionately low degrees of chemotaxis, and are resistant to intracellular killing (106,107). Whether these characteristics are shared in common has not been established.

Very likely, the most significant virulence factor of the anginosus streptococci is their ability to generate superantigens. These immunomodulators are able to nonspecifically activate lymphocytes without prior processing by macrophages. This accelerated course produces a huge outburst of inflammatory cytokines that markedly augment the severity of their tissue invasion (108). There is some evidence that the hemolysin (intermedilysin) of *S. intermedius* may act as a super-antigen (103). *S. anginosus* bacteremia may be secondary to a valvular infection. In turn, BSI, usually arising from the intestinal tract, may lead to the infection of the valves or myocardium. It might also arise from one of the several organs that have been infected usually from an intestinal focus. The anginosus group causes 3% to 15% of cases of streptococcal IE (109). They usually infect previously damaged valves. Its clinical manifestations truly reflect its pathogenic potential. Its suppurative complications are both intracardiac (myocardial abscesses and purulent pericarditis) and extracardiac. The most common metastatic infection appears to be brain abscesses (110).

Streptococcus anginosus group, clinically and experimentally, behaves like *S. aureus* much more than it does like the other members of the viridans streptococci. Although these micro-organisms produce only about 6% of total cases of IE (109), they are worthy of our attention as they have the potential of joining the forefront of nosocomial pathogens. They already are becoming more involved in HCBSI, especially among neutropenic cancer patients (111).

Nutritionally variant streptococci (NVS) were first identified as a species distinct from the closely related *S. mitior (mitis)* in 1961 (112). They have been found to be taxonomically unrelated to other members of the viridans group (113), and have been recently placed in a new genus *Abiotrophia,* species *Abiotrophia defectiva.* During this discussion, the older nomenclature will be employed. The colonies are small, and the organisms exhibit alpha or gamma hemolysis. They often are pleomorphic with a variable gram stain appearance. Like the viridans streptococci, they are residents of the oropharynx, GI, and genitourinary tracts. They are responsible for 5% of streptococcal IE. These cases usually are subacute in nature.

The term NVS describes the need of these organisms for supplemental vitamin B6 for growth in various types of media. The media must contain the thiol compounds, L-cysteine, or the active forms of vitamin B6 (pyridoxal or pyridoxamine—not pyridoxine). Human blood contains enough pyridoxal for NVS to grow in most types of blood culture media except for trypticase soy broth (114,115). The solid media that is used for subculture of positive blood cultures lacks the essential thiol compounds, and must be supplemented with 0.0001% pyridoxal for growth of NVS to occur. Another method, employed to facilitate the subculture of NVS, making use of the fact that *S. aureus* and some streptococci and Enterobacteriaceae "leak" the essential thiols into the immediate environment. The plated NVS will form colonies surrounding the preplaced *S. aureus*; the phenomenon of satelletism (116). Nutritionally variant streptococci used to be a major cause of culture-negative endocarditis (117). Modern bacteriological methods have lessened its role. When the gram stain of a blood culture demonstrates pleomorphic cocci, which fail to grow out on solid media, the clinician should be alerted to the likelihood that NVS is present.

Nutritionally variant streptococci IE exhibit a much higher mortality and morbidity rate than the corresponding figures for viridans streptococci, including the Anginosus group (118–121). Valve replacement surgery does not completely reverse the increased mortality and morbidity of NVS IE. One possible explanation for this differential in therapeutic response is the prolonged generation time for NVS as compared with the viridans streptococci (two to three hours compared with 50 minutes for the latter). Other slowly growing pathogens, such as *Haemophilus aphrophilus*, demonstrate similar resistance to antimicrobial eradication on the basis of their being relatively insensitive to the effects of cell wall–active antibiotics.

An important factor in the pathogenesis of IE caused by both viridans streptococci and NVS is their growing resistance to penicillin and other beta-lactam antibiotics. Antimicrobial prophylaxis of rheumatic fever has decreased the sensitivity of the oral streptococci to penicillin (122). The American Heart Association's Council on Cardiovascular Disease in the Young defines penicillin-susceptible viridans streptococci as having an MIC of <0.1 µg/mL; relatively resistant isolates, MIC >0.01 µg/mL and <0.5 µg/mL; and resistant examples have an MIC >0.5 µg/mL (123). Moellering defined the breakpoint of MIC resistance to penicillin to be 1.0 µg/mL (124). The MIC of all isolates of NVS to penicillin is currently >0.5 µg/mL, with at least 33% of the IE patients' isolates having an MIC >1.0 µg/mL (125). Occasionally, NVS with an MIC >4.0 µg/mL have been retrieved from blood culture (117). Resistance appears to be the result of alterations in the penicillin-binding proteins (126). All isolates of NVS exhibit tolerance if not high-grade resistance to penicillin (127). Tolerance is the situation in which the MBC of an antibiotic for a given organism exceeds the MIC by at least a factor of 10. Approximately 20% of viridans streptococci [*S. mutans, S. mitior (mitis)*] exhibit tolerance. Tolerance does not appear to be associated with a higher mortality rate. Patients who are infected with tolerance streptococci exhibit failure to respond to the initial antibiotic treatment and require a longer period of treatment (128,128a). Significant synergy between cell wall–active antibiotics and gentamicin has been demonstrated in cases of IE caused by tolerant and nontolerant NVS (129). Because the in-vitro susceptibility tests of NVS, performed by the clinical laboratory do not accurately predict a given patient's bacteriologic response, it is recommended that all patients receive a synergistic antibiotic combination. A more in-depth discussion of the antibiotic treatment of viridans streptococci and NVS is found in Chapter 14 entitled Medical Management.

Group D Streptoccoci

Prior to the 1980s, enterococci were classified as Lancefield group D streptococci with *Streptoccocus bovis* and *Streptoccocus equinus* as the nonenterococcal members of this group. Enterococci now are classified, not as streptococci, but as members of the genus Enterococcus (129). *S. bovis* and *S. equinus* remain in the streptococcal genus, and will be discussed later in this chapter. Enterococci produce small and smooth, cream-colored colonies on 5% sheep blood agar. They may produce either alpha, beta, or gamma hemolysis. They are the most common aerobic gram-positive cocci of human intestinal flora. All human-associated enterococci hydrolyze pyrrolidonyl arylamidase (PYR) and leucine aminopeptidase. They grow at 45°C and in 6.5% NaCl. Although many enterococcal species are capable of producing human infections, the clinician, in reality, will be only dealing with *Enterococcus faecalis* and *Enterococcus faecium* (130). In the past, *E. faecalis* has constituted the vast majority of isolates (90%) from a variety of infections—*E. faecium* less than 10%. Other types of enterococci have been recovered from cases of IE. The strains of enterococci accounted for 2% of endocardial infection at the Massachusetts General Hospital between 1944 and 1958. During the period between 1958 and 1964, this figure increased to 6% and 8% between 1964 and 1973. Currently, these two strains account for between 10% and 20% of all the categories of IE (131,132). Enterococci have become the second most common cause of nosocomial infections (133). In part, this increase in the incidence of enterococcal IE may be attributed to a decrease in that of viridans streptococcal IE. More likely, the dramatic rise, over the last 20 years, of serious enterococcal infections is related to the large amount of third-generation cephalosporins administered to acutely ill patients. These antibiotics have no activity against the members of this genus, and eradicate potential bacterial competitors of the enterococci from various bodily locations. Especially important in the normal suppression of enterococcal overgrowth are the intestinal anaerobes (134). Many other classes of antibiotics have been associated with the "fertilizing" of the intestinal enterococci (135). The third generation cephalosporins also appear to promote newer types of resistance, such as vancomycin-resistant enterococci (VRE) (136,137). These same factors may well account for the rise in multiresistant *E. faecium*. More than 35% of enterococcal bacteremias, currently, may be caused by *E. faecium* (138). The third-generation cephalosporins also lead to enterococcal infection of organs that were previously spared involvement with these organisms. Enterococcal pneumonia has been documented in patients receiving broad-spectrum antibiotics, especially in combination with tube feedings (139).

Approximately 5% of all positive blood cultures grow out enterococci. A very small percentage of enterococcal bacteremias are complicated by valvular infection. Risk factors for enterococcal bacteremia/IE include urinary tract infections, abdominal and pelvic infections, various types of wounds (pressure ulcers and diabetic foot ulcerations), intravascular catheters and biliary tract infections. The most prominent source of enterococcal bacteremias are various types of infections of the genitourinary tract of older men (i.e., prostatitis) (140). Eight percent of intravenous drug abuser IE is produced by this group of pathogens (141). Forty percent of enterococcal BSIs have no definable source (primary bacteremias). Usually these occur in the immunosuppressed, and most likely arise from the intestinal tract (142). Many enterococcal HCBSIs are polymicrobial. These are much less likely to be associated with enterococcal IE than monomicrobial HCBSIs. Other features that differentiate uncomplicated enterococcal bacteremia from enterococcal endocarditis are acquisition of infection in the community, primary bacteremia, and pre-existing valvular disease (143).

Enterococcal IE is a disease of older men (>60 years of age) who have undergone instrumentation for obstructive uropathy, and adult women have experienced various obstetrical/gynecological intervention (140). It is twice as common in males as females. Enterococcal IE is usually subacute affecting previously damaged valves. The disease may be present for up to six months prior to its diagnosis. Symptoms are quite nonspecific. However, acute disease has been well described. Forty percent of individuals have had previously healthy hearts. The reason for this clinical dichotomy is not known (144–146).

Although they play a significant role in healthcare-associated infections, there is relatively little known regarding enterococcal virulence factors as compared with those of *S. aureus*, CoNS, or even other streptococci. Serious enterococcal infections seldom affect the normal host (135). Enterococcal bacteremia is associated with extremely high rates of mortality (up to 68%) (147). No study has clearly demonstrated that enterococcal BSIs are nothing more than a reflection of a severely ill population of patients. The dermal and mucosal barriers to infection of these individuals already had been breached by intravascular and urinary catheters (148) and being damaged by malnourishment and chemotheraputic agents. Their virulence may depend in great deal on the organism's intrinsic ability to exchange extrachromosomal particles that code for several potential virulence factors, and probably more importantly, various types of antibiotic resistance. Indeed, resistance to vancomycin appears to be an independent risk factor for mortality from enterococcal bacteremia (149). There are several, potential virulence factors of enterococci (150–155). The first recognized and probably the most established of these is fibronectin-binding protein, which accounts for the fact that *Streptococcus faecalis* attaches more strongly in vitro to the valvular endothelial than any other organism, either gram-positive or gram-negative (156–157). The occurrence rates of these virulence factors among the strains of enterococci recovered from patients with endocarditis/bacteremia were as follows: esp (72.4%) (58.6%), aggregation substance (48.3%), and cytolysin (17.2%). Not surprisingly, as fibronectin-binding protein was not assayed, pathogenic adherence was not associated with any of the examined substances (158). Probably second in importance of potential virulence factors is the capacity of enterococci to produce biofilm. Strains of *E. faecalis*, isolated from human cases of IE, were found to be significantly greater generators of biofilm than nonendocarditis associated examples (39% vs. 6%) (159).

The current "bottom line" regarding the contribution of all of these to the development of enterococcal IE is that extended hospitalization, extensive exposure to multiple antibiotics, and especially decreased host defenses significantly outrank them as causative factors of valvular infection (160). Indeed, it has been demonstrated that oral antibiotics can promote extraintestinal translocation through intact gut cells of *E. faecalis* without the need of aggregation substance or any binding factors (161).

Enterococci have achieved a prominent place in nosocomial infections, primarily by their intrinsic resistance to penicillin. Additionally important is their unique facility to acquire resistance to ampicillin, gentamicin, and vancomycin through bacterial conjugation by means of the extrachromosomal elements, plasmids, and conjugative transpons. Transpons can cross the gram-positive/gram-negative barrier although infrequently.

Since the beginning of the antibiotic era, enterococci have been recognized as being markedly less sensitive to penicillin G than other streptococci, on the basis of the tolerance phenomenon (see earlier) (162). This tolerance prevents the use of a single beta-lactam agent in the treatment of serious enterococcal infections. Intrinsically, all enterococci are relatively or absolutely resistant to many antibiotics (163). The inability of aminoglycosides to penetrate the cell wall of enterococci makes them useless against these bacteria when used singly. Hunter in 1947 observed that the combination of penicillin and streptomycin was highly effective in treating enterococcal IE (164). Moellering and Weinberg uncovered the mechanism behind this synergistic effect (165). Certain penicillins, especially ampicillin and vancomycin, by damaging the integrity of the enterococcal cell wall, permit the aminoglycoside component to reach its ribosomal target. It is the aminoglycoside that is lethal to the enterococcus (166). Further discussion of the specifics of synergism in the treatment of enterococcal IE will be presented in Chapter 14.

Over the last 20 years, enterococci have become more resistant to the penicillins on the basis of the decreasing affinity of penicillin-binding proteins, especially PBP-5 (167–169). This has been most striking in the case of *E. faecium* (170). Enterococci are clinically resistant to all the cephalosporins and to the antistaphylococcal isoxazolyl penicillins (oxacillin, nafcillin) and the carboxypenicillins (ticarcillin). Neither are they synergistic with the aminoglycosides (171–173). The reasons for this inactivity are: (*i*) for intrinsic activity against enterococci; (*ii*) increased protein binding of both classes of antibiotics; and (*iii*) in vivo production of inactive metabolites that interfere with antimicrobial activity (174,175).

In vitro, rifampin is quite active against enterococcal species. However, they quickly develop resistance to this agent. Rifampin should never be used in combination with a cell wall–active antibiotic because of its antagonism to the latter (176). Enterococci are frequently quite sensitive to trimethoprim-sulfamethoxazole in vitro. They in vivo are able to circumvent the antimicrobial action of this compound by the uptake of exogenous preformed folic acids which are present in mammals (177). Enterococci exhibit low-level resistance to clindamycin on the basis of an ATP-binding reflux protein (178).

The fluoroquinolones possess variable activity against most clinical isolates of enterococci, and cannot be regarded as first-line agents against enterococcal IE (179). Enterococci gain resistance to ampicillin in several distinctive ways. Enterococci, usually *E. faecalis,* may acquire from *S. aureus* a gene regulating the production of penicillinase (180). The amount of enzyme produced is small, and is not easily detected in clinical laboratories. It becomes significant when there is a large bacterial inoculum. *E. faecium* may become highly resistant to ampicillin on the basis of an extremely low-affinity penicillin-binding protein, PBP5 (181); increased expression of PBP 5 (182); or an altered type of transpeptidase (183). In these situations, the MIC of the organisms may increase from 32 µg/mL to >256 µg/mL (170).

In the 1960s, enterococci began to exhibit widespread resistance to streptomycin and then to kanamycin (184). In 1979, isolates of *E. faecalis,* highly resistant to kanamycin, amikacin, and gentamicin, were first encountered (185). Twenty-five of these remain sensitive to streptomycin (186). Combined high-level resistance to gentamicin and streptomycin has developed (187). For these strains, there is no synergistic combination available.

Low-level resistance of enterococci to vancomycin has been described in some infrequently encountered strains of enterococci (*Enterococcus gallinarium* and *Enterococcus casseliflavus*) (167). True VRE (MIC >64 µg/mL) were first described in Europe in the mid-1980s (188). It is encoded by various clusters of genes (van A, van B, and van D). These clusters direct the replacement of D-ALA-D-ALA sequence of peptidoglycan with D-ALA-D-lactate. The vancomycin binds much less avidly to the altered sequence. The most common of these gene clusters is van A, which is also responsible for the greatest degree of resistance (189). It also encodes resistance to the antibiotic teicoplanin. The van B phenotype is the second most common variety, and is usually susceptible to teicoplanin. The versatility of this pathogen in mounting defenses against antibiotics is nowhere better demonstrated than in the case of two new agents that have great potential for treating multiple resistant enterococci.

Linezolid is the first available oxazolidinone. It is distinctive because of its wide gram-positive activity, including effectiveness against the emerging highly resistant examples, such as VRE and MRSA (190). Vancomycin-resistant enterococci IE has responded to linezolid, administered either orally or intravenously (191). Linezolid is bacteriostatic against most pathogens. Its mechanism of action is the inhibition of protein synthesis at the level of 23S rRNA (192).

Vancomycin-resistant enterococci that are naturally resistant to linezolid, have been isolated from patients without any exposure to this drug (193). Usually, resistance develops in individuals treated with this agent for more than 21 days, more often than not with previous exposure to multiple antibiotics (194). The basis of this resistance is mutation of 23S ribosomal RNA; the more copies of t 23S ribosome RNA that are altered, the higher is the MIC of the enterococcus (195).

Quinpristin-dalfopristin (QD) is a combination of two members of the streptogramin class of antibiotics. Bacterial protein synthesis is inhibited by confirmational changes at two different targets on the rRNA 23S (196). Synergy is achieved because dalfopristin produces irreversible attachment of quinpristin to the ribosome (197). All isolates of E. faecalis are naturally resistant to QD, as they possess the Isa gene, which causes efflux of QD (198). E. faecium may become resistant on the basis of enzymatic modifications, efflux, and modifications of the ribosomal targets. Resistance to dalfopristin blocks the synergistic effect of this combination. Resistance to QD in E. faecium, isolated from human stool, is approximately 2%. Approximately 1% of patients would develop resistance during treatment (199).

Daptomycin, a lipopeptide antibiotic, shows promise for treating resistant enterococcal and other resistant gram-positive IE, even VRE valvular infections (200). Its mechanism of action is to disrupt the bacterial cell membrane (201). Early data indicates a very low potential for the development of resistance to this antibiotic by enterococci and other gram-positive organisms (202).

Streptococcus bovis

As S. bovis reacts with Lancefield group D antiserum, it had long been classified as the other major member of group D enterococci. They both multiply in 40% bile and hydrolyze esculin. Five percent of S. viridans (usually S. salivarius) share these properties. Classically, S. bovis may be differentiated from the enterococci by its failure to grow in either sodium azide or 6.5% NaCl or react to PYR. The ability of S. bovis to ferment lactose separates it from S. equinus. The latter is a true member of group D streptococci, but unusually causes infection in humans (203). Currently, the API Rapid Strep test (API System S.A., Montalieu-Vercien, France) not only accurately identifies S. bovis, but also differentiates into its two major biotypes (biotypes I and II/1, II/2) (204) (see later for the significance of biotyping). Unlike enterococci, clinical isolates of S. bovis are sensitive to the semisynthetic penicillins (oxacillin, nafcillin) and clindamycin.

The GI tract is the most common source of *S. bovis* bacteremia, followed by the genitourinary tract (205). Valvular infection may complicate up to 50% of bacteremias caused by *S. bovis* (206,207). In some series, *S. bovis* causes up to 25% of all cases of IE (208). This figure appears to be country specific. Typically, this organism produces subacute IE on previously damaged valves. At times, it may present as an acute process. Its rate of morbidity and death, and its response to treatment is very similar to that caused by the viridans streptococci (209). Moellering observed that 12/13 individuals with *S. bovis* IE survived as compared with only 8/15 patients with enterococcal valvular infection (205).

A striking characteristic of *S. bovis* bacteremia is its association with the manipulation of the GI tract or a variety of colonic lesions. These range from carcinoma of the large intestine to intrinsic bowel disease (210–212). An early retrospective study of 36 patients with *S. bovis* bacteremia (210) described either GI procedures or abnormalities in 22 individuals. Nine of these had colon cancer. Esophageal carcinoma has also been associated with *S. bovis* BSI (212). The presence of bacteremic *S. bovis* mandates a thorough GI workup. An underappreciated characteristic of *S. bovis* is its significant association with chronic, advanced liver disease (213,214). The triad of *S. bovis* bacteremia, liver disease, and colonic pathology is overwhelmingly associated with biotype I (213). This biotype also appears to be connected with both aseptic and purulent meningitis that results from *S. bovis* bacteremia (215,216). There is no established reason to explain the predominance of *S. bovis* I in these various conditions. *S. bovis* does not appear to be involved in IVDA IE (213).

The virulence factors of this organism are incompletely identified. Patients are older with more associated diseases, such as diabetes (208) than those with most other types of IE. The adherence of *S. bovis* to epithelial and endothelial cells, and to extracellular matrix, results in a cytokine-mediated inflammatory response (217). Frequently, this process produces luxuriant valvular vegetations >10 mm more frequently than any other micro-organisms (218). It is not certain whether these thrombi have a higher-than-average rate of embolization (208,213). Fourteen percent of infections involve multiple valves (208). *S. bovis* may be extremely invasive and destructive of valvular leaflets. Abscesses both of the septum and valvular rings (219) may occur.

S. bovis is usually quite sensitive to penicillin G, in addition to most other beta-lactam antibiotics (205). It is not necessary to administer a synergistic combination of penicillin and an aminoglycoside. Isolates tolerant to penicillin have been retrieved from cases of IE with an MBC 100-fold greater than the MIC (220). Streptomycin resistance has also been documented (221). Moellering et al. observed that 12/13 individuals with *S. bovis* IE survived as compared with only 8/15 patients with enterococcal valvular infection (205).

Group B Streptococci (GBS, *Streptococcus agalactiae*)

Group B streptococcus, a gram-positive coccus, is a frequent colonizer of the GI and genital tracts (approximately 10% of the population) (222,223). It produces small white colonies on blood agar that are beta-hemolytic (224). The Lancefield group B antigen is a distinctive carbohydrate that is contained in the cell wall of the organism (see later for virulence factors). Group B streptococcus is itself beta-hemolytic, and also augments the beta-hemolysis of *S. aureus* by its production of the cAMP factor. Demonstration of cAMP activity along with failure to hydrolyze bile esculin agar and sensitivity to bacitracin provides adequate screening for group B streptococci. Confirmation is obtained by the use of commercially available antisera.

Long recognized as an obstetrical and pediatric pathogen, GBS is becoming a more frequent cause of invasive disease in older patients, especially in those with significant underlying diseases (e.g., diabetes, cancer, and hepatic diseases). In the community, the risk of GBS infections progressively increases past age 65 (222–225). There is an association of GBS BSI and IE with the presence of villous adenomas (226). In the preantibiotic era, GBS IE was seen almost exclusively associated with pregnancy. Rheumatic heart disease was usually present (227). Its course was rapidly progressive. Currently, IE may be either acute or subacute. Although the median age of patients is 50, it still occurs in women of child bearing age either during the peripartum period or following a therapeutic abortion. Most have underlying cardiac abnormalities, usually those of rheumatic heart disease (228). Younger patients share the same risk factors for invasive GBS infections with older individuals, with the addition of HIV disease (226). Diabetes is the premier risk factor for GBS invasive disease for all age groups. African Americans appear to be at greater risk for GBS invasive disease from IE prosthetic valves, pacemakers, and intravenous catheters that may become infected. Group B streptococcus is an increasing cause of IVDA IE (229), and GBS HCBSI is well documented (229). Twenty-five percent of these are polymicrobial, usually with *S. aureus* as the second pathogen (228). Less than 2% of primary GBS bacteremias are complicated by valvular infection (226). Approximately 3% of all cases of IE are caused by GBS (230).

Group B streptococcus IE primarily involves the mitral valve (48% of cases) (231). Tricuspid valve disease is exclusively seen in IVDA IE (232). Various cardiac conditions (rheumatic heart disease, calcific valvular disease, and mitral valve prolapse) underly 50% of cases (233). Major systemic emboli occur in 40% of cases often early in the course of the disease. These arise from large friable vegetations that are quite similar to those of *S. bovis* and *S. aureus* (233). Another distinctive characteristic of GBS-invasive disease, including IE, is its high rate of recurrence of approximately 4% (234,235). There have been case reports of three bouts of recurrent valvular infection despite apparently adequate antibiotic therapy. Infective endocarditis, owing to this organism, may be associated with a greater risk of embolic endophthalmitis (236). Capsular polysaccharides, which are composed of repeating oligosaccharides, determine the type specificity of GBS (237). There are nine recognized serotypes (238). Serotype V accounts for 30% of adult infections with serotype Ia/c, Ib/c, and III are the next most common (239). The capsular material of GBS is a major contributor to its virulence (240). Siliac acid, which is located in the terminal end of polysaccharide sidechain, inhibits the activation of the alternative complement pathway. The particular structure of the capsule probably determines the relative degree of invasiveness of the nine serotypes (refer to the earlier paras for the distribution of serotypes in adult GBS disease). Type III appears to have greater cellular invasive power than other serotypes.

Low levels of maternal-derived antibodies to type III capsular antigen and abnormalities of the complement system appear to put newborns at risk for invasive GBS disease (241). Both of these are required for phagocytosis and intracellular killing of GBS. Among adults, this humoral protection may not be as all encompassing. Non protective levels of serotype V capsular antibody have been documented among healthy adults (242). Functional activity of the white cells of these individuals to ingest and kill GBS was found to be deficient on opsinophagocytosis assay.

Addition of specific antibodies to type V corrected this dysfunction in vitro. It would be for future studies to determine whether case type V PBS vaccine would produce specifically active antibodies in older or debilitated people.

There is evidence that invasive GBS disease of nonpregnant adults may occur in the setting of high levels of IgG capsular antibody (243). Therefore, other factors may contribute to the susceptibility of older, especially chronically ill adults, to GBS IE. Expression of beta-hemolysin/cytolysin confers greater potential for tissue invasion and cellular injury (244,245). The inability of GBS to produce fibrolysin may contribute to its characteristic large valvular vegetations and increased embolic potential (245).

Other extracellular virulence factors of GBS include beta 1-integrin, C-5a peptidase, hyaluronate lyase, cAMP factor, and carotenoid pigment (246–249). Unlike the aforementioned organisms, GBS appears uniformly susceptible to the penicillins, cephalosporins, vancomycin, the carbapenems, and daptomycin (250,251). Penicillin G is the antibiotic of choice. However, the MIC of this antibiotic for GBS is significantly greater than that of group A streptococci (average 0.04 µg/mL) (222). Although approximately 5% of isolates are tolerant to penicillin G, there has been no need established for adding gentamicin to overcome potential relative resistance (252). There is growing resistance to erythromycin and clindamycin among GBS. In Spain, 17.4% and 20.1% strains are resistant to erythromycin and clindamycin, respectively. These resistant isolates appear quite susceptible to telithromycin. There is little experience using the fluoroquinolones to treat GBS IE. Resistance to the fluoroquinolones has been reported (253). Mortality has been reported as high as 50% (254). There may be a wide spectrum of outcomes. There are case reports of quite favorable outcomes with appropriate antibiotic therapy without a need for valvular replacement. This variation may well reflect differences in the infecting serotypes (255) with a high rate of relapse (236). Relapse may be attributed to the inability of penicillin to eradicate GBS from mucosal surfaces.

Other Beta-Hemolytic Streptococci (Group A Beta-Hemolytic, Group C, and Group G Streptococci)

Group A beta-hemolytic streptococci (GABHS) are found on the skin, oral pharynx, and anal mucosa (129). They currently are quite infrequent causes of valvular infection (256). This was not always the case. In the preantibiotic era, this organism had a "one-two cardiac punch." Its ability to cause rheumatic valvulitis set the stage for the development of valvular thrombi, which then could be infected by bacteremia with GABHS (257). This change can be ascribed to the reduction by antibiotics of the traditional sources of GABHS BSI (pneumonia, erysipelas cellulites, and pharyngitis). Group A beta-hemolytic streptococci bacteremia currently is seen in patients with chronic debilitating diseases, such as neoplasms, renal failure, and alcoholism. Corticosteroid usage and diabetes mellitus (33% of cases of GABHS IE) are other important predisposing factors. This organism has also been involved in IVDA IE (258). In addition, the ratio of the cases of IE to those of GABHS BSI is the lowest of any of the streptococci (86). This ratio appears to be correlated with the production of dextran by a particular species of streptococcus (259). Group A beta-hemolytic streptococci IE resembles in many respects that of *S. aureus* in that it may cause rapid valvular distraction, myocardial abscesses, and metastatic infection owing to septic emboli.

The particular virulence factors of GABHS that are involved in valvular infection are not understood. M protein enables GABHS to avoid phagocytosis by several mechanisms (260). It interferes with the deposition of C3b on the surface of these streptococci. M protein–like factors can bind to the immunoglobulins, IgG, IgA, and to fibrinogen, plasmin, and factor H (261). C5a peptidase is another surface protein that by splitting C5a interferes with the activation of PMNL (262). Group A beta-hemolytic streptococci produce substances that lead to the invasion and destruction of several types of tissues. Among these are the streptolysins O and S, streptokinase, DNAase, and hyaluronidase (129).

Groups C (*Streptococcus dysgalactiae*) and G streptococci are normal inhabitants of the skin nasopharynx, genitourinary, and GI tracts (129,263). The following discussion pertains only to the large colony size of beta-hemolytic streptococci (>0.5 mm in diameter). The smaller colony variants are classified as belonging to the *S. anginosus* group (129). Groups C and G are unusually retrieved from the cases of IE. From 150,000 blood cultures collected at the Mayo Clinic over 10-year period to the 1970s, group C was isolated in only eight individuals. One of these had IE (264). In one series, these two appear to cause IE more frequently than group A or group B beta-hemolytic streptococci (265). In a more recent survey, the Emerging Infectious Network of the Infectious Diseases Society of America identified 31 cases of IE caused by the beta-hemolytic streptococci. Group B was retrieved from 21; group A from five and group G from three individuals (266). In the author's experience, GBS is a much more frequent cause of IE than these other beta-hemolytic streptococci. Group C streptococci isolates that infect humans are divided into three subgroups (*Streptococcus equisimilis, Streptococcus zooepidemicus, Streptococcus equi*). Clinical series vary in that they document that group C IE can present as "semi acute," with a mean duration of symptoms of 17.4 days (267) or acute (268). However, they are consistent in that they find that valvular infection with this organism is characterized by macroemboli to the central nervous system, legs, spleen, kidneys, myocardium, and lung. There is a high rate of rapid valvular destruction, resulting in congestive heart failure, which requires emergent valvular replacement. Myocardial abscesses and intracardiac infection delays are also reported. Both normal native and prosthetic valves may be affected. Among those infected, there is a high rate of occupational contact with animals, such as farmers, cattle truck drivers, butchers, and those who process animal hides (264). Mortality runs between 30% and 50%.

Group G IE differs from valvular infection owing to group C in that it typically effects older patients (56 years of age) with multiple underlying diseases, such as diabetes mellitus, alcoholism, squamous cell carcinoma of the oropharynx, and alcoholism (269–272). The rate of embolization, valvular destruction, intracardiac complications, and death are essentially the same as for the cases of group C (273).

Groups C and G isolates produce streptolysins, streptokinase, and hemolysins to varying degrees. They also have antiphagocytic defenses (hyaluronic capsule and surface M proteins). All of these closely resemble their counterparts found in GBS (129). Although these streptococci are generally quite sensitive to penicillin, there is a good body of evidence indicating that a penicillin/aminoglycoside combination should be used in the treatment of IE (273).

Group F rarely causes IE. These organisms cause about 2% of all beta-hemolytic streptococcal bacteremias (274,275). Most group F BSI arise from a variety of GI lesions. They are often polymicrobial (39%), quite understandable given their intestinal origin. Similar to the valvular infections of other beta-hemolytic streptococci, group F IE has a high rate of suppurative complications. Its course is usually acute.

Streptococcus suis primarily involves swine. It possesses Lancefield antigens R, S, and T. Rarely, it can produce IE in humans (276). The cardiac infection often presents as meningitis or endophthalmitis. A history of ingesting of pork or some other type of exposure to swine can be elicited.

Groups I and L streptococci have been reported to cause valvular infection (277,278). There are several gram-positive cocci species that resemble viridans streptococci, and which occasionally are involved in IE (225). *Aerococcus viridans* differs from other streptococci in being weakly catalase positive. It forms tetrads in broth rather than chains. Like an enterococcus, it tolerates exposure to 40% of bile. However, it does not possess the group D streptococcal antigen, and is susceptible to many types of antibiotics. In clinical course, it is very similar to the viridans streptococci (279).

On Gram stain, *Gemella haemolysans* resembles diphtheroids because of its gram-variable staining reaction and its pleomorphism. Its clinical characteristics closely resemble those of the viridans streptococci in that it is sensitive to penicillin and many other antibiotics (280,281). *Leuconostac* spp. morphologically resembles diphtheroids. Little is known of their epidemiology and pathogenesis. They have been mostly documented as nosocomial bacteremias among immunocompromised patients or newborns (282). They are intrinsically resistant to vancomycin.

Streptococcus pneumoniae

Streptococcus pneumoniae are gram-positive organisms that are alpha-hemolytic and require catalase for growth in vitro. They are sensitive to optochin discs and to bile salts (225). In 1931, 15% of all cases of IE were attributed to *S. pneumoniae* (283). In the modern era, they are responsible for less than 3% of cases (284). Infection with *S. pneumoniae* occurs most frequently in those less than four years of age and in those >60 years of age (285). The incidence of pneumococcal bacteremia has almost tripled over the last two decades (286). Infective endocarditis is more common in patients with multilobar pneumonia, especially when treatment is delayed. This scenario is especially true for type 12S. pneumoniae. The strain is responsible for only 3% of pneumococcal pneumonias, but is responsible for 20% of pneumococcal IE (25,287). Pneumococcal IE follows a very acute course. In respect to its acute course, intra- and extracardiac complications, and mortality rates (up to 60%), it closely resembles the valvular infections of *S. aureus* (284,286,288). A recent series (289) demonstrated that 67% of patients had no predisposing cardiac factors and 13.3% had bioprosthetic valves. The aortic valve is the most frequently involved. In one-third of the affected individuals, the primary source of infection was pneumonia. Meningitis was present in 40%. The most frequent complications were congestive heart failure, macroemboli, and focal abscesses. Ninety-seven percent had vegetations by echocardiography; 20% had valvular perforation; and 13.3% had valvular ring abscesses on echocardiography. Forty percent were alcoholics; 16% were infected with pneumococcal strains that were penicillin resistant; 66.7% underwent valvular replacement, most occurring during the first month of infection; and 24% of patients died. The authors attributed this lower-than-average rate of death (50%) to the high rate of early valve replacement. Subacute cases of pneumococcal IE that resemble those of the viridans streptococci do occur (290).

HIV predisposes patients, especially African Americans, to invasive pneumococcal disease (291) and to recurrent bacteremia with *S. pneumoniae*. There appears to be a re-emergence of the Austrian syndrome (*S. pneumoniae* IE, meningitis, and rupture of the aortic valve) in patients with AIDS. These individuals also have a high rate of penicillin-resistant organisms. Those that respond to highly active antiretroviral therapy (HAART) show a decline in these cases (292).

Streptococcus pneumoniae possess a wide range of virulence factors. The major protective factor of *S. pneumoniae* is the ability of its polysaccharide capsule to interfere with effective phagocytosis (293). There are no receptors on phagocytes that recognize these polysaccharides. The capsule appears to be able to inactivate the complement. By means of electrochemical forces, it is able to repel phagocytic cells. The organism does not use any fibrillar structures to adhere to human cells. They make use of several types of proteins that connect to human cellular carbohydrates or to platelet activating factor (PAF) receptors (294). *S. pneumoniae* employ different ligands specific to a given organ. Disaccharides are the specific receptors of the lower respiratory tract for *S. pneumoniae* (295). Preceding the infection with the influenza virus increases the risk for invasive pneumococcal disease by upregulating pneumococcal cellular receptors (296,297).

S. pneumoniae have diminished invasive capacity as compared with other gram-positive cocci (298). In addition, there is a great variability for invasive potential that is dependent upon the serotype (299). Serotypes 3, 6A, and 15 have the highest rates of invasive disease. Choline, which is a unique component of the pneumococcal cell wall, promotes protein binding to the host cell and to the PAF receptor (300). Having done so, the bacteria enter the cytoplasm in an endocytic vacuole. Pneumolysin, a cytotoxin, both facilitates cellular invasion and promotes penetration into the bloodstream (301). Antibiotic resistance has become a major virulence factor of *S. pneumoniae*. A Centers for Disease Control (CDC) surveillance program documented that from 1995 to 1998, the rate of resistance of pneumococcal isolates involved in invasive disease in the United States increased from 21% to 25%. The isolates that were resistant to vancomycin increased from 9% to 14% during this period (302). Alterations in the PBPs account for both intermediate- and high-level resistance to penicillins (303). Resistance to other classes of antibiotics is associated with penicillin resistance (see Chapter 14). Especially notable is the development of vancomycin tolerance by *S. pneumoniae* (304).

GRAM-POSITIVE BACILLI

In the past, gram-positive bacilli seldom have been implicated in cases of IE. Although still unusual valvular pathogens, they are frequently recovered from cases of IE of patients with prosthetic valves, intravascular devices, and various types of immunosuppression.

Erysipelothrix rhusiopathiae and *Lactobacillus* sp. are catalase-negative nonforming gram-positive rods (305). *E. rhusiopathiae* are carried by fish, shrimp, birds, and many other types of wild and domestic animals. Men, especially fishermen, are especially affected because of their greater exposure to these veterinary sources. Thirty-three percent of individuals with IE are alcoholics, and 26% exhibit a skin lesion, characteristic of erysipeloid (306,307). Most cases of IE arise from primary bacteremias. Most likely, many of these arise from GI infections with *E. rhusiopathiae* (308). Sixty percent of cases of IE involve normal native valves (309). The organism is able to infect prosthetic ones as well (310). The aortic valve is involved in 70%. The course of this type of IE is quite acute and is complicated by myocardial abscesses, congestive heart failure, and meningitis (311). A distinctive characteristic of *E. rhusiopathiae* valvular infection is the high rate of acute renal failure secondary to proliferative glomerulonephritis (312). The mortality rate ranges from 33% to 50%. Thirty-three percent require valvular replacement.

The virulence factors of *E. rhusiopathiae* are not well known. The presence of SpaA surface antigen contributes in some way to its lethal effect (313,314). The most virulent isolates possess a capsule with antiphagocytic properties. In some way, this organism is able to increase its intracellular survival by reducing the stimulation of the oxidative respiratory burst (315,316). The beta-lactams, especially penicillin G and imipenem, are the agents of choice (317). As *E. rhusiopathiae* is naturally resistant to vancomycin, it is important to recognize its presence to avoid using this antibiotic that is so frequently employed in empiric coverage of gram-positive BSIs. Lactobacilli are normal members of the microflora of the intestinal tract and vagina (305). Three species (*Lactobacillus casei, Lactobacillus acidophilus, Lactobacillus plantarum*) have been involved in subacute cases of IE (318,319). The mitral valve is the most often involved. Eighty-three percent of patients have valvular pathology that was not recognized prior to the development of IE. Dental procedures are the most frequently recognized inciting factors. The rate of embolization is high (55% of cases). Although sensitive to penicillin G in vitro, there is a high rate of relapse when this drug is used as monotherapy (24 million units a day). This appears to be the result of the tolerance of the organism to this antibiotic. Combining gentamicin with penicillin is probably the best therapeutic option.

Listeria monocytogenes, Corynebacteria sp., and *Kurthia* spp. are nonspore-forming, catalase-positive, gram-positive rods. Listeria may appear as a coccobacillus, and so be confused with diphtheroids, streptococcal disease, or even *Hemophilus influenzae*. Cold enrichment growth techniques select out this organism. *Listeria* spp. are widely distributed in nature. *Listeria monocytogenes* is the only one that is involved in human infections. It is found in soil water and the GI tracts of many animals. Currently, *Listeria* infections are primarily foodborne (320,321). There is no good evidence of the passage of this pathogen from animal to human. *Listeria* IE occurs most frequently in the pregnant and in those >55 years of age (322). The incidence of endocardial infection is on the increase probably owing to the growing numbers of individuals with various types of immunodeficiencies, especially those treated with large dose corticosteroids (323,324). However, most cases still occur among the immunocompetent (325). The profile of a typical patient resembles that of one with IE owing to viridans streptococci. The mean age is 51. It usually follows a subacute course. However, the rate of embolization and death is greater for cases of *Listeria* IE. This may be attributed in part to the delay in establishing the correct etiologic diagnosis.

The major virulence factor of *L. monocytogenes* is the fact that it is intracellular not only in phagocytic, but also nonphagocytic cells (326). In this environment, it is sheltered from the host's defenses especially from the lymphokines (327). The manner in which *L. monocytogenes* gain access to their cytoplasmic haven is quite complex. First, it attaches to a heparin peptidoglycan receptor on the host cell's surface. The pathogen then secretes a surface protein (internalins) that facilitate entry into the cell. In order to survive intracellularly, *Listeria* makes use of a hemolysin (listeriolysin O) that lyses the phagosome's membrane. After this escape, it rapidly replicates and gathers around itself acting of the host cell. The bacterial product (ActA) then assembles the actin into filaments around the terminal end of the pathogen. This contractile protein moves the bacteria through the cell membrane to the surface of the neighboring cells (328). Resistance to commonly used antibiotics is not an important virulence factor (329). Isolates are usually quite sensitive to ampicillin or trimethoprim-sulfamethoxazole (330).

Several species of corynebacteria are involved in cases of IE. Among these are *Corynebacteria pseudodiphtheriticum* (formerly *Corynebacteria hofmanni*), *Corynebacteria xerosis*, and *Corynebacteria jeikium*, which is the most frequently recovered. Diphtheroid is a term that represents nondiphtheritic corynebacteria. They are found on the skin and mucus membranes of debilitated hospitalized patients (331). Diphtheroids (*C. hofmanni*) may infect previously damaged native valves, especially among the immunosuppressed (332). They more often infect prosthetic ones, usually causing early PVE. Nontoxigenic *Corynebacteria diphtheriae* have been documented to cause IE. Its course can be quite acute with frequent embolization and septic arthritis (333). Many of these cases occurred in patients who have been immunized. This observation emphasizes that immunization protects against the toxin-mediated effects of *C. diphtheriae*, but not against the invasive ones (334,335). The antibiotic sensitivity of diphtheroids is variable. Many are sensitive to penicillin G. The combination of penicillin and gentamicin are synergistic against some strains (336). *Kurthia bessoni* has been documented to cause IVDA IE. Often a combined medical and surgical approach is required for cure (337).

Rothia dentocariosa and *Rothia mucilaginosus* are nonacid-fast aerobic actinomycetes that are normal residents of the oral cavity (338). They appear to be coccobacilli on Gram stain. Rothia BSIs arise from carous teeth and gingivitis. They usually produce subacute disease (339,340). There is an association between the IE of *R. mucilaginosus* and cardiac catheterization or previous cardiac surgery (341). The valvular infection of *R. dentocariosa* is frequently complicated by perivalvular abscesses and vertebral osteomyelitis (342). Both prosthetic valves and native valves may be involved (343). Penicillin is the drug of choice for treating Rothia infections. *Bacillus* spp. are gram-positive, facultatively anaerobic spore-forming bacilli that may infect the cardiac valves that are either previously damaged or prosthetic ones. Infection of either type is much more common in IVDA with tricuspid valve (345); there is a high rate of septic pulmonary emboli and/or thrombosis brought about by an extracellular toxin that is manufactured by these organisms. A pan-endophthalmitis is often a presentation of IE caused by *Bacillus* spp. Additionally, they can adhere to prosthetic material of intravascular devices, such as pacemakers and prosthetic valves in a layer of glycocalyx (346). Antibiotic therapy with vancomycin or clindamycin is often adequate for cure (347).

REFERENCES

1. Lerner D, Weinstein L. Infective endocarditis in the antibiotic era. N Engl J Med 1966; 274:199.
2. Role of microscopy in the diagnosis of infectious diseases. In: Forbes BA, Sahm DF, Weissfeld AS, eds. Bailey and Scott's Diagnostic Microbiology. Chap. 9. 11th ed. St. Louis: Mosby, 2002:119.
3. Finland M, Barnes MW. Changing etiology of bacterial endocarditis in the antibacterial era: experiences at Boston City Hospital 1933–1955. Ann Intern Med 1970; 72:341.
4. Wilson LM. Etiology of bacterial endocarditis: before and since introduction of antibiotics. Ann Intern Med 1963; 58:946.
5. Bouza E, Menasalvas A, Munoz P, et al. Infective endocarditis—a prospective study at the end of the twentieth century. Medicine 2001; 88:298.
6. Friedland G, von Reyn CF, Levy BS, et al. Nosocomial endocarditis. Infect Control 1984; 5:284.
7. Thompson R. Staphylococcal infective endocarditis. Mayo Clin Proc 1982; 57:106.

8. Projan SJ, Novick RP. The molecular basis of pathogenicity. In: Crossley KB, Archer GL, eds. The Staphylococci in Human Disease. New York: Churchill Livingstone, 1997: 55–81.
9. Weidenmaier C, Peschel A, Xiong YQ, et al. Lack of wall teichoic acids in *Staphylococcus aureus* leads to reduced interactions with endothelial cells and to attenuated virulence in a rabbit model of endocarditis. J Infect Dis 2005; 191:1771.
10. Lowy FD. *Staphylococcus aureus* infections. N Eng J Med 1998; 339:520.
11. Roche FM, Masey R, Peacock SJ, et al. Characterization of novel LPXTG-containing proteins of *Staphylococcus aureus* identified from genome sequences. Microbiology 2003; 149:643
12. Kornblum J, Kreiswirth BN, Projan SJ, et al. Agr: a polycistronic locus regulating protein synthesis in *Staphylococcus aureus*. In: Novick RP, ed. Molecular Biology of the Staphylococci. New York: UCH Publ, 1990:373.
13. Cheung AL, Projan SJ. Cloning and sequencing of sar A of *Staphylococcus aureus*, a gene required for the expression of agr. J Bacteriol 1994; 176:4168.
14. Cheung Al, Koomey JM, Butler CA, et al. Regulation of exoprotein expression in *Staphylococcus aureus* by a locus (sar) distinct from agr. Proc Natl Acad Sci USA 1992; 89:6462.
15. Moreillon P, Entenza JM, Francioli P, et al. Role of *Staphylococcus aureus* coagulase and clumping factor in pathogenesis of experimental endocarditis. Infect Immun 1995; 63:4738.
16. Kuypers JM, Proctor RA. Reduced adherence to, tie to that heart valves by a little fibronectin-binding mutant of *Staphylococcus aureus*. Infect Immun 1989; 57:2306.
17. Donlan RM. Biofilm formation: a clinically relevant microbiological process. Clin Infect Dis 2001; 33:1387.
18. Noble WC, Somerville DA. Microbiology of human skin. London: W.B. Saunders, 1974.
19. Tuazon CU, Sheagren JN. Staphylococcal endocarditis in parenteral drug abusers: source of the organism. Ann Intern Med 1975; 82:790.
20. Vehoef J. Host defense against infection. In: Crossley KB, Archer GL, eds. The Staphylococci in Human Disease. New York: Churchill Livingstone, 1997:213.
21. Karakawa WW, Sutton A, Schneerson R, et al. Capsular antibodies induce type-specific phagocytosis of encapsulated *Staphylococcus aureus* by human polymorphonuclear leukocytes. Infect Immun 1988; 56:1090.
22. Baddour LM, Lowrance C, Albus A, et al. *Staphylococcus aureus* microcapsule expression attenuates bacterial virulence in a rat model of experimental endocarditis. J Infect Dis 1992; 165:749.
23. Peterson PK, Verhoef J, Sabatk LD, et al. Effect of protein A on staphylococcal opsonization. Infect Immun 1977; 15:760.
24. Iannini P, Crossley K. Therapy of *Staphylococcus aureus* bacteremia associated with a removable focus of infection. Ann Int Med 1976; 81:558.
25. Lee AH, Levinson AI, Shoemaker HR Jr. Hypogammaglobulinemia and rheumatic disease. Semin Arthritis Rheum 1993; 22:252.
26. Weike T, Schiller R, Fehrenbach FJ, et al. Association between *Staphylococcus aureus* nasopharyngeal colonization and septicemia in patients infected with the human immunodeficiency virus. Eur J Clin Microbiol Infect Dis 1992; 11:95.
27. Smith KJ, Wagner KF, Yeager J, et al. Staphylococcus aureus carriage and HIV-1 disease: association with increased mucocutaneous infection as well as deep soft-tissue infections and sepsis. Arch Dermatol 1994; 130:521.
28. Pos O, Stevenhagen A, Meenhorst PL, et al. Impaired phagocytosis *Staphylococcus aureus* by granulocytes and monocytes of AIDS patients. Clin Exp Immunol 1992; 88:23.
29. Aarestrup FM, Scott NL, Sordillo LM. Ability of *Staphylococcus aureus* coagulase genotypes to resist neutrophil bactericidal activity and phagocytosis. Infect Immun 1994; 62:5679.
30. Verhoef J, Visser MR. Neutrophil phagocytosis and killing: normal function and microbial evasion. In: Abramson JS, Wheeler JG, eds. The Neutrophil. Oxford: IRL Press, 1993:109.
31. Cheung A, Fuchetti L. The role of fibrinogen staphylococcal adherence to catheters in vitro. J Infect Dis 1990; 161:1177.

32. Gillet Y, Issartel B, Vanhems P, et al. Association between *Staphylococcus aureus* strains carrying gene for Panton-Valentine leukocidin and highly lethal necrotizing pneumonia in young immunocompetent patients. Lancet 2002; 359:753.

33. Mortensen JE, Shryock TR, Kapral FA. Modification of bactericidal fatty acids by an enzyme of *Staphylococcus aureus*. J Med Microbiol 1992; 36:293.

34. Fowler VG Jr, Sakoulas G, McIntyre LM, et al. Persistent bacteremia due to methicillin-resistant Staphylococcus aureus infection is associated with agr dysfunction and low-level in vitro resistance to thrombin-induced platelet microbicidal proteins. J Infect Dis 2004; 190:1140.

35. Cosgrove SE, Sakoulas G, Perencevich EN, et al. Comparison of mortality associated with methicillin-resistant and methicillin susceptible *Staphylococcus aureus* bacteremia: a meta-analysis. Clin Infect Dis 2003; 36:53.

36. Sabath L, Wheeler N, Lauerdiere M, et al. A new type of penicillin resistance of *Staphylococcus aureus*. Lancet 1977; 1:445.

37. Vann J, Hamill J, Albrecht R, et al. Immunoelectron microscopic localization of fibronectin in adherence of *Staphylococcus aureus* to cultured bovine endothelial cells. J Infect Dis 1989; 160:538.

38. Beile M. Vascular endothelial immunology and infectious disease. Rev Infec Dis 1989; 11:273.

39. Sheagren J. *Staphylococcus aureus*, the persistent pathogen. N Engl J Med 1984; 310:1368.

40. Bayer JS. New concepts in the pathogenesis and modalities of the chemoprophylaxis of native valve endocarditis. Chest 1989; 96:893.

41. Veltrop MH, Bancsi MJ, Bertina RM, et al. The role of monocytes and experimental *Staphylococcus aureus* endocarditis. Infect Immun 2000; 68:4818.

42. Sullam PM, Bayer AS, Foss WM, et al. Diminished platelet binding in vitro by *Staphylococcus aureus* is associated with reduced virulence in a rabbit model of infective endocarditis. Infect Immun 1996; 64:4915.

43. Bayer AS, Prasad R, Chandra J, et al. In vitro resistance of *Staphylococcus aureus* to thrombin-induced platelet microbicidal protein is associated with alterations in cytoplasmic membrane fluidity. Infect Immun 2000; 68:3548.

44. Bhakdi S, Tranum-Jensen J. Alpha-toxin of *Staphylococcus aureus*. Microbiol Rev 1991; 55:733.

45. Choudhuri KK, Chakrabarty AN. Hyaluronate lysis activity of staphylococci. Indian J Exp Biol 1969; 7:183.

46. Chu VH, Cabell CH, Abrutyn E, et al. Native valve endocarditis due to coagulase-negative staphylococci: report of 99 episodes from the international collaboration on endocarditis merged database. Clin Infect Dis 2004; 39:1527.

47. Rupp ME. Coagulase-negative staphylococcal infections: an update regarding recognition and management. Curr Clin Top Infect Dis 1997; 17:51.

48. Wisplinghoff H, Bischoff T, Tallent SF, et al. Nosocomial bloodstream infections in U.S. hospitals: analysis of 24,179 patients from a prospective nationwide surveillance study. Clin Infect Dis 2004; 39:309.

49. Malanoski GJ, Samore MH, Pefanis A, Karchmer AW. *Staphylococcus aureus* catheter-associated bacteremia. Minimal effective therapy and unusual infectious complications associated with arterial sheath catheters. Arch Intern Med 1995; 55:1161.

50. Schulin T, the Voss A. Coagulase-negative staphylococci as a cause of infections related to intravascular prosthetic devices. Limitations present therapy. Clin Microbiol Infect 2001; 7:1.

51. Kloss WE. Taxonomy and systematics of staphylococci indignous to humans. In: Crossley KB, Archer GL, eds. The Staphylococci in Human Disease. New York: Churchill Livingstone, 1997:113.

52. Peters G, von Eiff C, Herrmann M. The changing pattern of coagulase-negative staphylococci as infectious pathogens. Curr Opin Infect Dis 1995; (suppl 8):S12.

53. Khatib R, Riederer KM, Clark JA, et al. Coagulase-negative staphylococci in multiple blood cultures: strain relatedness in the determinants of same-strain bacteremia. J Clin Microbiol 1995; 33:816.

54. Baddour LM, Christensen GD, Hester MG, Bisno AL. Production of experimental endocarditis by coagulase-negative staphylococci: variability in species virulence. J Infect Dis 1984; 150:721.
55. Deighton M, Pearsons S, Capstick J, et al. Phenotypic variation of *Staphylococcus epidermidis* isolates from a patient with native valve endocarditis. J Clin Microbiol 1992; 30:2385.
56. Baddour LM, Simpson WA, Weems JJ Jr, et al. Phenotypic selection of small-colony variant forms of *Staphylococcus epidermidis* in the rat model of endocarditis. J Infect Dis 1988; 157:751
57. Vesga O, Groeschel MC, Otten MF, et al. In *Staphylococcus aureus* small colony variants are induced by the endothelial cell intracellular milieu. J Infect Dis 1996; 173:739.
58. Koo SP, Bayer AS, Sahl HG, et al. Staphylococcal action of thrombin-induced platelet microbicidal protein is not solely dependent on transmembrane potential. Infect Immun 1996; 64:1070.
59. von Heiff C, Bettin RA, Proctor C, et al. A site directed *Staphylococcus aureus* hemB mutant is a small colony variant which persists intracellularly. J Bacteriol 1997; 179:4706.
60. Worms R, Roujeau J, Dubuit H. The effect of a foreign body on the histological response to staphylococcal infection. In: Jeljaszewicz J, ed. Contributions to Microbiology and Immunology (vol. 1), Staphylococci and Staphylococcal Infections. Basel: Karger, 1973:258.
61. Pascual A, Fleer A, Westerdaal NAC, et al. Modulation of adherence of coagulase-negative staphylococci to Teflon catheters in vitro. Eur J Clin Microbiol 1986; 5:518.
62. Tojo M, Yamashita N, Goldmann DA, et al. Isolation and characterization of a capsular polysaccharide adhesion of *Staphylococcus epidermidis*. J Infect Dis 1988; 157:713.
63. Hartford O, O'Brien L, Schofield K, et al. The Fbe (SdrG) protein of *Staphylococcus epidermidis* HB promotes bacterial adherence to fibrinogen. Microbiology 2001; 147:2545.
64. Mack D, Fischer W, Krokotch A, et al. The intercellular adhesion involved in biofilm accumulation of *Staphylococcus epidermidis* is a linear b-1,6 linked glucosaminoglycan: purification and structural analysis. J Bacteriol 1996; 178:175.
65. McKenney D, Hubner E, Muller Y, et al. The ica locus of *Staphylococcus epidermidis* encodes production of the capsular polysaccharide/adhesin. Infect Immun 1998; 66:4711.
66. Gotz F, Peters G. Colonization of medical devices by coagulase negative staphylococci. In: Waldvogel FA, Bisno AL, eds. Infections Associated with Indwelling Medical Devices. Washington D.C.: ASM Press, 2000:5.
67. Rupp ME, Hamer KE. Effect of subinhibitory concentrations of vancomycin, cefazolin, ofloxacin, L-ofloxacin and D-ofloxacin on adherence to intravascular catheters and biofilm formation by *Staphylococcus epidermidis*. J Antimicrob Chemother 1998; 41:155.
68. Boussard P, Pithsy A, Devleeschouwer MJ. Relationship between slime production, antibiotic sensitivity and the phagetype of coagulase-negative staphylococci. J Clin Pharm Ther 1993; 18:271.
69. Williams I, Venables D, Lloyd F, et al. The effects of adherence to silicon surfaces on antibiotic susceptibility and *Staphylococcus aureus*. Microbiology 1997; 143(Pt 7):2407.
70. Yao Y, Sturdevant DE, Otto M. Genomewide analysis of gene expression in *Staphylococcus epidermidis*. Biofilms and the role of of phenol-soluble modulins in the formation of biofilms. J Infect Dis 2005; 191:289.
71. Kochinova S, Vvong C, Yao Y, et al. Key role of poly-gamma-D,L-glutamic acid in immune evasion and virulence of Staphylococcus epidermidis. J Clin Invest 2005; 115:688.
72. Rupp ME, Archer GL. Hemagglutination and adherence to plastic by Staphylococcus epidermidis. Infect Immun 1992; 60:4322.
73. Gemmell CG. Virulence characteristics of *Staphylococcus epidermidis*. J Med Microbiol 1986; 22:287.
74. Archer GL, Climo MW. Antimicrobial susceptibility of coagulase-negative staphylococci. Antimicrob Agent Chemother 1994; 38:2231.
75. Kernodle DS, Barg NL, Kaiser AB. Low-level colonization of hospitalized patients with methicillin-resistant coagulase-negative staphylococci and emergence of the organisms during surgical antimicrobial prophylaxis. Antimicrob Ag Chemother 1988; 32:2002.
76. Archer GL, Dietrick DR, Johnston JL. Molecular epidemiology of transmissible gentamicin resistance among coagulase-negative staphylococci in a cardiac surgery unit. J Infect Dis 1985; 151:243.

77. Anguera I, Del Rio A, Miro JM, et al. *Staphylococcus lugdunensis* infective endocarditis: description of 2 cases and analysis of native valve, prosthetic valve and pacemaker lead endocarditis clinical profiles. Heart 2005; 91:e10.

78. Lessing MPA, Crook DWM, Bowler ICJ, et al. In native valve endocarditis caused by *Staphylococcus lugdunensis*. QJM 1996; 89:855.

79. Etienne J, Brun Y, Flurette J. *Staphylococcus lugdunensis* endocarditis. J Clin Pathol 1989; 42:892.

80. Facklam R. What happened to the streptococci: overview of taxonomic and nomenclature changes. Clin Microbiol Rev 2002; 15:613.

83. Baddour LM, Bisno AL. Infective endocarditis complicating mitral valve prolapse: epidemiologic, clinical and microbiologic aspects. Review Infect Dis 1986; 8:117.

81. Lerner PI, Weinstein L. Infective endocarditis in the antibiotic era. N Engl J Med 1966; 274:323.

82. Hoen B, Alla F, Selton -Suty C, et al. Changing profile of infective endocarditis: results of a 1-year survey in France. JAMA 2002; 288:75.

84. Facklam RR, Washington JA II. Streptococcus and related catalase-negative Gram-positive cocci. In: Bellows A, Hausler WJ Jr, Hermann KL, et al., eds. Manual of Clinical Microbiology. 5th ed. Washington DC: American Society for Microbiology, 1991:237.

85. Kawamura Y, Hou XG, Sultana F, et al. Transfer of *Streptococcus adjacens* and *Streptococcus defectivus* to Abiotrophia gen. nov. as Abiotrophia adjacens comb nov. and Abiotrophia defectiva comb. nov., respectively. Int J Syst Bacteriol 1995; 45:798.

86. Parker MT, Ball LC. The streptococci and aerococci associated with systemic infection in man. J Med Microbiol 1976; 9, 275.

87. Colman G, Williams R. Taxonomy of some human viridans streptococci. In: Wannamaker C, Matsen J, eds. Streptococci and Streptococcal Disease: Recognition, Understanding and Management. New York: Academic Press, 1972:281.

88. Moreillon P, Que YA, Bayer AS. Pathogenesis of streptococcal and staphylococcal endocarditis. In: Durack DT, ed. Infective Endocarditis. Philadelphia: W.B. Saunders, 2002:297.

89. Pulliam L, Dall L, Inokuchi S, et al. Effect of exopolysaccharide production by viridans streptococci on penicillin therapy of experimental endocarditis. J Infect Dis 1985; 151:153.

90. Larsen T, Fiehn NE, Gutschik E, et al. Current status of taxonomic groups of streptococci in endocarditis. Can virulence factors discriminate between endocarditis and non-endocarditis strains? Clin Microbiol Infect 1999; 5:73.

91. Scheld WM, Strunk RW, Balian G, et al. Microbial adhesions to fibronectin in vitro correlates with production of endocarditis and rabbits. Proc Soc Exp Biol Med 1985; 180:474.

92. Lowrance JH, Baddour LM, Simpson WA. The role of fibronectin binding in the rat model of experimental endocarditis caused by *Streptococcus sanguis*. J Clin Invest 1990; 86:7.

93. Herzberg MC, MacFarlane GD, Gong K, et al. The platelet interactivity phenotype of *Streptococcus sanguis* influences the course of experimental endocarditis. Infect Immun 1992; 60:4809.

94. Schou C, Bog-Hansen TC, Fiehn NE. Bacterial binding to extracellular matrix proteins-in vitro adhesion. APMIS 1999; 107:193.

95. Stinson MW, Alder S, Kumar S. Invasion and killing of human endothelial cells by viridans group streptococci. Infect Immun 2003; 71:2365.

96. Ruoff KL, Whiley RA, Beighton D. Streptococcus. In: Murray PR, Baron EJ, Jorgensen JH, et al., eds. Manual of Clinical Microbiology. 8th ed. Washington: American Society for Microbiology Press, 2003:413.

97. Kitada KA, Inoue M, Kitano M. Experimental endocarditis infection in platelet aggregation by *Streptococcus anginosus*, *Streptococcus constellatus* and *Streptococcus intermedius*. FEMS Immunol Med Microbiol 1997; 19:25.

98. Shales D, Lerner P, Nolonsky D, et al. Infections due to Lancefield group and related streptococci (*S. milleri, S. anginosus*). Medicine 1981; 60:197.

99. Allen BL, Katz B, Hook M. *Streptococcus anginosus* adheres to vascular endothelium, basement membrane and purified extracellular matrix proteins. Microb Pathog 2002; 32:191.

100. Osawa R, Whiley RA. Effects of different acidulants on growth of "Streptococcus milleri group" strains isolated from various sites of the human body. Lett Appl Microbiol 1995; 20:263.
101. Young KA, Allaker RP, Hardie JM, et al. Interactions between Eikenella corrodens and "Streptococcus milleri-group" organisms: possible mechanisms of pathogenicity in mixed infections.
102. Quinlivan D, Davis TM, Daly FJ, et al. Hepatic abscess due to Eikenella corrodens and *Streptococcus milleri*: implications for antibiotic therapy. J Infect 1996; 33:47.
103. Maggume H, Whiley RA, Goto T, et al. Distribution of intermedilysin gene among the anginosus group streptococci and correlation between Med Lysholm production and deep-seated infection with *Streptococcus intermedius*. J Clin Microbiol 2000; 38:220.
104. Jacobs JA, Stobberingh EE. Hydrolytic enzymes of *Streptococcus anginosus*, *Streptococcus constellatus* and *Streptococcus intermedius* in relation to infection. Eur J Clin Microbiol Infect Dis 1995; 14:818.
105. Murray H, Gross K, Mazur H, et al. Serious infections caused by *Streptococcus milleri*. Am J Med 1970; 64:759.
106. Toyoda K, Kusano N, Saito A. Pathogenicity of the *Streptococcus milleri* group in pulmonary infections—effect on phagocytic killing by human polymorphonuclear neutrophils. Kansenshokagu Zasshi 1995; 69:308.
107. Wanahita A, Goldsmith EA, Musher DM, et al. Interactions between human polymorphonuclear leukocytes and *Streptococcus milleri* group bacteria. J Infect Dis 2002; 185:85.
108. Proft T, Fraser J. Superantigens: just like peptides only different. J Exp Med 1998; 187:819.
109. Gossling J. Occurrence and pathogenicity of the *Streptococcus milleri* group. Rev Infect Dis 1988; 10:257.
110. Libertin CR, Hermanns PE, Washington JA II. Beta-hemolytic group F streptococcal bacteremia: a study and review of the literature. Rev Infect Dis 1985; 7:498.
111. Pfaller MA, Jones RN, Marshall SA, et al. Nosocomial streptococcal bloodstream infections in the SCOPE Program: species, occurrence and antimicrobial resistance. Diag Microbiol Infect Dis 1997; 29:259.
112. Stein D, Nelson K. Endocarditis due to nutritionally-deficient streptococci: a therapeutic dilemma. Rev Infect Dis 1987; 90:1908.
113. Kawamura Y, Hou XG, Sultana F, et al. Transfer of *Streptococcus adejacens* and Streptococcus defectivus due Abiotrophia gen nov. at Abiotrophia adiacens comb. nov., respectively. Int J Syst Bacteriol 1995; 45:798.
114. Levine J, Hummer B, Pollock A, et al. Penicillin-sensitive nutritionally variant streptococcal endocarditis. Relapse after penicillin therapy. Am J Med Sci 1983; 31:202.
115. Tillitson GS. Evaluation of 10 commercial blood culture systems to isolate pyridoxal-dependent streptococcus. J Clin Pathol 1981; 34:930.
116. Ruoff KL. Nutritionially variant streptococci. Clin Microbiol Rev. Clin Microbiol Rev 1991; 4:184.
117. Robert RB, Krieger AG, Schiller NI, et al. Viridans streptococcal endocarditis: the role of various species, including pyridoxal-dependent streptococci. Rev Infect Dis 1979; 1:955.
118. Bouvet A. Human endocarditis due to nutritionally variant streptococci: Streptococcus adjacens and Streptococcus defectivus. Eur Heart J 1995; 16(suppl B):24.
119. Roberts RB. Streptococcal endocarditis: the viridans and beta-hemolytic streptococci. In: Kay D, ed. Infective Endocarditis. 2d ed. New York: Raven Press, 1992:191.
120. Corey R, Gross K, Roberts R. Vitamin B6 dependent *S. mitior* (*mitis*) isolated from patients with systemic infection. J Infect Dis 1975; 117:722.
121. Ginsberg F, Forbes B, Singh A, et al. Case report: prosthetic valve endocarditis due to a nutritionally variant streptococcus. Am J Med Sci 1988; 289:299.
122. Naimann R, Barrow J. Some-resistant bacteria in mouths and throats of children receiving continuous prophylaxis against rheumatic fever. Ann Int Med 1963; 58:768.
123. Wilson WR, Karchmer AW, Dajani AS, et al. Antimicrobial treatment of adults with infective endocarditis due to streptococci, enterococci, staphylococci and HACEK microorganisms. JAMA 1995; 274:1706.
124. Moellering R Jr. Treatment of endocarditis caused by resistant streptococci. In: Horstkotte B, Bodnar E, eds. Infective Endocarditis. London: ICR publishers, 1991:102.

125. Cooksey R, Swenson J. In-vitro antimicrobial inhibition patterns of nutritionally variant streptococci. Antimicrob Agent Chemother 1979; 16:514.

126. Karchmer AW, Moellering RC Jr, Maki DC, et al. Single-antibiotic therapy for streptococcal endocarditis. JAMA 1979; 241:1801.

127. Holloway Y, Dankert J. Penicillin tolerance in nutritionally variant streptococci. Antimicrob Agent Chemother 1982; 22:1073.

128. Hanslik T, Hartig C, Jurand C, et al. Clinical significance of tolerant strains of streptococci in adults with infective endocarditis. Clin Microbiol Infect 2003; 9:852.

128a. Bouvet A, Cremieux AC, Contrepois A, et al. Comparison of penicillin vancomycin, individually and in combination with gentamicin amikacin in the treatment of experimental endocarditis induced by nutritionally variant streptococci. Antimicrob Agent Chemother 1985; 28:607.

129. *Streptococcus, Enterococcus* and similar organisms. In: Forbes BA, Sahm DF, Weissfeld AS, eds. Bailey and Scott's Diagnostic Microbiology. Chap. 20. 11th ed. St. Louis: Mosby, 2002:298.

130. Ruoff KL, de la Maza L, Murtagh MJ, et al. Species identities of enterococci isolated from clinical specimens. J Clin Microbiol 1990; 28:435.

131. Karchmer A, Moellering R Jr, Maki D, et al. Unpublished data.

132. Cabell CH, Abrutyn E. Progress toward a global understanding of infective endocarditis. Lessons from the International Collaboration of Endocarditis. Cardiol Clin 2003; 21:147.

133. Schaberg DR, Culver DH, Gaynes RP. Major trends in the microbial etiology of nosocomial infection. Am J Med 1991; 91(suppl 3B):3B72S.

134. Donskey CJ, Chowdhry TK, Hecker MT, et al. Effect of antibiotic therapy on the density of vancomycin-resistant enterococci in the stool of colonized patients. N Engl J Med 2002; 343:1925.

135. Nichols RL, Muzik AC. Enterococcal infections in surgical patients: the mystery continues. Clin Infect Dis 1992; 15:72.

136. Evans Patterson J, Sweeney AH, Simms M, et al. An analysis of 110 serious enterococcal infections; epidemiology, antibiotic susceptibility and outcome. Medicine 1995; 74:191.

137. Vergis EN, Heyden MK, Chow JW, et al. Determinants of vancomycin resistance and mortality rates in enterococcal bacteremia. Ann Intern Med 2001; 135:484.

138. Qin X, Singh KV, Weinstock GM, et al. Effects of Enterococcus faecalis *fsr* genes on production of gelatinase and serine proteinase virulence factors. Infection Immunity 2000; 68:25.

139. Berk S, Verghle A, Hockslaw S. In enterococcal pneumonia occurrence in patients receiving broad-spectrum antibiotic regimens and enteric feeding. Am J Med 1983; 711:133.

140. Weinstein LW, Brusch JL. Gram-positive organisms. In: Infective Endocarditis. New York; 1996:44.

141. Levi D, Reiner N, Gopalkrishna KV, Lerner PI. Enterococcal endocarditis in heroin addicts. JAMA 1976; 235:1861.

142. Brusch JL. Cardiac infections in the immunosuppressed patient. In: Cunha, ed. Infections in the Compromised Host. Infect Dis Clin NA, 2001; 15:613.

143. Maki D, Agger WA. Enterococcal bacteremia: clinical features, the risk of endocarditis and management. Medicine 1988; 64:248.

144. Scheld W, Mandell G. Enigmatic enterococcal endocarditis. Ann Intern Med 1984; 100:816.

145. Megram D. Enterococcal endocarditis. Clin Infect Dis 1992; 15:63.

146. Mandell G, Kaye D, Levin C, et al. Enterococcal endocarditis: an analysis of 38 patients observed at the New York Hospital-Cornell Medical Center. Arch Intern Med 1970; 125:250.

147. Hoffman SA, Moellering RC Jr. The enterococcus: "Putting the bug in our ears." Ann Intern Med 1987; 106:757.

148. McDonald JR, Olaison L, Anderson DJ, et al. Enterococcal endocarditis: 107 cases from the International Collaboration on Endocarditis merged database. Am J Med 2005; 118:759.

149. Garbutt JM, Ventapragada M, Littenberg B, et al. Association between resistance to vancomycin and death in cases of *Enterococcus faecium* bacteremia. Clin Infect Dis 2000; 30:466.

150. Jett BD, Hucyke MM, Gilmore MS. Virulence of enterococci. Clin Microb Rev 1994; 7:462.
151. Guzman CA, Pruzzo C, Lipira G, et al. Role of adherence in pathogenesis of *Enterococci faecalis* urinary tract infections and endocarditis. Infect Immun 1989; 57:1834.
152. Shankar V, Baghdayan AS, Hucyke MM, et al. Infection-derived *Enterococcus faecalis* strains are enriched in *esp*, a gene and including a novel surface protein. Infect Immun 1999; 67:193.
153. Pillai SK, Sakoulas G, Gold HS, et al. Effect of glucose on *fsr*-mediated catabolic repression of biofilm formation in *Enterococcus faecalis*. J Infect Dis 2004; 190:967–970.
154. Qin X, Singh KV, Weinstock GM, et al. Characterization of *fsr*, a regulator controlling expression of gelatinase and serines protease in *Enterococcus faecalis* OGIRF. J Bacteriol 2001; 183:3372–3382.
155. Ike Y, Hashimoto H, Clewell DB. High incidence of hemolysin production by *Enterococcus (Streptococcus) faecalis* strains associated with human parenteral infections. J Clin Microbiol 1987; 25:1524.
156. Gould H, Ramirez-Rouch C, Holmes P, et al. Adherence of bacteria to heart valve in vitro. J Clin Invest 1975; 56:1364.
157. Drake T, Rodgers C, Sande M. Tissue factor is a major structure for vegetation formation in endocarditis in rabbits. J Clin Invest 1984; 73:1750.
158. Archimbaud C, Shankar N, Forestier C, et al. In vitro adhesive properties and virulence factors of *Enterococcus faecalis* strains. Res Microbiol 2002; 153:75.
159. Mohamed JA, Huang W, Nallapareddy SR, et al. Influence of origin of isolates, especially endocarditis isolates, and various genes on biofilm formation by *Enterococcus faecalis*. Infect Immun 2004; 72:3658.
160. Baldassarri L, Creti R, Arciola CR, et al. Analysis of virulence factors in cases enterococcal endocarditis. Clinical Microbial Impact 2004; 10:1006.
161. Krueger WA, Krueger-Ramcek S, Koch S, et al. Assessment of the role of antibiotics and enterococcal virulence factors in a mouse model of extraintestinal translocation. Crit Care Med 2004; 32:48.
162. Krogstad DJ, Parquette AR. Defective killing of enterococci: a common property of antimicrobial agents acting on the cell wall. Antimicrob Agent Chem 1980; 17:965.
163. Williamson R, Le Bourguenec C, Gutmann L, et al. One or two low affinity penicillin-binding proteins may be responsible for the range of susceptibility of *Enterococcus faecium* to benzylpenicillin. J Gen Microb 1985; 131:1933.
164. Hunter TH. Use of streptomycin in the treatment of bacterial endocarditis. Am J Med 1947; 2:436.
165. Moellering RC Jr, Weinberg AN. Studies on antibiotic synergism against enterococci. II effect of various antibiotics on the uptake of 14 C-labeled streptomycin by enterococci. J Clin Invest 1971; 50:2580.
166. Murray B. The life and times of the enterococcus. Clin Microb Rev 1992; 3:46.
167. Murray B. Antibiotic resistance among enterococci: current problems and management strategies. In: Remington K, Swartz M, eds. Current Clinical Topics in Infectious Diseases. Cambridge, MA: Blackwell Scientific, 1991:94.
168. Report on the Rockefeller University Workshop. Multiple-antibiotic-resistant pathogenic bacteria. N Engl J Med 1994; 330(17):1247.
169. Rice LB, Bellais S, Carias LL, et al. Impact of specific pbp5 mutations of expression of beta-lactam resistance in *Enterococcus faecium*. Antimicrob Agent Chemother 2004; 48:3028.
170. Grayson ML, Eliopoulos GM, Wennersten CB, et al. Increasing resistance to beta-lactam antibiotics among clinical isolates of *Enterococcus faecium*: a 22-year review at one institution. Antimicrob Agent Chemother 1991; 35:2180.
171. Watanakunakorn C, Glotzbecker C. Comparative in vitro activity of nafcillin, oxacillin and methicillin in combination with gentamicin and tobramycin against enterococci. Antimicrob Agent Chemother 1977; 11:88.
172. Glew RH, Moellering RC Jr, Wennestern C. Comparative synergistic activity of mass alone, oxacillin and methicillin in combination with gentamicin against enterococci. Antimicrob Agent Chemother 1975; 7:828.

173. Marier RL, Joyce N. Andriole to the life. Synergism of oxacillin and gentamicin against enterococci. Antimicrob Agent Chemother 1975; 8:571.
174. Glew RH, Moellering RC Jr. Effect of protein binding on the activity of penicillin in combination with gentamicin against enterococci. Antimicrob Agent Chemother 1979; 15:87.
175. Weinstein AJ, Moellering RC Jr. Studies of cephalothin: aminoglycoside synergism against enterococci. Antimicrob Agent Chemother 1975; 7:522.
176. Iannini PB, Ehret J, Eickhoff TC. Effect of ampicillin-amikacin and ampicillin-rifampin on enterococci. Antimicrob Agent Chemother 1976; 9:448.
177. Grayson ML, Thauvin C, Eliopoulos GM, et al. The failure of trimethoprim-sulfamethoxazole therapy in experimental enterococcal endocarditis. Antimicrob Agent Chemother 1990; 34:1792.
178. Chow JW, Zervos MJ, Lerner SA, et al. A novel gentamicin resistance gene in Enterococcus. Antimicrob Agent Chemother 1997; 41:511.
179. Martinez-Martinez L, Joynas P, Pascual A, et al. Activity of eight fluoroquinolones against enterococci. Clin Microbiol Infect 1997; 3:497.
180. Murray BE. Beta lactamase producing enterococci. Antimicrob Agent Chemother 1992; 36:2335.
181. Fontana R, Ligozzi P, Pittaluga F, Satta G. Intrinsic penicillin resistance in enterococci. Microbial Drug Resist 1996; 2:209.
182. Rice LB, Bellais S, Carias LL, et al. Impact of specific pbp mutations on expression of beta-lactam resistance in *Enterococcus faecium*. Antimicrob Agent Chemother 2004; 48:3028.
183. Mainardi JL, Legrand R, Arthur M, et al. Novel mechanism of beta-lactam resistance due to bypass of DD-transpeptidastion in *Enterococcus faecium*. J Biol Chem 2000; 275:16490.
184. Havard CW, Garrod LP, Waterworth PM. Deaf or dead? A case of subacute bacterial endocarditis treated with penicillin and neomycin. Br Med J 1959; 15:688.
185. Horodniceanu T, Bouquelert L, El-Solh N, et al. High level, plasmid-borne resistance to gentamicin in *Streptococcus faecalis* subsp. zymogens. Antimicrob Agent Chemother 1979; 16:686.
186. Nachamkin I, Axelrod P, Talbot CH, et al. Multiple high level aminoglycoside resistant enterococci isolated from patients in a university hospital (Abstr 120). Abstracts of the Eighty-Sixth Annual Meeting of the American Society for Microbiology. Washington DC, American Society for Microbiology, 1986.
187. Mederski-Samoraj BD, Murray BE. High-level resistance to gentamicin in clinical isolates of enterococci. J Infect Dis 1983; 147:751.
188. Uttley AHC, Collins CH, Naidoo K, et al. Vancomycin-resistant enterococci. Lancet 1988; 57:8.
189. Arthur M, Courvalin P. Genetics and mechanisms of glycopeptide resistance in enterococci. Antimicrob Agent Chemother 1993; 37:1563.
190. Bain KT, Wittbrodt ET. Linezolid for the treatment of resistant gram-positive cocci. Annals of Pharmacotherap 2001; 35:566.
191. Babcock HM, Ritchie DJ, Christiansen E, et al. Successful treatment of vancomycin-resistant Enterococcus endocarditis with oral linezolid. Clin Infect Dis 2001; 32:1373.
192. Shinabarger DL, Marotti KR, Murray RW, et al. Mechanisms of action of oxazolidineones; effects of linezolid and eperzolid on translation reactions. Antimicrob Agent Chemother 1997; 41:2132.
193. Rahim S, Pillai SK, Gold HS, et al. Linezolid-resistant, vancomycin-resistant *Enterococcus faecium* infection in patients without prior exposure to linezolid. Clin Infect Dis 3; 36:E146.
194. Meka VG, Gold HS. Antimicrobial resistance to linezolid. Clin Infect Dis 2004; 39:1010.
195. Prystowsky J, Siddiqui F, Chosay J, et al. Resistance to linezolid: characterization of mutations in rRNA and comparison of their occurrences in vancomycin-resistant enterococci. Antimicrob Agent Chemother 2001; 45:2154.
196. Heshberger E, Donabedian S, Konstantinou K, Zervos MJ. Quinpristin-dalfoprastin resistance in the gram-positive bacteria: mechanism of resistance and epidemiology. Clin Infect Dis 2004; 38:92.

197. Canu A, Leclerq R. Overcoming bacterial resistance by dual target inhibition: the case of streptogramins. Current Drug Targets Infect Disord 2001; 1:215.

198. Singh KV, Weinstock GM, Murray BE. An *Enterococcus faecalis* ABC homologue (Lsa) is required to the resistance of the species to clindamycin and Quinpristin-dalfoprastin. Antimicrob Agent Chemother 2002; 46:1845.

199. McDonald LC, Rossiter S, Mckinson C, et al. Quinpristin-dalfoprastin-resistant *Enterococcus faecium* infection in chicken and human stool specimens. N Engl Med 2001; 345:1155.

200. Critchley IA, Blosser-Middleton RS, Jones ME, et al. Baseline study to determine in vitro activities of dactinomycin against gram-positive pathogens isolated the United States 2000–2001.

201. Barry AL, Fuchs PC, Brown SD. In vitro activities of dactinomycin against 2,789 clinical isolates from 11 North American medical centers. Antimicrob Agent Chemother 2001; 45:1919.

202. Silverman JA, Oliver N, Andrew T, et al. Resistance studies with daptoomycin. Antimicrob Agent Chemother 2001; 45:1799.

203. Facklam R. Recognition of group D streptococcal species of human origin by biochemical and physiological tests. Appl Microbiol 1972; 23:1131.

204. Facklam R, Cooksey RC, Wortham EC. Evaluation of commercial latex agglutination reagent for grouping streptococci. J Clin Microbiol 1979; 10:641.

205. Moellering RC, Watson BK, Kunz L. Endocarditis to group D streptococci. Comparison of disease caused by *Streptococcus bovis* with that caused by the enterococci. Am J Med 1974; 57:239.

206. Maki D, Gazi N. Enterococcal bacteremia clinical features: the risk of endocarditis and management. Medicine 1988; 67:243.

207. Raverby W, Bottone E, Keusch G. Group D streptococcal bacteremia with emphasis on the incidence and presentation of infections due to *Streptococcus bovis*. N Engl J Med 1973; 289:1400.

208. Hoen B, Chirouze C, Cabell CH, et al. Emergence of endocarditis due to group D streptococci: findings derived from the verge database of the International Collaboration on Endocarditis. Eur J Clin Microbiol Infect Dis 2005; 24:12.

209. Hoopes WL, Lerner PI. Non-enterococcal group-D streptococcal endocarditis, caused by *Streptococcus bovis*. Ann Intern Med 1974; 81:588.

210. Murray H, Roberts R. *Streptococcus bovis* bacteremia and underlying gastrointestinal disease. Arch Int Med 1974; 81:588.

211. Duval X, Papastamopoulos V, Longuet P, et al. Definite *Streptococcus bovis* endocarditis: characteristics in 20 patients. Clin Microbiol Infect 2001; 7:3.

212. Klein R, Catalano M, Edberg S, et al. Streptococcus bovis septicemia in carcinoma of the colon. Ann Intern Med 1977; 97:800.

213. Tripodi MF, Adinolfi LE, Ragone E, et al. The *Streptococcus bovis* endocarditis and its association with chronic liver disease: an underestimated risk factor. Clin Infect Dis 2004; 38:1394.

214. Zarkin BA, Lillemoe KD, Cameron JL, et al. The triad of *Streptococcus bovis* erythremia, colonic pathology and liver disease. Ann Surg 1990; 211:786.

215. Gergaud JM, Breux JP, Robolot P, et al. Neurologic complications of infectious endocarditis. Ann Med Interne (Paris) 1995; 146:413.

216. Cohen LF, Dunbar SA, Sirbasku DM, et al. The *Streptococcus bovis* infection of the central nervous system: report of two cases and review. Clin Infect Dis 1997; 25:819.

217. Ellmerich S, Djouder N, Scholler M, Klein JP. Production of cytokines by monocytes, epithelial and endothelial cells activated by *Streptococcus bovis*. Cytokine 2000; 12:26.

218. Pergola V, DiSalvo G, Habib G, et al. Comparison of clinical and echocardiographic characteristics of Streptococcus bovis endocarditis with that caused by other pathogens. Am J Cardiol 2001; 88:871.

219. Ballet M, Gevigney G, Gare JP, et al. Infective endocarditis due to *Streptococcus bovis*. A report of 53 cases. Eur Heart J 1995; 16:1975.

220. Savitch C, Barry A, Hoperich P. Infective endocarditis caused by *Streptococcus bovis* resistant to the lethal effect of penicillin G. Arch Intern Med 1978; 138:931.

221. Enzler M, Rouse M, Henry N, et al. In vitro and in vivo studies of streptomycin-resistant penicillin susceptible streptococci in patients with infective endocarditis. J Infect Dis 1987; 155:951.
222. Baker CJ. Group B streptococcal infections. Adv Intern Med 1980; 25:475–501.
223. Colford JM, Mohle-Boetani J, Vosti KL. Group B streptococcal bacteremia in adults. Medicine 1995; 74:176.
224. Schwartz B, Schuchat A, Oxtoby MJ, et al. Invasive group B streptococcal disease in adults; a population based study in metropolitan Atlanta. JAMA 1991; 266:1112.
225. Cheng Q, Carison B, Pillai S, et al. Antibody against surface bound C5a peptidase is opsonic and initiates macrophage killing of group B streptococci. Infect Immun 2001; 69:2302.
226. Wiseman A, Rene P, Crelinsten GL. *Streptococcus agalactiae* endocarditis: an association with those adenomas of the large intestine. Ann Intern Med 1985; 103:893.
227. Farley MM, Harvey RC, Stull T, et al. A population-based assessment of invasive disease due to group B streptococcus in non-pregnant adults. N Engl J Med 1993; 328:1807.
228. Bayer A, Chow A, Anthony B, et al. Serious infections in adults due to group B streptococci. Am J Med 1976; 61:498.
229. Jackson LA, Hilsdon AS, Farley M, et al. Risk factors for group B streptococcal disease in adults. Ann Intern Med 1995; 123:415.
230. Opal SM, Cross A, Palmer M, Almazan R. Group D streptococcal sepsis and adults in infants. Contrast and comparisons. Arch Intern Med 1988; 148:641.
231. Rollan MJ, San Roman JA, Vilacosta I, et al. Clinical profile of *Streptococcus agalactiae* native valve endocarditis. Am Heart J 2003; 146:1095.
232. Lerner P, Gopalkrishna K, Wolinsky E, et al. Group B streptococcus (*S. agalactiae*) bacteremia in adults: analysis of 32 cases and review of the literature. Medicine 1977; 56:457.
233. Scully BE, Spriggs D, Neu HC. *Streptococcus agalactiae* (group B) endocarditis: a description of twelve cases and review of the literature. Infection 1987; 15:169.
234. Gallagher P, Watanakunakorn C. Group B streptococcal endocarditis: report of seven cases and review of the literature 1962–1985. Rev of Infect Dis 1986; 8:175.
235. Harrison LH, Ali A, Dwyer DM, et al. Relapsing invasive group B streptococcal infection in adults. Ann Intern Med 1995; 123:421.
236. Kiiveri KM, Pederson G, Berning J, Schonheyder HC. Recurrent endocarditis caused by beta-haemolytic streptococci group B. Scand J Infect Dis 2004; 36:488.
237. Chihara S, Siccion E. Group B streptococcus endocarditis with endophthalmitis. Mayo Clin Proc 2005; 80:74.
238. Jennings HJ, Katzenellenbogen E, Lugowski SEA, Kasper DL. Structure of native polysaccharide antigens of type Ia and type Ib group B Streptococcus. Biochemistry 1983; 22:1258.
239. Verghese A, Mireault K, Arbeit RD. Group B streptococcal bacteremia in men. Rev Infect Dis 1986; 8:912.
240. Harrison LH, Elliot JA, Dwyer DM, et al. Serotype distribution of invasive group B streptococcal isolates in Maryland: implications for vaccine formulation. J Infect Dis 1998; 177:998.
241. Baker CJ, Kasper DL. Correlation of maternal antibody deficiency with susceptibility to neonatal group B streptococcal infection. N Engl J Med 1976; 294:753.
242. Baker EJ, Edwards MS, Kasper DL. Role of antibody to native type III polysaccharide of group B Streptococcus in infant infection. Pediatrics 1981; 68:544.
243. Amaya RA, Baker CJ, Keitel WA, Edwards MS. Healthy elderly people lack neutrophil-mediated functional activity to type V group B Streptococcus. J Am Geriatr Soc 2004; 52:46.
244. Wessels MR, Kasper DL, Johnson KD, et al. Antibody responses in invasive group B streptococcal infections in adults. J Infect Dis 1998; 178:569.
245. Gibson RL, Nizet V, Rubens CE. Group B streptococcal beta-hemolysin promotes injury of lung microvascular endothelial cells. Pediatr Res 1999; 45:626.
246. Nizet V, Gibson RL, Chi EY, et al. Group B streptococcal beta-hemolyosin expression is associated with injury of lung epithelial cells. Infect Immun 1996; 64:3818.

247. Lione VO, Santos GS, Hirata Junior R, Mattos-Guaraldi AL, Nagao PE. Involvement of intracellular adhesion molecule-1 and beta 1 integrin in the internalization process to human endothelial cells of group B streptococcus clinical isolates. Int J Mol Med 2005; 15:153.

248. Liu GY, Doran KS, Lawrence T, et al. Sword and shield: like to group B streptococcal beta-hemolysin/cytolysin and carotenoid pigment function to subvert host phagocyte defense. Proc Natl Acad Sci USA 2004; 101:14491.

249. Liu GY, Nizet V. Extracellular virulence factors of group B streptococci. Front Biosci 2004; 9:1794.

250. Pietrocola G, Schubert A, Visai, et al. FbsA, a fibrinogen-binding protein from Streptococcus agalactiae, mediates platelet aggregation. Blood 2005; 105:1052.

251. Fernandez M, Hickman ME, Baker CJ. Antimicrobial susceptibility of group B streptococci isolated between 1992 and 1996 from patients with bacteremia or meningitis. Antimicrob Agent Chemother 1998; 42:1517.

252. Kim KS. Antimicrobial susceptibility of GBS. Antibiot Chemother 1985; 35:83.

253. Betriu C, Culebras E, Gomez M, et al. Erythromycin and clindamycin resistance and telithromycin susceptibility in Streptococcus agalactiae. Antimicrob Agent Chemother 2003; 47:1112.

254. Munoz P, Llancaqueo A, Rodriguez-Creixems M, et al. Group B streptococcus bacteremia in nonpregnant adults. Arch Intern Med 1997; 157:213.

255. Chen SC, Lin MF. Favorable outcome of infective endocarditis due to Streptococcus agalactiae after conservative treatment. J Microbiol Immunol Infect 2004; 37:307.

256. Savage D, Brown J. The endocarditis caused by group A streptococcus. Am J Med Sci 1991; 202:921.

257. Keefer C, Ingelfinger FS, Pink W. Significance of hemolytic streptococcic bacteremia: a study of 246 patients. Arch Intern Med 1937; 60:1084.

258. Barz N, Kish M, Kaufman C, et al. Streptococcal bacteremia in intravenous drug abusers. Am J Med 1985; 785:569.

259. Scheld WM, Valone JA, Sande MA. Bacterial adherence in the pathogenesis of endocarditis: interaction of bacterial dextran, platelets and fibrin. J Clin Invest 1978; 62:805.

260. Robinson JH, Kehoe MA. Group A streptococcal M proteins: virulence factors and protective antigens. Immunol Today 1992; 13:362.

261. Ohnishi R, Tomai M, Aelion J, et al. A family of streptococcal superantigen represented by rheumatic genetic serotypes of M proteins sharing specificity for human TCR-VO4 elements. In: Totolian A, ed. Pathogenic streptococci: present and future. St. Petersburg, Russia: Lorca, 1994:462.

262. Bisno AI. Alternative complement pathway activation by group A streptococci; role of M protein. Infect Immun 1979; 26:1172.

263. Duma RJ, Weinberg AN, Medrek JF, Kunz LJ. Streptococcal infections. Medicine 1969; 48:87.

264. Mohr D, Feist D, Washington J II, et al. Infections due to group C streptococci in man. Am J Med 1979; 66:450.

265. Aukenthaler R, Hermans PE, Washington JA II. Group G streptoccocal bacteremia: clinical study and review of the literature. Rev Infect Dis 1983; 5:196.

266. Baddour LM, and the Infectious Diseases Society of America's Emerging Infections Network. Infective endocarditis caused by beta-hemolytic streptococci. Clin Infect Dis 1998; 26:66.

267. Bradley SF, Gordon JJ, Baumgartner DD, et al. Group C streptococcal bacteremia: analysis of 88 cases. Rev Infect Dis 1991; 13:270.

268. Salata RA, Lerner PI, Shlaes DM, et al. Infections due to Lancefield group C streptococci. Medicine (Baltimore) 1989; 68:225.

269. Bouza E, Meyer RD, Busch DF. Group G streptococcal endocarditis. J Clin Pathol 1978; 70:108.

270. Smyth E, Pallett A, Davidson R. Group G streptococcal endocarditis: two case reports, a review of the literature and recommendations for treatment. J Infect 1988; 16:169.

271. Vartian C, Lerner PI, Shlaes D, et al. Infection due to group G streptococci. Medicine 1985; 65:75.

272. Ralston K, Chandrasekar P, Lefrock J. Clinical features and antimicrobial therapy of infection caused by Group G streptococci. Infection 1985; 13:203.
273. Erdem I, Goktas P, Dmirtunc R, Erdem A. Infectious endocarditis caused by group G streptococcus with multiple cerebral emboli. Acta Medica (Hradec Kralove) 2003; 46:125.
274. Tiverton C, Herman P, Washington JA II. Beta-hemolytic group F streptococcal bacteremia, a case study and review of the literature. Rev Infect Dis 1985; 7:498.
275. Shlaes P, Lerner PI, Wolinsky E, et al. Infection due to Lancefield group F and related streptococci (S. milleri, S. anginosus). Medicine 1981; 60:197.
276. Ho AKC, Woo KS, Tse KK, et al. Infective endocarditis caused by *Streptococcus suis* serotype 2. J Infect 1990; 21:209.
277. Bevanger L, Stamnes T. Group A streptococci as the cause of bacteremia and endocarditis. Acta Pathol Microbiol Scand (sect B) 1979; 87:301.
278. Dismukes W, Karchmer A, Buckley M, et al. Prosthetic valve endocarditis. Circulation 1973; 48:365.
279. Pein E, Wilson W, Kunz K, et al. *Aercoccus viridans* endocarditis. Mayo Clin Proc 1984; 59:47.
280. Buu-Joi A, Sapoetra A, Brangerr C, et al. Antimicrobial susceptibility of *Gemella haemolysans* isolated from patients with subacute endocarditis. Eur J Clin Microbiol 1982; 1:102.
281. Fresard A, Michel VP, Rueda X, et al. *Gemella haemolysans* endocarditis. Clin Infect Dis 1993; 16:586.
282. Handwerger S, Horwitz H, Coburn K, et al. Infection due to *Leuconostoc* species: six cases and review. Rev Infect Dis 1990; 12:602.
283. Thayer W. Bacterial or infective endocarditis. Edinb Med J 1931; 38:237.
284. Uglioni V, Pacifico A, Smitherman TC, et al. Pneumococcal endocarditis update: analysis of 10 cases diagnosed between 1974 and 1984. Am Heart J 1986; 112:813.
285. Musher DM. Infections caused by *Streptococcus pneumoniae*: clinical spectrum, the pathogenesis, immunity and treatment. Clin Infect Dis 1992; 14:801.
286. Plouffe J, Breiman R, Facklam R, et al. Bacteremia with *Streptococcus pneumoniae* in adults: implications for therapy and prevention. JAMA 1996; 275:194.
287. Strauss A, Hamburger M. Pneumococcal endocarditis in the penicillin era. Arch Intern Med 1966; 118:190.
288. Preble H. Pneumococcus endocarditis. Am J Med Sci 1904; 128:782.
289. Sewall NH, Tikly M. Invasive pneumococcal infection presenting as septic arthritis and Austrian-like syndrome involving the tricuspid valve in a patient with underlying HIV infection. Joint Bone Spine 2005; 72:86.
290. Gelfand MS, Threkeld MG. Subacute bacterial endocarditis secondary to *Streptococcus pneumoniae*. Am J Med 1992; 93:91.
291. Nuorti JP, Butler JC, Gelling L, et al. Epidemiologic relation between HIV and invasive pneumococcal disease in San Francisco County, California. Ann Intern Med 2000; 132:182.
292. Turett GS, Blum S, Telzak EE. Recurrent pneumococcal bacteremia: risk factors and outcomes. Arch Intern Med 2001; 161:2141.
293. Angel CS, Ruzek M, Hostetter MK. Degradation of C3 by Streptococcus pneumoniae. J Infect Dis 1994; 170:600.
294. Tuomanen EI, Austrian R, Masure HR. The pathogenesis of pneumococcal infection. N Engl J Med 1995; 332:1280.
295. Cundell D, Masure HR, Tuomanen EI. The molecular basis of pneumococcal infection: a hypothesis. Clin Infect Dis 1995; 21(suppl 3):S204.
296. McCullers JA, Rehg JE. Lethal synergism between influenza virus and Streptococcus pneumoniae: characterization of a mouse model and the role of platelet-activating factor receptor. J Infect Dis 2000; 186:341.
297. McCullers JA, Bartmess KC. Role of neuraminidase in lethal synergism between influenza virus and *Streptococcus pneumoniae*. J Infect Dis 2003; 187:1000.
298. Ring A, Weiser JA, Tuomanen EI. Pneumococcal trafficking across the blood brain barrier. Molecular analysis of a novel bidirectional pathway. J Clin Invest 1998; 102:347.

299. Brueggemann AB, Peto TE, Crook DW, et al. Temporal and geographic stability of the serogroup-specific invasive disease potential of *Streptococcus pneumoniae* in children. J Infect Dis 2004; 190:1203.
300. Cundell D, Gerard N, Gerard C, et al. *Streptococcus pneumoniae* anchors to activated eukaryotic cells by the receptor for platelet activating factor. Nature 1995; 377:435.
301. Rubins JB, Charboneau D, Paton JC, et al. Dual function of pneumolysin in the early pathogenesis of murine pneumococcal pneumonia. J Clin Invest 1995; 95:142.
302. Whitney CG, Farley MM, Hadler J, et al. Increasing prevalence of multidrug resistant *Streptococcus pneumoniae* in the United States. N Engl J Med 2000; 343:1917.
303. Tomasz A. Antibiotic resistance in *Streptococcus pneumoniae*. Clin Infect Dis 1997; 24(suppl 1):S85.
304. Novak R, Henriques B, Charpentier E, et al. Emergence of vancomycin tolerance in *Streptococcus pneumoniae*. Nature 1999; 399:590.
305. *Erysipelot hrix, Lactobacillus*, and similar organisms. In: Forbes BA, Sahm DF, Weissfeld AS, eds. Bailey and Scott's Diagnostic Microbiology. Chap. 23. 11th ed. St. Louis: Mosby, 2002:343.
306. Morris G, Shawbacher H, Lynch P, et al. Two fatal cases of septicemia due to *Erysipelothrix insidiosa*. J Clin Pathol 1965; 18:614.
307. Woodbine M. Erysipelothrix rhusiopathiae: bacteriology and chemotherapy. Bacteriol Rev 1950; 14:161.
308. Gorby GL, Peacock JE Jr. Erysipelothrix rhusiopathiae endocarditis: microbiologic, epidemiologic and clinical features of an occupational disease. Rev Infect Dis 1988; 10:317.
309. Grandsen WR, Eyken SJ. *Erysipelothrix rhusiopathiae* endocarditis. Rev Infect Dis 1988; 10:1228.
310. Hayek LJ. *Erysipelothrix endocarditis* affecting a porcine heart valve. J Infect 1993; 27:203.
311. Artz AL, Szabo S, Zabel LT, Hoffmeister HM. Aortic valve endocarditis with paravalvular disease caused by *Erysipelothrix rhusiopathiae*. Eur J Clin Microbiol Infect Dis 2001; 20:587.
312. Fernandez-Crespo P, Serra A, Bonet J, Gimenez M. Acute oliguric renal failure in a patient with *Erysipelothrix rhusiopathiae* bacteremia and endocarditis. Nephron 1996; 74:231.
313. Shimoji Y. Pathogenicity of *Erysipelothrix rhusiopathiae*: virulence factors and protective immunity. Microb Infect 2000; 2:965.
314. Cheun HI, Kawamoto K, Hiramatsu M, et al. Protective immunity of SpaA-antigen producing *Lactococcus lactis* against *Erysipelothrix rhusiopathiae* infection. J Appl Microbiol 2004; 96:1347.
315. Shimoji Y, Yokomizo Y, Sekizaki T, et al. Presence of a capsule in *Erysipelothrix rhusiopathiae* and its relationship to virulence for mice. Infect Immun 1994; 62:2806.
316. Shimoji Y, Yokomizo Y, Mori Y. Intracellular survival of *Erysipelothrix rhusiopathiae* within murine macrophages: failure of the induction of the oxidative burst of macrophages. Infect Immun 1996; 64:1789.
317. Vendetti M, Gelfusa V, Tarasi A, et al. Antimicrobial susceptibilities of *Erysipelothrix rhusiopathiae*. Antimicrob Agent Chemother 1990; 34:2038.
318. Griffiths J, Daly J, Dodge R. Two cases of endocarditis due to *Lactobacillus* species: antimicrobial susceptibility-review and discussion of therapy. Clin Infect Dis 1992; 15:250.
319. Sussman JI, Baron EJ, Goldberg SM, et al. Clinical manifestations and therapy of *Lactobacillus endocarditis*: report of a case and review of the literature. Rev Infect Dis 1986; 8:771.
320. *Listeria, Corynebacterium,* and similar organisms. In: Forbes BA, Sahm DF, Weissfeld AS, eds. Bailey and Scott's Diagnostic Microbiology. Chap. 22. 11th ed. St. Louis: Mosby, 2002:325.
321. Linnan M, Veda F. Epidemic listeriosis associated with Mexican-style cheese. N Engl J Med 1988; 319:823.
322. Ganz N, Myerowitz R, Medeiros H, et al. Listeriosis in immunocompromised patients: a cluster of 8 cases. Am J Med 1975; 58:637.
323. Annaissie E, Kotoyiannis DP, Kantarjian H, et al. Listeriosis in patients with chronic lymphocytic leukemia were treated with fludarabine and prednisone. Ann Intern Med 1992; 117:466.

324. Lorber B. Listeria monocytogenes. In: Mandell GL, Bennrett JE, Dolin R, eds. Principles and Practice of Infectious Diseases, 6th ed. Philadelphia PA: Churchill Livingstone, 2005:2478.
325. Lorber B. Listeriosis. Clin Infect Dis 1997; 24:1.
326. Southwick FS, Purich DL. Intracellular pathogenesis of listeriosis. N Engl J Med 1996; 334: 770.
327. Vasquez-Boland JA, Kuhn M, Berche P, et al. Listeria pathogenesis and molecular virulence determinants. Clin Microbiol Rev 2001; 14:584.
328. Alvarez-Domingues C, Vasquez-Boland JA, Carrasco-Marin E, et al. Host cell heparin sulfate proteoglycans mediate attachment and entry of *Listeria monocytogenes*, and the *Listeria* surface protein Act A is involved in heparin sulfate receptor recognition. Infect Immun 1997; 65:78.
329. MacGowan AP, Holt AJ, Bywater MI, Reeves DS. In vitro and a microbe susceptibility of *Listeria monocytogenes* isolated in the UK and other *Listeria* species. Eur J Clin Microbiol Infect Dis 1990; 9:767.
330. Charpentier E, Gerbaud G, Jaquet C, et al. Incidence of antibiotic resistance in *Listeria* species. J Infect Dis 1995; 172:277.
331. Gerry J, Greenough W III. Diphtheroid endocarditis: report of nine cases and review of the literature. Johns Hopkins Hosp Bull 1976; 139:61.
332. Morris A, Guild I. Endocarditis due to *Corynebacterium pseudodiphthericum*: five case reports, review and antibiotic susceptibilities of nine strains. Rev Infect Dis 1991; 13:887.
333. Trepeta R, Edberg S. *Corynebacteria diphtheriae* endocarditis: sustained potential of a classical pathogen. Am J Clin Pathol 1987; 8:679.
334. Love J, Medina D, Anderson S, et al. Infective endocarditis due to *Corynebacterium diphtheriae*: report of a case and review of the literature. Johns Hopkins Med J 1981; 128:41.
335. Rasmussen V, Bremmelgard A, Korner B, et al. Case report: acute corynebacteria endocarditis causing aortic valve destruction: successful treatment with antibiotics and valve replacement. Scand J Infect Dis 1979; 11:89.
336. Coyle MB, Lipsky BA. Coryneform bacteria and infectious disease: clinical and laboratory aspects. Clin Microbiol Rev 1990; 3:227.
337. Pancoast S, Ellner P, Jahre J, et al. Endocarditis due to *Kurthia bessonni*. Ann Intern Med 1979; 90:936.
338. *Nocardia, Streptomyces, Rhodococcus, Oerskova*, and similar organisms. In: Forbes BA, Sahm DF, Weissfeld AS, eds. Bailey and Scott's Diagnostic Microbiology. Chap. 24. 11th ed. St. Louis: Mosby, 2002:351.
339. Shands J. *Rothia dentocariosa* endocarditis. Am J Med 1988; 85:280.
340. Sudduth E, Rozich J, Farrar W. *Rothia dentocariosa* endocarditis complicated by periosteal abscess. Clin Infect Dis 1993; 17:772.
341. Ascher DP, Zpick C, White C, et al. Infections due to *Stomatococcus mucilaginosus*: 10 cases and review. Rev Infect Dis 1991; 13:1048.
342. Llopis F, Carratala J. Vertebral osteomyelitis complicating *Rothia dentocariosa* endocarditis. Eur J Clin Microbiol 2002; 19:562.
343. Binder D, Zbinden R, Widmer U, et al. Native and prosthetic valve endocarditis caused by *Rothia dentocariosa*: diagnostic and therapeutic considerations. Infection 1997; 25:22.
344. Sliman R, Rehm S, Shlaes D. Serious infections caused by *Bacillus* species. Medicine 1987; 66:218.
345. Steen Bruno-Murtha F, Chaux G, et al. *Bacillus cereus* endocarditis: report of a case and review. Clin Infect Dis 1992; 14:945.
346. Banerjee C, Bustmante CI, Wharton R, et al. *Bacillus* infections in patients with cancer. Arch Inter Med 1988; 128:1769.
347. Weber D, Javiteer S, Rinfalen W, et al. In vitro susceptibility of *Bacillus cereus* to selected antimicrobial agents. Antimicrob Agent Chemother 1988; 32:6412.

3 Microbiology of Infective Endocarditis and Clinical Correlates: Gram-Negative and Other Organisms

John L. Brusch
Harvard Medical School and Department of Medicine and Infectious Disease Service, Cambridge Health Alliance, Cambridge, Massachusetts, U.S.A.

GRAM-NEGATIVE ORGANISMS

Gram-negative aerobic bacteria have been responsible for only a small portion of the total cases of infective endocarditis (IE) (3%) (1). More recently, this figure has increased from 7% to 15% (2). They are involved in 10% of the cases of polymicrobial endocarditis (3). The essential epidemiological paradox of gram-negative IE is that despite the high incidence of gram-negative bacteremia, the incidence of valvular infection with these organisms remains quite low. For example, *Pseudomonas aeruginosa* is the fifth most common cause of bloodstream infections (BSI) in the intensive care unit (ICU). It causes 5% of total bacteremias (4,5). However, a very small percentage of gram-negative BSI results in valvular infection. One explanation for this is that *Escherichia coli* and *Klebsiella pneumoniae*, the most common bacteremic gram-negatives, adhere to the endothelium of native valves much less avidly than do the *Streptococcus viridans*, enterococci, *Staphylococcus aureus*, or even *P. aeruginosa* (6). Gould et al. (6) documented that this latter group of pathogens had adherence ratios (proportion of bacteria from surrounding media that adhered in vitro to human aortic valve leaflets) that ranged from 0.0003 to 0.017. Corresponding values for *E. coli* and *Klebsiella* were significantly less (0.00002–0.00004). *Staphylococcus aureus* is most frequently the cause of IVDA IE (7) with the gram-negative bacilli responsible for 13% of these cases. Of these, *Ps. aeruginosa* accounts for 60% (8). There has been gradual increase in catheter-associated infections, caused by gram-negative organisms, with a corresponding increase in valvular infections (9,10). The retrieval of certain gram-negatives (i.e., *Burkholderia cepacia*, *Citrobacter* spp.) from the bloodstream is consistent with a contaminated infusate (11).

Additionally, cirrhosis, because of a variety of reasons, increases the risk of gram-negative IE by threefold (12,13). *P. aeruginosa* is involved in approximately 7% of these cases.

Greater than three decades ago, the association of gram-negative IE with gram-positive infections was recognized by Finland and Barnes (3). Ten percent of the 400 cases of IE, which occurred at Boston City Hospital from 1933 to 1965, were because of gram-negatives. A variety of gram-positive infections preceded almost 66% of them. This relationship may reflect the decreased adherence of most gram-negative to normal valvular tissue or to the increased use of intravascular devices in acutely ill patients. These same principles may underlie the high rate of polymicrobial IE (both gram-negative and gram-positive organisms) that occurs in up to 30% of IVDA IE. Nonaddicts have a corresponding rate of 2% (14,15). By damaging a previously normal valve, the gram-positive component (especially *S. aureus*) may permit secondary invasion by gram-negative isolates (16).

The review of gram-negative endocarditis, by Cohen et al., published more than 25 years ago, remains quite relevant as regards the clinical presentations and epidemiology of gram-negative IE (17). The mean age of patients with gram-negative IE (39 years) is significantly less than those with IE due to *S. viridans*. Gram-negative healthcare-associated IE (HCIE) usually involves prosthetic valves; either early or late after implantation. In the review of Cohen et al., only 25% of infected native valves had been previously normal. In more recent reports, 66 to almost 100% of these valves exhibited no underlying pathology (18,19). Rapidly progressive congestive heart failure (CHF) occurs in greater than 50% of the patients with gram-negative IE. However, it occurs in only 14% of all individuals with *P. aeruginosa* IE. Thirty-seven percent of IVDA with left-sided gram-negative IE develop cardiac decompensation whereas only 3% of those with right-sided involvement do so. Heart failure occurs most frequently in cases of prosthetic valve endocarditis (PVE) usually those involving the aortic valve. Large vegetations may lead to valvular obstruction, systemic, and pulmonary emboli (50% of cases). The gram-negative IE of IVDA exhibits distinctive features: panophthalmitis (10% of cases) and an increased incidence of cerebral mycotic aneurysms that are prone to rupture (17).

GRAM-NEGATIVE RODS
Pseudomonas Species, *Burkholderia*, and Similar Organisms
At one time, all of these species belonged to the genus *Pseudomonas*. Because of their clinical similarities, they will be discussed as a group. These slender bacilli are non-lactose fermenters. They are colorless on MacConkey agar and are oxidase-positive (20). Many are quite adept at persisting in the hospital environment especially in contaminated medical solutions and devices. In doing so, they position themselves to infect the most vulnerable patients.

Pseudomonas aeruginosa
The current epidemiology of *P. aeruginosa* IE may be summarized as "in recent years, venous access (usually illicit) has been major predisposing factors to this infection and abuse of pentazocaine and tripelennamine has been particularly associated with endocarditis due to this organism. This infection involves previously damaged as well as normal valves" (21). In the past, IVDA are the most frequently effected with *P. aeruginosa* valvular infection. *P. aeruginosa* is involved in 88% of polymicrobial IVDA IE (22). However, we no longer see the outbreaks in major urban areas of IVDA IE with this pathogen (23) (Chapter 7). The incidence of *P. aeruginosa* IE has almost doubled over the period 1984–1993 (24). This significant increase is due in the, in great part, to the rise in pseudomonal HCIE.

P. aeruginosa is widely distributed throughout nature. Its ability to flourish in all types of watery environments, including hospital respirator equipment, dialysis fluid, and even disinfectant solutions, significantly contributes to making it a superb nosocomial pathogen (25). Outside the hospital, the most common significant watery reservoir is that used to dilute the illicit drug prior to injection. The pathogen's growth characteristics are quite important in its opportunistic successes. It can flourish throughout a wide range of temperatures; it requires little in the way of nutrients; and it has widespread resistance to many classes of antibiotics (Table 1) (26).

TABLE 1 Virulence Factors Involved in *Pseudomonas aeruginosa* Infective Endocarditis

Factor	Activity
Pili/fimbriae	Adhesion factor
Exopolysaccharide capsule (alginate)	Adhesion factor, decrease in penetration of antibiotics, and suppresses polymorphonuclear leukocyte function
Neuramidase	Promotes pili-mediated adhesion
Exotoxin A	Disruption of protein synthesis, inhibition of phagocytosis
Exoenzyme S	Adhesion factor
Pyocyanin	Breaks down the elastin layer of blood vessels, inhibits mitochondrial function, and interferes with white cell function and lymphocytic proliferation
Proteinases Alkaline proteinases Metalloproteinases	Damage elastin, collagen, and fibrin
Elastases	Damage the elastin layer of blood vessels and breaks down C3b and C5a
Phospholipases	Disrupt the phospholipid components of cell membranes
Leukocidins	Damages polymorphonuclear leukocytes
Ability to penetrate endothelial cells	Produces endotheliosis
Antibiotic inactivating enzymes	Resistance to beta-lactams and aminoglycosides

Colonization with *P. aeruginosa* occurs significantly in hospitalized patients owing to their exposure to a variety of contaminated solutions and the use of broad-spectrum antibiotics (27). In the 1990s, the pathogen was responsible for 13.6% of healthcare-associated BSIs (HCBSI), making it the eighth most common cause of nosocomial bacteremias and the sixth most frequent in those acquired in the ICU (28). Currently, *Pseudomonas* species cause 4% of nosocomial BSIs (29–31). *P. aeruginosa* may cause up to 10% of cases of IE acquired in the ICU setting (32).

Table 2 presents the clinical characteristics of *P. aeruginosa* IE. Left-sided valvular infection with *P. aeruginosa* presents with frequent complications, such as CHF, septic emboli, conduction abnormalities, splenic abscesses, neurological involvement, and ring abscesses (33). Right-sided disease usually follows a subacute course with right-sided heart failure and/or manifestations of septic emboli. These include cough, pleuritic chest pain, and hemoptysis. On chest X-ray, there may be evidence of septic emboli, which may eventually cavitate. The diagnosis of *P. aeruginosa* IE is usually clinically evident within a few weeks of the onset of symptoms. Left-sided IVDA IE may take a prolonged but ultimately fatal course despite intensive appropriate antibiotic therapy. The mortality rate is high (50–89%) despite vigorous antibiotic therapy. Valvular replacement is often required for cure. This should probably be performed as soon as the diagnosis of left-sided *P. aeruginosa* is made (33). Right-sided disease has a better prognosis with a fatality rate of 20%. Removal of the tricuspid valve should be considered in right-sided disease if blood cultures remain positive after two weeks of appropriate therapy or relapse after six weeks of medical therapy (34). A possible explanation for this difference in outcomes is the higher oxygen tension of the left ventricle, which enhances the production of exopolysaccharides and leads to increased resistance to the antibacterial effect of aminoglycosides (35). The more oxygen-rich chamber also promotes the production of beta-lactamases by this organism (36).

There is a distinctive pathological pattern that is quite characteristic of infections caused by *P. aeruginosa*. Infrequently, other gram-negatives may produce

TABLE 2 Clinical Features of *Pseudomonas aeruginosa* Endocarditis

Item	Value
Mean age	31.8 years
Underlying heart disease	36%
Predisposing conditions	
Drug addiction	64%
Recent cardiac surgery	15%
Cardiac angiography	5%
Urinary tract infection	4%
Other infections	9%
Polymicrobial bacteremia	24%
Splenomegaly	13%
Peripheral stigmata	18%
Congestive heart failure	14%
Embolization	
Pulmonary	49%
Arterial	20%
Myocardial abscesses	9%
Central nervous system involvement	23%
Infected valve	
Tricuspid	41%
Pulmonic	3%
Aortic	11%
Mitral	14%
Aortic and mitral	10%
Right and left sided infection	7%
Ventricular septal defect	9%
Other/not determined	5%
Mortality rate	
Left-sided infection	50–89%
Right-sided infection	20%

Source: From Ref. 17.

a similar pattern. *Pseudomonas vasculitis* has four distinct processes: (*i*) tissue necrosis; (*ii*) a large amount of bacilli especially found in the medial layers of blood vessels; (*iii*) extensive hemorrhage; and (*iv*) all of these three features are centered around the smaller arteries and veins (a vasocentric pattern) (37). Few polymorphonuclear cells are present. When the left side of the heart is affected, *pseudomonas vasculitis* is visibly manifest as the dermal lesion, ecthyma gangrenosum (38). This signal lesion may be present in up to 28% of bacteremic individuals with *pseudomonas bacteremias*. These same histological findings are characteristic of *Ps. aeruginosa* IE (38). These organisms have a tropism for the connective tissue of heart valves (6). Specifically, it deforms the valve, produces necrosis of the valvular rings, and generates septic emboli. The ongoing bacteremia can bring this necrotizing process to the walls of larger blood vessels. Ultimately, mycotic aneurysms may result.

Most cases of *P. aeruginosa* IE are right-sided owing to contaminated injection diluent of IVDA or nosocomial by right-sided intravascular catheters (33). The septic pulmonary emboli that arise from infected tricuspid valves histologically closely resemble the findings of ecthyma gangrenosum.

In any discussion of the virulence factors of *Ps. aeruginosa*, it is important to emphasize that this organism is a true "hyena" of bacterial pathogens (39). Impressive that they are in number and quality, these factors are seen to be effective only in significantly impaired hosts such as the immunosuppressed; those with prolonged stays in ICUs especially in the presence of intravascular catheters; those with extensive burns and those implanted with various prosthetic materials such as cardiac valves and pacemakers. It is important to bear in mind that the end product of these pathogenic substances is an area of infection characterized by necrosis with very little polymorphonuclear leukocytes response. In a sense, this process produces a dry "gangrene" of the infected valve. The virulence factors of *P. aeruginosa* can be divided into those that act at the site of infection and those that function away from the area of infections. Those that act locally include the adhesin factors, exoenzyme S, pili, and alginate (40). Those that have systemic effects include lipopolysaccharide, cytotoxins, and exotoxin A. It is important for the clinician to appreciate the high degree of redundancy of the pathogenic properties of *P. aeruginosa*. Many of these substances have multiple functions. This brief review will focus on the primary properties of each. Table 1 summarizes the best characterized of these. However, no one factor appears supreme in producing human infection.

The chief adherence components of this organism are its pili/fimbriae. Mucoid strains of *Pseudomonas* also make use of their exopolysaccharide capsule to attach to the host's tissues. Both mechanisms dock with the sialic acid molecules of the patient's cells. These attachment sites need to be uncovered either by bacteria's neuramidase, in the case of pili attachment, or by the alginite component of its exopolysaccharide (41). The alginite component also seems to decrease intracellular penetration of aminoglycosides. In an animal model, inactivation of alginite has been shown to markedly decrease the concentration of *Pseudomonas* within the valvular thrombus (42). Exoenzyme S also can function as an adhesin and can also be involved in tissue invasion (43).

The ability of *P. aeruginosa* to adhere to a variety of intravascular catheters is a key component of the rise of catheter-related bloodstream infections (CR-BSI) (44). It does this by means of its ability to form biofilms. Formation of this extracellular "slimy" matrix depends on several factors: (*i*) how long the catheter has been in place; (*ii*) the composition of the catheter; (*iii*) and the ability of the organism to adhere to that material. Eighty-eight percent of central venous catheters (CVC) that are placed in the ICU have evidence of biofilms formation. *Pseudomonas* biofilm formation on CVC consists of three phases: attachment, colony formation, and differentiating into a structure that resembles a multicellular organism. The members of this colony communicate with each other and coordinate their function by means of quorum sensing (45). This bacterial aggregate differs functionally from the usual colony of the same species in many respects especially in being resistant to many of the antibiotics to which individual bacteria would be susceptible. Biofilm resistance is based on several mechanisms including: (*i*) antibiotic efflux mechanisms; (*ii*) decreased diffusion of the antibiotic through the biofilm; and (*iii*) decreased penetration into the biofilm. This matrix provides to certain bacteria, not only the means of adhering to native tissues and prosthetic materials, but also shielding them from phagocytes and the host's antibodies. Even a concentration of an antibiotic, which is 1000 times greater than its minimum bactericidal concentration (MBC), against a free-living form of *P. aeruginosa*, is unable to kill the same strain when it is living within a biofilm (46,47). Central venous catheter biofilms are most frequently produced by *S. aureus*, *Candida albicans*, coagulase-negative staphylococci, and anaerobic gram-negative rods (48). Normal flagellar functioning, on the part of *P. aeruginosa* isolate, seems necessary for its production of biofilm.

The multiple invasive factors of *P. aeruginosa* are extracellular products with a variety of functions (39,40). Exotoxin A and exoenzyme S are adenosine diphosphate ribosyl transferases similar in function to diphtheria toxin. Exotoxin A damages tissue and inhibits phagocytosis and protein synthesis (49). Exoenzyme S not only is an adhesion (see previous para) but can be lethal to several types of tissue by damage to the cytoskeleton. To activate this cytotoxic property, it is necessary that exoenzyme S be actively transported within the cell to be activated by the cytoplasmic protein, FAS (50,51). Production of exotoxin A and exoenzyme S is inhibited by elevated serum iron levels but stimulated by quorum sensing (the interplay between the residents of the multicellular biofilm) (52). Pyocyanin is a phenazine pigment that imparts the characteristic greenish fluorescent hue to the organism. It also has multiple toxic effects on the host's cells by interfering with mitochondrial function by binding to cytochrome B. It also acts as a defensin by interfering with polymorphonuclear leukocytes generation of superoxide and lymphocyte proliferation (53). Alkaline proteinases and the metalloproteases damage the elastin and collagen components of tissues as well as digesting antibodies (39,40). The elastases not only damage the elastin layer of blood vessels but also destroy the C3b and C5a components of complement (51). The phospholipases disrupts the phospholipid components of mammalian cell membranes (40). The proteinases, the elastases, and the phospholipases are the major necrosis-generating factors of this pathogen.

Leukocidin seems to be specific for inducing injury to polymorphonuclear leukocytes (54). The exopolysaccharide capsule of *Pseudomonas* also exhibits significant virulence factors by its ability to suppress lymphocytic and neutrophilic functions (55).

A distinctive property of *P. aeruginosa*, which it shares with few other bacteria, that is quite significant in its role in producing gram-negative IE, is its ability to cause endotheliosis (Chapter 2, discussion of *S. aureus* IE). The organism is able to adhere to, penetrate, and internally damage human endothelial cells. This function explains a great deal of its ability to infect normal heart valves especially among IVDA. One does not have to postulate that *Pseudomonas* requires an adulterant, within the injected drug, to scar and damage the endothelium before it can produce valvular infection (56).

Stenotrophomonas maltophilia

Stenotrophomonas maltophilia has successively belonged to *Pseudomonas* group, to the *Xanthomonas* group, and now to the *Stenotrophomonas* one. The organism is essentially nonpathogenic for the normal host. It is widely found throughout nature and in the hospital environment. Its epidemiology is quite similar to that of *P. aeruginosa*. It is an increasingly important opportunistic infection. Patients with cancer, lymphoma, and cystic fibrosis are its prime targets (57). It may infect native and prosthetic valves although probably more frequently the latter (58). Fifty percent of PVE occur within two weeks of implantation of the valve. The source of bacteremia is usually hospital equipment. Central venous catheter BSI is the second most frequent type of *S. maltophilia* infections. There seems to be a significant association between vacutainer tubes, contaminated with *S. maltophilia*, and either real or Pseudobacteremia. It appears that reflux from the collecting tubes is the source of *S. maltophilia* in these instances (17,59). The use of fluoroquinolones and other broad-spectrum antibiotics appear to increase the risk of *S. maltophilia* infection (60). Because many of the BSIs with *S. maltophilia* are polymicrobial, the significance of this organism has been in question. Despite isolation of several types of proteolytic enzymes, lipases, and DNAse (57), none of them were established as a bona fide virulence factor. Through its production of highly effective beta-lactamases, it has the potential to enable the overgrowth of *Serratia* or *P. aeruginosa* (61).

By 2002, 24 cases of *S. maltophilia* IE had been reported (62). The clinical course of *S. maltophilia* IE is usually acute. Arterial embolization is a major complication. Ecthyma gangrenosum has been described (63).

The initial challenge to the clinician and treating BSI/possible IE with this organism is to decide the significance of its retrieval from the bloodstream. Pseudobacteremia, owing to contaminated collection devices, must be considered especially in normal hosts. When it is part of a polymicrobial BSI, it is difficult to attribute significance to *S. maltophilia*. The sensitivity patterns of this organism make empiric choices antibiotics difficult especially when it is associated with other more classic pathogens (61).

Stenotrophomonas maltophilia is resistant to many classes of antibiotics owing to multiple factors (chromosomal resistance, disruption of antibiotic permeability, and the ability to produce many types of activating enzymes) (64). Its slow growth and high rate of mutation contributes to inconsistencies between in vitro sensitivity patterns and clinical outcomes (65). Empiric antibiotic therapy usually consists of trimethoprim-sulfamethoxazole (20 mg/kg/day) and 3.1 g of ticarcillin-clavulanate every four hours; both given intravenously (66). Although they are the most reliable and effective agents, there is a high rate of resistance to them, (67,68). Sixty-three percent of patients who have *S. maltophilia* IE Live 47% of these underwent valve replacement; 60% of those treated medically survived (62%) (62).

Burkholderia cepacia

Burkholderia cepacia, like *S. maltophilia* and *P. aeruginosa*, is an environmental organism. Because it does not require many nutrients, it can survive in antiseptic solutions, dialysis fluid, and in any watery environment for long periods of time (20). The majority of *B. cepacia* IE has been reported in IVDA. It may be also seen in patients with normal native valve or prosthetic ones (17,69). Infective endocarditis, because of this organism, is usually subacute. Some cases have followed an acute course marked by the skin lesion, ecthyma gangrenosum.

The virulence factors of *B. cepacia*, which pertain to the development of IE, are poorly characterized (70). It appears that, similar to *P. aeruginosa*, quorum-sensing by *B. cepacia*, residing in a biofilm, may be significant in this area (71).

B. cepacia is sensitive to trimethoprim-sulfamethoxazole, chloramphenicol, the third-generation cephalosporins, azteonam, and meropnem (72). The most well-established of these for treatment of *B. cepacia* valvular infection is trimethoprim-sulfamethoxazole (73). The role of combination antibiotic therapy in treating this type of IE has not been established. Use of combination antibiotics must be individualized. The greatest experience in using two more drugs has been to treat patients with cystic fibrosis and *B. cepacia* respiratory infections.

The non-*P. aeruginosa* species, most commonly involved in bacteremia/IE, are *P. stutzeri*, *P. fluorescence*, and *P. putida* (74). They share many properties in that they are ubiquitous in the hospital environment; occasionally cause BSI or pseudo-BSI/valvular infection among debilitated/immunosuppressed patients or those with prosthetic valves. They have been reported to cause contamination of blood products as they can grow at 4°C (75). *P. stutzeri* is the most frequently isolated example.

Salmonella

It is quite interesting, that for such a well-established pathogen, the first cases of *Salmonella* IE were recognized in late 1940s (76). They used to be the most frequently isolated Enterobacteriaceae in cases of IE. Any *Salmonella* sp. may produce IE. *Salmonella typhi* is the least often isolated. Unlike other gram-negatives, bacteremia/ IE is usually acquired in the community. This inability to take advantage of the hospital environment to produce HCIE has led to its being eclipsed as a frequent cause of gram-negative IE. Formerly most patients were older than 50 years. Few were IVDA. These organisms may infect damaged native valves or prosthetic ones. The chief predisposing condition was and is gastroenteritis. However, less than 4% of competent hosts have bacteremia complicating their intestinal infection (77). *Salmonella* isolates have a stronger predilection to infect the damaged endothelium (78) in up to 25% of individuals greater than 50 years of age (79). Most of these infections involve the aorta and some involve the endocardium or valvular endothelium. Immunosuppression or nosocomial acquisition, each, were major predisposing factors in <4% of the cases (17,80–83). The course of disease was often acute. In non-HIV patients, right-sided IE is unusual. Complications include atrial thrombi (24% of cases), valvular perforation, pericarditis, and myocardial abscess. Progressive CHF is frequent. The peripheral stigmata of IE (Osler's nodes, petechiae, and subungual hemorrhages) occur in two-thirds of patients. Valvular vegetations are characteristically large.

The epidemiology of *Salmonella* IE has changed during the AIDS era. These individuals have up to 100 times the rate of *Salmonella* bacteremia than non-AIDS patients (84). They are also younger. The rate of recurrent *Salmonella* BSIs is also markedly elevated. This dual susceptibility reflects the AIDS virus ability to markedly impair cellular immunity which is very essential in limiting the course of *Salmonella* infections (85,86). Among those with both AIDS/IVDA, there is a marked increase in right-sided valvular infections especially about those with a previously abnormal tricuspid valve (87). In non-HIV IVDA patients, Salmonella is rarely a cause of valvular infection.

In *Salmonella* IE, usually all blood cultures are positive. Valvular infection with this organism may be cryptic when the valvular infection has evolved into an abscess that has burrowed into the myocardium and is no longer in direct communication with the bloodstream. *Salmonella* IE/mycotic aneurysm should be ruled out by echocardiography and computed tomography (CT) scan/magnetic resonance angiography (MRA) if appropriate therapy has failed to clear the bacteremia after 7 to 10 days (17), even in the absence of clinical findings.

The mortality rate of *Salmonella* IE is currently 10% (81). This is probably because of the availability of the third-generation cephalosporins and fluoroquinolones. In the past, chloramphenicol was felt to be the mainstay of treatment of *Salmonella* endovascular infections. However, despite in vitro sensitivity data there was a high clinical failure rate with this antibiotic (78). Even the need of valvular replacement has decreased with the availability of these newer antibiotics. However, mycotic aneurysms still generally require resection for cure (88).

HACEK Organisms

The HACEK group of bacteria includes *H. influenzae, H. parainfluenzae, H. aphrophilus, H. paraphrophilus, Actinobacillus actinomycetocomitans, Cardiobacterium hominis, Eikenell corrodens,* and *Kingella kingii.* This group does not represent a bacterial classification. The members have no common genetic bond (89,90). All are small gram-negative bacilli/coccobacilli that are normal inhabitants of the human oropharynx. All are slow-growing and are capnophiles (requiring incubation in CO_2 for their growth). All *Hemophilus* isolates require either X-factor (hemin) or V-factor (NAD). They are becoming a more frequent cause of IE (5% of the total cases) (91,92). Infection of native valves follows a subacute course. These organisms usually infect abnormal valves; the mitral being the most common. HACEK PVE usually occurs after one year following implantation. A variety of dental procedures is the common inciting event for almost all cases of HACEK IE. There have been recent case reports of *H. aphrophilus* endocarditis following body piercing in patients with congenital heart disease (93). Large valvular vegetations, which frequently embolize, are hallmarks of HACEK IE. Disease is usually present for longer than one month prior to diagnosis. Worsening of pre-existent cardiac failure may be the initial clinical manifestation. Peripheral stigmata of IE (Osler's nodes, Janeway lesions, or Roth's spots) are inconsistently present. On the average, these organisms require approximately seven days to grow out of blood cultures. For some species, this period may be up to 30 days. These organisms should be considered a cause of the culture-negative endocarditis. The correct diagnosis is made at autopsy or cardiac surgery. The particular virulence factors that are relevant to IE, have not been well characterized except for the growing problem of resistance to the beta-lactams, including ampicillin, and other antibiotics. Resistance results from their beta-lactamase production and other mechanisms (94). Their slow growth makes sensitivity testing problematic. Third-generation cephalosporins have become the therapeutic agents of choice while awaiting final sensitivity data. In addition, the large vegetations, so typical of this group, probably interfere with antibiotic effects. "Vegectomy" is sometimes required when appropriate antibiotics fail to eradicate these bacteria from the bloodstream.

H. aphropilus is the most common species of *Hemophilus* involved in endocarditis (89). The mean age of patients is less than 50 years (95). In addition to dental procedures, upper respiratory tract infection may be another source of valvular infection (96). Twenty percent of the cases involve prosthetic valves. Vegetations, usually quite large, are present in 70% of the cases. Formerly, the mortality rate was 50%. Death was usually because of intractable CHF or the effects of systemic embolization. Improved diagnostic approaches have lessened the death rate to <10% (Table 3).

A few cases of *H. paraphrophilus* IE have been recognized (97,98). This organism appears to have a particular proclivity for affecting prolapsed mitral valves (75% of the cases). Neither *H. aphrophilus* nor *H. paraphrophilus* are associated with IVDA IE.

H. influenzae remains an unusual cause of IE. This was the case even when bacteremia with this organism was quite common prior to the development of the *H. influenzae* vaccine (99). It usually attacks normal valves with a clinical spectrum that ranges from the subacute to acute.

H. parainfluenzae is far more frequently involved in valvular infections with 66 patients reported in the world's literature as of 2001 (100). *H. parainfluenzae* IE appear to be on the rise. This organism targets young adults. It attacks both normal and abnormal valves. Prosthetic valve endocarditis makes up 10% of the cases. *H. parainfluenzae* IE is typically subacute in its course. Advanced cardiac failure is unusual. However, macroembolization of giant vegetations is relatively common (85% of the cases). The diagnosis is often delayed because of the difficulty in isolating the organism in blood cultures owing to its strict growth requirement for the V-factor. Additionally, 10% of the cases are polymicrobial. In these ones, the recognition

TABLE 3   Clinical Features of *Haemophillus aphrophilus* Endocarditis

Item	Value
Mean age	43 years
Underlying heart disease	88%
Predisposing conditions	
Dental disease/oral surgery	60%
Upper respiratory infections	19%
Peripheral stigmata	63%
Congestive heart failure	50%
Arterial embolization	31%
Myocardial abscesses	15%
Infected valve	
Mitral	40%
Aortic	30%
Tricuspid	5.5%
Prosthetic	20%
Mortality rate	50%[a]

[a]Rate based on older studies. Current mortality rates approach zero (see text).
Source: From Ref. 17.

of *H. parainfluenzae* may be obscured by the presence of other organisms. It is not clear whether the high rate of macroembolization is owing to a particular property of this pathogen or the extended period of time before appropriate therapy is initiated. The death rate ranges from 10% to 35% (Table 4).

Cardiobacterium hominis is distinctive among the HACEK Group in its appearance (pleomorphic with bulbous swellings at its ends), in its growth in the form of chains or rosettes, and in its oxidase positivity (101–103). It may be part of the normal bowel flora. Up until 2001, 76 cases of *C. hominis* IE had been reported. The clinical course is subacute and nonspecific. Sixty-two percent and 13% of patients have underlying abnormal valves or prosthetic valves, respectively. Uniquely among this bacterial group, the organism most frequently infects the aortic valve. Embolization occurs in more than 50% of the patients. Valvular replacement is necessary in up to 30% of the cases. The death rate is 13% (Table 5).

TABLE 4   Clinical Features of *Hemophilus parainfluenzae* Endocarditis

Item	Value
Mean age	31 years
Underlying heart disease	52%
Predisposing conditions	
Oral infections/dental procedures	45%
Drug abuse	3%
Sinus infections	10%
Peripheral stigmata	59%
Congestive heart failure	10%
Arterial embolization	85%
Polymicrobial bacteremia	10%
Infected valve	
Aortic	17%
Mitral	67%
Mortality rate	10–35%

Source: From Ref. 17.

TABLE 5 Clinical Features of *Cardiobacterium hominis* Endocarditis

Item	Value
Mean age	49 years
Underlying heart disease	75%
Predisposing conditions	
Oral infection/dental procedures	44%
Upper respiratory infections	18%
Peripheral stigmata	81%
Congestive heart failure	62%
Arterial embolization	38%
Mycotic aneurysm	9%
Infected valve	
Mitral	36%
Aortic	44%
Aortic and mitral	7%
Prosthetic	13%
Mortality rate	13%

Source: From Ref. 17.

Actinobacillus actinomycetemcomitans was so named because it was considered a contributory pathogen in infections caused by *Actinomyces israelii* (104–106). On Gram stain, it resembles *Hemophilus* strains. Recovery from blood cultures may take as long as 25 days. This organism may spread within families. *Actinobacillus actinomycetemcomitans* is the most frequent cause of HACEK IE. Sixty-seven percent of patients have underlying valvular disease, 33% of native valves, and 34% of prosthetic valves. The course of this infection is quite insidious. It may present as polymyalgia rheumatica. In some series, 50% of patients have no significant fever. Peripheral manifestations of IE are often absent. Complications are the same ones common to all members of this group, CHF and embolization (39%). Twenty-eight percent of patients require valvular replacement. Mortality rates range up to 15%. Rates of complications and death are less in cases of PVE. This probably reflects the shorter time to diagnose this type of IE. Most likely, this reflects a higher degree of clinical suspicion of valvular infection when prosthetic material is in place (Table 6).

Eikenella corrodens rarely causes IE despite the fact that it is present in 16% of transient bacteremias associated with dental extraction (107–110). It is a facultative anaerobe. Its colonies have a distinctive "bleach-like" odor and pit the underlying agar. In addition to the usual oral sources of infection, IE caused by this organism, is associated with recreational drugs, especially amphetamines. Fifty percent of the IVDA IE of *E. corrodens* is polymicrobial usually with all *streptococci*. The association may arise from the IVDA habit of licking the needle before injection for good luck. There is also the evidence that it can affect intravascular catheters. The mortality rate is 15%. It is rarely necessary to replace the infected valve.

Kingella spp., *K. kingae* and *K. denitrificans*, have been reported to cause 33 cases of IE as of 2001 (111,112). Twenty-eight of these were due to *K. kingae*. The organisms frequently infect children and younger adults. In the pediatric age group, *Kingella* IE equally attacks normal and abnormal valves usually congenital abnormalities including mitral valve prolapse. In older patients, 33% of infections involved prosthetic valves. Twenty-five percent of cases of *K. kingae* IE are complicated by embolic strokes.

TABLE 6   Clinical Features of *Actinobacillus actinomycetemcomitans* Endocarditis

Item	Value
Mean age	47.4 years
Underlying heart disease	70%
Predisposing conditions	
Oral infection/dental procedures	46%
Thoracotomy	7%
Chest trauma	14%
Peripheral stigmata	50%
Congestive heart failure	57%
Arterial embolization	39%
Mycotic aneurysm	9%
Infected valve	
Aortic	46%
Mitral	31%
VSD	8%
Prosthetic	50%
Mortality rate	15%

Abbreviation: VSD, ventricular septal defect.
Source: From Ref. 17.

INFECTIVE ENDOCARDITIS CAUSED BY NON-*SALMONELLA* *ENTEROBACTERIACEAE*

The non-*Salmonella enterobacteriaceae* may be categorized into two groups: the opportunistic pathogens and the overt pathogens. *Salmonella* sp., *Shigella* sp., and *Yersinia pestis* are considered the overt pathogens. Their presence in a patient always represents disease. The opportunistic pathogens, such as *Citrobacter*, *Enterobacter*, *E. coli*, *Klebsiella*, *Proteus*, and *Serratia* take advantage of the impaired host.

Escherichia coli

Although *Escherichia coli* is a very prominent cause of community-acquired BSI and HCBSI especially in older individuals, cases of *E. coli* IE are unusual (113). *E. coli* bacteremia, arising in the community, is three times more frequent than pneumo-coccal bacteremia (114). The most common source of *E. coli* bacteremia is the urinary tract. In men, the risk factors for *E. coli* BSI include urinary catheterization and incontinence. Whereas for women, these are cancer, renal failure, cardiac failure, cor-onary artery disease, and incontinence. Even uncomplicated by valvular infection, *E. coli* BSI has a mortality rate of 20%. *E. coli* IE is seen most frequently in IVDA, vari-ous types of immunosuppressed individuals, and those with prosthetic valves (17,18,115). The association between IE and *E. coli* CR-BSI is not well documented. However, it is most likely becoming a major source of HCBSI/IE because of its ability to produce biofims (see previous discussion of *Pseudomonas* IE). Sixty-seven percent of cases have previously normal valves. The disease is quite acute. The pathological hallmark of *E. coli* and other types of Enterobacteriaceae IE is massive, obstructing vegetations with surprisingly minimal valvular destruction. Because of the lack of preceding valvular pathology, a murmur is not often present. This makes it difficult to determine whether the retrieval of *E. coli* in multiple blood cultures represents IE. Supportive of the diagnosis of *E. coli* IE are: (*i*) persistent bacteremia even in the absence of murmur; (*ii*) when an extracardiac source of infection is inadequately

TABLE 7 Clinical Features of *Escherichia coli* Endocarditis

Item	Value
Mean age	51 years
Underlying heart disease	33%
Predisposing conditions	
Urinary tract infections	57%
Other[a]	36%
Peripheral stigmata	43%
Congestive heart failure	62%
Arterial embolization	36%
Shock	14%
Infected valve	
Aortic	7%
Mitral	57%
Other[b]	36%
Mortality rate	68%–75%

[a]Many of these probably are infected intravascular catheters.
[b]Most are prosthetic valves.
Source: From Ref. 17.

controlled by appropriate antibiotics; or (*iii*) prolonged bacteremia in the absence of hypotension. Without valvular replacement, most patients will die (Table 7).

In addition to its ability to produce biofilms, *E. coli* possess several other potential extraintestinal virulence factors that may well play a role in the pathogenesis of valvular infection. *E. coli* has the ability to invade brain microvascular endothelial cells. The same mechanism may be applicable to the cardiac endothelium. *E. coli* that produce extraintestinal disease possess fimbriae. These structures may serve as an endothelial adhesion factor by binding to cellular fibronectin. The capsule of *E. coli* and other Enterobacteriaceae interferes with phagocytosis by inhibiting contact between the pathogen and the white cell (116). The K1 antigen of is not directly connected with cellular invasion. It does appear to enhance survival of the organism after invasion has taken place by protecting it from the alternative pathway of complement. Outer membrane porin (OMP) augments the invasive capability of *E. coli*. It does so by rearranging cellular actin. Certainly, lipopolysaccharide is important as a virulence factor in septicemia. The protein, cytotoxic necrotizing factor 1, by activating GTPase leads to cellular death (117,118). The increase in extended spectrum beta-lactamases (ESBLs) are the most recent of the gram-negatives' virulence factors (119) and are becoming a progressively therapeutic challenge (Table 8).

TABLE 8 Virulence Factors Involved in *Escherichia coli* Infective Endocarditis[a]

Factor	Activity
K1 capsular antigen	Protective against host antibodies
OMP	Augmentation of invasive capability
Cytotoxic necrotizing factor of 1	Cellular death
Lipopolysaccharide	Sepsis
Extended spectrum beta-lactamases	Resistance to beta-lactam antibiotics

[a]Refer to text.
Abbreviation: OMP, outer membrane porin.

Klebsiella/Enterobacter/Proteus

Bloodstream infections with these three species most often arise from a urinary tract focus (120–122). Although they produce >11% of HCBSIs (123) they seldom cause infections of either native or prosthetic valves. Prosthetic valve endocarditis, owing to these organisms, usually occurs soon after valvular surgery. The peripheral stigmata of IE occur more frequently in valvular infections, owing to this group of organisms, than in cases produced by *E. coli*. The mortality rate is approximately 50% even in those treated medically and surgically.

The virulence factors, pertinent to the development of valvular infection, of the non-*E. coli* enterobacteriaceae are not well described. *Klesilla* sp. posses fimbriae that may act as adhesion factors (124). The capsule of polysaccharides of *Klebsiella* are similar in functioning to those of *E. coli* (116). In the case of *Proteus mirabilis*, the possession of ESBLs significantly increased the mortality rate (50% of the cases). Risk factors for the presence of ESBLs include the use of the Foley catheter and recent residence in a nursing home (125).

Serratia

Serratia marcescens is truly an opportunistic pathogen that primarily infects the hospitalized (126–128). In the past, there was an interesting association between this organism and IE. Between 1969 and 1974, there was an outbreak of *Serratia* IVDA IE in the San Francisco/Oakland Bay area (128). Currently, its involvement in IVDA valvular infections is nil. It is responsible currently for about 2% of HCBSI (123). Radiation exposure increases the risk of invasion. Both native valves and prosthetic valves (early type) may be infected. The clinical course of *Serratia* IE is usually subacute. Complications include macroembolization, secondary to large, friable vegetations, myocardial abscesses, and valvular destruction. Because of the low rate of peripheral signs and symptoms and its subacute course, the infection is recognized only at autopsy/cardiac surgery in up to 45% of patients. Medical management achieves cure in approximately 30% of the patients (Table 9).

Yersinia enterocolitica

Yersinia enterocolitica primarily causes foodborne illnesses in humans. The organism rarely produces bacteremia/IE (129). It invades the bloodstream via Peyer's patches. Most patients have significant underlying immunosuppressed states such as being recipients of immunosuppressive therapy and HIV disease. There is a distinctive association of *Y. enterocolitica* bacteremia/IE with various iron-loading states such as hemoglobinopathies, hemolytic anemias, various types of cirrhosis, hemochromatosis, and iron therapy. The most common serotypes are 0:3, 0:9, and 0:9. This organism is one of the few that can cause transfusion-associated BSI with contaminated blood and blood products (130). This may be attributable to *Yersinia*'s ability to reproduce at 4°C. Only the nonsiderophore-producing serotypes (see next) have been involved in these cases. Both previously damaged native valves and prosthetic valves may become infected. The BSI of *Y. enterocolitica* may be complicated by metastatic abscesses, development of mycotic aneurysms, and endocarditis (131). The mortality rate approaches zero when the patient receives appropriate antibiotic therapy. This usually consists of a third-generation cephalosporin combined with gentamicin.

Y. enterocolitica posseses several important virulence factors. Strictly speaking, it is not an intracellular pathogen but an extracellular one owing to its ability to kill

TABLE 9 Clinical Features of *Serratia marcescens* Endocarditis

Item	Value
Mean age	41 years
Underlying heart disease	73%
Predisposing conditions	
Drug addiction	<5%[a]
Recent cardiac surgery	37%
Urinary tract infections	26%
Intravascular catheters	37%[a]
Peripheral stigmata	26%
Congestive heart failure	53%
Arterial embolization	53%
Myocardial abscesses	26%
Infected valve	
Aortic	11%
Mitral	22%
Tricuspid	27%
Prosthetic	37%
Mortality rate	63%

[a]Estimations of current values.
Source: From Ref. 17.

phagocytic cells of all types by means of toxins directly into these cells. These are products of the Yop virulon (132), which is a type III secretion apparatus that injects these lethal substances directly into the scavenger cell. The details of this process are beyond the scope of this text. In addition, components of the Yop virulon inhibit the immune system of the host by suppressing tumor necrosis factor, interfering with platelet aggregation, and inhibiting the activation of the complement (133). Yersiniabactin, an iron-binding siderophore, appears to be important in the early stages of the infection (Table 10) (132).

Other Enterobacteriaceae

Citrobacter species are opportunistic pathogens. *Citrobacter diversus* appears to be the most invasive owing to its outer membrane (134). *C. freundi* has been involved in IVDA IE (135). The aortic valve is most commonly involved. They are sensitive to the cephalosporins and aminoglycosides.

    Edwardsiella tarda is normally found in the gastrointestinal tract of reptiles. In humans, it primarily causes gastroenteritis, which is unusually complicated by bacteremia/IE (136).

TABLE 10 Virulence Factors of *Yersinia enterocolitica* Endocarditis[a]

Item	Factor
Unknown	Cold tolerance
Yersiniabactin	Potentiates early stages of infection
Type III secretion system	Injects toxins into a variety of cells especially phagocytes
Yersinia adhesion A (Yad A)	Adhesion factor and anticomplement factor
Yersinia outer proteins	Antiphagocytic, anticomplement effects

[a]Refer to text.

Non-Enterobacteriaceae

Brucella

Members of the genus *Brucella* are small, nonmotile, anaerobic gram-negative coccobacilli. They require supplemental CO_2 for culture. *B. abortus*, *B. melitensis*, *B. suis*, and *B. canis* are the species pathogenic to humans. Of these, *B. melitensis* and *B. suis* are the most virulent. Valvular infection complicates brucellosis in <0.6% of the cases. Infective endocarditis is the leading cause of death in *Brucella* infection. Worldwide, the incidence of *Brucella* IE is <1% of all the cases. In endemic areas (Spain, Saudi Arabia, and Italy), this value may approach 10%. Persistence of positive blood cultures after appropriate antibiotic therapy is an important clue that valvular infection has complicated the course of brucellosis. Native mitral valves are most frequently affected. Prosthetic valve endocarditis, due to *Brucella*, has been reported. *Brucella* valvular infections usually follow a subacute to chronic course. Because of its insidious onset, it often takes more than three months to make the diagnosis. This delay contributes significantly to the high mortality rate, of the past, of cases treated solely with antibiotics. Extracardiac manifestations are common because of embolization of the massive vegetations. They may ulcerate or fibrose or become nodular and calcific. Complications include mycotic aneurysms of the aortic sinus and brain, diffuse myocardial abscess, cardiac granulomas, pericarditis, myocarditis, disseminated intravascular coagulation, and. The ring abscesses of *Brucella* PVE often lead to catastrophic detachment of the valve. At times, the infection may follow a very acute course manifested by valvular perforation resulting in intractable cardiac failure with associated deep venous thrombosis. Diagnosis is made by culturing the organisms from the blood or cardiac tissue. Incubation times may extend up to six weeks (Chapter 12) (Table 11) (137–139).

Most cases require a combination of appropriate antimicrobial therapy combined with valvular replacement. Preferred antibiotic therapy consists of doxycycline and either rifampin or streptomycin for eight weeks following valvular replacement. Because the correct diagnosis is being arrived at earlier, medical therapy, by itself, is achieving cures. This probably reflects the fact that the mass of the vegetations is less; therefore allowing improved antibiotic penetration (140,141). Those individuals who have not yet developed CHF, myocardial abscess, or severe

TABLE 11   Clinical Features of *Brucella* Endocarditis

Item	Value
Mean age	41 years
Underlying heart disease	88%
Predisposing conditions	
Exposure to un-pasteurized dairy products	25%
Abattoir workers/farmers	34%
Peripheral stigmata	75%
Congestive heart failure	91%
Arterial embolization	88%
Infected valve	
Aortic	75%
Mitral	8.3%
Prosthetic	8.3%
Mortality rate[a]	83%

[a]With earlier diagnosis, this rate may be significantly less.
Source: From Ref. 17.

valvular damage and who do not have a prosthetic valve in place would be candidates for therapy with antibiotics alone.

Brucella organisms are both extracellular and intracellular pathogens. There are four routes of human infection: (*i*) ingestion of contaminated dairy products; (*ii*) penetration of the oral mucosa or conjunctiva; (*iii*) direct penetration into the bloodstream by trauma; and (*iv*) inhalation. Once within the host, the organisms are phagocytized by neutrophils. Within the white cells, they survive, multiply, and eventually kill these cells. Leukocytes containing *Brucella* are taken up by the reticuloendothelial system. *Brucella* with smooth lipopolysaccharides (LPS) in their cell walls are more resistant to killing by polymorphonuclear leukocytes than those with rough LPS. These pathogens also inhibit the myeloperoxidase pathway of phagocytes as well as producing superoxide dismutase, which blocks the oxidative system of these cells. *Brucellae* can also prevent the fusion of the phagosome with the lysosome of the white cell. Eventually granulomas are formed. Clearance of the infection by the host depends on the particular species producing the infection, the route of the infection, the size of the inoculum, and development of cellular immunity (142). The reader is referred to an excellent review of all aspects of brucellosis including pathogenesis and host response to these organisms (143).

Bordetella spp.
Bordetella spp. are zoonoses that rarely effect humans. *Bordetella bronchiseptica* is a straight gram-negative rod. *Bordetella holmesi* can present as a coccobacillus or a short or a straight gram-negative rod. Little is known regarding their virulence factors. *B. bronchiseptica* and *B. holmesi* have been documented to produce human IE (144,145). There are no well-established guidelines for the treatment of these species. Generally, the aminoglycosides, piperacillin, third-generation cephalosporin, imipenem, and the quinolones show favorable in vitro effect (146).

Francisella tularensis
Infective endocarditis owing to *F. tularensis* is extremely rare. It may be underdiagnosed because of the lengthy incubation time. In the one case report available, the pathogen was retrieved after nine days of incubation in a Bactec blood culture system (147). *Francisella* isolates are generally susceptible to the aminoglycosides. The fluoroquinolones are becoming the antibiotics of choice for all types of tularemia (148,149).

Pasturella spp.
Pasturella spp. are short, nonsporulating gram-negative bacilli. On Gram stain, they sometimes appear like coccobacilli and so may be confused with *H. influenzae* or *Acinetobacter*. Contact with animals, especially their teeth, is the major documented source of human infection (37–44% of the cases) (91,150). The oropharynx is secondary only to cellulitis, as a portal of entry of the organism into the human circulation. However, there are many cases with no known exposure to animals. Of all the *Pasteurella* sp., *P. multocida* most frequently produces valvular infections. Other species (*P. pneumotropica*, *P. hemolytica*, *P. gallinarum*, and *P. dagmatis*) have been documented as causing IE (151,152). There are some evidences that IE, due to nonmultocida *Pasteurella*, are less likely to have a history of animal exposure. The incidence of infection, involving previously damaged valves, is approximately 50%. Most patients suffer from one or more severe comorbidities. Thirty-four percent have significant underlying cirrhosis of varying etiologies. *Pasteurella* PVE is well

documented (153). Often, infection has been present from three to six months before the correct diagnosis is made. This delay is because of the indolent course of *Pasteurella* IE and not because of any difficulty in culturing the organism. Mortality is high at 31% and is attributable, in great part, to this delay. All species of *Pasteurella* are quite sensitive to penicillin (154), a quite unusual situation for a gram-negative organism. All the beta-lactam antibiotics and macrolides are effective against the *Pasteurella* sp.

The major virulence factor of *P. multocida* is its polysaccharide capsule. The larger the capsule; the more resistant the isolate is to phagocytosis. The capsule also appears to mediate adherence and resistance to killing by the complement system (155).

Campylobacter fetus

Campylobacter fetus is a comma-shaped, gram-negative rod. Unlike *C. jejuni*, it is capable of producing extraintestinal infections primarily BSI. *C. fetus* has a significant tropism for vascular sites including cardiac valves; large-size arteries leading to development of mycotic aneurysms and veins resulting in septic thrombophlebitis. The histological hallmark of *C. fetus* vascular infections is widespread necrosis. Seventy percent of the cases involve normal cardiac structures. These organisms are able to infect prosthetic valves. Dental procedures, systemic lupus erythematosus, and alcoholism are some of the predisposing factors of *C. fetus* IE. The mortality rate is 25%. The antimicrobial treatment regimen of choice is a combination of imipenem and gentamicin (156–158). The major virulence factor of *C. fetus* is a surface protein that, by preventing binding of C3b, protects the organism from opsonization and eventual death within phagocytes (159).

Aeromonas hydrophilia

Aeromonas hydrophilia is a gram-negative bacillus found in freshwater. They are facultative anaerobes that produce beta-hemolysins on blood agar. It has rarely caused IE. A typical case history would be the development of IE in a cirrhotic exposed to floodwater. Because of its increasing involvement in HCBSI, *A. hydrophilia* valvular infections may become more common. Sanguivorous leeches that are employed in graft surgery may transmit this organism. A distinctive characteristic of these infections is ecthyma gangrenosum owing to Aeromonas' ability to cause widespread muscle necrosis. *Aeromonas* sp. produce a wide spectrum of beta-lactamases including carbapenemases. Third-generation cephalosporins, tetracyclines, aminoglycosides, fluoroquinolones, and trimethoprim/sulfamethoxazole are generally effective (160–165).

Acinetobacter spp.

The primary human pathogens of this genus, *A. baumanni* and *A. calcoaceticus*, have been reclassified as *Acinetobacter* spp. saccharolytic, nonhemolytic (166). Examples are found throughout nature in soil and water. In the stationary phase, they are gram-negative rods but may appear as gram-positive cocci on direct smear of positive blood cultures. Because they are most often colonizers, they are frequent causes of pseudobacteremia because of poorly collected blood cultures (167). *Acinetobacter* spp. are generally regarded as nonpathogenic for the healthy individual. The modern hospital has provided an ideal ecological niche for nosocomial transmission to patients. A hospital's moist areas (ventilatory equipment, sinks, and humidifiers) serve as reservoirs of these pathogens, which are also able to survive on dry areas

TABLE 12 Clinical Features of *Acinetobacter* Endocarditis

Item	Value
Mean age	31 years
Underlying heart disease	56%
Predisposing conditions	>50%
Immunosuppression of all types	
Malignancies, burns, and major surgeries	
Intravascular catheters	
Peripheral stigmata	67%
Congestive heart failure	33%
Arterial embolization	67%
Infected valve	
Aortic	67%
Mitral	22%
Prosthetic	11%
Mortality rate[a]	56%

[a]Estimated value.
Source: From Ref. 17.

such as mattresses. (Into this environment, we, with the best of intentions, place our most debilitated patients.) Additionally, these pathogens are the most common gram-negative organisms to persist on the skin of healthcare workers (168). Risk factors for infection include intravascular catheters, mechanical ventilation, wide-spectrum antibiotic use, and surgery (169). *Acinetobacter* spp. produce three varieties of IE (17). In the first, the patient has underlying cardiac pathology (rheumatic heart disease or congenital heart disease). The clinical course is subacute. Congestive heart failure and massive embolization have led to the fatal outcome in 50% of the patients. The second type involves normal valves and follows an acute course. It is often associated with IVDA. Seventy-five percent of the patients die. The third represents PVE caused by HCBSI with *Acinetobacter* sp. (Table 12). Quinolones, tri-methoprim/sulfamethoxazole, ampicillin/sulbactam, ticarcillin/clavulanate, dox-ycycline, and imipenem are generally effective against most isolates of *Acinetobacter* (170). There is enough variation among isolates that susceptibility testing is required for final choice of antibiotic regimen. The carbapenems offer the highest degree of activity against these organisms. However, up to 11% of isolates have been tested to be resistant to this class. Many strains are at least partially resistant to most of the aminoglycosides. However, combinations of various beta-lactam antibiotics with the aminoglycosides are least additive in many cases (171).

The virulence factors of *Acinetobacter* are not well understood. Candidates include the polysaccharide capsule, several enzymes that damage tissue lipids, the lipopolysaccharide component of the cell wall, and poorly defined adhesins (172).

Streptobacillus moniliformis and *Spirillum minus*

Streptobacillus moniliformis is a pleomorphic facultative anaerobe that lives in the upper respiratory tract of rats. Culture medium has to be enriched with blood or other supplements. Sodium polyanethol sulfonate (SPS) that is employed in commercial blood culture bottles, impedes the growth of this pathogen. In broth cultures, the organism produces "puffballs" that settle at the bottom of the bottle. Successful incubation often requires up to six days. The organism may revert to an L form. This transformation may explain its persistence in the host. When *S. moniliformis* is transmitted to humans through rat bites, the resultant disease appropriately is called rat bite fever. When the organism is acquired by ingesting contaminated dairy products or other foods, the infectious process is termed Haverhill fever. Clinically both illnesses are almost identical. They begin abruptly with chills, fever, and headache. After three to four days, a rash appears on the palms and soles. This can range in appearance from maculopapular to vesicular or pustular or petechial. Eventually desquamation occurs. Fifty percent of patients develop asymmetric polyarthritis; most often involving the knees. The arthritis usually resolves in a few days but may relapse. Haverhill fever exhibits a greater frequency of gastrointestinal symptoms and of pharyngitis. This symptom complex may last for weeks or months. Endocarditis is an unusual complication. It usually involves valve damage by rheumatic fever or calcific degeneration. Treatment regimens are based on anecdotal experience. Most likely, the most successful therapeutic approach is the administration intravenously of 20 million units of penicillin G daily with or without the use of streptomycin or doxycycline. These latter two may be effective against the L form (173–176).

Spirillum minus is a gram-negative spiralar bacteria that is strictly anaerobic. It produces a form of rat bite fever (termed "sodoku" in Japan) that is usually without arthritic symptoms but marked by generalized lymphadenopathy. It may produce a false-positive reagin test for syphilis. Very few cases of IE as a result of this organism have been described. It usually follows a subacute course (177).

Alcaligenes and Achromobacter spp.

Alcaligenes and *Achromobacter* spp. may be normally found in the human upper respiratory and gastrointestinal tracts. Their nosocomial epidemiology is quite similar to that of *Pseudomonas* in that they only colonize and infect the most debilitated of the individuals. In the hospital, they are recovered from a variety of medical devices such as intravenous solutions, intravascular devices, respiratory, and hemodialysis equipment and even in disinfectants. Outbreaks arise from reservoirs of water within patient care units. Rarely do these two produce IE. *Achromobacter xylosoxidans* is the species most frequently isolated from valvular infections. All reported cases have involved exclusively the aortic valve. Both of these pathogens produce a variety of beta-lactamases and cephalosporinases. *Achromobacter xylosoxidans* is sensitive to trimethoprim/sulfamethoxazole, the carbapenems, ticarcillin/clavulanate, piperacillin/tazobactam, certain cephalosporins (ceftazadime, cefoperazone), and colistin. They are generally resistant to most of the cephalosporins, aztreonam, and the aminoglycosides with variable sensitivity to the quinolones. *Alcaligenes faecalis* has a sensitivity pattern similar to that of *Achromobacter* sp. with the exception that they are sensitive to most of the cephalosporins. Although, neither produce any definable virulence factors, their ability to survive in disinfectants and their high degree of antibiotic resistance does contribute to the ability to produce healthcare associated infections (178–182).

Chryseobacterium spp.

Chryseobacterium (formerly *Flavobacterium*) spp. are similar epidemiologically to *Alcaligenes* and *Achromobacter* spp. in that they are widely distributed throughout the hospital environment especially in watery environments such as ice machines, humidifiers, and solutions used to flush intravascular catheters. These organisms are able to survive in chlorinated tap water. *Chryseobacterium meningosepticum* is the species most commonly involved with human infections. In adults, infections with this organism are usually acquired in the hospital by significantly immunocompromised individuals often through infected intravascular lines. *C. meningosepticum* bacteremia may be complicated by native valve endocarditis (NVE) and PVE. *Chryseobacterium* are resistant to the aminoglycosides, third-generation cephalosporins, and most penicillins unless combined with beta-lactamase inhibitors. The most active compounds are clindamycin and rifampin. Ciprofloxacin, trimethoprim/sulfamethoxazole, and vancomycin may be effective against some strains. Possible virulence factors of *C. meningosepticum* include its capsule and its production of proteases and gelatinases that have potential to damage human cells (183–186).

Capnocytophaga spp.
Capnocytophaga canimorsus (formerly CDC classification DF2) is a dysgonic fermenter that normally inhabits the mouths of dogs, cats, and other animals. It is a fusiform bacillus with a tapered and a rounded end. It grows out well on blood agar (90). The mean age of patients with IE is 53 years with males predominating (78% of the patients). A history of dog bite was present in 33% of the cases and additional 33% had close contact with dogs. Major risk factors include splenectomy and alcoholism. Valvular infection, due to *C. canimorsus*, most frequently is subacute. At times, it may follow rapidly progressive course with complications of disseminated intravascular coagulation occurring most often, but not limited to, splenectomized individuals. An important clinical clue sign of possible acute *C. canimorsus* BSI/IE is the onset of symmetrical peripheral gangrene (187,188). The penicillins and cephalosporins are the most effective antibiotics. Clindamycin and the quinolones, but not the aminoglycosides, also have good activity. Susceptibility to trimethoprim/sulfamethoxazole is variable (189). Up to 25% of the patients may die despite appropriate treatment. The only virulence factor, so far identified, has been a powerful cytotoxin (190).

   C. cynodegmi is also another inhabitant of the canine mouth. It closely resembles *C. capnocytophaga* in all respects except that it produces a far milder disease (191). This may be because of its inability to produce cytotoxins (190).

Gram-Negative Cocci
Neisseria spp.
Neisseria gonorrhea formerly was responsible for 5% to 10% of all cases of IE. Currently <1% of IE is caused by this organism. There have been <100 cases reported in the English literature since 1942. This drastic reduction reflects the effectiveness of our microbial therapy even in the age of increasing gonorrhea resistance. Infective endocarditis complicates 1% to 2% of disseminated gonococcal infection (DGI). Young men without pre-existing heart disease are the most commonly affected. Many patients have deficiencies of the terminal components of the complement. Fifty percent of cases involve the aortic valve. Valvular infection usually begins within three weeks of the start of genital gonorrhea. However, not all suffer from proximate genital infection. Genitourinary discharge is present in 35% of the cases. Symptoms of pharyngitis are commonly observed. Congestive heart failure and septic arthritis are evident at the time presentation in 33% and 50% of patients, respectively. Dermal signs of DGI/IE are documented in only 20% of the individuals. The clinical course remains acute resembling that of pneumococcal IE with valvular destruction and ring abscess formation. Ninety-five percent of the cases have significant vegetations detected in the antibiotic era, and subacute cases have been reported. In the past,

TABLE 13 Virulence Factors of *Neisseria gonorrhea*

Item	Factor
Lipoligosaccharides	Limits complement binding and blocks phagocytosis
Rmp (protein III)	Blocks binding of antibodies to the cell wall
IgA proteases	Cleaves IgA
POR and Opa proteins	Facilitate cellular and bloodstream invasion
POR proteins	Interfere with phagolysome fusion
Opa proteins	Interfere with phagocytosis and killing
Yop-like substances	Toxic to the cytoskeleton of host cells
Lipoligosaccharides and peptidoglycan	Trigger the production of tumor necrosis factor (cause of local inflammatory response)

Abbreviations: IgA, immunoglobulin A; Yop, *Yersinia* outer proteins.
Source: From Ref. 196.

right-sided IE was relatively common. Double quotidian fever was recorded in 50% of the cases. Neither finding is currently common. There is a high rate of renal failure often due to glomerulonephritis. It is the cause of death in 40% of the patients. Other complications due to circulating immune complexes occur. Ceftriaxone remains the most useful antibiotic; however, resistance to it is growing. Valvular replacement is eventually required in 50% of the patients. The mortality rate, despite appropriate therapy, remains approximately 20% (192–195).

Table 13 lists the properties of *N. gonorrhea* that may serve as virulence factors for the organism's invasion of cardiac valves (196). *N. meningitidis* is an extremely rare cause of IE. Valvular infection is secondary to meningococcemia. Therefore its course is quite acute even eclipsing that of *S. aureus*. Death is usually because of overwhelming circulatory collapse. If the patient survives this cataclysmic phase, several types of intracardiac complications develop. These include myocardial abscesses, myocarditis, and pericarditis. The last two of these are probably because of immunological process. Meningococcal PVE has been reported (197). Its polysaccharide capsule blocks effective phagocytosis. Many of its complications are mediated by endotoxin.

The "nonpathogenic" *Neisseria* spp. colonize the upper human respiratory tract. This group includes: *N. lactamica, N. cinerea, N. polysaccharea, N. sicca, N. subflava, N. flavescens, N. mucosa,* and *N. elongata.* Of these, *N. mucosa, N. flavescens, N. sicca,* and *N. sublava* are the most frequently isolated from cases of IE. They primarily infect either abnormal native valves or prosthetic ones (198). Twenty percent of the patients have had a variety of dental procedures just prior to the onset of IE. Many of them had received standard antibiotic prophylaxis use of intravenous recreational drugs in the background of many cases. This may be because of the fact that many IVDA lick their needles for purposes of lubrication or for good luck prior to injecting themselves. A wide variety of the immuno-suppressive diseases, such as AIDS, diabetes mellitus, and asplenia, are predisposing factors for this type of valvular infection. The course is usually quite acute because of the rapid progression of valvular destruction and the extreme size of the vegetations. Significant embolization occurs in all patients. These nonpathogenic *Neisseria* spp. are usually quite sensitive to the penicillins and tetracyclines. *Neisseria mucosa* is an exception in the fact that it is resistant to penicillin but sensitive to chloramphenicol (91,198,199).

Moraxella catarrhalis

Moraxella catarrhalis (formerly *Branhamella catarrhalis*) is an unusual etiologic agent of IE. The majority of cases arise from pneumonia-associated bacteremia in patients with a variety of comorbid conditions. This pathogen used to be quite sensitive to penicillin. In recent years, it commonly produces a wide spectrum of beta-lactamases. Current treatment is the use of a third-generation cephalosporin or the penicillins combined with clavulanic acid or sulbactam (200,201). Infective endocarditis-related virulence factors for this organism are unknown.

Organisms of Blood Culture-Negative Endocarditis

Culture-negative IE (CNIE) denotes the situation in which the diagnosis of valvular infection is made on a clinical basis but the blood cultures remain negative for growth of any pathogen. Prior to the development of strict diagnostic criteria and modern microbiological methods, CNIE exceeded 30% of the cases. Currently, blood cultures are negative in 5% of the presumed cases. There are many causes of CNIE, both infectious and non-infectious (see discussion subsequently in this chapter). Many of the fastidious and slow-growing organisms that have been already presented (members of the HACEK group, *Brucella* spp. *Abiotrophia* spp.) often take greater than one week to grow on standard blood culture medium. Presently, we will focus our discussion on those microorganisms that require serological studies on blood or valvular tissue; or special staining of tissue or special blood cultures medium for diagnosis (Chapter 12) (202,203).

Coxiella burnetii

Coxiella burnetii is a gram-negative, pleomorphic rickettsia that is the agent of Q (Queensland)-fever. It is an obligate intracellular (monocytes and macrophages—especially alveolar macrophages) organism that lives within the acidic (pH 4.8) phagolysozymes of eukaryotic cells. This organism exhibits phase variation brought about by changes in its lipopolysaccharide component. Phase I organisms are more virulent than associated with acute disease; phase II ones are of much lower virulence. Q-fever is a zoonosis with worldwide distribution. Farm animals (goats, sheep, and cattle) are the chief reservoirs. Infected pets may give rise to disease acquired in urban areas. Infected animals shed organisms in their body fluids that resist environmental extremes. There have been approximately 400 cases of Q-fever IE documented. Proven cases remain quite rare in the United States. It is becoming more frequently recognized in other parts of the world. This may be because of the increased sensitivity and specificity of current diagnostic methods (204,205).

Q-fever may be either acute or chronic. Valvular infection is the most common manifestation of the chronic form. Most patients are male and older than 60. Ninety percent have some valvular abnormality (congenital, degenerative, and rheumatic). There is a high rate of various forms of cancer and other immunosuppressive diseases (pregnancy) in those patients without pre-existing valvular disease. Prosthetic valves are present in >50% of the patients.

Q-fever is usually a self-limited illness that results from inhaling the metabolically inactive small cell variant of this rickettsia. Most acute infections resolve within three weeks. A small percentage of cases go on to the chronic stage when the intracellular replication of *C. burnetii* leads to a persistent bacteremia (see subsequent discussion of pathogenesis). It has been estimated that 39% of chronic *C. burnetii* infections develop IE (203). There is a wide range of symptoms of *C. burnetii* IE (206).

Occasionally, they focus directly on the heart with the development of cardiac failure as a result of valvular insufficiency. Aneurysms of the aortic wall, located at the base of the leaflets common are well described. More often, noncardiac-related constitutional symptoms of intermittent low-grade fever, fatigue anorexia, and weight loss occur. It is said that the fever is well tolerated. Eventually 67% of the patients will develop CHF. Significant splenomegaly exists in 50%. This form of valvular infection is known for its high rate of clubbing and purpuric rash of the arms, legs, and mucosa (39% and 20%, respectively). The rash is because of immune complex vasculitis. Immune complex disease also causes the proliferative glomerulonephritis of this disease. Hepatomegaly with elevated liver function tests is common. The liver is reported to be quite hard. Emboli occur in 20% of the patient; most frequently involving the cerebral circulation. As in most cases of subacute IE, anemia, and thrombocytopenia, elevated sedimentation rate and positive rheumatoid factor are quite common. Additional distinctive laboratory findings include elevated liver function tests, hypergammaglobulinemia, immune complexes (89% of patients), and cryoglobulins (Table 14). Hematuria, hepatosplenomegaly, and laboratory findings of hepatitis are much less common in Q-fever PVE.

The nonspecific nature of its symptoms and the presence of hepatosplenomegaly, the aforementioned laboratory tests and the low rate of valvular thrombi detectable by echocardiography, have led to significant delays in diagnosis of *C. burnetii* IE. Duration of disease until diagnosis is made extends from one to as long as 20 years. The valvular vegetations are quite small, with a smooth surface and are nodular. Such configuration tests the limits of clinically available echocardiographic techniques. The major "clues" to the diagnosis of Q-fever endocarditis include valvular heart disease, such as valvular dysfunction, in association with an unexplained infectious or inflammatory syndrome (91) in the setting of CNIE. Serological tests have become the primary means of diagnosis. The most frequently utilized of these is the microimmunofluorescence test. In chronic disease, antibodies to phases I and II are quite high. IgG antibody levels to phase I antigen of >1/800 and an IgA titer of >1/100 indicates chronic infection/IE (207). The Duke criteria have been modified, for the diagnosis of Q-fever IE, so that a positive serological test has been upgraded to a major criteria (208). Polymerase chain reaction (PCR)

TABLE 14 Clinical Features of *Coxiella burnetii* Endocarditis

Item	Value
Mean age	Approximately 60 years
Underlying heart disease	90%
Predisposing conditions	
Animal exposure	59.6%
Consuming raw milk	9.6%
Immunosuppressive states	9%
Peripheral stigmata	At least 60%
Congestive heart failure	89%
Arterial embolization	20%
Infected valve	
Aortic	Approximately 50%
Mitral	Approximately 50%
Mortality rate[a]	24%

[a]With earlier diagnosis, this rate may be significantly less.
Source: From Ref. 91.

assays appear promising for the early diagnosis of IE. Isolation of *C. burnetii* from various tissues (valvular, liver, and emboli) or demonstration of the organism in the same tissues by various staining techniques or by electron microscopy is quite specific but less available then serological techniques (91).

Although tetracyclines have been the antibiotics of choice, it appears that they are able to suppress but not cure the infection in many patients. After four years of doxycycline, organisms were inhibited by culture from resected valves. The combination of hydroxychloroquine (200 mg, three times a day) with doxycycline (200 mg per day), administered for >18 months, appears to be the best of the medical regimens. Surveillance of phase I antibodies is useful in the following response. Treatment may be discontinued when phase-I IgG antibodies become <1/800 and IgA antibodies decrease to <1/50. Pairing of doxycycline with rifampin or a quinolone is more effective than doxycycline alone (209). Valvular replacement should be employed only when hemodynamic instability is documented. Mortality rate is approximately 24%. Recently, fatalities appear to be lessening probably because of more expeditiously arrived-at diagnoses as well as more effective treatment regimens (210).

Virulence factors of *C. burnetii* include an acid phosphatase that protects it from attack by phagolysosomal enzymes (211). Surface proteins are also potential virulence factors. Those that are encoded by plasmid QpRs are highly associated with valvular infection (212). However, infection with *C. burnetii* appears to be, in major part, dependent on the host's response. Abnormalities in cytokine production appear to have a positive effect on intracellular survival replication of *C. burnetii*. Tumor necrosis factor and interleukin-10 levels are significantly higher in patients with valvular infection than in those with acute Q-fever (213).

Bartonella spp.

Bartonella spp. are gram-negative rods that are the most recently recognized causes of valvular infections (3% of all cases of IE). As they often require more than a month to grow out of specially enriched blood cultures, these pathogens have become an increasingly important cause of CNIE (10% of the cases) (214,215). Although human *Bartonella* valvular infections may be produced by any one of five species (*B. quintana, B. hensellae, B. elizabethae, B. vinsonii,* and *B. koehlerae*), but the vast majority of cases are produced by either *B. quintana* or *B. henselae*. The reservoir for *B. henselae* are chronically bacteremic cats. Humans become infected by either cat fleas or by bites or scratches from these felines. The sources of *B. quintana* are homeless and/or alcoholic men (70% of the cases). Human body lice transmit the organism to like individuals that usually live in shelters. Eighty-seven percent of the cases of *B. henselae* IE involve previously abnormal valves. The corresponding figure for *B. quintana* is 30%.

Bartonella NVE follows a clinical course that is typically subacute with quite nonspecific signs and symptoms of low-grade fever malaise and weight loss (91). Infected individuals however are considerably younger (mean age 48 years) than others suffering from subacute disease. Also, there is a greater interval between the start of the infection and its diagnosis than is seen in *S. viridans* IE (more than three months vs. six weeks) (216,217). The homeless condition of many patients with *B. quintana* IE impedes their access to healthcare. Because of this delay, most cases exhibit significant cardiac failure at the time of their presentation. Bartonella PVE often is much more acute with rapid development of valvular perforation (218). Echocardiography demonstrates luxuriant vegetations with calcifications in 96% to

100% of cases (219). This is quite unlike the minimal valvular changes detected in cases of *C. burnetii*. At this point of the patient's evaluation, IE becomes the most likely diagnosis. The clinical challenge then shifts to establishing the pathogen involved.

Only 25% of the cases ever have positive blood cultures (214) and these often require more than eight weeks to grow in modified blood cultures. *Bartonella* IE is one of the major exceptions to the rule of continuous bacteremia as an essential part of valvular infection. Definitive diagnosis is made by one of more than the following methods: (*i*) positive serologies, (*ii*) detection of the organism in valvular tissue by Warthin-Starry staining, and (*iii*) a positive PCR probe of valvular tissue that is based on primers for the 16S rRNA gene of Bartonella. IFA and enzyme-linked immunosorbent assay (ELISA) are the most frequently used serologic tests. They have a 0.88 positive predictive value (214). Because cross-reactions may occur between *Bartonella* and *Chlamydia* spp., a positive assay must be studied by cross-adsorption techniques (incubating the patient's serum with the organism most likely to cause cross-reactions). A PCR test may be performed on valvular tissue that has been obtained at the time of surgery. This test may be 95% sensitive even when the patient has been receiving antibiotics (220). The Wharthin-Starry staining reveals large amounts of extracellular bacteria with large amounts of calcification and fibrosis (215).

It is quite important to establish a specific etiology of the valvular infection as the specifics of treatment very significantly among the different possible agents. The generic treatment of suspected *Bartonella* IE would consist of ceftriaxone (2 g IV for six weeks and gentamicin 1 mg/kg IV every eight hours for 14 days) ± doxycycline (100 mg IV/PO every 12 hours for six weeks). In proven cases of *Bartonella* valvular infection, doxycycline should be substituted for the ceftriaxone. If necessary, rifampin can be used instead of gentamicin. Most experts would administer doxycycline therapy for a total of three to six months taken orally for the last several months. If the patient undergoes valvular removal (80% of cases), then antibiotics are administered for six weeks postvalvulectomy (221,222). The mortality rate is approximately 20% (Table 15).

TABLE 15   Clinical Features of *Bartonella* Endocarditis

Item	Value
Mean age	48 years
Underlying heart disease	In *Bartonella henselae* cases 88%
	In *Bartonella quintana* cases 30%
Predisposing conditions	
Exposure to cats—*B. henselae*	
Alcoholism, homelessness,	
lice infestation—*B. quintana*	
Peripheral stigmata	Frequent
Congestive heart failure	>90%
Arterial embolization	41%
Infected valve	
Aortic	55%
Mitral	40%
Prosthetic	<5%
Mortality rate[a]	20%

[a]With earlier diagnosis, this rate may be significantly less.
Source: From Ref. 91.

Little is known regarding the virulence factors of *Bartonella* data relevant to endocarditis. The lipopolysaccharide component is known to affect certain chemokines (IL-8) as well as delaying the apoptotic course of human white cells (223).

Chlamydophilia psittaci

Chlamydophilia psittaci is customarily listed as a cause of CNIE. Usually there is a history of exposure to psittacine birds. Cats are another potential vector. Most cases follow a subacute course. Patients usually have underlying heart disease especially aortic valve disease. On occasion, the course is more acute with rapid destruction of the aortic valve (224,225). Mortality rate approaches 40% despite prolonged antibiotic therapy (usually doxycycline) and surgical replacement of the infected valve. This pathogen has also been connected with human cases of myocarditis and pericarditis (226). The evidence supporting its role in these cases is not well established (227). It is an obligate intracellular organism that can only be grown in tissue culture. Serological techniques are the mainstay of diagnosis. There is a well described cross-reactivity between *Chlamydia* and *Bartonella* using the standard rapid polyclonal antibody test. In one series, 80% of the cases, initially diagnosed being because of Chlamydia, were, on re-examination, found to be caused by *Bartonella*. Interestingly epidemiologically, these cases had many attributes of IE as result of *B. quintana* (homeless alcoholics). There is at least one well-documented case in which *C. psittiaci* was detected in valvular tissue by staining with an antibody specific for the organism (228). Cases of IE, attributable to *C. trachomatis* and *C. pneumoniae*, have been described (229,230). In summary, *C. psittaci* is a very rare cause of CNIE. There are no well-established chlamydial virulence factors that are relevant to the pathogenesis of IE.

Mycobacteria

Mycobacterium tuberculosis is a very unusual cause of IE. As of 2001, there have been only 16 cases reported (91). These included infections of congenitally abnormal aortic valves, prosthetic valves, and ventriculoatrial shunts (231). Infection usually arises as a complication of miliary disease but also may have spread from adjacent sites of tuberculous pericarditis or myocardial abscess. Six of 800 patients who had received homograft valves developed miliary tuberculosis secondary to contamination of the valve prior to its implantation (232).

Atypical mycobacteria are quite an infrequent cause of IE. Usually, they infect implanted valves both mechanical and bioprosthetic valves. *M. chelonei, M. fortuitum*, and *M. gordonae* are the primary species involved (233). There are only two documented cases of NVE involving these rapid growers. Organisms may infect the valves during manufacture secondary to inadequate sterilization. It is recommended that porcine grafts be cultured in thioglycolate broth for at least three weeks prior to surgery. Nosocomial outbreaks, as a result of contaminated bone wax or water baths that lead to sternal infections, have been reported. Both these types of mycobacterial PVE become clinically evident about five to six months after implantation. Indeed, there are cases of pseudo-mycobacterial PVE in which the valve has become contaminated after it was removed and stored in a nonmycobacteriacidal solution of 2% glutaraldehyde (234–236). Symptoms of mycobacterial PVE are typically that of any type of subacute valvular infection (237).

Diagnosis of mycobacterial IE is chiefly made by culturing the patient's blood either on Middlebrook, a solid medium, or in the Bactec 9000 system (238,239). Pathologic examination with Ziehl Nielsen stain of the affected valve is quite specific (236).

Prolonged (more than six months) antituberculous therapy is indicated in proven cases of mycobacterial IE. Because IE complicates such a small percentage of infections with *M. tuberculosis* or atypical mycobacteria, antimycobacterial therapy should only be started when a definitive diagnosis has been reached. There are no controlled studies indicating the role of surgical resection of the infected valve. Because of the slow-growing nature of the tubercle bacillus, extirpation of the focus of infection must strongly be considered (240). The virulence factors of *M. tuberculosis* and atypical mycobacteria that are involved in producing valvular infection are not well defined.

Legionella spp.

Legionella are small gram-negative intracellular bacteria that inhabit watery sites. It is transmitted most commonly to humans by aerosolization of contaminated potable hot water or air conditioning systems. Eighty-five percent of all types of human infections are a result of *Legionella pneumophilia*. Extrapulmonary sites of infection are unusual (241). Most individuals with extrapulmonary *Legionella* are surgical patients, usually without serious underlying diseases. Twenty-three percent are on immunosuppressive agents. The source of infection in these cases is most likely topical exposure of wounds to contaminated water. This mode of transmission has given rise to mini-epidemics within hospitals. *Legionella* PVE follows a chronic course (3 to 19 months after surgery) of fever, weight loss, anemia, and thrombocytopenia. Leukocytosis is usually not present. Embolization is rare. There are no reports of immune complex disease. Patients who suffered from post-cardiotomy syndrome had a significantly greater chance of developing *Legionella* PVE (242). Both *Legionella pneumophilia* and *Legionella dumoffi* have been involved.

Although it appears that the rate of *Legionella* infection of prosthetic valves seemingly has decreased in recent years, it should be suspected in patients with apparent culture-negative PVE. The organism may be diagnosed by culturing the excised valve (90% of cases) or the patient's blood (40% of cases) (242,243). *Legionella* spp. can be grown in automated blood culture systems. Because the concentration may be below that necessary to be detected by the system, subcultures should be obtained periodically and plated on buffered charcoal yeast extract (BCYE). Similar to cases of Q-fever IE, echocardiography usually fails to demonstrate any valvular vegetations because of their small size. Only 33% of the patients are diagnosed as having valvular involvement by this imaging technique. Serological testing and PCR assays appear to offer little in addition to blood tissue cultures (244). Urinary antigen testing for *L. pneumophilia*, type 1 (the most common strain), may be a reasonable first step in evaluating a patient for this rare cause of PVE.

Most patients survive their infections. Sixty-seven percent require replacement of the prosthetic valves for cure. Erythromycin and rifampin, ciprofloxacin, or doxycycline have all been administered for at least five months with apparent equal success (242).

Legionella has become the paradigm for intracellular pathogens surpassing *Salmonella* and *Mycobacteria* in this role. It has an impressive repertoire of virulence factors. The natural habitats of this organism are bodies of freshwater and other moist environments. They are resistant to the chlorination process for water supplies. They are found in the biofilms of various types of hot water and airconditioning systems (245). They are able to penetrate and multiply within free-living protozoans. This intracellular environment helps the pathogen meet its complex nutritional requirements. *Legionella* binds to macrophages by means of complement receptors

TABLE 16 Virulence Factors of *Legionella*

Item	Factor
Biofilm production	Promotes infection of prosthetic valves
Fimbria/pili	Facilitates entry into macrophages
Macrophage infectivity promoter	Facilitates entry into macrophages
icm genes	Promotes intracellular multiplication
Unknown	Prevents intracellular killing of *Legionella* by preventing fusion of phagolysozymes
Cytotoxins	Promotes lysis of host cells

Source: From Ref. 247.

and pili. Cellular entry is facilitated by macrophage infectivity promoter. *Legionella* is then taken up by phagosomes. The pathogen is protected from being killed because of interference, by unidentified factors, with normal phagoysozyme fusion. When the organism senses deficiencies of certain proteins (thiamine and thymidine), it activates expression of its virulence genes (flagella and cytotoxic compounds). Zinc metalloproteases act as cytolysins to give a host cell and promote spread of infection (246,247). Its ability to flourish in biofilms most likely explains its proclivity for infecting prosthetic valves (Table 16). *Legionella*'s virulence factors provide great potential for it to become a more common cause of HCIE.

Mycoplasma spp. and Cell Wall-Deficient Organisms
There are few reports of IE as a result of *Mycoplasma*. These cases are usually more suggestive then definitive in establishing the role of *Mycoplasma* in producing valvular infection (248). *Mycoplasma hominis, M. pneumoniae,* and *Ureaplasma parvum* have been implicated (249). *Mycoplasma* cannot grow in regular blood cultures nor they cannot be stained by Gram stain. Specific *Mycoplasma* media must be employed for their culture. Serologic testing is the most commonly used diagnostic technique. Polymerase chain reaction tests may eventually prove to be more sensitive and specific. There is evidence that *Mycoplasma* damage eukaryotic cells. This is probably produced by membrane glycoproteins that can trigger release of various cytokines. Additionally cytokines may interfere with phagocytic functioning by nonspecifically stimulating B-cells and hence subvert the host's immune response (250).

Organisms, such as spheroplasts, *L. forms*, protoplasts, may be the result of conversion from their normal structure to a cell-wall deficient one owing to exposure to penicillins (251). These are called *persisters* as they may remain dormant in the infected tissue indefinitely. Case reports of IE as a result of these organisms exist. In these, electron microscopy detected not only morphologically normal bacteria but also cell wall-deficient forms in the valvular vegetations (252). It is still not clear whether these forms produce prolonged fever in patients with negative blood cultures. Four criteria have been proposed for establishing their role-specific infections: (*i*) usual appearance on stained preparations of tissue; (*ii*) failure to grow on routine media; (*iii*) evidence of reversion to usual morphology; and (*iv*) consistency of the isolate with the patient's disease.

Tropheryma whippelii
Tropheryma whippeli is a gram-positive bacterium that is related to Actinomycetes. It can only be grown in tissue culture. This organism is the causative agent of

Whipple's disease, which is a systemic bacterial infection that is characterized by arthritis, abdominal pain malabsorption syndrome with diarrhea, and central nervous system manifestations. Cardiac involvement (myocarditis, endocarditis, and pericarditis) occurs in approximately 33% of the patients. Endocardial involvement can occur without any of the arthritic or gastrointestinal symptoms of the disease. In comparison with positive blood culture and Q-fever and *Bartonella* IE, individuals with Whipple's IE often exhibit minimal systemic symptoms. It has a lower incidence of fever, history of previous valvular disease, and CHF than the other three types of IE (253).

Because of lack of systemic reaction of the host, the Dukes criteria may not be pertinent for diagnosing Whipple's IE. Diagnosis is based on the histologic findings of PAS positive macrophages in surgically resected valves and/or by PCR testing of the valve. This is the same appearance that a duodenal biopsy would have from a patient with gastrointestinal symptoms of Whipple's disease (254). Recommended treatment for *T. whippelii* IE is ceftriaxone 2 g IV daily ± gentamicin for four weeks with follow-up of trimethoprim/sulfamethoxazole (one double strength tablet twice a day) for one year (255).

The cause of Whipple's disease is unknown. Wherever the bacterium is taken up in the host's body, there is little inflammatory response. By unknown mechanisms, the pathogen downregulates the immune system of the host (256,257).

Other Bacteria
Nocardia spp.
Nocardia are partially acid-fast, gram-positive aerobic Actinomycetes. They have a typical branching appearance on the Gram stain. The most cases of *Nocardia* IE involve prosthetic valves (258,259). *Nocardia bacteremia* and probably valvular infection has been associated with CVC. Most media will support the growth of *Nocardia* spp. Trimethoprim/sulfamethoxazole is the standard treatment. Usually extirpation of the infected valve is required for cure.

They are facultatively intracellular organisms that are able to grow up within various types of human cells. Virulence factors that may be pertinent to the pathogenesis of valvular infection include their ability to avoid intracellular killing by inhibiting phagolysozyme fusion. Production of catalase also helps prevent their intracellular death (260).

Anaerobic Bacteria
Actinomyces spp.
Actinomyces spp. are gram-positive, higher bacteria that seldom cause valvular infection. The most commonly involved is *Actinomyces israeli*. Less than 2% of the cases of actinomycosis affect the heart (261). The incidence of cardiac involvement in thoracic actinomycosis is 75%. Pericarditis is the most common cardiac manifestation (79%) and is the most common source of endocardial infection. The aortic valve is involved in 35%. Less often actinomycotic IE arises from primary bloodstream infection. There is no well-defined virulence factor for *Actinomyces* spp. (262).

Other Anaerobes
Probably the most common cause of anaerobic IE are the anaerobic cocci. They often are found in combination with other anaerobes. The remaining anaerobic pathogens

have accounted for less than 2% of the total cases of IE. There is evidence that the incidence of anaerobic IE has increased to 7% to 10% of all cases of valvular infection (263). Of the nonanaerobic cocci, *B. fragilis* is the most commonly isolated (35.8%) followed by *Fusobacterium* spp. (22.4%), *Clostridial* spp. (13.4%), *Propionibacterium acnes* (7.5%) with *Bacteroides oralis* and *Provatella* (Bacteroides) *melaniogenicus* each responsible for 3% of the cases. It is commonly held that up to one-third of unidentified pathogens are *B. fragilis*. However, proof of this concept remains lacking. Twenty-five percent of cases are polymicrobial usually with other anaerobes (264–267). The cases of IE, because of multiple anaerobes, are most frequently seen among IVDA. This may well be because of the patient's habit of licking the needle just prior to injection either to judge the strength of illicit drug to be administered or for "good luck." A typical case report of this situation describes right-sided endocarditis caused by usually at least three anaerobes. Generally, the source of the pathogen depends on the particular anaerobe involved and so can give a clue to the disease process triggering the infection. The gastrointestinal tract is the usual wound source of *B. fragilis* IE. Other *Bacteroides* spp. Fusobacteria arise from the head and neck. Peptostreptococcus IE usually are associated with genitourinary tract infection/colonization. The clinical picture of anaerobic IE resembles closely that of anaerobic disease except for the fact that underlying heart disease is less common and the incidence of thromboembolic disease is higher (up to 67% of the patients). Other recognized complications include growing cartilage destruction from aortic ring abscesses and multiple mycotic aneurysms. This is a usually anaerobic IE that follows a subacute course except for those cases caused by *F. necrophorum* in which massive valvular destruction with resulting refractory CHF and major embolic phenomenon may occur within a matter of days of onset of the infection. *P. acnes* is strongly associated with anaerobic PVE (268). The fatality rate ranges from 21% to 46%. Recently, the vast majority of fatal cases have been caused by *B. fragilis*. With early detection and more effective antibiotics, the death appears to be decreasing (Table 17).

It is important to remember that there is a significant and growing resistance of anaerobes to currently employed antibiotics. This is especially true for *B. fragilis*. For anaerobes as a whole, resistance was found in 12.4%, 9.8%, and 17% for imipenem, amoxicillin/clavulanic acid, metronidazole, and clindamycin, respectively (269). With increasing exposures to broad-spectrum antibiotics, beta-lactamases are being

TABLE 17   Clinical Features of *Bacteroides* Endocarditis

Item	Value
Mean age	50.3 years
Underlying heart disease	78%
Predisposing conditions	>50%
Appendicitis, gastroenteritis	46%
Peripheral stigmata	91%
Congestive heart failure	36%
Arterial embolization	64%
Infected valve	
Aortic	64%
Mitral	36%
Mortality rate[a]	<46%

[a]Is continuing to decrease.
Source: From Ref. 17.

produced by many of the anaerobes that were formerly quite sensitive to this class of antibiotics. In vitro, linezolid appears to be quite promising. In one series reported in 2003, there were no anaerobic strains resistant to this antibiotic (270).

The infrequency of anaerobic IE may be because of the oxygen-rich nature of the vascular space and difficulties in adhering to the endocardium (91). However, the anaerobes, which are most commonly involved in valvular infections, possess several significant virulence factors. Among these are adherence factors, immunoglobulin proteases, thrombotic factors (heparinases), bacterial capsules and pili (271,272).

Fungal Endocarditis

In 1950, Zimmerman quite accurately predicted a marked increase in the incidence of all types of fungal infections (273). He attributed this rise to the increasing employment of antibiotics and cytotoxic drugs. Before 1945, there had only been three case reports of candidal IE. Two of these occurred in IVDA. The number of cases of fungal IE had followed this overall trend. In the 1970s, the risk factors for disseminated fungal infections/fungal IE included: (*i*) administration of broad-spectrum antibiotics and corticosteroids; (*ii*) cardiac surgery; (*iii*) IVDA; (*iv*) gynecological and urological procedures; (*v*) oral surgery; and (*vi*) burns (274). In that era, 46% of the patients with fungal IE were IVDA and 27% had undergone cardiac surgery (275). *Candida, Aspergillus*, and *Histoplasma* were primarily responsible for fungal valvular infections. Other fungi have been identified as sporadic causes of fungal IE. Among these are *Blastomyces, Coccidioides, Cryptococcus*, and *Mucormycosis* (7).

Intensive care medicine has generated fundamental changes in the incidence, risk factors, and organisms involved in fungal IE. Twenty-five percent of cases of fungal IE are acquired within healthcare facilities. Cases of the sepsis syndrome, produced by fungal infections, increased to almost 300% between 1980 and 2000 (276). Currently (1995–2000), only 4.1% of the cases occurred in IVDA. In 47.3% there were underlying cardiac abnormalities. Prosthetic valves and CVC were present, respectively in 44.6% and 30.4% of the patients (277). About 20.3% had received prolonged broad-spectrum antibiotics. Surprisingly, parenteral nutrition was involved in less than 1% of the cases. Underlying immunosuppressive states (solid organ transplants, diabetes mellitus, AIDS, corticosteroid use, and bone marrow transplants) were documented in approximately 7%. Many patients had >1 risk factor. In one series, the average number of risk factors of those with fungal IE was 2.5 (278). *Candida* spp. constitute 62% of the cases; 50% of these are *C. albicans*. Nineteen percent are due to *Aspergillus* and 6% are due to histoplasmosis. Recently, emerging fungi (e.g., *Trichosporin* spp., *Fusarium, Saccharomyces, Pseudoallescheria boydii*) are implicated in 25% (Table 18). Many of these occurred in the severely immuno-suppressed or in those with prosthetic valves in place.

In their review, Ellis et al. identified 34 symptoms that were evident at the time of the patient's presentation (Table 19) (278). The mean number of symptoms per patient was 6. Eighty-two percent of patients had symptoms for several weeks before admission to the hospital (mean 32 days ± standard deviation of 39 days). Overall mortality rate approaches 60%. This is because of a number of factors including delay in diagnosis; macrovegetations that interfere with access of the antifungals to their targets; and the presence of biofilms (see later) and antifungal compounds that possess significant toxicities. Fifteen to twenty-five percent of blood cultures may be negative in cases of *C. albicans* IE and higher in valvular infections produced by other *Candida* spp. Fifty percent of *Aspergillus* spp. IE may have negative blood cultures.

TABLE 18 Clinical Manifestations of Fungal Endocarditis

Item	Value
Mean age	44 years
Underlying heart disease	47.3%
Predisposing conditions (see text)	100%
Congestive heart failure	16%
Embolization	61%
Valves infected[a]	
Aortic valve alone and with other valves	44%
Mitral valve alone and with other valves	26%
Tricuspid valve alone and with other valves	7%
Mortality rate[a]	56.6%

[a]54% of patients had previous valve surgery.
Source: From Refs. 277, 278.

Survival rates have increased since the 1980s primarily because of the diagnostic contribution of echocardiography as well as due to an increase in suspicion of the possibility of fungal IE. Currently, 72% are diagnosed prior to surgery as compared with only 43% in the past. Newer agents such as capsofungin and voriconazole may contribute to a continuing lowering of the mortality rate. Valve replacement surgery is recommended for both native and prosthetic valve fungal IE except for cases of *Histoplasma* IE (279). This type of valvular infection appears to be able to be cured by amphotericin alone. Thirty percent of patients relapse (Chapter 14).

Candida spp.

The particular species of *Candida* isolated from an infected valve is closely associated with the patient's background. In fungal IVDA IE, *C. albicans* is infrequently isolated whereas *C. parapsilosis* (>50% of cases) and *C. tropicalis* predominate. An exception is found in those patients who use brown heroin. In these cases, *C. albicans* predominates because lemon juice use is employed in cutting the heroin and promotes the growth of this candidal species (280). *C. albicans* is the overwhelming species in candidal PVE (281). *C. guilliermondi*, *C. krusei*, and *C. stellatodiae* can also produce candidemia/IE. Valvular infections are a complication of candidemia that may arise from the gastrointestinal tract, a variety of other sites, and probably most commonly infected intravascular lines. It is important to remember that there is a high risk of prosthetic valvular infections following nosocomial candidemia (282). The risk of infection is approximately 25%. The presentation of candidal IE is very similar to that of bacterial IE with the major exception of the high rate of macroembolization.

TABLE 19 Presenting Features of Fungal Endocarditis

Item	Value
Fever	75%
Changing/new heart murmurs	51%
Major embolization	36%
Focal or generalized neurological abnormalities	31%
Heart failure	24%
Dyspnea	23%

Source: From Ref. 278.

Fifty percent of these involve the intracranial vessels. Myocardial abscesses that involve the conducting system have been documented (283). Infection of a left atrial myxoma has been reported (284). *Candida* IE may be present for up to 10 weeks prior to its diagnosis. The mainstay for the diagnosis of candidal IE remains the blood culture. Sometimes the detection of candidal forms in retrieved peripheral emboli is the sole positive finding when pathogen fails to grow out of multiple blood cultures. A variety of serological tests for various components of the organism have not proven clinically useful (Chapter 12).

Candidal virulence factors include the ability to attach themselves to epithelial cells of many sites (gastrointestinal, dermis) and produce lipases and proteinases that facilitate invasion of the bloodstream (285). *Candida* isolates (especially *C. albicans*) possess the ability to produce biofilms on implanted materials; especially on intravascular lines, prosthetic valve, and pacemakers; have contributed markedly to the rise in candidemia/IE. The candidal biofilms adhere to intravascular lines in a bilayer structure with a basal yeast layer and an overlying hyphal layer (286–288). In various types of models of biofilms, *C. albicans* isolates are highly resistant to fluconazole and amphotericin B. It is not clear whether this resistance is a result of decreased penetration by antifungals into the biofilm or because of acquired resistance of the organisms when they reside in the plankton form or because of a combination of these factors. This bestowed resistance makes it mandatory that the host prosthetic material be removed in the face of candidemia/IE.

Candida species also possess intrinsic resistance to a variety of antifungal agents (Table 20) (279). The development of newer agents such as voriconazole and capsofungin are proving to be superior to amphotericin preparations because of increased efficacy and decreased amount of side-effects (289,290).

Aspergillus spp.

Aspergillus spp. are the second most common cause of fungal IE (278). The most frequently isolated *Aspergillus* species are *A. fumigatus* (56%), *A. flavus* (16%), and *A. niger* (12%) (291). The majority of cases are associated with cardiac surgery. The heart is infected in the operating room owing to the contaminated air. The presence of foreign body (prosthetic valve) may well interfere with the ability of the patient to eradicate the organisms before the state of contamination becomes one of active infection. *Aspergillus* IE also occurrs in immunosuppressed patients, especially those with AIDS, as well as those with uremia and gram-negative bacterial sepsis (292,293). In these patients, the route of entry is most likely intravascular catheters.

TABLE 20 Sensitivity of *Candida* Species to Various Antifungals

Candida species	Amphotericin B	Fluconazole	Itraconazole	Voriconazole	Capsofungin
C. albicans	S	S	S	S	S
C. parapsilosis	S	S	S	S	S/R
C. tropicalis	S	S	S	S/I	S
C. krusei	S/I	R	R[a]	S	S
C. glabrata	S/I	R[a]	R[a]	S	S
C. lusitaniae	S/R	S	S	S	S

[a]For some isolates, resistance may be overcome by increased serum level of the antifungal achieved by optimizing dosage and bioavailability of the drug.
Abbreviations: I, intermediately sensitive to antifungal; R, resistant to antifungal; S, sensitive to antifungal.
Source: From Ref. 279.

Aspergillus may also cause IVDA IE. Several cases of *A. mural* IE have been recognized (294). *Aspergillus* spp. are quite invasive and may cause pericarditis. Resultant myocardial abscesses may produce a variety of cardiac arrhythmias. Macroemboli are fairly common. It is unusual to isolate the organism from blood cultures. Pathological study of a peripheral embolus will often reveal characteristic hyphae. Detection of the galactomannan antigen which is released during hyphal growth is promising for diagnosing invasive aspergillosis (295) *Aspergillus* IE is usually subacute and almost invariably fatal even with combination of antifungal agents and surgery. Voriconazole appears to be the most effective agent against *Aspergillus* (296).

Aspergillus produces several possible virulence factors including gliotoxin, phospholipases, hemolysins, and elastase. The most important of these appears to be gliotoxin. This compound interferes with macrophage ingestion of *Aspergillus* as well as with the activation of phagocytic NADPH oxidase. The organism is distinctive in its ability to invade the wall of the blood vessels and produce massive infarction (297).

Histoplasma capsulatum

Histoplasma capsulatum is a dimorphic fungus, which is found in the soil of the Ohio-Mississippi Valley. In the last two decades, its incidence has markedly decreased perhaps owing to the availability of amphotericin B (278). It may infect both native and prosthetic valves. The distinctive features of *H. capsulatum* IE include significant splenomegaly (50% of cases), leukopenia (10% of cases), and macroemboli (58%). The aortic valve is involved in 66% of the infections (298–300). The disease is usually subacute. Less than 20% of the blood cultures are positive for the organism. The diagnosis is usually made by serological titers (complement fixation antibody, or immunodiffusion test for precipitins) or measurement of urinary antigen. Sometimes culture/histopathological studies of bone marrow, valvular tissue, or embolic material are required to make the diagnosis. Prolonged treatment with amphotericin B is usually quite successful. The role of other antifungals is not well established. Secondary prophylaxis as in the case of *Candida* is seldom required. *H. capsulatum* IE is distinctive in the fact that it is the one fungal valvular infection for which valve surgery is usually not necessary (301). The indications for valvular replacement are almost identical to those for bacterial IE.

The major virulence factor of *H. capsulatum* is its ability to survive within the macrophage by a calcium-dependent process in nonimmune animals (302).

Pseudallescheria boydi and *Trichsporon beigellii* have become increasingly more important as causes of IE in severely immunosuppressed patients and those with prosthetic valves in place (303,304).

Polymicrobial Endocarditis

Polymicrobial IE (PMIE) has been recognized since the 1960s (305). Over the years, it has caused between 5% and 6% of cases of IE. In the initial reports, streptococci were involved in almost every case of PMIE (306). Saravolatz was the first to document the importance of IVDA IE as an underlying cause (307). In his series, eight of nine patients who had PMIE were addicted to heroin. Some of them had undergone previous cardiac surgery. All were young adult males. The mean duration of symptoms prior to diagnosis was 16 days. Two patients had evidence of septic pulmonary emboli. Mitral and tricuspid valve insufficiency were common. Until the 1990s, *P. aeruginosa* have been the pathogen most often involved in PMIE.

Staphylococcus aureus had always played a prominent role (50% of the cases). Other causative organisms included *S. faecalis, S. aureus, H. influenzae, S. epidermidis,* and *Candida* spp. The most common combination had been *S. faecalis* and *P. aeruginosa.* During the 1980s, *P. aeruginosa* became somewhat less prominent and *S. aureus* more prominent (90% of the cases) (308). The vast majority of cases are both IVDA- and HIV-positive, 50% of whom have AIDS. As would be expected, most have infection of the tricuspid valve. Over half of these developed septic pulmonary emboli. The next major group of patients at risk of PMIE are those who undergo cardiac surgery. The most common combination is *S. aureus* and *S. pneumoniae* followed by *S. aureus* and *P. aeruginosa.* The signs and symptoms of PMIE cannot be distinguished from cases of IE caused by a single organism. Fifty-two percent of patients have required cardiac surgery despite appropriate medical treatment. Individuals with PMIE have a higher mortality rate (32%) than those infected by a single agent. It appears that the outlook for cases of PMIE is dependent primarily on the particular pathogen and not simply on the number of organisms involved. Left-sided disease and older age groups are associated with poorer outcomes.

Culture-Negative Endocarditis

Culture-negative infective endocarditis has been defined as "definite infective endocarditis in which aerobic and anaerobic blood cultures of three sufficiently sized samples drawn over 24 to 48 hours remain negative" (309). It is important to emphasize that cases of CNIE represent active valvular infection and are not mimics of valvular infection. Currently, the incidence of CNIE is approximately 5% (310–313). This has markedly decreased to rates as low as 30% due both to the availability of improved microbiological methods and stricter case definitions of IE as provided by the modified Dukes criteria. Table 21 presents the major causes of apparently CNIE. The most common cause of this syndrome is prior treatment with antibiotics (40% to 70% of cases of CNIE). The antibiotic is usually given when the patient's signs and symptoms are ascribed to a more mundane process than IE. In my experience, this usually occurs in subacute IE. In streptococcal IE, administration of penicillin

TABLE 21   Causes of Culture-Negative Infective Endocarditis

Causes
Prior antimicrobial treatment
Difficult to culture (fastidious) organisms
Fungal infections
Rickettsial infections
Mycobacteria
Chlamydia
Mycoplasma
L forms
Viruses
Right-sided endocarditis
Uremia
Mural endocardial infection in the presence of a ventricular septal defect
Prosthetic valve endocarditis
Infected pacemaker wires
Blood cultures obtained three months after the onset of disease

for more than a few days could suppress bacterial growth in blood cultures for up to two weeks (314). In a large recent series of 348 cases of CNIE (313), 48% were associated with *C. burnetii*; 28% with *Bartonella* spp. and 1% with a group of unusual organisms, *T. whipplei*, *Abiotrophia* spp., *Legionella pneumophila*, and *Mycoplasma hominis*. The remaining 73 cases, 58 had received antibiotics prior to obtaining blood cultures (28% of the total). It is important to emphasize that this study is from a French referral hospital. Most likely the rate of patients treated with antimicrobial agents prior to drawing blood cultures would be significantly higher in an American community hospital owing to geographic prevalence of this series of most frequent causes of CNIE. Prolonged subacute IE (more than three months untreated) can lead to the persistently negative blood cultures of the bacterial-free stage (315). This is because of the suppression of bacterial growth by excess of antibody. There were no differences found in the clinical presentations between those pretreated with antibiotics and the other causes of CNIE. The diagnosis of endocarditis was based usually on the modified Dukes criteria. Paradoxically, CNIE appears to have at least as many complications. Many of these patients experience significant embolic events and CHF (316). This may be especially true in cases of prosthetic valve CNIE (317). Pesanti detailed two cases of PVE in which blood cultures were consistently negative. Because it was felt that fever may be because of a postcardiotomy syndrome corticosteroids were administered. The patients overall improved but the blood cultures became positive for *S. epidermidis* after the anti-inflammatory agent was begun. It appears that outcomes of patients with CNIE because of previous antibiotic treatment are better than those with CNIE due to other causes (318,319). This may be a result of the earlier use of transesophageal echocardiography (TEE) in those recognized to have recently received a course of antibiotics. However, it is almost impossible for TEE to differentiate between CNIE, valvular sclerosis, and a sterile platelet/fibrin thrombus.

Despite the availability of PCR analysis and other sophisticated techniques (Chapter 12), the ongoing diagnostic challenge of CNIE is the fact that the only gold standard is examination of the excised valve. The specificity of PCR approaches 100% with a sensitivity of less than 40%.

REFERENCES

1. Cherubin C, Neu H. Infective endocarditis at the Presbyterian Hospital in New York City from 1938–1967. Am J Med 1977; 51:83.
2. Kim EL, Ching DL, Pien FD. Bacterial endocarditis at a small community hospital. Am J Med Sci 1990; 299:87.
3. Finland M, Barnes M. Changing etiology of bacterial endocarditis in the antibacterial era: experience at Boston City Hospital 1933–1965. Ann Intern Med 1972; 72:341.
4. Richards MJ, Edwards JR, Culver DH, et al. and the NISS System. Nosocomial infections in medical ICUs in the United States. Crit Care Med 1999; 27:887.
5. Gales AC, Jones RN, Turnidge J, et al. Characterization of *Pseudomonas aeruginosa* isolates: occurrence rates, antimicrobial susceptibility patterns and molecular typing in the global SENTRY Antimicrobial Surveillance Program, 1997–1999. Clin Infect Dis 2001; 32(suppl 2):S146.
6. Gould K, Ramirez-Ronda CH, Holmes RK, et al. Adherence of bacteria to heart valves in vitro. J Clin Invest 1975; 56:1364.
7. Weinstein L, Brusch JL. Gram-negative and other organisms. In: Infective Endocarditis. New York: Oxford University Press, 1996:73.
8. Reisberg B. Infective endocarditis in the narcotic addict. Prog Cardiovasc Dis 1977; 56:287.

9.   Pelletier L, Petersdorf R. Infective endocarditis: a review of 125 cases from the University of Washington Hospitals, 1953–1972. Medicine 1977; 56:287.
10. Elting LS, Bodey GP. Septicemia due to Xanthomonas species and non-aeruginosa Pseudomonas species: increasing incidence of catheter-related infections. Medicine 1990; 69:296.
11. Thadepalli H, Francis CK. Diagnostic clues and metastatic lesions of endocarditis in addicts. West J Med 1978; 128:1.
12. Snyder N, Allerbury C, Correira J, et al. Increased occurrence of cirrhosis and bacterial endocarditis. Gastroenterology 1977; 73:1107.
13. Hsu RB, Chen RJ, Chu SH. Infective endocarditis in patients with liver cirrhosis. J Formos Med Assoc 2004; 103:355.
14. Castagnola E, Garaventa A, Viscoli C, et al. Changing pattern of pathogens causing Broviac catheter-related bacteremias in children with cancer. J Hosp Infect 1995; 29:129.
15. Castagnola E, Conte M, Venzano P, et al. Iliac catheter-related bacteremias due to unusual pathogens in children with cancer: case reports with literature review. J Infect 1997; 34:215.
16. Archer G, Fekety F, Supena R. *Pseudomonas aeruginosa* endocarditis in drug addicts. Am Heart J 1974; 88:570.
17. Cohen P, Maguire J, Weinstein L. Infective endocarditis caused by Gram-negative bacteria: a review of the literature, 1945–1977. Prog Cardiovasc Dis 1980; 22:205.
18. Carruthers M. Endocarditis due to enteric bacilli other than Salmonella: case reports and literature review. Am J Med Sci 1977; 273:203.
19. Cooper R, Mills J. Serratia endocarditis: a follow-up reports. Arch Intern Med 1980; 140:199.
20. Forbes BA, Sahm DF, Weisfeld AS, Trevino EA. *Pseudomonas, Burkholderia* and similar organisms. In: Forbes BA, Sahm DF, Weissfeld AS, eds. Bailey and Scott's Diagnostic Microbiology. 11th ed. St. Louis: Mosby, 2002:85.
21. Wieland M, Lederman MM, Kline-King C, et al. Left-sided endocarditis due to *Pseudomonas aeruginosa*. A report of 10 cases and review of the literature. Medicine (Baltimore) 1986; 65:18.
22. Banks T, Fletcher R, Ali N. Infective endocarditis in heroin addicts. Ann Intern Med 1973; 55:444.
23. El Khatib, Wilson MR, Lerner AM. Characteristics of bacterial endocarditis in heroin addicts in Detroit. Am J Med Sci 1976; 271:197.
24. Benn M, Hagelskjaer LH, Tvede M. Infective endocarditis, 1984 through 1993: a clinical and microbiological survey. J Intern Med 1997; 242:15.
25. Botzenhart K, Doring G. Ecology and epidemiology of *Pseudomonas aeruginosa*. In: Campa M, Bendinelli M, Friedman H, eds. *Pseudomonas Aeruginosa* as an Opportunistic Pathogen. New York: P lenum Press, 1993:1.
26. Sewell DL. Pseudomonas infections. In: Wentworth BB, ed. Diagnostic Procedures for Bacterial Infections in Washington DC: American Public Health Association, 1987:455.
27. Morrison AJ, Wenzel RP. Epidemiology of infections due to *Pseudomonas aeruginosa*. Rev Infect Dis 1984; 6(suppl):S627.
28. Jarvis WR, Martone WJ. Predominant pathogens in hospital infections. J Antimicrob Chemother 1992; 29(suppl A):19.
29. Wisplinghoff H, Bischoff T, Tallent SM, et al. Nosocomial bloodstream infections in U.S. hospitals: analysis of 24,179 cases from a prospective nationwide surveillance study. Clin Infect Dis 2004; 39:309.
30. Chatzinkolaou I, Abi-Said D, Bodey GP, et al. Patient experienced to *Pseudomonas aeruginosa* bacteremia in patients with cancer: retrospective analysis of 245 episodes. Arch Intern Med 2002; 160:501.
31. Komshian SV, Tablan OC, Palutke W, Reyes MP. Characteristics of left-sided endocarditis due to *Pseudomonas aeruginosa* in the Detroit Medical Center. Rev Infect Dis 1990; 12:693.
32. Gouello JP, Asfar P, Brenet O, et al. Nosocomial endocarditis in the intensive care unit: an analysis of 22 cases. Crit Care Med 2002; 28:377.
33. Reyes MP, Lerner AM. Current problems in the treatment of infective endocarditis due to *Pseudomonas aeruginosa*. Rev Infect Dis 1983; 5:314.
34. Middlemost S, Wisenbaugh T, Meyerowitz C. A case for early surgery and native left-sided endocarditis complicated by heart failure: results in 203 patients. J Am Coll Cardiol 1991; 18:663.

35. Bayer AS, O'Brien T, Norman DC, et al. Oxygen dependent differences in E polysaccharide production and aminoglycoside inhibitory bactericidal interactions with *Pseudomonas aeruginosa*: implications for endocarditis. J Antimicrob Chemother 1989; 23:21.
36. Letendre ED, Mantha R, Turgeon PL. Selection of resistance by piperacillin during *Pseudomonas aeruginosa* endocarditis. J Antimicrob Chemother 1988; 22:557.
37. Teplitz C. Pathogenesis of *Pseudomonas vasculitis* and septic lesions. Arch Pathol 1965; 80:297.
38. Baltch Al Griffin PE. *Pseudomonas aeruginosa* bacteremia. A clinical study of 75 patients. Am J Med Sci 1977; 274:119.
39. Fick RB Jr. *Pseudomonas aeruginosa*. The microbial hyena and its role in disease. In: Fick RB Jr, ed. *Pseudomonas aeruginosa*, the Opportunist, Pathogenesis and Disease. Boca-Raton, Florida: CRC Press, 1993:1.
40. Salyers AA, Whitt DD. *Pseudomonas aeruginosa*. In: Salyers AA, Whitt DD, eds. Bacterial Pathogenesis: A Molecular Approach. Washington DC: American Society for Microbiology, 1994:260.
41. Irvin RT. Attachment and colonization of *Pseudomonas aeruginosa*: role of the surface structures. In: Campa M, Bendinelli M, Friedman H, eds. *Pseudomonas aeruginosa* as an Opportunistic Pathogen. New York: Plenum Press, 1993:19.
42. Bayer AS, Park S, Ramos MC, et al. Effects of alginase on the natural history and antibiotic therapy of experimental endocarditis caused by mucoid *Pseudomonas aeruginosa*. Infect Immun 1992; 60:3979.
43. Galloway PR. Role of exotoxin in the pathogenesis of *Pseudomonas aeruginosa* infections. In: Campa M, Bendinelli M, Friedman H, eds. *Pseudomonas aeruginosa* as an Opportunistic Pathogen. New York: Plenum Press, 1993:107.
44. Nicastri E, Petrosillo N, Viale P, Ippolito G. Catheter related bloodstream infected patients. Ann NY Acad Sci 2001; 946:274.
45. O'Toole GA, Pratt LA, Watnick DK, et al. Biofilm formation as microbial development. Ann Rev Microbiol 2000; 54:49.
46. Schwartzmann S, Boring JR III. Antiphagocytic effect of slime from a mucoid strain of *Pseudomonas aeruginosa*. Infect Immun 1971; 3:762.
47. Stewart PS, Costerton JW. Antibiotic resistance of bacteria in biofilms. Lancet 2001; 358:135.
48. Mermel LA, B Farr M, Sherertz MJ, et al. Guidelines for the management of intravascular catheter-related infections. Clin Infect Dis 2001; 32:1249.
49. Li J. Bacterial toxins. Curr Opin Struct Biol 1991; 2:545.
50. Coburn J. *Pseudomonas aeruginosa* exoenzyme S. Curr Top Microbiol Immun 1992; 175:133.
51. Mechanisms of cell and tissue damage. In: Mims C, Nash A, Stephen J, eds. Mims' Pathogenesis of Infectious Disease. 5th ed. London: Academic Press, 2001:216.
52. Passador L, Iglewski BH. Quorum sensing and virulence gene regulation in *Pseudomonas aeruginosa*. In: Roth JA, Bolin CA, Brogden KA, et al., eds. Virulence Mechanisms of Bacterial Pathogens. 2nd ed. Washington DC: American Society for Microbiology, 1995:65.
53. Sorensen RU, Klinger JD. Biological effects of *Pseudomonas aeruginosa* phenazine pigments. Antibiot Chemother 1987; 39:113.
54. Baltch AL, Hammer MC, Smith RP, et al. Effects of *Pseudomonas aeruginosa* cytotoxin on human serum and granulocytes on their microbicidal, phagocytic and chemotactic functions. Infect Immun 1985; 48:498.
55. Mai GT, Seow WK, Pier JG, et al. Suppression of lymphocytes and neutrophil functions by *Pseudomonas aeruginosa* and mucoid exopolysaccharide (alginate): reversal by physicochemical, collagenase and specific antibody treatments. Infect Immun 1993; 61:559.
56. Plotowski MC, Saliba AM, Pereira SH, et al. *Pseudomonas aeruginosa* selective adherence to an entry into endothelial cells. Infect Immun 1994; 62:5456.
57. Marshall WF, Keating MR, Anhalt JP, et al. *Xanthomonas maltophilia*: an emerging nosocomial pathogen. Mayo Clin Proc 1989; 64:1097.
58. Khan IA, Mehta NJ. *Stenotrophomonas maltophilia* endocarditis: a systematic review. Angiology 2002; 53:49.
59. Semel JD, Trenholme GM, Harris AA, et al. *Pseudomonas maltophilia* pseudosepticemia. Am J Med 1978; 64:403.

60. Krupova Y, Novotny J, Sabo A, et al. Aetiology, cost of antimicrobial therapy and outcome in leukopenic patients who developed bacteremia during antibiotic prophylaxis: A case-controlled study. Int J Antimicrob Agents 1998; 10:313.
61. Sattler CA, Mason EO, Kaplan SL. Nonrespiratory *S. maltophilia* infection at a childrens hospital. Clin Infect Dis 2000; 21:1321.
62. Jae-Han K, Shin-Woo K, Hye-Run K, et al. Two episodes of *Stenotrophomonas maltophilia* endocarditis of a prosthetic mitral valve: report of a case and review of the literature. J Korean Med Sci 2002; 17:263.
63. Mehta NJ, Khan IA, Mehta RN, Gulati A. *Stenotrophomonas maltophilia* endocarditis prosthetic aortic valve: report of a case and review of literature. Heart Lung 2000; 29:351.
64. Alonso A, Martinez JL. Multiple antibiotic resistance in *Stenotrophomonas maltophilia*. Antimicrob Agents Chemother 1997; 41:1140.
65. Garrison MW, Anderson DE, Campbell DM, et al. *Stenotrophomonas maltophilia*: emergence of multidrug-resistant strains during therapy and an in-vitro pharmacodynamic chamber model. Antimicrob Agents Chemother 1996; 40:2859.
66. Friedman ND, Korman TM, Fairley CK, et al. Bacteremia due to *Stenotrophomonas maltophilia*: an analysis of 45 episodes. J Infect 2002; 45:47.
67. Barbier-Frebour N, Boutiba-Boubak I, Nouvello M, et al. Molecular investigation of *Stenotrophomonas maltophilia* isolates exhibiting rapid emergence of ticarcillin-clavulanate resistance. J Hosp Infect 2002; 45:35.
68. Crispino M, Boccia MC, Bagattini M, et al. Molecular epidemiology of *Stenotrophomonas maltophilia* in a university hospital. J Hosp Infect 2002; 52:88.
69. Noriega ER, Rubinstein E, Simberkoff MS, Rahal JJ. Subacute and acute endocarditis due to *Pseudomonas cepacia* in heroin addicts. Am J Med 1975; 59:29.
70. Mohr CD, Tomich M, Herfst CA. Cellular aspects of *Burkholderia cepacia* infection. Microbes Infect 2001; 3:425.
71. Lutter E, Lewenza S, Dennis JJ, et al. Distribution of quorum-sensing genes in the *Burkholderia cepacia* complex. Infect Immun 2001; 69:4661.
72. Bhakta DR, Leader I, Jacobson R, et al. Antimicrobial properties of investigational and seldom, used antibiotics against isolates of *Pseudomonas cepacia* isolates in Michigan. Chemotherapy 2003; 47:400.
73. Street A, Durack D. Experience with trimethoprim-sulfamethoxazole in treating infective endocarditis. Rev Infect Dis 1988; 10:915.
74. Pitt TL, Barth AL. *Pseudomonas aeruginosa* and other medically important pseudomonads. In: Emmerson AM, Hawkey PM, Gillespie SH, eds. Principles and Practice of Clinical Bacteriology. Chichester, England: John Wiley and Sons, 1997:494.
75. Hsueh PR, Teng LJ, Pan HJ, et al. Outbreak of *Pseudomonas fluorescence* bacteremia among oncology patients. J Clin Microbiol 1998; 36:2914.
76. Swiet J. Medical memorandum: subacute bacterial endocarditis due to *Salmonella typhimirium*. Brit Med J 1949; 2:1155.
77. Buchwald DS, Blaser MJ. A review of human salmonellosis: II. Duration of excretion following infection with non typhi Salmonella. Rev Infect Dis 1984; 6:345.
78. Cohen P, O'Brien T, Schoenbaum S, et al. Risk of endothelial infection in adults with *Salmonella bacteremia*. Ann Intern Med 1978; 89(6):931–932.
79. Cohen JI, Bartlett JA, Corey GR. Extra-intestinal manifestations of Salmonella infections. Medicine (Baltimore) 1987; 66:349.
80. Schneider PK, Nernoff J, Gold JA. Acute salmonella endocarditis: report of a case and review. Arch Intern Med 1967; 120:478.
81. Doraiswami S, Friedman S, Kagan A, et al. Salmonella endocarditis complicated by a myocardial abscess. Am J Cardiol 1970; 26:102.
82. Yamamoto N, Magidson O, Posner C, et al. Probable Salmonella endocarditis treated with prosthetic valve replacement: a case report. Surgery 1974; 76:678.
83. Choo PW, Gantz NM, Anderson C, Maguire JH. Salmonella prosthetic valve endocarditis. Diagn Microbiol Infect Dis 1992; 15:273.
84. Celum CL, Chaisson RE, Rutheford GW. Incidence of salmonellosis in patients with AIDS. J Infect Dis 1987; 156:998.

85. Guerrero F, Ramos MLJM, Nunez A, de Gorgolas M. Focal infection due to non-typhi Salmonella in patients with AIDS: report of 10 cases and review. Clin Infect Dis 1997; 25:690.

86. Guerrero F, Torres Perea MLR, Rodrigo JGS, et al. Infectious endocarditis due to non-typhi Salmonella in patients infected with human immunodeficiency virus: report of two cases and review. Clin Infect Dis 1996; 22:853.

87. duPlessis JP, Govendrageloo K, Levin SE. Right sided endocarditis due to Salmonella typhi. Pediatr Cardiol 1997; 18:443.

88. Hsu RB, Tsay YG, Chen RJ, Chu SH. Risk factors for primary bacteremia and endovascular infection in patients without acquired immunodeficiency syndrome who have non-typhoid salmonellosis. Clin Infect Dis 2003; 36:829.

89. Das M, Badley AD, Cockerill FR, et al. Infective endocarditis caused by HACEK microrganisms. Annu Rev Med 1997; 28:25.

90. *Actinobacillus, Kingella, Cardiobacterium, Capnocytophaga* and similar organisms. In: Forbes BA, Sahm DF, Weissfeld AS, eds. Bailey and Scott's Diagnostic Microbiology. 11th ed. St. Louis: Mosby, 2002:385.

91. Brouqui P, Raoult D. Endocarditis due to rare and fastidious bacteria. Clin Microbiol Rev 2001; 14:177.

92. Darras-Jolly C, Lortholary O, Mainardi JL, et al. Haemophilus endocarditis: report of a 42 cases in adults and review. Haemophilus Endocarditis Study Group. Clin Infect Dis 1997; 24:1087.

93. Hossein A, Rahimi AR. *Haemophilus aphrophilus* endocarditis after tongue piercing. Emerg Infect Dis 2002; 8:850.

94. Kugler KC, Biedenbach DJ, Jones RN. Determination of the antimicrobial activity of 29 clinically important compounds tested against fastidious HACEK organisms. Diagn Microbiol Infect Dis 1999; 34:73.

95. Huang ST, Lee HC, Lee NY, et al. Clinical characteristics of invasive *Haemophilus aphrophilus* infections. J Microbiol Immunol Infect 2005; 38:271.

96. Elster SK, Mattes BR, Meyers BR, Jurado RA. *Haemophilus aphrophilus* endocarditis: review of 23 cases. Am J Cardiol 1975; 35:72.

97. Coll-Vinent BX, Suris A, Lopez-Soto J, et al. *Haemophilus paraphrophilus* endocarditis: case report and review. Clin Infect Dis 1995; 20:1381.

98. Lynn D, Kane J, Parker R. *Haemophilus parainfluenzae* and *Haemophilus influenzae* endocarditis: a review of forty cases. Medicine 1977; 56:115.

99. Geraci JE, Wilkowske CJ, Wilson WR, Washinton WA. *Haemophilus* endocarditis. Report of 14 patients. Mayo Clin Proc 1977; 52:209.

100. Blair D, Walker W, Doseman T, et al. Bacterial endocarditis due to *Haemophilus parainfluenzae*. Chest 1977; 71:146.

101. Raucher B, Tobkin J, Mandel L. Occult polymicrobial endocarditis with *Haemophilus parainfluenza* in intravenous drug abusers. Am J Med 1983; 143:18.

102. Geraci J, Greipp P, Wikowske C, et al. *Cardiobacterium hominis* endocarditis: four cases with clinical and laboratory observations. Mayo Clin Proc 1978; 53:49.

103. Savage DD, Kagan RL, Young NA, Horvath AE. *Cardiobacterium hominis* endocarditis: description of two patients and characterization of the organism. J Clin Microbiol 1977; 5:75.

104. Wormser G, Bottone E, Tudy J, et al. Case report: *Cardiobacteriium hominis*: review of prior infections and report of endocarditis on a fascia lata prosthetic heart valve. Am J Med Sci 1987; 276:117.

105. Chen YC, Chang SC, Luh KT, Hsieh WC. *Actinobacillus actinomycetemcomitans* endocarditis: a report of four cases and review of the literature. Q J Med 1991; 81:871.

106. Kaplan AH, Weber DJ, Oddone EZ, Perfect JR. Infection due to *Actinobacillus actinomycetemcomitans*: 15 cases and review. Rev Infect Dis 1989; 11:46.

107. Grace CJ, Levitz RE, Katz-Pollak H, Brettman LR. *Actinobacillus actinomycetemcomitans* prosthetic valve endocarditis. Rev Infect Dis 1988; 10:677.

108. Landis SJ, Korver J. *Eikenella corrodens* endocarditis: case report and review of the literature. Can Med Assoc J 1983; 128:822.

109. Sobel J, Carrizola J, Ziobrowski T, et al. Case report: polymicrobial endocarditis involving *Eikenella corrodens*. Am J Med Sci 1981; 282:41.

110. Deber M, Graham B, Hunter E, et al. Endocarditis and infection of intravascular devices due to *Eikenella corrodens*. Am J Med Sci 1986; 292:209.
111. Jenny D, Letendre P, Iveson G. Endocarditis due to Kingella species. Rev Infect Dis 1988; 10:1065.
112. Swann R, Holmes B. Infective endocarditis caused by *Kingella denitrificans*. J Clin Pathol 1984; 37:1384.
113. Grandsen WR, Elykyn SJ, Phillips I, Rowe B. Bacteremia due to *Eschericia coli*: a study of 861 episodes. Rev Infect Dis 1990; 12:1008.
114. Jackson LA, Benson P, Neuzil KM, et al. Burden of community-onset *Escherichia coli* bacteremia in seniors. J Infect Dis 2005; 191:1523.
115. Hansing C, Allen V, Cherry J. *Escherichia coli* endocarditis: a review of the literature and a case study. Arch Intern Med 1967; 120:472.
116. Moxon ER, Kroll JS. The role of bacterial polysaccharide capsules as virulence factors. Curr Top Microbiol Immunol 1990; 150:65.
117. *Escherichia coli*—extraintestinal infections. In: Saylers AA, Whitt DD, eds. Bacterial Pathogenesis. A Molecular Approach. 2nd ed. Washington DC: ASM Press, 2002:343.
118. Yersin B, Glauser MP, Guze PA. Experimental *Escherichia coli* endocarditis in rats: roles of serum bactericidal activity of catheter placement. Infect Immun 1988; 56:1273.
119. Sanders CC, Sanders WE. Beta-lactam resistance in Gram-negative bacteria—global trends and clinical impact. Clin Infect Dis 1992; 15:824.
120. Anderson MJ, Janoff EN. Klebsiella endocarditis: report of two cases and review. Clin Infect Dis 1998; 26:468.
121. Weinstein L, Rubin R. Infective endocarditis—1973. Prog Cardiovasc Dis 1973; 16:239.
122. Rosen P, Armstrong D. Active endocarditis in patients treated for malignant neoplastic diseases: a post-mortem Study. Am J Clin Pathol 1973; 59:241.
123. Wisplinghoff H, Bischoff T, Tallent SM, et al. Nosocomial bloodstream infections in U.S. hospitals: analysis of 24,179 cases from a prospective nationwide surveillance study. Clin Infect Dis 2004; 39:309.
124. Tarkkanen AM, Allen BL, Williams PH, et al. Fimbriation, capsulation and iron-scavenging systems of Klebsiella strains associated with urinary tract infection. Infect Immun 1992; 60:1187.
125. Endimani A, Luzzaro F, Brigante G, et al. *Proteus mirabilis* bloodstream infections: risk factors and treatment outcome related to the expression of extended-spectrum beta-lactamases. Antimicrob Agents Chemother 2005; 49:2598.
126. Yu V. *Serratia marcescens*: historical perspective and clinical review. N Engl J Med 1979; 300:887.
127. Cooper R, Mills J. *Serratia endocarditis*: a follow-up report. Arch Intern Med 1980; 140:99.
128. Mills J, Drew D. *Serratia marcescens* endocarditis: a regional illness associated with intravenous drug abuse. Ann Intern Med 1976; 84:29.
129. Giamarellou H, Atoniadou A, Kanavos C, et al. *Yersinia enterocolitica* endocarditis: case report and literature review. Eur J Clin Microbiol Infect Dis 1995; 14:126.
130. Centers for Disease Control and Prevention. Red blood cell transfusions contaminated with *Yersinia enterocolitica*—United States, 1991–1996 and initiation of a national study of detecting bacteria-associated transfusion reactions. Morbid Mortal Wkly 1997; 46:617.
131. Bottone EJ. *Yersinia enterocolitica*: the charisma continues. Clin Microbiol Rev 1997; 10:257.
132. *Yersinia pestis*, the cause of plague, and its relatives. In: Saylers AA, Whitt DD, eds. Bacterial Pathogenesis. A Molecular Approach. 2nd ed. Washington DC: ASM Press, 2002:202.
133. Cornelis GR, Boland A, Boyd AP, et al. The virulence plasmid of *Yersinia*, an anti- host genome. Microbiol Mol Biol Rev 1998; 62:1315.
134. McCullough D, Menzies R, Corhere B. Endocarditis due to *Citrobacter diversus* developing resistance to cephalothin. NZ Med J 1977; 85:182.
135. Plantholt SJ, Trofa AF. *Citrobacter freundi* endocarditis in an intravenous drug abuser. South Med J 1987; 80:1439.
136. Le Frock J, Klainer A, Zuckerman K. *Edwardsiella tarda* bacteremia. South Med J 1976; 69:188.
137. Young EJ. An overview of human brucellosis. Clin Infect Dis 1995; 21:283.

138. Al-Harthi SS. The morbidity and mortality patterns of Brucella endocarditis. Intern J Cardiol 1989; 25:321.

139. Delvecchio G, Fracassetti O, Lorenzi N. Brucella endocarditis. Intern J Cardiol 1991; 33:328.

140. Jacobs F, Abramowicz D, Vereerstraeten P, et al. Brucella endocarditis: the role of combined medical and surgical treatment. Rev Infect Dis 1990; 12:740.

141. Flugelman M, Galun E, Ben-Chetrit J, et al. Brucellosis in patients with heart disease: when should endocarditis be diagnosed? Cardiology 1990; 77:313.

142. Smith LD, Ficht TA. Pathogenesis of Brucella. Crit Rev Microbiol 1990; 17:209.

143. Pappas G, Akeritidis N, Bosilkovski M, Tsianos E. Brucellosis. N Engl J Med 2005; 352:2325.

144. Tang YW, Hopkins CP, Kolbert PA, et al. *Bordetella holmsei* like organisms associated with septicemia, endocarditis and respiratory failure. Clin Infect Dis 1998; 26:389.

145. Dale A, Geraci J. Mixed cardiac valvular infections: report of case and review of the literature. Staff Meet Mayo Clin 1961; 36:288.

146. Lindquist SW, Weber DJ, Magnum ME, et al. *Bordetella holmesii* sepsis in an asplenic adolescent. Pediatr Infect Dis J 1995; 14:813.

147. Tancik CA, Dillaha JA. *Francisella tularensis* endocarditis. Clin Infect Dis 2000; 30:399.

148. Enderlin G, Morales L, Jacobs RF, et al. Streptomycin and alternative agents for the treatment of tularemia: review of the literature. Clin Infect Dis 1994; 19:42.

149. Limaye AP, Hooper CJ. Treatment of tularemia with fluoroquinolones: two cases and review. Clin Infect Dis 1999; 29:922.

150. Raffi F, Barrier J, Baron D, et al. Castro almost as the bacteremia: report of 13 cases over 12 years and review of the literature. Scand J Infect Dis 1987; 19:385.

151. Sorbello AF, O'Donnell J, Kaiser-Smith J, et al. Infective endocarditis due to *Pasteurella dagmatis*: case report and review. Clin Infect Dis 1994; 18:336.

152. Weber P, Wolfson J, Schwarz M, et al. *Pasteurella multocida* infections: report of 34 cases and review of the literature. Medicine 1989; 63:133.

153. Nettles RE, Sexton DJ. *Pasteurella multocida* prosthetic valve endocarditis: case report and review. Clin Infect Dis 1997; 25:920.

154. Holst E, Roloff J, Larsson L, et al. Characterization in distribution of Pasteurella species recovered from infected humans. J Clin Microbiol 1992; 30:2984.

155. Boyce JD, Chung JY, Adler B. *Pasteurella multocida* capsule: composition, function and genetics. J Biotechnol 2000; 83:153.

156. Farrugia DC, Eykyn SJ, Smyth EG. *Campylobacter fetus* endocarditis: two case reports and review. Clin Infect Dis 1994; 18:443.

157. Loeb H, Bettag J, Young N, et al. Vibrio fetus endocarditis: report. Am Heart J 1966; 71:381.

158. Dzau V, Shur P, Weinstein L. *Vibrio fetus* endocarditis in a patient with systemic lupus erythematosus. Am J Med Sci 1976; 272:331.

159. Blaser MJ, Smith PF, Repine JE, et al. Pathogenesis of *Campylobacter fetus* infections. Failure of C3b to bind explains serum and phagocytosis resistance. J Clin Invest 1988; 81:1434.

160. Davis W II, Kane J, Garagusi V. Human *Aeromonas* infections: a review of the literature and the case report of endocarditis. Medicine 1978; 57:267.

161. Fenollar F, Fournier PE, Legre R. Unusual case of *Aeromonas sobria* cellulitis associated with the use of leeches. Eur J Clin Microbiol Infect Dis 1999; 18:72.

162. Janda JM. Recent advances in the study of the taxonomy, pathogenicity and infectious syndromes associated with the genus *Aeromonas*. Clin Microbiol Rev 1991; 4:397.

163. Janda JM, Guthertz LS, Kokka RP, et al. *Aeromonas* species in septicemia: laboratory that characteristics and clinical observations. Clin Infect Dis 1994; 19:77.

164. Jones PL, Wilcox MH. Aeromonas infections and their treatment. J Antimicrob Chemother 1995; 35:453.

165. Balotescu C, Israil A, Radu R, et al. Aspects of constitutive and acquired and antibioresistance in *Aeromonas hydrophilia* strains isolated from water sources. Roum Arch Microbiol Immunol 2003; 62:179.

166. *Acinetobacter, Chrysemonas, Flavemonas* and *Steotrophomonas*. In: Forbes BA, Sahm DF, Weissfeld AS, eds. Bailey and Scott's Diagnostic Microbiology. 11th ed. St. Louis: Mosby, 2002:378.

167. Ristuccia P, Cunha B. Acinetobacter. Infect Cont 1983; 4:226.
168. Retailleau H, Hightower A, Dixon R, et al. *Acinetobacter calcoaceticus*: a nosocomial pathogen with an unusual seasonal pattern. J Infect Dis 1979; 139:371.
169. Ayaz M, Durmaz R, Atkas E, Durmaz B. Bacteriological, clinical and epidemiological characteristics of hospital-acquired *Acinetobacter baumanni* infection in a teaching hospital. J Hosp Infect 2003; 54:39.
170. Gales A, Jones RN, Forward J, et al. Emerging importance of multidrug-resistant Acinetobacter species and *Stenotrophomonas maltophilia* as pathogens in seriously ill patients: geographic patterns, epidemiological features and trends in the SENTRY antimicrobial surveillance program (1997–1999). Clin Infect Dis 2001; 32(suppl 2):104.
171. Marques MB, Brookings ES, Moser SA, et al. Comparative in vitro antimicrobial susceptibilities of nosocomial isolates of *Acinetobacter baumanni* and synergistic activities of nine antimicrobial combinations. Antimicrob Agents Chemother 1997; 41:881.
172. Avril JL, Mesnard R. Factors influencing the area was Acinetobacter. In: Towner KJ, Bergogne-Berezin E, Fewson CA, eds. The Biology of Acinetobacter. New York: Plenum Publishing, 1991:77.
173. Rupp ME. *Streptobacillus moniliformis* endocarditis: case report and review. Clin Infect Dis 1992; 14:769.
174. Freundt EA. Experimental investigations into the pathogenicity of the L phase variant of *Streptobacillus moniliformis*. Acta Pathol Microbiol Scand 1956; 38:246.
175. Wullenweber M. *Streptobacillus moniliformis*—a zoonotic-pathogen: taxonomic considerations, host species, diagnosis, therapy, geographic distribution. Lab Anim 1995; 29:1–15.
176. Berger C, Altwegg M, Meyer A common, et al. Broad range polymerase chain reaction for diagnosis of rat-bite fever caused by *Streptobacillus moniliformis*. Pediatr Infect Dis J 2001; 20:1181.
177. Hitzig WM, Liebesman A. Subacute endocarditis associated with a Spirillum. Arch Intern Med 1994; 73:415.
178. Cole A, Marchall C. Infective endocarditis due to *Bacillus faecalis* alcaligines. Br Med J 1952; 2:867.
179. McKinley KP, Laundry TJ, Masterson RG. Achromobacter group B replacement valve endocarditis. J Infect 1990; 20:262.
180. Cieslak TJ, Raszka WV. Catheter-associated sepsis due *Alcaligines xylosoxidans* in a child with AIDS. Clin Infect Dis 1993; 16:592.
181. Bizet C, Tekaia F, Philippon A. In vitro susceptibility of *Alcaligenes faecalis* compared with those of other *Alcaligines* spp. Two microbial agents including seven beta-lactams. J Antimicrob Chemother 1993; 32:907.
182. Knippschild M, Schmid EN, Uppenkamp M, et al. Infection by *Alcaligenes xylosoxidans* subsp. xylosoxidans in neutropenic patients. Oncology 1996; 53:258.
183. Brunn B, Tvenstrup, Jensen JE, Lundstrom K, Andersen GE. *Flavobacterium meningosepticum* infection. Eur J Clin Microbiol Infect Dis 1989; 8:509.
184. Ratner H. *Flavobacterium meningosepticum*. Infect Control 1984; 52:37.
185. Raimondi, Moosden F, Williams JD. Antibiotic resistance patterns of *Flavobacterium meningosepticum*. Eur J Clin Microbiol 1986; S461.
186. *Chryseobacterium*, *Sphingobacterium*, and similar organisms. In: Forbes BA, Sahm DF, Weissfeld AS, eds. Bailey and Scott's Diagnostic Microbiology. 11th ed. St. Louis: Mosby, 2002:406.
187. Sandoe J. *Capnocytophaga canimorsus* endocarditis. J Med Microbiol 2004; 53:245.
188. Medfield S, Young E. Native valve endocarditis caused by dysgonic fermenter bacilli. Am J Sci 1988; 296:69.
189. Verghese A, Hamati F, Berk S, et al. Susceptibility of dysgonic fermenter 2 to antimicrobial agents in vitro. Antimicrob Agents Chemother 1988; 32:78.
190. Fischer LJ, Weyant RS, White EH, et al. Intracellular multiplication and toxic distruction of cultured macrophages by *Capnocytophaga canimorsus*. Infect Immun 1995; 63:3484.
191. Brenner DJ, Hollis DG, Fanning R, et al. *Capnocytophaga canimorosus* sp. nov (formerly CDC group DF2), a cause of septicemia following dog bite and *C. cynogemi* sp nov, a cause of localized wound infection following dog bite. J Clin Microbiol 1989; 27:23.

192. Berberi EF, Cockerill FR III, Steckelberg J. Infective endocarditis due to unusual or fastidious microorganisms. Mayo Clin Proc 1997; 72:532.
193. Wall TC, Peyton RB, Corey GR. Gonococcal endocarditis: a new look at an old disease. Medicine (Baltimore) 1989; 68:375.
194. Ebright J, Komorowski R. Gonococcal endocarditis associated with immune complex glomerulonephritis. Am J Med 1980; 68:793.
195. Jurica JV, Bomzer CA, England AC. Gonococcal endocarditis: a case report and review of the literature. Sex Transm Dis 1987; 14:231.
196. *Neisseria* species. In: Saylers AA, Whitt DD, eds. Bacterial Pathogenesis. A Molecular Approach. 2nd ed. Washington DC: ASM Press, 2002:437.
197. Sternberg R, Smith J. Meningococcal endocarditis in an Ionescu-Shiley aortic valve prosthesis: successful treatment with intravenous penicillin. South Med J 1989; 82:1314.
198. Dankert J. Neisseria. In: Cohen J, Powderly WG, eds. Infectious Diseases. 2nd ed. New York: Mosby, 2004:2173.
199. Ghoneim A, Tandor A. Prosthetic valve endocarditis due to *Neisseria sicca*: a case report. Indian Heart J 1979; 31:246.
200. Doem G, Miller M, Winn R. *Branhamella* (*Neisseria*) *catarrhalis* systemic disease in humans. Arch Intern Med 1981; 141:1690.
201. Ionnidis JPA, Worthington M, Griffiths JK, Snyderman DR. Spectrum and significance of bacteremia due to *Moraxella catarrhalis*. Clin Infect Dis 1995; 21:390.
202. Van Scoy RE. Culture-negative endocarditis. Mayo Clin Proc 1982; 57:150.
203. Houpakian P, Raoult D. Blood culture negative endocarditis in a reference center: etiologic diagnosis of 348 cases. Medicine (Baltimore) 2005; 84:162.
204. Raoult D, Tissot-DuPont H, Foucault C, et al. Q-fever 1985–1998. Clinical and epidemiologic features of 1383 infections. Medicine 2000; 79:109.
205. Fenollar F, Fournier PE, Carrieri MP, et al. Risk factors and prevention of Q-fever endocarditis. Clin Infect Dis 2001; 33:312.
206. Stein A, Raoult D. Q-fever endocarditis. Eur Heart J 1995; 16(suppl B):19.
207. DuPont HT, Thirion X, Raoult D. Q-fever serology: cut off determination for microimmunofluorescence. Clin Diagn Lab Immunol 1994; 1:189.
208. Fournier PE, Casalta JP, Habib G, et al. Modification of the diagnostic criteria proposed by the Duke endocarditis service to permit improved diagnosis of Q-fever endocarditis. Am J Med 1996; 100:629.
209. Raoult D, Houpikian P, Tissot-DuPont, et al. Treatment of Q-fever endocarditis: comparison of two regimens containing doxycycline and ofloxacin or hydrochloroquine. Arch Intern Med 1999; 159:167.
210. Houpakian P, Habib G, Mesana T, Raoult D. Changing clinical presentation of Q-fever endocarditis. Clin Infect Dis 2002; 34:E28.
211. Baca OG, Roman MJ, Glew RH, et al. Acid phosphatase activity in *Coxiella burnetii*: a possible virulence factor. Infect Immun 1993; 61:4232.
212. Mason PR, Kelly PJ. Rickettsia and Rickettsia like organisms. In: Cohen J, Powderly WG, eds. Infectious Diseases. 2nd ed. New York: Mosby, 2004:2317.
213. Honstettre A, Imbert G, Ghigo E, et al. Dysregulation of cytokines in acute Q-fever: role of interleukin-10 and tumor necrosis factor in chronic evolution of Q-fever. J Infect Dis 2003; 187:956.
214. Raoult D, Fournier PE, Drancourt M, et al. Diagnosis of 22 new cases of Bartonella endocarditis. Ann Intern Med 1996; 125:646.
215. Spach DH, Kanter AS, Dougherty MJ, et al. *Bartonella* (Rochalimaea) *quintana* bacteremia in inner city patients with chronic alcoholism. N Engl J Med 1995; 332:424.
216. Albrich WC, Kraft C, Fisk T, Albrecht H. A mechanic with a bad valve: blood-culture-negative endocarditis. Lancet Infect Dis 2004; 4:777.
217. Starkebaum M, Durack D, Beeson P. "The incubation period" of subacute bacterial endocarditis. Yale J Biol Med 1977; 50:49.
218. Kreisel D, Pasque MK, Damiano RJ, et al. The *Bartonella* species-induced prosthetic valve endocarditis associated with rapid progression of valvular stenosis. J Thorac Cardiovasc Surg 2005; 130:567.

219. Raoult D, Fournier PE, Vandenesch F, et al. outcome and treatment of *Bartonella* endo-carditis. Arch Intern Med 2003; 163:226.
220. Fournier PE, Lelievre H, Eykyn SJ, et al. Epidemiologic in clinical characteristics of *Bartonella quintana* and *Bartonella henselae* endocarditis: a study of 48 patients. Medicine (Baltimore) 2001; 88:245.
221. Maurin M, Gasquet S, Ducco C, Raoult D. MICs of 28 antibiotic compounds for 14 *Bartonella* (formerly Rochalimaea) isolates. Antimicrob Agents Chemother 1995; 39:2387.
222. Rolain JM, Broqui P, Koehler JE, et al. Recommendations for treatment of human infec-tions caused by *Bartonella* species. Antimicrob Agents Chemother 2004; 48:1921.
223. Matera G, Liberto MC, Quirino A, et al. *Bartonella quintana* lipopolysaccharide effects on leukocytes, CXC chemokines and apoptosis: a study on human whole blood and a rat model. Int Immunopharmacol 2003; 3:853.
224. Birkhead JS, Apostolov K. Endocarditis caused by a psittacosis agent. Br Heart J 1974; 36:728.
225. Jones RB, Priest JB, Kuo C-C. Subacute chlamydial endocarditis. JAMA 1982; 247:655.
226. Odeh M, Oliven A. Chlamydial infections of the heart. Eur J Clin Microbiol Infect Dis 1992; 11:885.
227. Maurin M, Eb F, Etienne J, Raoult D. Serological cross-reactions between *Bartonella* and *Chlamydia* species: implications for diagnosis. J Clin Microbiol 1997; 35:2283.
228. Jariwalla A, Davies B, White J. Infective endocarditis complicating psittacosis: response to rifampin. Br Med J 1980; 19:155.
229. Brearley BF, Hutchinson DN. Endocarditis associated with *Chlamydia trachomatis* infec-tion. Br Heart J 1981; 46:220.
230. Marrie TJ, Harczy M, Mann OE, et al. Culture-negative endocarditis probably due to *Chlamydia pneumoniae*. J Infect Dis 1990; 161:127.
231. Cope A, Heber M, Wilkins E. Valvular tuberculous endocarditis: a case report and review of the literature. J Infect 1990; 21:293.
232. Anyanwy C, Nassau E, Yacoub M. Miliary tuberculosis following homograft valve replacement. Thorax 1976; 31:101.
233. Laskowski L, Marr J, Spernoga J, et al. Fastidious mycobacteria grown from porcine prosthetic heart valves cultures. N Engl J Med 1977; 297:101.
234. Rumisek JD, Albus RA, Clarke JS. Late *Mycobacteria chelonei* bioprosthetic valve endocarditis: activation of the implanted contaminant. Ann Thorac Surg 1985; 39:277.
235. Alvarez-Elcoro S, Mateos-Mora M, Zajarias A. *Mycobacterium fortuitum* endocarditis after mitral valve replacement with a bovine prosthesis. South Med J 1985; 78:865.
236. Lohr DC, Goeken A, Doty DB, Donta ST. *Mycobacterium gordonae* infection of a prosthetic aortic valve. JAMA 1978; 239:1528.
237. Chow WH, Leung WH, Tai YT, et al. Echocardiographic diagnosis of an aortic root abscess after *Mycobacterium fortuitum* prosthetic valve endocarditis. Clin Cardiol 1991; 14:273.
238. Wallace RJ Jr, Musser JM, Hull SI, et al. Diversity and sources of rapidly growing mycobacteria associated with infections following cardiac surgery. J Infect Dis 1985; 52:500.
239. Jacomo V, Musso D, Gevaudan MJ, Drancourt M. Isolation of blood-borne Mycobacterium avium by using the non-radioactive Bactec 9000 MB system and comparison with a solid-culture system. J Clin Microbiol 1998; 36:3703.
240. Wallace RJ Jr, Swenson JM, Silcox VA, Bullen MG. Treatment of nonpulmonary infec-tions due to *Mycobacterium fortuitum* and *Mycobacterium chelonei* on the basis of in vitro susceptibilities. J Infect Dis 1985; 152:500.
241. Lowry PW, Tompkins LS. Nosocomial legionellosis: a review of pulmonary extrapul-monary syndromes. Am J Infect Control 1993; 21:21.
242. Tompkins LS, Roessler BJ, Redd SC, et al. Legionella prosthetic-valve endocarditis. N Engl J Med 1988; 318:530.
243. McCabe RE, Baldwin JC, McGregor CA, et al. Prosthetic valve endocarditis caused by *Legionella pneumophilia*. Ann Intern Med 1984; 100:525.
244. Stout JE, Yu VL. Legionellosis. N Engl J Med 1997; 337:682.
245. Fields BS. The role of amoebae in legionellosis. Clin Microbiol Newslett 1991; 13:92.
246. Cianciotto NP. Pathogenicity of *Legionella pneumophilia*. Int J Microbiol 2001; 291:331.

247. *Legionella pneumophilia* and Legionnaires' disease. In: Saylers AA, Whitt DD, eds. Bacterial Pathogenesis. A Molecular Approach. 2nd ed. Washington DC: ASM Press, 2002:311.
248. Popat K, Barnado D, Webb-Peploe M. *Mycoplasma pneumoniae* endocarditis. Br Heart J 1980; 44:111.
249. Fenollar F, Gauduchon V, Casalta JP, et al. Mycoplasma endocarditis: two case report and a review. Clin Infect Dis 2004; 38:21.
250. Rosengarten R, Citti C, Glew A, et al. Host-pathogen interactions in Mycoplasma pathogenesis: virulence and survival strategies of minimalist prokaryocytes. Int J Med Microbiol 2000; 290:15.
251. Feingold D. Biology and pathogenicity of microbial spherplasts and L-forms. N Engl J Med 1969; 281:1149.
252. Charache P. Atypical bacterial forms in human disease. In: Guze LB, ed. Protoplasts, Spherplasts and L-forms. Baltimore: Williams and Wilkins, 1967:484.
253. Raoult D, Birg ML, LaScola B, et al. Cultivation of the bacillus of Whipple's disease. N Engl J Med 2000; 342:620.
254. Durand DV, Lecomte C, Cathebras P, et al. Whipple disease. Clinical review of 52 cases. The SNMFI Research Group On Whipple Disease. Societe Nationale Fracaise de Medecine Interne. Medicine (Baltimore) 1997; 76:170.
255. Lepidi H, Fenollar F, Dumler JS, et al. Cardiac valves in patients with Whipple's endocarditis. J Infect Dis 2004; 190:935.
256. Fenollar F, Lepidi H, Raoult D. Whipple's endocarditis: review of the literature and comparisons with Q-fever, *Bartonella* infection, and blood culture-positive endocarditis. Clin Infect Dis 2001; 33:1309.
257. Marth T, Roux M, von Herbay A, common et al. Persistent reduction of complement receptor 3 alpha-chain expressing mononuclear blood cells and transient inhibitory serum factors in Whipple's disease. Clin Immunol Immunopathol 1994; 72:217.
258. Vlachakis N, Gazes P, Hairston P. Nocardial endocarditis following mitral valve replacement. Chest 1975; 63:276.
259. Lui WY, Lee AC, Que TL. Central venous catheter-associated Nocardia bacteremia. Clin Infect Dis 2001; 33:1613.
260. Beaman BL, Beaman L. Nocardia species: host parasite relationships. Clin Microbiol Rev 1994; 7:213.
261. Dutton W, Inclan H. Cardiac actinomycosis. Chest 1968; 54:65.
262. Lam S, Samarj J, Rahman S, Hilton E. Primary actinomycotic endocarditis: case report and review. Clin Infect Dis 1993; 16:481.
263. Nastro SL, Sarma RJ. Infective endocarditis due to anaerobic and microaerophilic bacteria. West J Med 1982; 137:18.
264. Bisharat N, Goldstein L, Raz R, Elias M. Gram-negative anaerobic endocarditis: two case report and review of the literature. Eur J Clin Microbiol Infect Dis 2001; 20:651.
265. Brook I. Endocarditis due to anaerobic bacteria. Cardiology 2002; 98:1.
266. Jackson R, Dopp A. *Bacteroides fragilis* endocarditis. South Med J 1988; 81:781.
267. Oh S, Havlen PR, Hussain N. A case of polymicrobial endocarditis caused by anaerobic organisms in an injection drug user. Gen Intern Med 2005; 20:958.
268. Guthard H, Hany A, Turina M, Wust J. *Proprionobacterium acnes* as a cause of aggressive aortic valve endocarditis and importance of tissue grinding: case report and review. J Clin Microbiol 1994; 32:3043.
269. Behra-Miellet J, Calvet L, Dubreuil L. Activity of Linezolid against anaerobic bacteria. Int J Antimicrob Agents 2003; 22:28.
270. Lortholary O, Buu-Hoi A, Podglajen I, et al. Endocarditis caused by multiply resistant *Bacteroides fragilis*: case report and review. Clin Microbiol Infect 1995; 1:44.
271. Brook I, Myhal LA, Dorsey HC. Encapsulation and pilus formation of Bacteroides sp. J Infect 1991; 25:251.
272. Hofstad T. Virulence determinants in non-spore forming bacteria. Scand J Infect Dis 1989; 62(suppl):15.
273. Zimmerman L. Candida and Aspergillus endocarditis. Arch Pathol 1950; 50:591.
274. Seelig M, Goldberg P, Kozinn P, et al. Fungal endocarditis: patients at risk and their treatment. Postgrad Med J 1979; 55:632.

275. Rubinstein E, Noriega E, Simberkoff M, et al. Fungal endocarditis: analysis of 24 cases and review of the literature. Medicine (Baltimore) 1975; 54:331.
276. Martin GS, Mannino DM, Eaton S, et al. The epidemiology of sepsis in the United States from 1979 through 2000. N Engl J Med 2003; 348:1546.
277. Pierrotti LC, Baddoural M. Fungal endocarditis, 1995–2000. Chest 2002; 122:302.
278. Ellis ME, Al-Abdely H, Sandridge A, et al. Fungal endocarditis: evidence in the world literature, 1965–1995. Clin Infect Dis 2001; 32:50.
279. Pappas PG, Rex JH, Sobel JD, et al. Guidelines for treatment of candidiasis. Clin Infect Dis 2004; 38:161.
280. Bisbe J, Miro JM, Latorre X, et al. Disseminated candidiasis in addicts who use brown heroin: report of 83 cases and review. Clin Infect Dis 1992; 15:910.
281. Nguyen MH, Nguyen ML, Yu VL, et al. Candida prosthetic valve endocarditis: prospective study of six cases and review of the literature. Clin Infect Dis 1996; 22:262.
282. Melgar GR, Nasser RM, Gordon SM, et al. Fungal prosthetic valve endocarditis in 16 patients. An eleven year experience in a tertiary care hospital. Medicine (Baltimore) 1997; 76:94.
283. Scully R, Galdabini J, McNeely B. Case Records of the Massachusetts General Hospital. N Engl J Med 1979; 301:34.
284. Joseph P, Himmelstein D, Mahowald J, et al. Atrial myxoma infected with Candida: first survival. Chest 1980; 78:340.
285. Mathews RC. Pathogenicity determinants of *Candida albicans*: potential targets for immunotherapy? Microbiology 1994; 140:1505.
286. Baille GS, Douglas LJ. Matrix polymers of Candida biofilms and their possible role in biofilm resistance to antifungal agents. J Antimicrob Chemother 2000; 46:397.
287. Douglas LJ. *Candida albicans* biofilms and their role in infection. Trends Microbiol 2003; 11:30.
288. Crump JA, Collington PJ. Intravascular catheter-associated infections. Eur J Clin Microbiol Infect Dis 2000; 19:8.
289. Mora-Duarte J, Betts R, Rotstein C, et al. Comparison of capsofungin and amphotericin B for invasive candidiasis. N Engl J Med 2002; 347:2020.
290. Barchiesi F, Spreghini E, Maracci M, et al. In vitro activities of voriconazole in combination with three other antifungal agents against antimicrobe AB chemotherapy 2004; 48:3317.
291. Carrizosa J, Levison ME, Lawrence T, et al. Cure of *Aspergillus ustus* endocarditis of a prosthetic valve. Arch Intern Med 1974; 133:486.
292. El-Hamamsy I, Durrleman N, Stevens LM, et al. *Aspergillus* endocarditis after cardiac surgery. Ann Thorac Surg 2005; 80:359.
293. Sergi C, Weitz J, Hofmann WJ, et al. *Aspergillus* endocarditis, myocarditis and pericarditis complicating necrotizing fasciitis: case report and subject review. Virchows Arch 1996; 29:177.
294. Walsh T, Hutchins G. *Aspergillus* mural endocarditis. Am J Clin Pathol 1979; 71:640.
295. Maertens J, Van Eldere J, Verhaegen J, et al. Use of circulating galactomannan screening for early diagnosis of invasive *Aspergillus* in allogenic stem cell transplant recipients. J Infect Dis 2002; 186:129.
296. Walsh TJ, Pappas P, Winston DJ, et al. Voriconazole compared with liposomal amphotericin B for empirical antifungal therapy in patients with neutropenia and persistent fever. N Engl J Med 2002; 346:225.
297. Denning DW. Aspergillosis: diagnosis and treatment. Intern J Antimicrob Agents 1996; 6:168.
298. Blair T, Waugh R, Pollock M, et al. *Histoplasma capsulatum* endocarditis. Am Heart J 1980; 99:783.
299. Alexander W, Mowry R, Cobbs G, et al. Prosthetic valve endocarditis caused by *Histoplasma capsulatum*. JAMA 1979; 22:1399.
300. Bhatti S, Vilenski L, Tight R, Smego RA, Jr. The Histoplasma endocarditis: clinical and mycological features and outcome. J Infect 2005; 51:2.
301. Horstkotte D, Schulte H, Bircks W. Factors influencing prognosis and indication for surgical intervention native valve endocarditis. In: Horstkotte D, Bodner E, eds. Infective Endocarditis. London: ICR Publishers, 1991:187a.

302. Sebghati TS, Engle JT, Goldman WE. Intracellular parasitism by *Histoplasma capsulatum*: fungal virulence and calcium dependence. Science 2000; 290:1368.
303. Welty FK, McLeod GX, Ezratty C, et al. *Pseudallescheria boydii* pulmonic valve endocarditis in a liver transplant recipient. Clin Infect Dis 1992; 15:858.
304. Keay S, Denning DW, Stevens DA. The endocarditis due to *Trichosporon bigelii*: in vitro susceptibility of isolates and review. Rev Infect Dis 1991; 13:383.
305. Pankey G. Acute bacterial endocarditis at the University of Minnesota Hospitals 1939–1959. Am Heart J 1962; 64:583.
306. Baddour Q, Meyer J, Henry B. Polymicrobial infective endocarditis in the 1980s. Rev Infect Dis 1991; 13:913.
307. Saravolatz L, Burch K, Quinn E, et al. Polymicrobial infective endocarditis. Am Heart J 1978; 95:163.
308. Valencia-Ortega ME, Enriquez Crego A, Guinea Esquerdo J, Gonzalez Lahoz J. Polymicrobial endocarditis: a clinical and evolutive study of 2 of cases diagnosed during a 10-year. Rev Clin Esp 1997; 197:245.
309. Lepidi H, Durack DT, Raoult D. Diagnostic methods: current best practices and guidelines for histologic evaluation in infective endocarditis. Infect Dis Clin North Am 2002; 16:339.
310. VanScoy R. Culture-negative endocarditis. Mayo Clin Proc 1982; 57:149.
311. Lamas CC, Eykyn SJ. Blood culture negative endocarditis: analysis of 63 cases presenting over 25 years. Heart 2003; 89:258.
312. Albrich WC, Kraft C, Fisk T, Albrecht H. A mechanic with a bad valve: blood-culture-negative endocarditis. Lancet 2004; 4:777.
313. Houpikian P, Raoult D. Blood culture-negative endocarditis in a reference center. Medicine 2005; 84:162.
314. Weinstein L. Infective endocarditis. In: Braunwald E, ed. Heart Disease: A Textbook of Cardiovascular Medicine. 3rd ed. Philadelphia: WB Saunders, 1988:1113.
315. Libman E. The clinical features of cases of subacute bacterial endocarditis that have spontaneously become bacteria free. Am J Med Sci 1913; 146:625.
316. Pesanti E, Smith I. Infective endocarditis with negative blood cultures: an analysis of 52 cases. Am J Med 1979; 66:43.
317. Hilton E, Lerner C, Lowry F, et al. "Culture-negative" prosthetic valve endocarditis. Arch Intern Med 1984; 144:2083.
318. Kupferwasser LI, Darius H, Muller AM, et al. Diagnosis of culture-negative endocarditis: the role of the Duke Criteria and the impact of transesophageal echocardiography. Am Heart J 2001; 142:146.
319. Zamorano J, Sanz J, Almeira C, et al. Differences between endocarditis with true negative blood cultures and those with previous antibiotic treatment. J Heart Valve Dis 2003; 12:256.

4   Pathology of Infective Endocarditis

Richard L. Kradin
Departments of Pathology and Medicine, Massachusetts General Hospital,
Boston, Massachusetts, U.S.A.

INTRODUCTION

The true incidence of infective endocarditis (IE) is uncertain, but it has been estimated to account for one out of every 1000 hospital admissions (1). The morbidity of this disorder is substantial, as it can cause cardiac valvular insufficiency, congestive heart failure, and cardiac conduction system abnormalities. Embolization of infected vegetations can damage vital organs, including brain, kidney, and lung. Circulating immune complexes that develop in response to endovascular infection can yield microvascular injury, arthritis, and renal failure.

Revised diagnostic criteria for IE have improved diagnostic accuracy (2), although cases of IE continue to be discovered at the time of valve surgery and at autopsy. The emergence of fastidious microorganisms has led to increased recognition of the microbiologic spectrum of this disease. The widespread use of endovascular prosthetic devices and bioprosthetic grafts has expanded the scope of IE and complicated its management (3). Finally, research into bacterial interactions with vascular endothelium, and recognition of the importance of bacterial biofilms promise to change the mode of treatment of IE in the future.

The pathology of IE is complex; it reflects the virulence of the organism, host immunity, the biology of the endocardial surface, and the topography of infection. For example, infection of a cardiac valve by *Staphylococcus aureus* in a patient with AIDS is more likely to produce a rapidly progressive syndrome of valvular incompetence and acute heart failure than endocarditis, owing to an organism of low virulence in a normal host. Whereas IE can affect an ostensibly normal endocardial surface, it far more commonly targets anatomically distorted valves (4) (Table 1). The site of infection is critical with respect to the spectrum of possible complications, so that the IE on the left side of the heart is more likely to result in acutely life-threatening embolic events, including cerebral and myocardial emboli, than right-heart endocarditis. Extension of aortic valve infection into the heart can produce myocardial abscess and complete heart block. Infected fistulous tracts forming between cardiac chambers can lead to intracardiac shunting of blood, depending on the anatomy of the involved valve. For these reasons, IE must always be approached nongenerically, as specific pathology determines both potential complications and the optimal therapeutic approach in each case.

THE CARDIAC VALVES

Most cases of IE involve the cardiac valves. The normal atrioventricular mitral and tricuspid valves of the cardiac inflow tracts and the semilunar aortic and pulmonary valves of the outflow tracts share a common structure. They consist of a dense avascular collagenous core, termed the valvular fibrosa that is contiguous with the fibrous skeleton of the heart, surrounded by a spongiosa that consists of a loose

TABLE 1   Conditions Associated with Infective Endocarditis

Rheumatic valvular disease	Mechanical prosthetic valves
Bioprosthetic valve	Swan–Ganz catheter
Post-traumatic valvulitis	Pacemaker leads
Annular calcifications	Internal defibrillators
Atherosclerotic degeneration	Left ventricular assist devices
Mural thrombi	Intravenous catheters
Hypertrophic cardiomyopathy	Intravenous hyperalimentation
	Hemodialysis shunts

matrix of collagen, elastic fibers, and glycosaminoglycans. The valve surfaces are lined by endothelium. This topographic arrangement is critical to the normal function of the valves during the cardiac cycle. The cardiac ventricles are filled with blood that passes through the open leaflets of atrioventricular valves during diastole, and the valves must remain tightly apposed during systole. Conversely, the semilunar valves must open during systole, and remain competently closed during diastole. This is achieved by the elastic and deformable properties of the valves. As the normal cardiac valve is normally avascular, stromal cells that contribute to both the valvular fibrosa and spongiosa must dynamically maintain valvular structure.

With the mechanical wear and tear that accompanies age—the valves must open and close almost three million times in the course of a 75-year lifetime—the normal configuration of the valve changes. Fibrosis is the most common complication of aging, whereas myxomatous change can result from either altered hemodynamics, for example, the functional insufficiency that follows dilatation of a valve ring, or genetically encoded defects, like Marfan's syndrome.

Mechanical degeneration leads to increased collagen deposition by valvular mesenchymal cells, and to a relative decrease in the size of the spongiosa. In addition, shear forces produce focal endothelial denudation of the valvular surface, leading to the deposition of a platelet–fibrin coagulum that signals subendothelial fibrogenesis.

Valvular calcifications complicate both age-related fibrosis and postinflammatory valvulitis. The structural distortions produced by scarring are further enhanced by calcifications that grow by accretion to be nodular and bulky, leading to valvular stenosis and insufficiency (5). In some cases, concomitant foci of ossification also develop.

Rheumatic fever, an immunologic complication of group A *Streptococcal* infection, is the most common cause of valvulitis. Rheumatic fever causes a pancarditis that affects the cardiac valves, myocardium, and pericardium. Histiocytic inflammation is accompanied by neovascularization and fibrosis. In the case of the atrioventricular valves, the chordae tendinae become scarred and foreshortened, promoting the late hemodynamic consequences of valvular distortion. The end result is a scarred valve that is predisposed to further deformation by dystrophic calcification, and functionally to both stenosis and insufficiency (6).

INFECTIVE ENDOCARDITIS

Infective endocarditis results from the growth of microorganims on the endocardial surfaces of either the cardiac valves or vascular endothelium. Most infections are caused by bacteria that have been entrapped in a mesh of fibrin and platelets, previously deposited along an injured endocardial surface. These deposits are termed *vegetations*. They are friable, and grow by accretion to be potentially bulky, depending on the cause, location, and duration of the infection. In the absence of antimicrobial treatment, effective healing of vegetations does not occur, and the risk of infected platelet–thrombi dislodging and traveling into the circulation is substantial.

In the past, IE was termed bacterial endocarditis, but with increased recognition that nonbacterial species, including fungi and rickettsia can also cause endocarditis, the term infective endocarditis is currently preferred. Modifiers, such as acute, subacute, or chronic, refer to the clinical course of the disease; however, they are imprecise and do not correlate well with the underlying pathology. Instead, IE should be considered a spectral disorder that can exhibit either an aggressive or indolent course, depending on the circumstances of infection.

The once universal mortality of IE has been substantially reduced by improved diagnosis, antimicrobial treatment, and aggressive surgical intervention. The current mortality ranges from 10% to 30% (7). In the first half of the twentieth century, the vast majority of cases of IE complicated rheumatic mitral valvular disease. However, with decreased prevalence of rheumatic valvular disease and increased aging of the population, the senile fibrocalcific aortic valve has become an increasingly common target (8). New sources of infection include intravenous drug use and the widespread iatrogenic use of intravenous catheterization (9). Host immunosuppression, in patients receiving corticosteroids and other immunosuppressant agents, HIV-1 infection (10), diabetes, renal failure, alcoholism, and cirrhosis all substantially increase the risk for developing IE (11).

Cardiac and vascular prostheses are potential niduses for infection, and remain at continued risk for IE following implantation (12). Right-heart pacemaker implantation can lead to infection along the pacemaker leads and the tricuspid valve. *Staphylococcus aureus* and *Staphylococcus epidermidis* are the most common early (the first 60 days) and late pathogens, respectively, following implantation (13). Left ventricular assist devices are currently used in the treatment of intractable left ventricular failure and as a "bridge" to cardiac transplantation. The prevalence of IE associated with these devices ranges from 15% to 44%, and the diagnosis can be difficult to establish noninvasively. *Enterococcus* sp. and *Staphylococcal* sp. are the most common infections, but fungi and low virulence organisms also cause disease (14).

Pathogenesis of Infective Endocarditis

Experimental models have demonstrated that a catheter introduced into the right heart of rabbits or rats, can cause endothelial injury of the tricuspid valve (15). Endocardial injury greatly increases the risk of developing IE when coupled with subsequent exposure to circulating bacteria (Fig. 1). Endothelial injury exposes basement membrane proteins, including laminin, fibronectin, and vitronectin, which serve as adhesion molecules for bacteria. Activation of platelets and thrombus formation further promote bacterial adhesion. Bacterial binding to thrombus is followed by a lag period of several hours before bacterial proliferation is detected (16).

The risk of developing experimental disease is a function of the virulence and size of the bacterial inoculum, and whether the injurious catheter is left in place or removed. When a bacterial inoculum is introduced after catheter removal, the risk

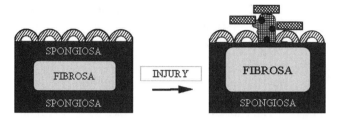

FIGURE 1 Pathogenesis of infective endocarditis. The figure shows the sequence of events leading from the configuration of a normal cardiac valve to a scarred valve, with increased valvular *fibrosa*, endothelial (▨) denudation, and the deposition of fibrin (■) with platelets (▩) and bacteria (▦).

of developing IE decreases progressively with time. The histopathology of the valve shows healing of the catheter-induced lesion by re-endothelialization, which appears to protect against subsequent bacterial colonization.

Other animal models of IE that do not require an indwelling catheter have been developed. In the guinea pig, electrocoagulation of the aortic valve, followed by inoculation with *Staphyloccocal aureus* or *Coxiella burnetti* yields IE. In addition, electrical stimulation of the cervical vagus nerve can result in the injury of the mitral valve, and predisposes to IE with subsequent bacterial challenge.

Specific microbial factors have been examined in the pathogenesis of IE (17). Resistance by an *S. aureus* species to a thrombin-induced microbiocidal protein protects against IE. Fibronectin-binding proteins expressed by *S. aureus* facilitate binding to fibronectin, and act as invasins. Organisms that do not bind fibronectin show decreased propensity to cause IE. Gelatinase/type IV collagenase enhances the virulence of *Streptococcus gorgoni*, and an aggregation substance expressed by *Enterococcus fecalis* increases virulence in the catheter-injury model.

Biofilm formation plays a critical role in the pathogenesis of IE and has important consequences with respect to its treatment (18). Bacteria can survive as isolated free-living planktonic organisms or as stationary colonies associated with a substratum. Four criteria have been proposed for the biofilm etiology of infection. These include the adherence of pathogenic bacteria to a substratum; the presence of bacteria in clusters or colonies associated with either an endogenous or host-derived matrix; localized infection; and resistance to antibiotic therapy despite sensitivity of the planktonic organism. Most, if not all, cases of IE associated with prosthetic surfaces, meet these criteria. Bacteria within biofilms produce extracellular polymeric substances—slime-producing glycocalices that limit the accessibility of host humoral and cellular defenses and antibiotics to those organisms that are matrix embedded. Biofilms confer other advantages to the bacterial colonies as well. When the availability of growth requirements is limited, biofilm bacteria can convert to a slow-growing stationary state, so-called "persisters." Water channels form within the biomass, and serve as a circulatory system via which nutrients are shared and waste products are released. The activities of the biofilm are coordinated by redundant interbacterial genetic signals. The properties of the biofilm make it virtually impossible to eradicate infection as long as the stationary phase persists. Organisms can spread along surfaces via a "ripple" effect, or alternatively, as detached clumps of organisms that can break free of the substratum matrix and travel to distant sites via the circulating blood. These mechanisms explain the local and distant spread of infection in IE.

Hemodynamic Factors that Predispose to the Development of Infective Endoarditis

Structural deformation of a cardiac valve can lead to local shear stresses and injury (16). Jet lesions, produced by critically stenotic valves or shunts from the systemic to pulmonary circulation, increase the risk of IE. Bicuspid aortic valves are at risk owing to their propensity to cause both stenosis and insufficiency (19). Aortic insufficiency of the aortic valve also increases the risk of mitral valve endocarditis, as regurgitant flow through an incompetent aortic valve causes fluttering and superficial injury of the anterior mitral leaflet. A comparable mechanism accounts for mural endocarditis along the ventricular septum in aortic insufficiency. In mitral insufficiency, vegetations may develop along jet lesions formed in the left atrium (20).

In the absence of primary involvement of the cardiac valve, other conditions, including mitral annular calcification and mural thrombi, become important sites of infection in IE. Left-to-right shunts, owing to congenital heart disease, show a propensity to cause endocarditis at the maximum site of the jet stream. Ventricular septal defects are at high risk, whereas secundum atrial septal defects rarely develop IE. However, endocardial cushion or septum primum defects that involve the mitral apparatus and patent ductus lesions are at risk. Approximately 5% of patients with hypertrophic cardiomyopathy and asymmetric septal thickening (IHSS) will develop IE (21).

Microbiology of Infective Endocarditis

Virtually all bacterial and fungal pathogens have been reported to cause IE (Table 2). The most common cause of IE continues to be *Streptococcus viridans*, a low virulence organism that is a part of the normal oral flora (22). The classical clinical scenario for the development of IE is transient bacteremia, caused by dental manipulation in a patient with rheumatic valvular disease. However, any site of active infection with access to the bloodstream can yield IE. These include cellulitis, puncture wounds, sinus disease, bronchiectasis, pneumonia, surgery within an unsterile field, and urogenital instrumentation (23). Other oral flora β-hemolytic streptococci, including *Streptococcus sanguis*, *Streptococcus mitis*, *Streptococcus mutans*, and *Streptococcus milleri*, account for approximately half the cases of IE in the community. *Streptococcus pneumoniae* endocarditis is an unusual complication of a pyogenic pneumonia, otitis media, or meningitis (24). Patients with defects of opsonization, splenic insufficiency, and diminished phagocytotic capacity are at increased risk. Infective endocarditis owing to group D streptococci—enterococci, *Streptococcus bovis*, *Streptococcus fecalis*, and *Streptococcus faecium*—complicates bowel pathologies, including colon carcinoma

TABLE 2 Organisms that Cause Infective Endocarditis

Organism	Cases (%)
Streptococci[a]	6–80
Enterococci	5–18
Staphylococci[b]	20–35
Gram-negative bacilli	2–13
Fungi	2–4
Culture negative	5–24

[a]Includes *Streptococcus viridans* and other *Streptococci* sp.
[b]Includes coagulase-positive and coagulase-negative organisms.
Source: From Ref. 21.

and diverticulitis, and urogenital instrumentation. These organisms account for ~20% of cases of IE, and *S. aureus*, *Staphylococcus epidermidis*, gram-negative bacilli (25), culture-negative organisms, and fungi roughly account for the remainder.

Infective endocarditis of prosthetic valves is associated with a high rate of complications, including valvular incompetence, obstruction of blood flow, and embolic phenomena (26). In bioprosthetic valves, IE generally affects the valve cusps, whereas mechanical prosthetic valves develop infections primarily along their sewing rings. Most cases of endocarditis occur within the first six months of implantation, but there is a steady annual rate of infection of 2% to 4% (12). Early infection, within the first 60 days following implantation, is caused by *S. aureus*, gram-negative bacteria, including *Klebsiella* sp. and coliforms, or by fungi, most often *Candida* sp. Coagulase-negative *S. aureus* accounts for approximately half of the late cases of IE, and nonvirulent organisms, including *S. epidermidis* and *S. alba*, account for the majority of the remainder.

Intravenous drug users have a high incidence of IE (26). The organisms isolated from blood in these patients tend to be virulent, and include *S. aureus* and *Pseudomonas* sp. *Candida albicans* and other fungi account for 10% of the cases. Involvement of the tricuspid valve is most common, but mutivalvular disease also occurs. Embolic complications may involve both the lungs and the left side of the circulation.

Blood culture-negative endocarditis accounts for approximately 10% of the cases at most major medical centers (27). Slow-growing gram-negative bacilli can require several weeks before they are detected in culture, and it is optimal laboratory practice to save blood cultures at least three weeks before discarding them as negative. This group of bacteria has collectively been referred to by the acronym HACEK (*Hemophilus* spp., *Actinobacillus* spp., *Cardiobacterium hominis*, *Eikenella corrodens*, and *Kingella kingii*).

Coxiella burnetti, the cause of Q-fever endocarditis, often eludes diagnose (28). Blood cultures may be negative and vegetations difficult to detect. The noninvasive diagnosis rests on serological and polymerase chain reaction (PCR) results. Other uncommon culture-negative organisms must be considered in the differential diagnosis. *Trophyrema whipelli* (Whipple's bacillus) can cause culture-negative endocarditis, and the noninvasive diagnosis centers on PCR, as cross-reactivity with *C. burnetti* confounds serological testing (29). The diagnosis may require ultrastructural examination to detect characteristic *Whipple bodies*. The cases of IE owing to *Chlamydia* sp. are uncommon, and their clinical and pathologic features mimic those of *C. burnetti*.

Pathology of Infective Endocarditis
Gross Pathology
The sine qua non of IE is the vegetation. These are friable fibrinous excrescences that develop along the endocardial surface. Most vegetations in IE are polypoid, but they can alternatively be sessile. Vegetations vary in size, in part dependent on the causative organism, the length of infection, and whether they affect the right or left heart. In Q-fever, vegetations may be inconspicuous, exhibiting only a thin coating of fibrin along the valve surface. Bulky vegetations occur on the tricuspid valve reflecting the virulence of the organisms that tend to attack the valve in intravenous drug use, and the lower systolic pressures of the right ventricle. They are white or yellow, as opposed to the dark red vegetations that are usually present on the left

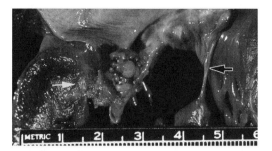

FIGURE 2 (*See color insert*) Vegetations along the mitral valve. The anterior leaflet of the mitral valve shows large polypoid vegetations owing to *Staphylococcus aureus* infection. Note the predominant involvement of the atrial surface of the leaflet. The valve was distorted by rheumatic valvular disease as evidenced by the thickened and shortened chordae tendinae (*white arrow*). Calcification of the mitral annulus is present (*outline arrow*).

side of the heart. Tricuspid vegetations have a propensity to involve the anterior leaflet of the valve, and to produce obstruction of the right ventricular outflow tract.

Vegetations along the mitral valve are dark tan or red (Fig. 2). They are distributed primarily along the atrial endocardial surfaces of the valve, but do not respect lines of closure. They can extend from the valve surface to involve the adjacent atrial endocardium, or spread inferiorly to infect the chordae tendinae. The continuity of the fibrous skeleton of the mitral and aortic valves allows extension of infection by direct contiguity. As the anterior leaflet of the mitral valve normally moves toward the aortic outflow tract during systole, infection can spread directly from one valve surface to the other, via the streaming of organisms at the surface of a biofilm. Infection may also extend directly into the adjacent valve annulus, and from there into the subjacent myocardium to produce a myocardial abscess and fistulous tracts to other cardiac chambers.

Vegetations of the aortic valve are generally smaller than those seen along the atrioventricular valves (Fig. 3). Infection weakens the valve cusps leading to aneurysmal dilatation of the sinuses of Valsalva or to tears and ruptures. Rupture of the chordal attachments of an atrioventricular valve may cause a sudden increase in valvular insufficiency, acute pulmonary edema or hepatic centrilobular necrosis, and peripheral congestion. If the disease is treated and arrested, healing of the valve takes place, but deformations can result in late hemodynamic complications. Local fibrosis or calcification may mark an area of healed endocarditis, and foci of limited rupture may persist as re-endothelialized fenestrations (Fig. 4).

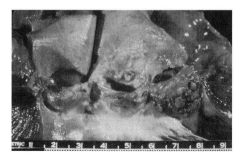

FIGURE 3 Aortic valve endocarditis. All three cusps of the aortic valve are involved by vegetations with the left coronary cusp (*right*) showing most severe disease. Note the relatively small size of the vegetations and the involvement of the ventricular surface of the cusps.

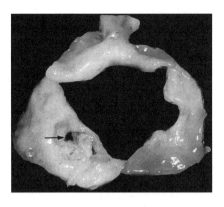

FIGURE 4 Healed aortic endocarditis. A healed vegetation is seen adjacent to a perforation of the noncoronary cusp (*arrow*). The left coronary cusp is also eroded along its free margin. The valve was resected owing to aortic insufficiency postantibiotic treatment.

Microscopic Pathology

The microscopic appearance of IE can vary from subtle to exuberant. In all cases of active IE, it is possible to discern fibrin deposition along the disrupted endocardial surface. Large polypoid excrescences of fibrin and platelets containing colonies of bacteria or fungi may be evident (Fig. 5). The vegetations may be paucicellular or acutely inflamed with areas of valvular and leukocyte necrosis. The valve cusp is edematous and commonly shows a heterogeneous infiltration of neutrophils and histiocytes. The extent and type of inflammation varies with the offending organism. Virulent pyogenic infections, for example those caused by *S. aureus* or *C. albicans,* show substantial acute neutrophilic inflammation, whereas less virulent organisms may show subtle leukocyte infiltration. Early inflammation is rapidly followed by neoangiogenesis and active fibroplasia (Fig. 6). In IE caused by *C. burnetti, Chlamydia* sp., and *T. whipelli,* fibrinous vegetations are scant, and the pathology primarily exhibits foamy histiocytes in areas of scarring (Fig. 7).

Demonstrating Microorganisms In Situ

The demonstration of microorganisms in situ is an essential part of the pathologic examination of IE. In most cases of IE that come to surgery, the diagnosis has previously been established by blood culture, and weeks of antibiotics have been administered prior to valve resection. It is incumbent upon the surgical pathologist to be certain that the surgeon has properly cultured the infected tissue at the time of surgical excision.

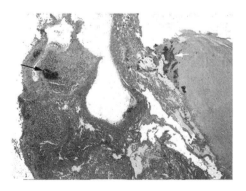

FIGURE 5 Histopathology of vegetation. A fibrotic and calcified aortic valve cusp (*white arrow*) shows vegetation composed of fibrin, platelets, neutrophils, and a colony of *Streptococcus viridans* (*black arrow*).

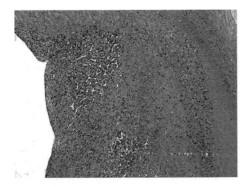

FIGURE 6 Histopathology of healing vegetation. Mitral valve in *Streptococcus viridans* endocarditis shows prominent neoangiogenesis and fibroplasia.

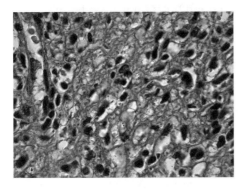

FIGURE 7 Histiocytic inflammation in *Coxiella burnetti* endocarditis. An area of scarring adjacent to an infected prosthetic aortic valve sewing ring with foamy histiocytic inflammation.

Rapid diagnosis may be enhanced by direct-touch preparations of the vegetations and appropriate histochemical or immunohistochemical staining of organisms.

Microscopic examination of the valve must include an assessment of inflammatory activity and whether there are local structural complications, including tears, perforations, and myocardial extension. The minimal battery of histochemical stains includes a tissue gram stain and a silver stain, such as Gomori methenamine silver (GMS). The tissue gram stain demonstrates most gram-positive and gram-negative organisms, but some gram-negative organisms, such as *Legionella* sp., require silver impregnation techniques. In addition, the phenomenon of variable staining of gram-positive organisms must not be overdiagnosed as polymicrobial infection (Fig. 8). In cases that have been treated, and where the underlying valvular pathology includes

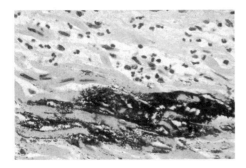

FIGURE 8 Tissue Gram stain of mitral vegetation. Tissue Gram stain (Brown–Hopps) shows a colony of gram-positive cocci consistent with *Staphylococcus aureus*. Note the area of Gram-variable staining that can be mistaken for polymicrobial (mixed gram-positive and -negative) infection.

dystrophic calcifications, it may be difficult to distinguish microcalcifiations from bacteria, as both can stain positive on both Gram and GMS stains. A positive Von Kossa stain for calcium phosphate can help to exclude the infection.

The GMS stain detects all gram-positive bacteria and some encapsulated gram-negatives, for example, *Klebsiella* sp. In cases that have received antibiotic treatment, residual organisms may fail to stain with the tissue gram stain, whereas they retain their GMS positivity. In those small numbers of cases where it is impossible to decide whether the putative organisms are real or artifactual, the area of interest can be removed from the paraffin block and processed for ultrastructural examination. Most fungi are well visualized on the hematoxylin and eosin (H&E) stain, but they are seen better with GMS. Screening of fungi should routinely include the GMS, as some fungal organisms, such as *Histoplasma capsulatum*, are not optimally visualized with periodic acid Schiff (PAS).

When a diagnosis of IE is clinically suspected but an organism has not been cultured, the pathologist must be prepared to demonstrate the presence of organisms by other methods. Mycobacteria can be demonstrated with routine or modified Ziehl–Nielsen stains. The modified acid-fast stain (Fite or Putts) also detects *Nocardia* sp., *Rhodococcus equii*, and *Legionella micdadei*.

Silver impregnation techniques, including the Warthin–Starry, Steiner, and Dieterle stains, decorate all eubacteria, including mycobacteria and actinomycetes. However, the high background in these stains can preclude a confident diagnosis. All culture-negative cases of endocarditis should be examined by silver impregnation (Fig. 9). Other special stains, like the Gimenez stain, have been used to demonstrate *C. burnetti*, and the Machiavello stain can assist in detecting *Rickettsiae* and *Chlamydia* sp.

Ultrastructural examination is useful when there is morphologic suspicion of infection by light microscopic examination. Most microbes withstand processing for routine paraffin sections, and can be identified with the electron microscope from the paraffin block (Fig. 10). Specific identification of microorganisms in situ can only be achieved by immunohistochemical or peptide nuclear agglutination techniques. Although antibodies to a wide variety of microbial agents have been developed, many are not commercially or widely available. In difficult cases, referrals to regional reference laboratories or to the Pathology Branch of the Centers for Disease Control, Atlanta, GA, U.S.A. can help establish the presence of an unusual pathogen.

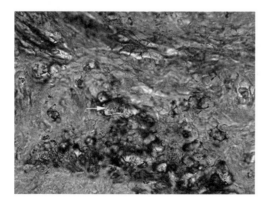

FIGURE 9 (*See color insert*) Silver impregnation (Warthin–Starry) in case of *Coxiella burnetti*. Warthin–Starry stain demonstrates small intracellular organisms that proved to be *Coxiella burnetti* by polymerase chain reaction assay.

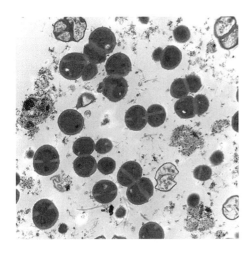

FIGURE 10 Ultrastructural appearance of gram-positive cocci from aortic valve endocarditis. The histologic appearance of a calcified infected valve was suspicious for bacteria, but a definitive diagnosis could not be established by light microscopy. Ultrastructural examination of a section of the paraffin block revealed diagnostic cocci.

Complications of Infective Endocarditis

Congestive heart failure is a major complication of IE. There are multiple pathways that lead to heart failure in IE, including (*i*) valvular insufficiency; (*ii*) valvular stenosis; (*iii*) rupture of an infected fistulous tract; and (*iv*) conduction system abnormalities.

Valvular insufficiency is the most common complication of IE. It reflects either destruction of the valve by tears or penetrations, or loss of structural support by tethering chordae or the valve ring. In mechanical prosthetic valves, direct involvement of Silastic balls, or metal discs and rings, is unusual, but paravalvular leaks secondary to dehiscence of the sewing ring are common (Fig. 11). Vegetations may

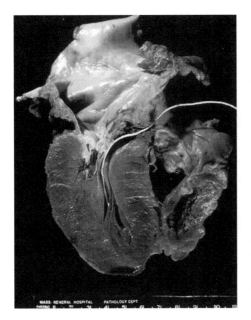

FIGURE 11 (*See color insert*) Fistulous tract complicating mitral valve endocarditis. Extension of infection from a vegetation of the mitral valve led to fistula formation between the left ventricle and right atrium. The patient died from acute right ventricular failure owing to a large left to right shunt. A small thread illustrates the fistula.

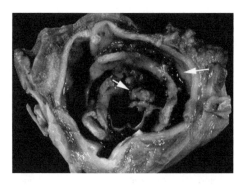

FIGURE 12 (*See color insert*) Infective endocarditis of a bioprosthetic valve. An aortic bioprosthesis shows vegetations bridging the cusps (*small arrow*) and involvement of the sewing ring that led to paravalvular insufficiency (*long arrow*).

interfere with the mechanics of the valve during the cardiac cycle leading to both stenosis and regurgitation.

Abscesses of the mitral valve can form fistulous tracts between the left ventricle and the right side of the heart (Fig. 12). Abscesses of the aortic sinuses of Valsalva can lead to fistulous tracts that communicate with the right atrium or right ventricle, leading to acute right heart failure owing to massive left-to-right shunting (Fig. 13). Periaortic valvular abscesses can extend directly into the adjacent atrioventricular (A-V) node causing conduction of A-V node and fascicular block (Fig. 14).

Embolic Complications

Embolic complications are common in IE. Involvement of the tricuspid valve by virulent organisms like *S. aureus* or *Candida* sp. is associated with bulky vegetations that fragment and travel to the lungs. As vegetations are composed of both infected and bland fibrin–platelet excrescences, the result is a potential mixture of bland pulmonary infarctions and septic pulmonary abscesses. Microthrombi can also travel through a patent foramen ovale (PFO) to produce embolic complications on the left side of the circulation (Fig. 15).

Emboli on the left side of the circulation may affect virtually any organ, but cerebral emboli are of greatest clinical concern (Fig. 16). Approximately 20% of

(A) **(B)** **(C)**

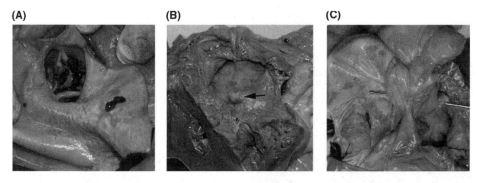

FIGURE 13 Rupture of sinus of Valsalva aneurysm (posterior noncoronary cusp). Patient with methicillin-resistant *Staphylococcus aureus*. (**A**) Aortic valve endocarditis developed aneurysm of the noncoronary sinus of Valsalva that ruptured acutely in the right atrium. (**B**) The area of rupture appears as a small nubbin on the right atrial surface. (**C**) The path of the fistulous tract is demonstrated by a probe.

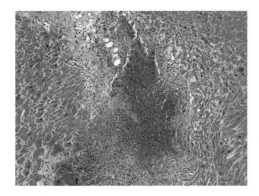

FIGURE 14 Myocardial abscess. Aortic valve endocarditis owing to *Streptococcus pneumoniae* extended into the adjacent myocardium leading to complete blockade of the atrioventricular node. Disrupted myocardial muscle cells surround a central abscess.

patients with IE develop cerebral emboli with an associated mortality of approximately 40% (8). Hemorrhages and cotton-wool Roth spots reflect septic emboli to the microcirculation of the retina. Splenic emboli (Fig. 17) can cause flank pain or diaphragmatic irritation, but may also be symptomatically silent. Renal microemboli produce a classic flea-bitten appearance of the cortex with focal segmental necrosis of the glomerular tuft. Janeway lesions are caused by microemboli to skin, whereas Osler's nodes are caused by arteriolar injury owing to immune complex deposition. Septic emboli to the skin must be distinguished from other

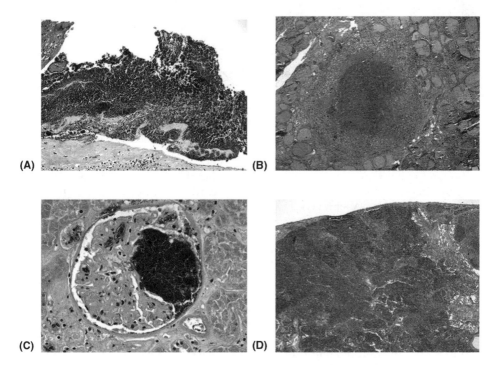

(A)　　　　(B)

(C)　　　　(D)

FIGURE 15 (*See color insert*) Tricuspid endocarditis in a patient with a patent foramen ovale. (**A**) Intravenous drug user with HIV-1 infection developed *Staphylococcus aureus* endocarditis of the tricuspid valve. At autopsy, infected lesions were found in (**B**) thyroid, (**C**) kidney, and (**D**) lung.

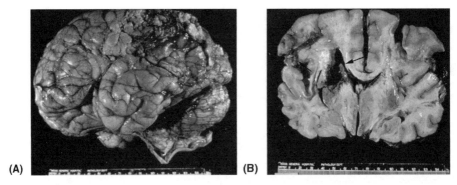

FIGURE 16 Bilateral acute cerebral embolic infarctions. Patient with *Staphylococcus aureus* aortic valve endocarditis developed acute hemiplegia, and then rapidly lapsed into coma and died. **(A)** The left cerebral hemisphere shows hemorrhagic infarction of parietal, temporal, and occipital lobes. **(B)** Coronal section shows hemorrhage in the left hemisphere with distortion of the lateral ventricles and die cephalic displacement.

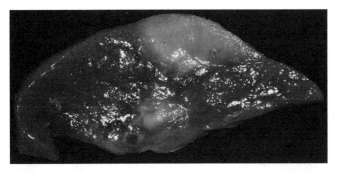

FIGURE 17 Splenic infarction. A pale subcapsular splenic infarction in a patient with *Streptococcus viridans* mitral endocarditis.

immune-mediated dermatoses like Sweet's syndrome (Fig. 18). Coronary artery emboli are uncommon, and are most often a complicated prosthetic aortic valve endocarditis (Fig. 19). Microemboli to the myocardium can produce patchy areas of necrosis (Bracht–Wachter bodies), leading to myocardial dysfunction and congestive heart failure.

Immune Complex Disease

Circulating immune complexes are detected in the vast majority of patients with IE. Rheumatoid factor can be demonstrated in 50% of patients with endocarditis after six weeks of infection (30). These circulating immune complexes include immunoglobulin, complement, and bacterial antigens (31). Immune complexes cause arthritis, subungual splinter hemorrhages, and skin lesions (32). In addition, the deposition of immune complexes leads to proliferative glomerulonephritis (Fig. 20) and renal failure. Mycotic aneurysms develop late in the course of IE, and most likely reflect a combination of infective emboli and immune complex deposition that predispose to aneurysmal dilatation and rupture of the affected vessel.

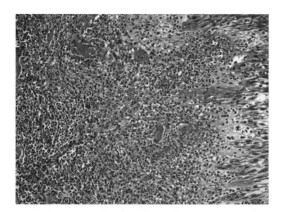

FIGURE 18 Neutrophilic dermatosis in a patient with aortic endocarditis. The patient was treated for *Staphylococcus aureus* aortic valve endocarditis for several weeks with clearance of bacteria from the blood and decreasing size of valvular vegetations by echocardiography. Subsequently, raised purpuric lesions developed on the extremities with hematuria and increased serum creatinine. Skin biopsy shows a neutrophilic infiltrate with no organisms, consistent with Sweet's syndrome. A kidney biopsy showed immunoglobumin A nephropathy, attributed to antibiotics (not shown).

Lesions that Mimic Infective Endocarditis

Other disorders can mimic both the clinical and pathologic findings of IE. Noninfective (bacterial) thrombotic endocarditis (NBTE) is caused by the presence of bland fibrin thrombi localized along the aortic and mitral valves. As opposed to the vegetations of IE that tend to involve any aspect of the valve cusp or ring, the lesions of NBTE are limited to the valve's lines of closure. On an average, the vegetations of IE are larger than those seen in NBTE, but these conditions cannot be distinguished based on size alone. NBTE represents a pathological syndrome that is associated with carcinomatosis owing to mucin-secreting malignancies, chronic infection, or in the later stages of other wasting diseases (marantic endocarditis). The pathogenesis appears to reflect a hypercoagulable state in the absence of bacteremia (33). The embolic complications of NBTE are comparable with those seen in IE (Fig. 21).

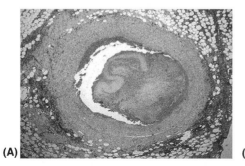
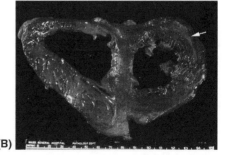

(A)   **(B)**

FIGURE 19 (*See color insert*) Coronary artery embolus from vegetation of aortic valve. (**A**) An infected embolus is seen in the circumflex artery. (**B**) The heart at autopsy shows an acute myocardial infarction of the lateral wall of the left ventricle caused by the embolus.

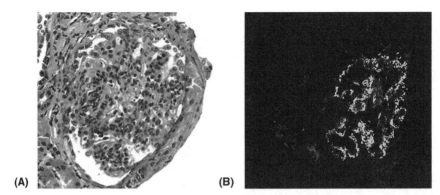

FIGURE 20 Immune-complex glomerulonephritis. A patient with *Streptococcus viridans* mitral endocarditis developed acute renal failure. (**A**) Kidney biopsy showed diffuse proliferative glomerulonephritis. (**B**) Direct immunofluorescence revealed granular deposition of immunoglobulin G and C3 (not shown).

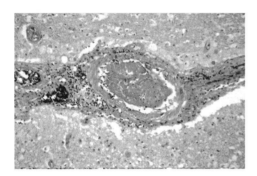

FIGURE 21 Cerebral embolus owing to noninfective thrombotic endocarditis of aortic valve. Patient with advanced carcinoma of the colon developed a lethal cerebral infarction. At autopsy, noninfective vegetations were seen along the lines of closure of the aortic valve, and a bland embolus was seen in the left carotid artery.

Other disorders, including rheumatic fever, Libmann–Sachs endocarditis, and carcinoid syndrome can produce lesions on the cardiac valves that mimic IE. Libmann–Sachs endocarditis affects the mitral valve, and is seen in 50% of fatal cases of systemic lupus erythematosus (SLE). The vegetations are flat, cover both surfaces of the valve cusp, and often extend to the adjacent atrial and ventricular myocardium. Histologically, the valve shows fibrinoid necrosis (Fig. 22). The

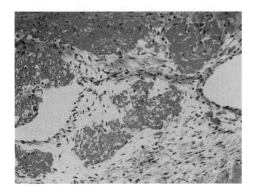

FIGURE 22 Libmann–Sachs Endocarditis. A 27-year-old woman died during an acute exacerbation of systemic lupus erythematosus. At autopsy, the mitral valve and surrounding endocardium showed small vegetations. The histology shows the fibrinoid necrosis of the valve cusp that is characteristic of Libmann–Sachs endocarditis.

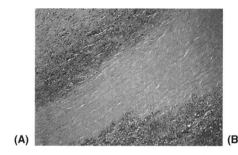 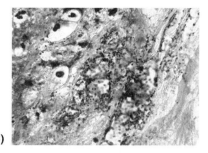

(A) **(B)**

FIGURE 23 Mycotic aortic aneurysm. A 75-year-old man died from rupture of mycotic thoracic aortic aneurysms. (**A**) The aortic media shows necrosis and abscess formation. (**B**) Gram stain revealed multiple lancet-shaped gram-positive diplococci, and cultures were positive for *Streptococcus pneumoniae.*

pulmonic and tricuspid valves may scar in response to a serotonin-secreting peripheral carcinoid. In the carcinoid syndrome, the pulmonic valve is either stenotic or incompetent, whereas insufficiency dominates with respect to the tricuspid valve. These findings are easily distinguished from vegetations, but can be difficult to distinguish from previously treated IE.

Mycotic Aortic Aneurysms
Infective endocarditis can complicate atherosclerotic aneurysms, and the outcome in the absence of aggressive medical and surgical intervention is invariably fatal. Infrarenal abdominal aortic aneurysms are most often affected, but any site is susceptible. Patients can present with the signs and symptoms of IE or the disease may be clinically silent. Pain in the region of the aneurysm is an ominous sign, as it often heralds imminent rupture. Efforts should be made to sterilize the lesion with antibiotics, but definitive treatment is surgical excision, and must not be unduly delayed.

Pathologically, the lesions show infection at the base of a mural thrombus with bacteria and acute inflammation that extends through the wall of the aneurysm (Fig. 23). Pseudoaneurysms may form in response to blood leaking from the vessel wall. Involvement of vascular grafts by IE mimics the features of prosthetic devices with infection primarily targeting the areas of graft anastomoses. Pseudoaneurysm and graft rupture are dreaded complications. Septic emboli may lodge at sites distal to the graft leading to infarction and abscess formation.

REFERENCES

1. Harris S. Definitions and demographic characteristics. In: Kaye D, ed. Infective Endocarditis. New York: Raven, 1990.
2. Durack D, Lukes A, Bright D. New criteria for diagnosis of infective endocarditis. Am J Med 1994; 96:200–209.
3. Romano G, Carozza F, Della Corte A, et al. Native versus primary prosthetic valve endocarditis: comparison of clinical features and long-term outcome in 353 patients. J Heart Valve Dis 2004; 13(2):200–208.
4. Davis WA, Kane JG, Gargusi VF. Human aeromonas infection: a review of the literature and a case report of endocarditis. Medicine (Baltimore) 1978; 57:267–277.
5. Pomerance A. Pathological and clinical study of calcification of the mitral valve ring. J Clin Pathol 1970; 23:354–361.

6.   Roberts W, Perloff J. Mitral valvular disease. A clinicopathological survey of the condi-
     tions causing the mitral valve to function abnormally. Ann Intern Med 1972; 77:939–975.
7.   Malquarti V, Saradariam W, Btienne J, et al. Prognosis of native valve infective endocar-
     ditis: a review of 253 cases. Eur Heart J 1984; 5:11–20.
8.   Chuangsuwanich T, Warnnissorn M, Leksrisakul P, et al. Pathology and etiology of 110
     consecutively removed aortic valves. J Med Assoc Thai 2004; 87(8):921–934.
9.   Reisberg B. Infective endocarditis in the narcotic addict. Prog Cardiovasc Dis 1979;
     22:193–204.
10. Bruno R, Sacchi P, Filice G. Overview on the incidence and the characteristics of
     HIV-related opportunistic infections and neoplasms of the heart: impact of highly active
     antiretroviral therapy. AIDS 2003; 17(suppl 1):S83–S87.
11. Devlin R, Andrews M-M, Fordham von Reyn C. Recent trends in infective endocarditis:
     influence of case definitions. Curr Opin Cardiol 2004; 19:134–139.
12. Watanakunakorn C. Prosthetic valve endocarditis. Prog Cardiovasc Dis 1979; 22:181–192.
13. Cacoub P, Leprince P, Nataf P, et al. Pacemaker infective endocarditis. Am J Cardiol 1998;
     82:480–484.
14. Herrmann M, Weyand M, Greshake B, et al. Left ventricular assist device infection is
     associated with increased mortality but is not a contraindication to transplantation.
     Circulation 1997; 95:814–817.
15. Freedman L, Valone J. Experimental infective endocarditis. Prog Cardiovasc Dis 1979; 22:
     169–180.
16. Durack D, Beeson P. Experimental bacterial endocarditis I. Colonisation of a sterile vege-
     tation. Survival of bacteria in endocardial vegetations. Br J Exp Pathol 1972; 53:44–53.
17. Moreillon P, Que Y. Infective endocarditis. Lancet 2004; 363:139–149.
18. Hall-Stoodley L, Costerton JW, Stoodley P. Bacterial biofilms: from the natural environ-
     ment to infectious disease. Nat Rev 2004; 2:95–105.
19. Sabet H, Edwards W, Tazelaar H, et al. Congenitally bicuspid aortic valves: a surgical
     pathology study of 542 cases (1991 through 1996) and a literature review of 2,715 addi-
     tional cases. Mayo Clin Proc 1999; 74:14–26.
20. MacMahon S, Hickey A, Wilcken D, et al. Risk of infective endocarditis in mitral valve
     prolapse with and without precordial systolic murmurs. Am J Cardiol 1986; 58:105–108.
21. Fowler VG, Scheld WM, Bayer AS. Endocarditis and intravascular infections. In: Mandell
     GL, Bennett GE, Dolin R, eds. Principles and Practice of Infectious Diseases. 6th ed.
     Philadelphia: Elsevier, 2005.
22. Bayliss R, Clarke C, Oakley C, sommerville W, Whitefield A, Young S. The microbiology
     and pathogenesis of infective endocarditis. Br Heart J 1983; 50:513–519.
23. Sullivan N, Sutter V, Mims M, et al. Clinical aspects of bacteraemia after manipulation of
     the genitourinary tract. J Infect Dis 1973; 127:49–55.
24. Wolff F, Regnier B, Witchitz S, et al. Pneumococcal endocarditis. Eur Heart J 1984; 5:77–80.
25. Cohen P, Maguire J, Weinstein L. Infective endocarditis caused by Gram-negative
     bacteria: a review of the literature 1945–1977. Prog Cardiovasc Dis 1980; 22:205–242.
26. Nahaas R, Weinstein M, Bartels J, et al. Infective endocarditis in intravenous drug users:
     a comparison of human immunodeficiency virus type 1-negative and -positive patients.
     J Infect Dis 1990; 162:967–970.
27. Bruneval P, Choucair J, Paraf F, et al. Detection of fastidious bacteria in cardiac valves in
     cases of blood culture negative endocarditis. J Clin Pathol 2001; 54:238–240.
28. Baca O. Pathogenesis of rickettsial infections—emphasis on Q fever. Eur J Epidemiol
     1991; 7:222–228.
29. Bouvet A, Acar J. New bacteriological aspects of infective endocarditis. Eur Heart J 1984;
     5:45–48.
30. Williams RC, Kunkel HG. Rheumatoid factors and their disappearance following
     therapy in patients with SBE. Arthritis Rheum 1965; 5:126–132.
31. Inhan R, Redecha P, Knechtle S, et al. Identification of bacterial antigens in circulating
     immune complexes of infective endocarditis. J Clin Invest 1982; 70:271–280.
32. Bayer A, Theofilopoulos A. Immunopathogenetic aspects of infective endocarditis. Chest
     1990; 97:204–212.
33. Kim H, Suzuki M, Lie J, et al. Non-bacterial thrombotic endocarditis (NBTE) and
     disseminated intravascular coagulation (DIC). Arch Pathol Lab Med 1977; 101:65–68.

5

Pathoanatomical, Pathophysiological, and Clinical Correlations

John L. Brusch
Harvard Medical School and Department of Medicine and Infectious Disease Service, Cambridge Health Alliance, Cambridge, Massachusetts, U.S.A.

INTRODUCTION

There are very few, if any, diseases whose pathogenesis is as well understood as that of infective endocarditis (IE). Over 150 years of basic and clinical research have defined most of the pathophysiological correlates of IE. Although there are many varieties of IE, they all share the same basic developmental steps. The goal of this chapter is to present the pathoanatomical, pathophysiological, and immunological events that are involved in the genesis of acute and subacute IE, and to correlate these with the clinical course of the disease.

Endocarditis has been studied by the giants of both pathology and clinical medicine. In 1847, Virchow first recognized the connection between bloodborne infections and IE in his description of a patient with valvular infection, complicated by embolization (1). Four years later, he examined valvular thrombi with a microscope and noticed "numerous granulosa, smaller than the nuclei of leukocytes, within many of the valvular thrombi" (2). In 1852, Luschka postulated that the heart valves became infected during the course of a bacteremia (3). The conclusion is correct, but it was based on the misconception that there was an extensive intravalvular vascular plexus feeding from the coronary arteries. What he was studying were not normal valves but those affected by rheumatic fever. Wadsworth, in 1914, described the role of immunological processes in the development of subacute IE (4). In 1885, William Osler presented the first complete account in English of IE in his three Goulstonian Lectures (5,6). In the early part of the twentieth century, both pathological and clinical knowledge of IE advanced rapidly (7). Weinstein and Lerner, in their landmark review (8), comprehensively summarized the state of IE two decades into the antibiotic era.

SETTING THE STAGE FOR VALVULAR INFECTION

Infective endocarditis may be classified according to its clinical course as acute or subacute; by the nature of the underlying cardiac pathology (native or prosthetic valve endocarditis); or by its epidemiology [intravenous drug abuser endocarditis (IVDA IE), healthcare-associated IE (HCIE)]. Although these entities are quite distinct clinically, they share a common pathogenesis (Table 1). All these varieties of IE have the development of a sterile platelet/fibrin thrombus, currently termed nonbacterial thrombotic endocarditis (NBTE), as the essential nidus for the development of endocardial infection (9). Since Osler's description of malignant endocarditis, explaining the distribution of infective vegetations became a challenge to students of this disease. The first valid explanation of the particular sites of endocardial infection was advanced by Lepesckin in 1952. He believed that mechanical and hydraulic forces played an important role in the development of IE. He based this conclusion on his study of 1024 autopsied cases of IE (10). This

TABLE 1 Steps in the Pathogenesis of Infective Endocarditis

Steps	Contributing factors
Damage to valvular endothelium or the endocardium	Endotheliosis Rheumatic valvulitis Degenerative valvular disease Trauma to the valve (vascular catheters) Hemodynamic turbulence Metabolic abnormalities Stress High output states Atrioventricular fistulas
Development of NBTE (platelet–fibrin thrombus deposition on endothelium)	Endothelial damage Hypercoagulable state Hydraulic forces
Bacterial adherence to NBTE	Bacteremia from a variety of sources Adherence factors Complement Antibody
Bacterial invasion of, and replication/ colonization within NBTE	Fibrin deposition and platelet aggregation that shelter the replicating bacteria Bacterial virulence factors

Abbreviation: NBTE, nonbacterial thrombotic endocarditis.

documented that 86% of cases involved the mitral valve; 55%, the aortic valve; 19.6%, the tricuspid valve; and 1.1%, the pulmonic valve. The resting pressures on the closed valves were 116, 72, 24, and 5 mmHg respectively. These findings suggested that the rate of valvular involvement was directly related to the hydraulic and mechanical stress to which it was exposed. In 1963, Rodbard documented the contribution of the Venturi effect to both the pathogenesis and the location of NBTE (11). He injected an aerosol of bacteria into a stream of air passing through an agar Venturi tube from a higher pressure source into a lower pressure sink (Fig. 1). This model replicated the characteristic pattern of IE with the maximum concentration of bacteria appearing in the lower pressure area immediately beyond an intracardiac constriction owing to decreased lateral pressure on the walls of the tube. In addition, the turbulence around the lower pressure side of the orifice is conducive to intravascular clotting that contributes to the formation of NBTE on the atrial side of the valve's surface. This one process produces the vegetations and a maximum concentration of bacteria to invade this platelet/ fibrin thrombus. For example, the IE of a regurgitant mitral valve involves the

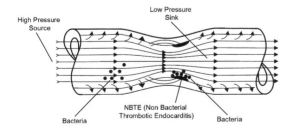

FIGURE 1 Localization of nonbacterial thrombotic endocarditis and maximum bacterial concentration as determined by the Venturi effect.

TABLE 2 Location of Infective Endocarditis Produced by the Venturi and Jet Effects

Lesion	Low-pressure sink	Location
Aortic insufficiency	Left ventricle	Ventricular surface of aortic valve and mitral chordae
Mitral insufficiency	Left atrium	Atrial surface of mitral valve and left atrium
Pulmonary insufficiency	Right ventricle	Ventricular surface of pulmonary valves
Tricuspid insufficiency	Right atrium	Atrial surface of tricuspid valve
Coarctation of the aorta	Distal aorta	Lateral wall of aorta distal to stenosis
Patent ductus arteriosus	Pulmonary artery	Pulmonary artery and pulmonary valve
Ventricular septal defect	Right ventricle	Right ventricular side of defect and pulmonary artery

atrial side of the valve and the adjacent atrial endocardium. During systole, the blood, being squeezed from the left ventricle through the nearly closed mitral valve into the atrium, impacts and damages the endocardium (Mac Callum's patch). Thus does this "jet" effect also produce areas of atrial NBTE (12). Infection of a regurgitant aortic valve develops in a similar way. The vegetations are present on the ventricular surface (low-pressure sink) of the aortic leaflets. Table 2 lists the various locations of IE that are related to hydraulic mechanisms. Both the jet and Venturi effects are lessened in the presence of congestive failure associated with atrial fibrillation. Subacute bacterial endocarditis occurs infrequently in these patients because of the decrease in the turbulence of their blood flow. Large ventricular defects and those that connect chambers of equal volume lead to equalization of pressures and blunting of the jet and Venturi effects. Small isolated septal defects are good examples of this.

Changes in the rheology of blood also affect the morphology and the function of endothelial cells (13–15). In areas of laminar flow, the nuclei of endothelial cells are aligned in parallel. In turbulent areas, this alignment is lost. These cells, especially along the lines of closure of the valve, become polygonal and assess an increased amount of cytoplasmic filaments. This disruption of the blood flow also produces functional changes of the endothelium. The turbulence increases the adhesion of leukocytes to the blood vessel walls into the surface of cardiac valves. There is an increase in the reactivity of platelets on the surface of those cells that are subject to low shear stress. These changes may result in the endothelial cells having a lower threshold for the development of a sterile platelet thrombus.

It had been long recognized that stress alone, in certain animals held in captivity (pigs and opossums), can produce valvular alterations that promote the development of NBTE. These are the only two species of the animals that can develop spontaneous endocarditis (16). Hormonal manipulation, exposure to extreme cold or to high altitude, or production of high cardiac output states by surgically created arterovenous (AV) fistulas lead to the deposition of sterile platelet–fibrin thrombi (17–19).

Nonbacterial thrombotic endocarditis has been found in 1.3% of all autopsies (20). It is more commonly seen in chronic inflammatory states (systemic lupus erythematosus, rheumatoid arthritis) and a variety of wasting disorders (uremia, carcinoma) (21). In one series, 19% of the patients with underlying tumors had echocardiographic evidence of valvular vegetations. These were most often seen in cases of pancreatic cancer, lung cancer, and lymphoma (22). The common denominator of this increased incidence of sterile platelet–fibrin thrombi appears to be hypercoagulability.

Although "marantic" signifies a wasting state, the affected individual may appear quite healthy. In this type of patient, marantic endocarditis may present with a macro-embolic event. The lesions of marantic endocarditis are most frequently located on the low-pressure side of the valve.

Damage to the endothelial layer exposes the underlying extracellular matrix (ECM) proteins and induces the production of various tissue factors (TFs) that lead to platelet and fibrin deposition (NBTE) as part of the healing process (23). This disruption of the "teflon" endothelium may be brought about by several processes including rheumatic heart disease and degenerative valvular lesions (calcific deposits or atherosclerotic lesions). Twenty-five percent of middle-aged individuals exhibit microscopic ulcerations and inflammatory lesions, characteristic of arteriosclerosis (24,25). *Chlamydia pneumoniae* has been involved, although unproven, as a cause of atherosclerosis (26). If true, it would be a unique situation in which one microorganism set the stage for another type of bacterial infection. Thromboplastin and TF that reside in the exposed subendothelial layer trigger locally the clotting process, which results in a thrombus made up of fibrinogen–fibrin, platelets, and fibronectin (27). In IVDA IE, the valvular endothelium may be injured through repeated injections of the types of adult trends present in the illicit drugs. One study demonstrated talc embedded in the valves of IVDA (28). Repetitive injections of foreign proteins also may lead to NBTE on the basis of various immunological processes (29).

Rivaling in importance in these natural processes is the iatrogenic damage done to the valvular endothelium by the direct trauma of long intravascular lines that extend to the right or left side of the heart (Swan–Ganz). Every day, in our intensive care units (ICUs), we recreate the rabbit model of endocarditis of Garrison and Freedman (30). These investigators threaded a catheter from the femoral vein to the right heart. The aortic valve was then traumatized by scraping it with back-and-forth motion. The resultant area of NBTE was then infected by injecting a solution of *Staphylococcus aureus* through the catheter. This technique was modified to produce left-sided lesions (31). These experimentally produced infected thrombi closely resemble the early pathological changes of human IE (32,33). Initially, the bacteria were found in the surface of the coagulum covering the area of trauma. Gradually, the organisms were covered by a layer of fibrin. The bacteria living on the surface were the most metabolically active whereas those that resided within the vegetations were relatively indolent (34). Healthcare-associated infective endocarditis now accounts for approximately 20% of all cases of endocarditis (35). The intravascular catheter has become the prime source of HC-associated bloodstream infections (HCBSI) and HCIE. The pathogenesis of HCIE closely resembles that of these animal models. Thirty-three to seventy-eight percent of *S. aureus* HCBI are attributed to intravascular devices (36).

It had been long recognized that endocarditis can occur without any preexisting valvular pathology that could induce the formation of NBTE. This apparent exception was most striking in cases of IVDA IE caused by *S. aureus* (see earlier discussion). This pathogen can adhere to and invade endothelial cells (endotheliosis). It shares this property with a few other bacteria (*Coxiella burnetii, Legionella* spp., *Chlamydia* spp., *Bartonella* spp.) (37). By means of its fibronectin-binding proteins (FnBPA and FnBPB), *S. aureus* binds to plasma fibronectin, which in turn gets attached to the endothelium by means of vascular cell adhesion (VCA) molecules. It appears that local inflammation, such as arteriosclerosis, may trigger cytokine production that can promote the endothelial binding of fibronectin. Bridging of the fibronectin proteins across the endothelium leads to the uptake of the pathogen by these cells (Chapter 2). In response to this invasion, the endothelium produces tissue factor activity (TFA) of the extrinsic clotting system. This response eventually leads to the formation of microthrombi that evolve into a typical platelet–fibrin vegetation. The capability of *S. aureus* to produce NBTE de novo is an important reason why this organism has become the premier pathogen of IE (38).

SOURCE OF ORGANISMS FOR INFECTING THE NONBACTERIAL THROMBOTIC ENDOCARDITIS

The role of bacteremia is critical to the development of all types of IE. The organisms enter the vascular space by several pathways, including (*i*) spontaneously from an extracardiac site of infection; (*ii*) following manipulation of the oral cavity, upper airway, intestinal tract, or genitourinary system; (*iii*) damage to the mucosa (mucositis); and (*iv*) breakdown of the dermal barrier owing to the insertion of intravascular catheters.

Spontaneous bacteremias from an extracardiac focus infection, except for dental/oral cavity infections, are currently unusual. Prior to the development of antibiotics, pneumococcal pneumonia was a frequent cause of acute IE. This association is seldom encountered currently. Other infections that may be complicated by IE are acute hematogenous osteomyelitis owing to *S. aureus*, pyelonephritis, brucellosis, and rat-bite fever (39). Spontaneous bacteremia has been documented in 9% to 11% of patients with significant gingival disease (40). This rate of spontaneous BSI is significant but clearly surpassed by that associated with dental extractions (18–85%) (41). If vigorous retrieval techniques, such as using filters to retrieve bacteria, are employed, 60% to 80% of healthy individuals may have a low level of bacteremia. The organisms involved in these silent bacteremias are generally considered nonpathogenic (40).

The concentrations and duration of organisms in the bloodstream during a procedure-related bacteremia are dependent on the degree of trauma associated with the intervention and the concentrations and the characteristics of the particular organism/organisms involved (41). There is a considerable variation in the data regarding the frequency of transient bacteremias. Most likely, this is caused by a lack of uniformity in the method of obtaining blood cultures. Optimal technique dictates that the quantity of blood for culture must be at least 10 mL. To detect postprocedural bacteremias, blood should be drawn at 5, 10, 15, and 30 minutes after the start time (42). The ideal ratio of blood to broth appears to be 1:10. The cultures are incubated at 37°C for at least four to six days. Longer periods are needed for fastidious organisms (refer Chapters 2 and 3). There are usually <10 colony-forming units (CFU)/mL. The bacteremia lasts less than 30 minutes, usually <15 minutes.

The importance of the degree of severity of gingival disease in determining the risk of procedure-related BSI and of IE is documented in the animal model of Overholser et al. These investigators induced gingivitis in rats by ligating their molars and then feeding them a diet rich in sucrose. When a catheter was placed into the carotid artery, 4% of the rats with gingival disease developed valvular infection. Seven percent of those not fed sucrose suffered this complication (43).

Transient BSI is documented in up to 85% of patients who have undergone extractions of teeth (41). The most common organisms are *Streptococcus viridans* and other streptococcal spp., diphtheroids, *Staphylococcus epidermidis*, various oral anaerobes and occasionally enterococci. When multiple teeth are removed, the bacteremia may last five to 10 minutes. The number of CFU is at the most 40/mL. Chewing hard candy (17–51%), various periodontal procedures (32–88%), an oral irrigation device (27–50%), and tooth brushing (0–26%) also cause transient BSI. Winslow and Kobernick studied in depth the connection between the severity of gum disease and the risk of developing a transient bacteremia and the concentration of organisms that made up the bacteremia. They stratified the patients into three groups based on the degree of gingival disease. All underwent removal of scale and curettage of the gums. Spontaneous bacteremias were seen in a few individuals with periodontitis and uncomplicated gingivitis. There was none in those with simple gingivitis (44). The CFU/ml was found to be directly proportional to the activity of gingival disease. The authors concluded that there is a significantly increased risk of BSI when prophylactic procedures are employed in patients with periodontitis. The significance of these types of transient bacteremias was questioned by the investigators in the comment that "the bacteremia produced by prophylaxis and other dental procedures have no clinical importance in the great majority of instances."

Other procedures performed on the upper airway and oral pharyngeal areas also have led to BSI. These include tonsilloadenoidectomy (28–38%) and rigid bronchoscopy (15%). The organisms recovered from these bacteremias are *S. aureus*, streptococci, *Hemophilus* spp., *Streptococcus pneumoniae*, and *S. epidermidis*. Sixteen percent of the patients who underwent nasotracheal suctioning, with or without intubation, developed BSI (45). *Escherichia coli*, *Klebsiella pneumoniae*, *Pseudomonas aeruginosa*, *Enterobacter aerogenes*, *Hemophilus influenzae*, *S. aureus*, viridans streptococci, and *Bacteroides* spp. were recovered in postprocedural blood cultures.

Table 3 illustrates the risk of bacteremia following several types of gastrointestinal (GI) procedures. In most studies, barium enemas seem to have a higher risk of bacteremia than colonoscopies. This may be attributed to (*i*) the trauma to the mucous membrane spot brought about by the pressure of this technique; (*ii*) abrasion of the wall of the rectum by the tip of the enema; and (*iii*) the increase in intraluminal pressure produced by the barium itself (41). Some indicate that there is no risk of bacteremia during colonoscopy (51).

TABLE 3 Characteristics of Transient Bacteremia Following Various Procedures on the Gastrointestinal Tract

Procedure	Rate of transient bacteremia (%)	Organisms involved
Fiber-optic endoscopy	8–12	*Propionibacterium aches*, *Acinetobacter calocoaceticus*, *Neisseria* spp., *Streptococcal* spp.
Sigmoidoscopy	9–13	Viridans streptococci, *Escherichia coli*, *Bacteroides* spp.
Barium enema	11	Viridans streptococci, *E. coli*, *Klebsiella* spp., *Bacteroides* spp.
Colonoscopy	2.5–5.3	Bacteremias occur less frequently than they do in barium enemas[a]
Liver biopsy	3–13	—
Sclerotherapy of esophageal varices	8–12	*Enterobacter cloacae*, coagulase-negative staphylococci

[a]See text for discussion.
Source: From Refs. 41, 46–53.

TABLE 4 Risk of Bacteremia Following Urological Procedures

Procedure	Risk of bacteremia (%)
Internal urethrotomy	75
Urethral dilatation	86
Transurethral prostatectomy	12–57.5 in the presence of bacteruria
Removal of Foley catheters in the presence of bacteruria	26.3
Retropubic prostatectomy with sterile urine	7.4–12.8
Cystoscopy in the presence of bacteruria	82.4

Source: From Ref. 41.

The presence of active viral or chronic hepatitis and cirrhosis due to any type may increase the risk of procedure-related BSI (52). Table 4 presents the risk of bacteremia following various urological procedures. Bloodstream infections may occur even in the presence of sterile urine (chronic prostatitis). In addition to infected urine, the primary sources of bacteremia include the urethral micro-flora, the prostate and contaminated instruments, or irrigation fluid (9). Table 5 presents the risk of bacteremia associated with a variety of gynecological/obstetrical procedures (54–58).

Prosthetic valve implantation is associated with two to four times the risk of infection as other open-heart procedures (59). Intraoperative BSI occurs in 20% of patients on cardiopulmonary bypass systems that are contaminated by airborne bacteria (60). The presence of infected wounds and urinary and respiratory infections contribute to the bacteremia of the postoperative period. Somewhat surprisingly, procedurally related BSI is a very unusual event during cardiac catheterizations or during other types of vascular angiographic studies when they are performed under strict conditions of sterility (61).

Bloodstream infections are common among individuals with burns involving >60% of their surface area (62). These patients are at high risk of developing IE. Nearly 1.5% to 2% of patients with significant burns develop IE (63,64). Fifty percent have right-sided involvement, 25% have left-sided disease, and 25% have both sides involved. Seventy-seven percent of the cases are attributed to *S. aureus* alone with 5% of them having a mix of *S. aureus* and gram negatives. Fourteen percent have gram negatives alone, often Providencia and Serratia. Sixty-one percent of the cases are acute. The diagnosis of IE in the burn patient is challenging because of a hyperdynamic nature of these individuals. They often have other causes of fever. Suppurative thrombophlebitis is common (1.4–4.2%) (65). Localized findings of the infection of the vein occur in only 35% of the cases. As a rule, multiply positive

TABLE 5 Risk of Bacteremia with Various Obstetrical/Gynecological Procedures

Procedure	Risk (%)	Organism
Natural childbirth	5	*Mycoplasma* spp.
Intrauterine device placement	0	—
Suction abortion	85	*Peptococcus, Peptosteptococcus, Lactobacillus, Veillonella,* viridans streptococci
Cervical biopsy	0	—

Source: From Refs. 54–58.

blood cultures, in the absence of suppurative thrombophlebitis, need to be considered the result of valvular infection. In this situation, echocardiography has proven to be very useful.

Infective endocarditis is present in 1.2% to 3.5% of patients with hepatic cirrhosis, especially those cases owing to alcohol (66). Valvular infection is unusual in other forms of chronic liver disease. It is speculated that the source of the bacteremia was primary peritonitis with the impaired reticuloendothelial system of the liver unable to clear the resultant BSI. Gram negatives, enterococci, other streptococcal species, and *S. aureus* have been isolated in these cases.

In 1978, Garvey and Neu were among the first who described cases of IE among immunosuppressed patients believed to be under no risk of developing IE. Among the underlying disorders were a variety of neoplastic processes—collagen vascular diseases, diabetes mellitus, renal failure, and treatment with corticosteroids and other immunosuppressive agents (67). A major source of bacteremia in these patients, which most likely causes damage to their mucous membranes (mucositis), is especially that of the GI tract (68). Mucositis of the GI tract is usually attributed to chemotherapy and radiation that may adversely affect the bowel's integrity. When this occurs, there is an increase in the transmigration of bowel flora into the bloodstream. The availability of hemopoietic growth factors and granulocyte colony–stimulating factor permits the use of high doses of radiation and chemotherapy with a corresponding increase in their cytotoxic effects (69). Concurrent defects in intestinal motility promote the overgrowth of *Candida* spp., *S. viridans* and gram-negative organisms. The various effective antibiotics on the normal flora of the GI tract promote excessive growth of organisms, such as *P. aeruginosa*, *Capnocytophaga* spp. and *S. mucilginosus* produced mucositis. The beta-lactam antibiotics, clindamycin and rifampin, have the most damaging effect on the mucosal barrier, and trimethoprim sulfamethoxazole and the quinolones the least.

Addiction to the use of parenteral drugs has become a major source of BSI. The intravenous drug abuser is the most common cause of IE in urban areas (70). Accurate determination of its incidence is hard to arrive at for several reasons (71). This population often has very irregular follow-up in the HC system. Right-sided IVDA IE, owing to the methicillin-sensitive *S. aureus* (MSSA), often can be treated for two weeks (72). There is anecdotal evidence that right-sided disease is amenable to much shorter courses, and is even treated by "on the street"-obtained antibiotics. In the United States, the best estimates indicate that 1% to 5% of IVDA develop valvular infection yearly. Up to 73% of individuals with IVDA IE have concurrent infection with HIV (73). The campaigns to decrease parenteral spread of HIV by clean needle-exchange programs and other methods appear to be decreasing the incidence of IVDA IE (74). *Staphylococcus aureus* produces at least 60% of cases of IVDA IE (75). The reservoir of these staphylococci is usually the nasal mucosa of the addict (76). From there, they transiently colonize the skin and enter the bloodstream during injection of the illicit materials (76). For other organisms, the source is usually the contamination of the injected substance or of the drug paraphernalia. Seventy percent of IVDA involves the right side of the heart with corresponding pulmonary symptoms of cough and pleuritic chest pain (70). For a more complete discussion of this topic refer to Chapter 7.

There are approximately 250,000 cases of HCBSI yearly in this country. The vast majority are attributed to intravascular catheters. Of these, 52% are caused by central venous catheters (CVC), 35% are caused by peripheral lines, and 3.7% secondary to arterial catheterization (77). Not surprisingly, more than half occur in

ICUs. The mean time of the onset of intravascular device–related bacteremias ranges from 12 to 26 days (78). Bloodstream infections are characterized as being primary or secondary in nature. Primary BSI (64% of all BSI) are infections that directly involve the bloodstream. Secondary BSI are the consequences of extravascular infections, such as pneumonia or urinary tract infections (79). The incidence of BSI may be affected by whether the surveillance definition or clinical definition is employed (80,81) (for further discussion refer to Chapter 4).

Until the 1980s, gram-negative aerobes were the primary cause of HCBSI. Currently, the gram positives, including coagulase-negative staphylococci (CoNS), *S. aureus* and enterococci, and Candida have become predominant (82). The rise in *S. aureus* and CoNS is attributed primarily to the increased placement of intravascular devices. Table 6 presents the pathogens currently isolated from cases of HCBSI. Approximately 25% of primary *S. aureus* bacteremia is complicated either by valvular infection or infection of other organs (83–85). Infected intravascular catheters produce 39% of *S. aureus* HCIE in patients hospitalized for other conditions. Infected ulcerations, wounds, or hemodialysis grafts were responsible for the remainder.

Gram-negative aerobes remain a significant factor in intravascular catheter infections, but unusually cause valvular infections. This situation is attributed to the inability of gram-negative aerobes to meet several requirements in the pathogenesis of valvular infection. First of these is for the organism to arrive at the target NBTE. To do so, it must be resistant to the bactericidal properties of serum that are primarily mediated by the complement system (86). The C5b-C9 components of complement (the membrane-attack complex) kill the gram-negative organisms by damaging their outer membrane. The plasma membranes of gram-positive bacteria are protected from the membrane-attack complex by the peptidoglycan layer. In an experimental rat model, these serum-sensitive organisms could produce valvular infection only as long as the induction catheter was present. Once removed, the infection clears spontaneously (87). Certain gram-negative isolates (*E. coli, Serratia marcescens*, and *P. aeruginosa*) are classified as serum resistant, in that they can produce experimental IE in the standard rabbit model. All of these experimentally resistant isolates, and the members of the HACEK (*Hemophilus* spp., *Actinobacillus* spp., *Cardiobacterium hominis, Eikenella corrodens*, and *Kingella kingii*) group, have been isolated from human cases of IE. The observation that Pseudomonas IVDA IE usually follows a subacute course supports the theory that preformed antibody may have some suppressive effect on the virulence of this extremely pathogenic organism.

Body piercing for cosmetic reasons is becoming increasingly common throughout the world (87a). It has been recently cited as a cause of IE from the

TABLE 6 Organisms Isolated from Cases of Health Care-Associated Bacteremia

Organism	Percentage of cases
Coagulase-negative staphylococci	31
Gram-negative aerobes[a]	22
Staphylococcus aureus	20
Enterococci	9
Candida spp.	9

[a]Include *Escherichia coli, Klebsiella* spp., *Pseudomonas* spp., *Enterobacter* spp., *Serratia* spp., and *Acinetobacter* spp.
Source: From Ref. 77.

resultant bacteremia. The particular pathogen is determined by the floor of the area of the body that is pierced—oral bacteria associated with lip piercing and *S. aureus* arising from skin piercing.

The role of preformed antibody in effecting the development of IE is unclear. Rabbits immunized against streptococcal species were relatively more resistant to the development of IE than their nonimmunized counterparts (88). This protective effect seems to hold for *Streptococcus sanguis*, *Streptococcus pneumoniae*, *Streptococcus mutans* and *Candida albicans* (89,90). The salutary effect of antibody appears to be organism specific. It did not hold true for *S. aureus* or *S. defectivus* (91,92). There is some evidence that specific preformed antibody may enhance the clearance of bacteremias by the reticuloendothelial system (93,94).

In contrast, agglutinating antibodies appear to have a vital role in the pathogenesis of subacute IE (4,16). This form of endocarditis is caused primarily by fully invasive organisms that depend on a pre-existent site of NBTE. The concentration of organisms in a spontaneous bacteremia is small, and does not reach the threshold that is necessary to initiate growth on the surface of the thrombus. High levels of agglutinating antibodies are the consequence of recurrent bacteremia with the oral streptococci. These agglutinating antibodies are not bactericidal (9,12). Over the years, they have achieved high enough levels to produce aggregates of bacteria (immune complexes) that are of sufficient size to initiate growth on the surface of the NBTE. These immune complexes play a key role in the progression and complications of subacute IE.

ADHERENCE OF ORGANISMS TO THE NONBACTERIAL THROMBOTIC ENDOCARDITIS

The stage is now set for the key step in the pathogenesis of IE, the adherence of the organisms to a preformed NBTE. Chapters 2 and 3 present in detail the virulence factors of individual organisms that promote adherence. Certain molecules on the surface of the circulating pathogen interact with corresponding molecules located on the NBTE. These are called microbial surface components recognizing adhesive matrix molecules (MSCRAMMs). The ECM molecules on the platelet/fibrin thrombus act as ligands for the various MSCRAMMs (95). Probably, the first MSCRAMMs identified are the surface glucans (dextrans) of streptococcal spp. Gould et al. noted that those organisms that adhere most readily to canine cardiac valves in vitro are the same as those most frequently involved in infecting an injured human valve (96). This ability correlates with the production of extracellular dextrans by several streptococcal spp. Parker and Ball demonstrated that the four streptococcal spp. with the greatest percentage of bacteremias, complicated by valvular infection, were also high producers of dextran (97). These were *S. mutans* (93%), *Streptococcus bovis* (86%), *Streptococcus mitior* (77%), and *S. sanguis* (75%). Only 45% of BSI with *Streptococcus faecalis* resulted in IE, whereas a comparable figure for *Streptococcus pyogenes* was 3%. The percentage of in vitro adherence was directly related to the amount of dextran produced in the system. The dextran MSCRAMM corresponding ligands, in vitro, are the platelet fibrin/thrombus and damaged cardiac valves. The addition of dextranase reversed the effect of dextran (98). This glucan also provides partial resistance of these streptococci to phagocytosis, and may be protective against a variety of antimicrobials (99).

As only a minority of organisms possess the capability of manufacturing dextran, there must be other means by which bacteria adhere to the platelet–fibrin thrombus (27,38,100). The most widely distributed ligand appears to be fibronectin. Fibronectin is a large matrix protein that is manufactured directly by injured endothelial cells and by fibroblasts and platelets that are recruited by the damaged endothelium. Many bacteria and *C. albicans* have MSCRAMMs complimentary to fibronectin (see later). Among the streptococci, *S. mutans*, *S. sanguis*, and probably enterococci and *S. pneumoniae* are able to adhere to fibronectin (101). Fim A is a MSCRAMM that is shared by many streptococci (*S. sanguis* and *S. pneumoniae*) and *Enteroccocus faecalis*. This MSCRAMM attaches to a variety of ECM substances. All streptoccocal fim A proteins are so similar in structure that there is a real possibility of producing cross-strain immunity. The ability of streptococcal spp. to bind to and then cause platelet aggregation has been best established for *S. sanguis* (102). This potential is not only important for initial adherence to the fibrin/platelet thrombus, but also for its propagation. As will be presented later, platelets act as a double-edged sword for the pathogenesis of IE. There appear to be many MSCRAMMs associated with viridans streptococci (Chapter 2). They remain incompletely characterized (103). Many bacteria are able to adhere to other ECM, such as laminin and type 4 collagen, by a variety of mechanisms (104).

Staphylococcus aureus adheres to fibronectin by means of fibronectin-binding proteins A and B and to fibrinogen/fibrin by means of clumping factor A (105). The functions of both MSCRAMMs support one another. Both adhere to NBTE. However, the fibronectin-binding proteins (FnbPs) are required for endothelial invasion which promotes thrombus proliferation through the release of TFA and various cytokines. Thus, FnbP becomes an important mediator for the persistence of *S. aureus*. The activity of the virulence factors of *S. aureus* is coordinated (Chapter 2) by the agr and sar genes (106). The production of the MSCRAMMs occurs during the phase of exponential growth. Secretion of the soluble virulence factors of *S. aureus* takes place during the postexponential growth phase (107). *Staphylococcus aureus* adheres to platelets rapidly and reversibly by means of an incompletely characterized adherence factor and ligand system (108). Adhesion-activated platelets may occur by means of thrombospondin and other factors (109). After the stage of platelet binding, *S. aureus* may trigger aggregation by bridging with fibrinogen (110).

Understanding the various components of the adherence phase is also important in developing strategies of prophylaxis against developing valvular infection. Early animal experiments indicated that bacteriostatic antibiotics are not very effective in preventing IE. These models used infecting innocula many times more concentrated than those of the transient bacteremias of humans (108 vs. 101–102) (111). When lower concentrations are employed, both bactericidal and bacteriostatic compounds appear effective (41,112). Even subinhibitory levels of antibiotics may be successful (113). It appears that antibiotic prophylaxis has dual mechanism interference with bacterial adherence to NBTE and bactericidal action on and within the platelet/fibrin thrombus (114). To decide the component which is more important depends on the particular pathogen involved, the specific antibiotic employed, and the state of development of NBTEs (Chapter 16).

BACTERIAL SURVIVAL AFTER ADHERENCE TO THE NONBACTERIAL THROMBOTIC ENDOCARDITIS

Moreillion calls this phase in the development of IE "in-situ bacterial persistence" (38). This terminology is somewhat misleading in that it is really quite an active one for the organisms. During this time, the bacteria shield themselves from the host's defenses, and set the stage for both local invasion and metastatic infection. Their primary defense is the enhancement of the platelet/fibrin thrombus. As cited earlier, antibody to adherence factors of *S. viridans* may be protective (115). Once they have made attachment to the thrombus and become embedded in the growing vegetation, they are protected against most of the host's defenses. In rabbits, induced antibody against enterococcal aggregation substance is not protective against IE. It cannot penetrate the clot adequately to reach the organisms within (116). Likewise, the thrombus denied them access to the invaders (117). Recognizing this failure of cellular and humoral immunity to change the course of experimental IE makes it easier to accept the observation that the incidence of IE is not significantly greater in many types of immunosupression. Curative therapy of IE is limited to the administration of antibiotics. As will be presented later and in Chapter 14, antimicrobial compounds face similar challenges in their penetration of the vegetation.

The NBTE matures into the classic vegetation of IE by enhancement of the localized production of TF, and by an increase in platelet aggregation. Tissue factor is a glycoprotein found in the membranes of endothelial cells, fibroblasts, and monocytes. In combination with activated factor VII, it activates factor X that in turn splits thrombin from prothrombin (118). Thrombin leads to the polymerization of fibrinogen to fibrin. Tissue factor also can activate platelets. Endothelial cells and fibroblasts are absent from the early infected vegetation (119). This leaves the monocyte as the source of TF at the start of IE. The binding of monocytes to fibrin and fibronectin triggers the production of TF (120). Unsuccesful attempts by these cells to take up streptococci that are already bound to fibrin induces TF production (121). *Staphylococcus aureus* and *S. epidermidis*, in combination with poorly defined ECM substances, are able to induce the production of TF (122).

As presented earlier, *S. aureus* can directly trigger TFA production by intact endothelium. This ability explains the production of TF in *S. aureus* IE, an infection which is generally devoid of monocytes. Other bacteria, *S. sanguis* and *S. epidermidis*, do so only in conjunction with monocytes (123).

Platelets play a dual role in the pathogenesis of IE. They both serve to grow the vegetation in addition to being the host's last line of defense. The ability of an organism to cause platelet aggregation, in general, is directly proportional to its involvement in IE. *Streptococcus sanguis* aggregates platelets in conjunction with plasma components adhering to protease-sensitive binding sites (124). By bridging with fibrin, *S. aureus* induces platelet aggregation (107). This process does not require the presence of plasma.

The alpha granules of platelets contain various antibacterial proteins [platelet microbicidal proteins (PMPs) in rabbits, thrombocidins in humans]. Isolates of *S. sanguis* that can trigger platelet aggregation had larger vegetations than those that did not have this ability (125). Platelet microbicidal proteins appear to kill *S. aureus* by damaging its cytoplasmic membrane (126). *Staphylococcus aureus*, isolated from human intravascular infections are more resistant to PMPs than the strains that caused other types of infections (127). To summarize the effect of the platelet on the course of IE, the platelet is the body's sole defensive weapon within the evolving vegetation which can be turned against the host by a pathogen that is resistant to its microbicidal proteins.

Aspirin appears to have beneficial effects in animal models of *S. aureus* IE (128). Aspirin and its principal metabolite, salicylic acid, decreased the amount of bacteria within the vegetation and reduced embolic events and bacterial adherence to fibrin. The parent compound works as an antiplatelet agent. Salicylic acid has a direct effect on the staphylococcus. Therapy with antiplatelet agents has an unproven role in the treatment of IE. Such an approach has potential risk of severe bleeding problems in the course of both acute and subacute disease.

Unlike aspirin, anticoagulants actually increase the degree of the secondary bacteremia arising from the infected valve (129). Fibrinolytic agents have similar negative effects (130).

Over time, the infected thrombus grows by successive deposition of platelets and fibrin. In subacute IE, numerous capillaries and fibroblasts migrate into the infected area in an eventually futile effort to repair the damage to the valve (131). These endothelial cells and fibroblasts become potential providers of TF. This is not the case in acute IE. There are no fibroblasts or capillaries present, only acute inflammatory cells (132). Shielded from the body's defenses, the organisms grow luxuriantly to reach concentrations of 109 to 1015 bacteria per gram of tissue (34). Those bacteria that lie deep within the vegetation are metabolically quite dormant (133). This combination of inactivity (lack of rapid growth phase) and the high number of organisms present a formidable challenge to the administered antibiotics.

PHASE OF LOCAL INVASION AND DISSEMINATION

The bacteria now are poised to invade the proximate cardiac structures and spread infection beyond the heart. This stage in valvular infections has gained so much attention owing to *S. aureus*. It is primarily FnBPA (Chapter 2) that enables *S. aureus* to invade the endothelial cells of the perivalvular tissues (134). Agr and sar genes are activated by quorum sensing of the increased bacterial growth. These genes control the release of exoenzymes, such as hemolysins and toxins (alpha toxin). These substances both harm the host and provide nutrients for further bacterial proliferation (135).

Dissemination of infection by means of bacteremia is dependent on the size of the vegetation and its fragility. These properties are related to the causative organism. Valvular vegetations that are infected by proteolytic strains of *S. faecalis*, are more friable than the those infected by many other types of organisms. The consequence of such a brittle thrombus is a higher density bacteremia, an increased incidence of septic emboli. All of these complications contribute to a decreased period of survival of the study animals (136). Although not thoroughly studied, the same sequence of events that resulted in the infection of the valve (adherence bacterial survival after adherence, and local invasion and dissemination) occur in the areas targeted by septic emboli.

CLINICAL PATHOPHYSIOLOGY OF INFECTIVE ENDOCARDITIS

The systemic clinical manifestations of IE, such as fever and malaise, are attributed most likely to several of the cytokines. Valvular infection impacts the various organ systems by one of three major mechanisms: (*i*) intracardiac damage; (*ii*) septic or sterile embolization; (*iii*) various immunological phenomenon (9,12,39,137). Many aspects of each will be discussed in detail in subsequent chapters. Table 7 summarizes the clinical impact of each.

TABLE 7 Mechanisms and Clinical Manifestations of Organ Damage
in Infective Endocarditis

Mechanism	Clinical manifestations
Intracardiac damage	Destruction of valvular leaflets
	Annular abcesses
	Myocardial or septal abcesses
	Suppurative pericarditis
	Papillary muscle rupture
	Aortocardiac and other fistula
	Mycotic aneurysm of sinus of valsalva
	Valvular outlet obstruction
Sterile or septic embolization	Stroke
	Metastatic infections
	Myocardial infarction
	Mycotic aneurysms
	Pulmonary infarcts
Immunological	Janeway lesions
	Roth spots
	Subungul hemorrhages
	Glomerulonephritis
	Various musculoskeletal manifestations

The intracardiac changes brought about by subacute disease are significantly different from those caused by the acute form (131,132,138). This is especially true for the valves themselves. The cusp, underlying the infected thrombus, is the site of destruction. In the subacute form, there are very few polymorphonuclear leukocytes and bacteria found in the valvular structures. Monocytes, lymphocytes, and histiocytes predominate. The repairative process is evidenced in the proliferation of capillaries and fibroblasts ("hypercapillarization"). These give a spongy texture to the vegetation. The repair efforts gradually lag behind the destructive ones. There is essentially no spread of infection beyond the valvular area. In acute IE, the vegetations are characterized by large amounts of bacteria and polymorphonuclear leukocytes within the ever-widening areas of necrosis. There are no areas of regeneration by "hyper capillarization." The destructive process inexorably spreads into the myocardium with a variety of suppurative complications (Chapter 4).

Embolization is second only to congestive heart failure as a complication of IE in both acute and subacute cases. Antibiotics have significantly reduced this process from >80% in the preantibiotic era to 15% to 43% currently. Corresponding figures, derived from postmortem examinations, are somewhat higher (45–65%) (9,39,139–141). Emboli most commonly travel to the kidney (56%), brain (33%), spleen (50%), and coronary arteries (56%). Splenic emboli are often of little clinical importance (9,139,142,143). Cerebral emboli occur in >33% of cases with the middle cerebral artery involved most frequently. Hemiplegia is the most common sequelae. In 1917, Jochmann observed "in hemiplegia in young adults or children always think of subacute bacterial endocarditis." This advice remains relevant in the current era. Cerebral emboli may occur for up to one year after microbiological cure has been achieved. Other embolic effects on the nervous system include cerebral microabcesses, cerebritis, and cranial nerve palsies. Paraplegia is the consequence of spinal artery embolization. Signs of typical peripheral neuropathy may result from embolic microinfarcts (142–146). Embolic brain abcesses are seen in acute disease. They are multiple and small in nature. Macroabcesses are most frequently seen in congenital heart disease (147).

Embolic occlusion of major blood vessels is uncommon. It most commonly occurs in cases of fungal IE, and less often in those of *S. aureus* or *Hemophilus* spp. Atrial myxoma or marantic endocarditis must be included in the differential diagnosis.

The consequences of embolization differ between those that occur during acute and subacute disease. Metastatic infection results from the emboli of acute IE, classically produced by *S. aureus*. Those of subacute disease are not capable of causing metastatic infection because of (*i*) lack of or limited virulence factors of the typical subacute organism (e.g., viridans streptococci); (*ii*) low concentration of organisms within the embolus; and (*iii*) presence of bactericidal antibody at the site of deposition (9).

Mycotic aneurysms occur more frequently in subacute IE. There are several mechanisms underlying their development (9): (*i*) occlusion of the vasa vasorum by microemboli; (*ii*) immune complex injury to the blood vessel wall; and (*iii*) direct bacterial invasion of the vessel's wall, the least common of these. They are located most frequently in the arteries of the brain, the abdominal aorta, the spleen, the sinus of Valsalva, the superior mesenteric artery, coronary arteries, pulmonary arteries, and a ligated ductus arteriosus. Of the cerebral arteries, the middle cerebral artery is involved the most often. Mycotic aneurysms typically develop at the point of bifurcation of the vessels. They usually are asymptomatic prior to their rupture (148,149).

In 1965, Cordeiro et al. presented the concept that a great deal of the clinical manifestations of subacute disease are caused by a variety of immunological processes (150). These investigators recognized the increase in 19S and 7S globulins, followed by a later rise in alpha-2 globulins in subacute IE. Some of these were found to bind specifically to glomerular basement membrane, vascular endothelium, and myocardium in vitro. These included agglutinating, bactericidal, and complement fixating antibodies and cryoglobulins. This distribution suggested that they played an important role in the pathogenesis of IE. In subacute IE, the immune system undergoes major changes. These include: (*i*) increased B-cell activity, leading to hypergammaglobulinemia; (*ii*) the appearance of circulating immune complexes; and (*iii*) stimulation of a generalized inflammatory response against the host tissue (151).

Subacute IE is the disease in which there is an ongoing stimulation of the cellular and humoral immune systems by an ongoing antigenemia. This process is quite similar to that seen in cases of malaria and leprosy. Immune complexes are detectable, by the Raji cell assay, in almost every patient with subacute endocardial infection. These are made up of immunoglobulins (Ig) G, A, and the components of the complement system. A prominent example is rheumatoid factor which consists most commonly of IgM, less often IgG, directed against IgG (152). This factor is present in approximately 50% of patients with subacute disease of more than two months' duration. It is not associated with any one particular organism, but its tide is most elevated when helping hemolytic streptococci are the inciting organisms. Extremely high levels of rheumatoid factor are found in patients with longstanding valvular infection and persistently sterile blood cultures. The more prolonged the course of IE, the higher are its levels. Titers decrease readily with antibiotic treatment. By two months after the start of therapy, they are undetectable (153). Serum levels of both IgG and IgM rheumatoid factor peak later than the circulating immune complexes. Administration of antibiotics clears the serum of circulating immune complexes more rapidly and completely than it does with the rheumatoid factors (154). Elevated levels of rheumatoid factor are also observed in acute IE (155). Approximately 25% of IVDA with *S. aureus* IE have circulating rheumatoid factor during the course of the disease. Its presence is positively correlated with the severity of the disease. At the end of therapy, failure to lessen the level of rheumatoid factor should strongly suggest the possibility of a relapse (156).

Rheumatoid factor also contributes to the pathogenesis of subacute IE. It interferes with the ability of polymorphonuclear leukocytes to phagocytize bacteria. It also interferes with opsonization by interfering with the Fc portion of 7s immunoglobulins. Both circulating immune complexes and rheumatoid factors can produce an Arthus-like reaction which produces an inflammatory response that turns on the chemotactic arm of the complement system (155).

Detection of circulating immune complexes by the Raji cell assay may distinguish simple bacteremia from that representing valvular infection (157). Ninety percent of those with IE, but only 50% of those without, had levels of circulating immune complexes. In the latter group, levels of these complexes were low.

Circulating immune complexes may cause many of the clinical findings of IE. The deposition of immune complexes on the glomerular basement membrane leads to the "lumpy-bumpy" of glomerulonephritis of IE (158). The deposition of immunoglobulins and complement has been detected by immunofluorescence studies. The location and size of the glomerular deposits is determined by the manner in which they are formed. Complexes that arise early in the course of IE tend to be small because they are formed during antigen excess and are deposited in the subepithelial area. Those that develop later are larger and are deposited in the subendothelial mesangium.

Although there are many different appearances by light microscopy of the glomerulonephritis of IE (focal, diffuse, and membranous), they arise from the same process. They may be, at least partially, cured by appropriate antibiotic therapy. Before the availability of antibiotics, 35% of patients with subacute IE developed significant renal failure. Repeatedly, blood cultures were sterile. This was described by Libman as bacteria-free stage of subacute disease. The current incidence of the bacteria-free stage is approximately 10% (159).

Many of the classic peripheral manifestations of subacute disease, such as purpura, Osler nodes, Roth spots, and subungual hemorrhages, may be attributed to circulating immune complexes. When these are deposited on the walls of small vessels, they can induce a localized leukocytoclastic vasculitis (160,161). Microscopy reveals a mixture of polymorphonuclear leukocytes, monocytes, and lymphocytes in these lesions. The pathogenesis of Osler nodes differs in patients with subacute and acute disease. Those that are associated with *S. aureus* IE are usually caused by septic emboli, as opposed to the sterile inflammatory reaction seen in IE caused by the organisms of subacute disease. Not all of the other, peripheral lesions of IE are caused by immunological mechanisms. Janeway lesions are almost always the result of septic microemboli (162). The pathogenesis of the various musculoskeletal manifestations of subacute IE, such as low back pain, is not well understood (163). Table 7 summarizes the mechanisms and clinical manifestations of organ damage owing to IE.

REFERENCES

1. Virchow F. Ueber die acute Entzundug der Arterien. Arch Pathol Anat Physiol Klin Med 1847; 1:272.
2. Virchow F. Gesammelte Abhandlugen zur wissenschschaftlichen Medicin, Frankfurt: Meidinger, 1856:709.
3. Luschka H. Das endocardium imd die endocarditis. Arch Pathol Anat Physiol 1852; 4:171.
4. Wadsworth AB. A study of the endocardial lesions developing pneumococcal infection in horses. J Med Res 1914; 39:279.
5. Cushing H. The Life of Sir William Osler. Vol. 1. Oxford; Clarendon Press, 1925.
6. Pruitt R. William Osler and his Goulstonian lectures on malignant endocarditis. Mayo Clin Proc 1982; 57:8.
7. Weinstein L, Brusch JL. The natural history of infective endocarditis prior to the availability of antimicrobial therapy. In: Weinstein L, Brusch JL. Infective Endocarditis. New York: the Oxford University Press, 1995:322.
8. Lerner P, Weinstein L. Infective endocarditis in the antibiotic era. N Engl J Med 1966; 274:199, 259, 307, 323.
9. Weinstein L, Schlesinger JJ. Pathoanatomic, pathophysiologic and clinical correlations in endocarditis (first of two parts). N Engl J Med 1974; 291:832.
10. Lepeschkin E. On the relation between the site of valvular involvement in endocarditis and the blood pressure resting on the valve. Am J Med Sci 1952; 224:318.
11. Rodbard S. Blood velocity and endocarditis. Circulation 1963; 27:18.
12. Weinstein L, Schlesinger JJ. Pathoanatomic, pathophysiologic and clinical correlations in endocarditis (second of two parts). N Engl J Med 1974; 291:1122.
13. Davies PF, Remuzzi A, Gordon EJ, et al. Turbulent fluid shear stress induces vascular endothelial turnover in vitro. Proc Natl Acad Sci USA 1986; 83:2114.
14. Langille BL. Integrity of arterial endothelium following acute exposure to high shear stress. Biotheology 1984; 21:333.
15. Dewey CF, Bossolari SR, Gimbrone MA, et al. The dynamic response of vascular endothelial cells to fluid shear stress. J Mech Eng 1981; 103:177.
16. Tunkel AR, Scheld WM. Experimental models of endocarditis. In: Kaye D, ed. Infective Endocarditis. New York: Raven Press, 1992:37.
17. Lee SH, Fisher B, Fisher ER, et al. Arteriovenous fistula and bacterial endocarditis. Surgery 1962; 52:463.
18. Oka M, Shirota A, Angrist A. Experimental endocarditis: endocrine factors in valve lesions on AV shunt rats. Arch Pathol 1966; 82:85.
19. Highman B, Altland P. Effect of exposure and acclimatization and cold on susceptibility of rats to bacterial endocarditis. Proc Soc Exp Biol Med 1962; 110:663.
20. Livornese L Jr, Korzeniowski OM. Pathogenesis of infective endocarditis. In: Kaye D, ed. Infective Endocarditis. New York: Raven Press, 1992:19.
21. Chino F, Kodama A, Otake M, et al. Nonbacterial thrombotic endocarditis in a Japanese autopsy sample: a review of 80 cases. Am Heart J 1975; 90:190.
22. Edoute Y, Haim N, Rinkevich D, et al. Cardiac valvular vegetations in cancer patients: a prospective echocardiographic study of 200 patients. Am J Med 1997; 102:252.
23. Gould K, Ramirez-Rhonda CH, Holmes RK, et al. Adherence of bacteria to heart valves in vitro. J Clin Invest 1975; 56:1364.
24. McKinsey DS, Ratts TE, Bisno AL. Underlying cardiac lesions in adults with infective endocarditis: the changing spectrum. Am J Med 1987; 82:681.
25. Stehbens WE, Delahunt B, Zuccollo JM. The histopathology of the endocardial sclerosis. Cardiovasc Pathol 2000; 9:161.
26. Maass M, Bartels C, Engel PM, et al. End of vascular presence of viable Chlamydia pneumoniae is a common phenomenon in coronary artery disease. J Am Coll Cardiol 1998; 31:827.
27. Moreillion P, Yok- Al Q. Infective endocarditis. The Lancet 2004; 363:139.
28. Cannon NJ, Cobbs NG. Infective endocarditis in drug addicts. In: Kaye D, ed. Infective Endocarditis. New York: Raven Press, 1992:11.

29. McGeown MG. Bacterial endocarditis: an experimental study of healing. J Pathol Bacteriol 1954; 67:179.

30. Garrison PK, Freedman LR. Experimental endocarditis. I staphylococcal endocarditis in rabbits resulted from placement of a polyethylene catheter in the right side of the heart. Yale J Biol Med 1970; 42:394.

31. Perlman BB, Freedman LR. Experimental endocarditis II. Staphylococcal infection of the aortic valve following placement of a polyethylene catheter in the left side of the heart. Yale J Biol Med 1971; 44:206.

32. McGowan D, Gillet R. Scanning electron microscopic observations on the initial lesions in experimental streptococcal endocarditis in the rabbit. Br J Exp Pathol 1980; 61:164.

33. Ferguson P, McColm A, Ryan D. Experimental staphylococcal endocarditis and aortitis: morphology of the initial colonization. Virchow's Arch (A) 1986; 410:93.

34. Durack DT, Beeson PB. Experimental bacterial endocarditis. II. Survival of bacteria in endocardial vegetations. Br J Exp Pathol 1972; 53:50.

35. Fowler V, Sanders L, Kong L, et al. Infective endocarditis due to Staphylococcus aureus. 59 prospectively identified cases with follow-up. Clin Infect Dis 1999; 28:106.

36. Gouello JP, Asfar P, Brenet O, et al. Nosocomial endocarditis in the intensive care unit: an analysis of 22 cases. Crit Care Med 2000; 28:377.

37. Broqui P, Raoult D. Endocarditis due to rare and fastidious bacteria. Clin Microbiol Rev 2001; 14:177.

38. Moreillion P, Que YA, Bayer AS. Pathogenesis of streptococcal and staphylococcal endocarditis. Infect Dis Clin NA 2002; 16:297.

39. Weinstein L, Brusch JL. Pathoanatomical, pathophysiological, and clinical correlations. In: Infective Endocarditis. New York: Oxford University Press, 1996:138.

40. Loesche WJ. Indigenous human flora and bacteremia. In: Kaplan EL, Taranta AV, eds. Infective Endocarditis. An American Heart Association Symposium. Dallas: American Heart Association, 1977:40.

41. Everett ED, Hirschman JV. Transient bacteremia and endocarditis: a review. Medicine 1977; 56:61.

42. Aronson M, Bor D. Blood cultures. Ann Intern Med 1987; 106:246.

43. Overholser CD, Moreillon P, Glauser MP. Experimental bacterial endocarditis after dental extractions in rats with periodontitis. J Infect Dis 1987; 155:107.

44. Winslow MB, Kobernick SD. Bacteremia after prophylaxis. J Am Dent Assoc 1960; 61:69.

45. LeFrock JL, Klainer AS, Wu WH, et al. Transient bacteremia associated with nasotracheal and orotracheal intubation. Anesth Analg 1973; 52:873.

46. Shull JH Jr., Greene BM, Allen SD, et al. Bacteremia with upper gastrointestinal endoscopy. Ann Intern Med 1975; 83:212.

47. LeFrock JL, Ellis CA, Turchik JB, et al. Transient bacteremia associated sigmoidoscopy. N Engl J Med 1975; 289:467.

48. LeFrock JL, Ellis CA, Klainer AS, et al. Transient bacteremia associated with barium enema. Arch Intern Med 1975; 135:835.

49. Schimmel DH, Hamelin LG, Cohen S, et al. Bacteremia and the barium enema. Amer J Roentgen 1977; 128:207.

50. Dickman MD, Farrell R, Higgs RH, et al. Colonoscopy associated bacteremia. Surg Gynecol Obstet 1976; 142:173.

51. Hartong WA, Barnes WG, Calkins WG. The absence of bacteremia during colonoscopy. Am J Gastroenterol 1977; 67:240.

52. Loludice T, Buhac I, Balint J. Septicemia as a complication of percutaneous liver biopsy. Gastroenterology 1977; 72:949.

53. Camara DS, Gruber M, Barde CJ, et al. Transient bacteremia following endoscopic infection. Sclerotherapy of esophageal varices. Arch Intern Med 1983; 143:1350.

54. Redlead PD, Fadell EJ. Bacteremia during parturition. JAMA 1959; 69:1284.

55. McCormack WM, Rosner B, Lee YH, et al. Isolation of genital mycoplasmas from blood obtained shortly after vaginal delivery. Lancet 1975; 1:596.

56. Everett ED, Reller LB, Droegemuller W, et al. Absence of bacteremia after insertion or removal of intrauterine devices. Obstet Gynecol 1976; 47:207.

57. Ritvo R, Monroe P, Andriole VT. Transient bacteremia due to suction abortion. Implications for SBE prophylaxis.Yale J Biol Med 1977; 50:471.
58. Regetz MJ, Starr SE, Dowell VR Jr., et al. The absence of bacteremia after diagnostic biopsy of the cervix. Chemoprophylactic implications. Chest 1974; 65:224.
59. Yeh TJ, Anabtani IN, Cornett VE, et al. Bacterial endocarditis following open-heart surgery. Ann Thorac Surg 1967; 3:29.
60. Blakemore WS, McGarrity GS, Thurer RJ, et al. Infection by airborne bacteria with cardiopulmonary bypass. Surgery 1971; 70:830.
61. Sande MA, Levision ME, Lucas DS, et al. Bacteremia associated with cardiac catheterization. N Engl J Med 1969; 281:1104.
62. Beard CH, Ribiero CD, Jones DM. The bacteremia associated with burns and surgery. Brit J Surg 1975; 62:638.
63. Baskin RW, Rosenthal A, Pruitt BA Jr. Acute bacterial endocarditis: a silent source of sepsis in the burn patient. Ann Surg 1976; 184:618.
64. Mozingo DW, Pruitt BA Jr. Infectious complications after burn injury. Curr Opin Surg Infect 1994; 2:69.
65. Pruitt BA Jr., McManus WF, Kim SH, Treat RC. Diagnosis and treatment of cannula-related intravenous sepsis in burn patients. Ann Surg 1980; 191:546.
66. Snyder N, Atterbury CE, Correia JP, et al. Increased concurrence of cirrhosis and bacterial endocarditis. Gastroenterology 1977; 73:1107.
67. Garvey GJ, Neu HC. Infective endocarditis, an evolving disease: a review of endocarditis at the Columbia-Presbyterian Medical Center, 1968–1973. Medicine 1978; 57:105.
68. Brusch JL. Cardiac infections in the immunosuppressed host. Infect Dis Clin NA 2001; 15:613.
69. Rubin RH. Infection in the organ transplant recipients. In: Rubin RH, Young LS, eds. Clinical Approach to Infection in the Compromised Host. 3d ed. New York: Plenum Medical Book Company, 1994:629.
70. Miro JM, del Rio A, Mestres CA. Infective endocarditis and intravenous drug abusers and HIV-1 infected patients. Infect Dis Clin NA 2002; 16:273.
71. Reisberg BE. Infective endocarditis in the narcotic addict. Progr Cardiovasc Dis 1979; 22:193.
72. Matthew J, Addai T, Anand A, et al. Clinical features, site of involvement, bacterologic findings and outcome of infective endocarditis in intravenous drug users. Arch Intern Med 1995; 155:1641.
73. Ribera E, Miro JM, Cortes E, et al. Influence of human immunodeficiency virus 1 infection and degree of immunosuppression in the clinical characteristics and outcome of infective endocarditis in intravenous drug users. Arch Intern Med 1998; 158:2043.
74. Currie PF, Sutherland GR, Jacob AJ, et al. A review of endocarditis in acquired immunodeficiency syndrome and human immunodeficiency virus infection. Eur Heart J 1995; 16(suppl B):15.
75. Hecht SR, Berger M. Right sided endocarditis in intravenous drug users: prognostic features and 102 episodes. Ann of Intern Medicine 1992; 17:560.
76. Tuazon CU, Sheagren JN. Staphylococcal endocarditis in parenteral drug abusers; source of the organism. Ann Intern Med 1975; 82:788.
77. Wiplinghoff H, Bischoff T, Tallent SM, et al. Nosocomial bloodstream infections in U.S. hospitals: analysis of 24,179 cases from a prospective nationwide surveillance study. Clin Infect Dis 2004; 39:309.
78. Raad II, Bodey GP. Infectious complications of indwelling vascular catheters. Clin Infect Dis 1992; 15:197.
79. Martone WJ, Gaynes RP, Horan TC, et al. National Nosocomial Infections Surveillance (NNIS) semi annual report, May 1995. A report from the National Nosocomial Infections Surveillance (NNIS) System. Am J Infect Control 1995; 23:377.
80. Garner JS, Jarvis WR, Emori TG, et al. CDC definitions for nosocomial infection. Am J Infect Control 1988; 16:28.
81. O' Grady NP, Alexander M, Dellinger EP, et al. Guidelines for the prevention of intravascular catheter-related infections. Centers for Disease Control and Prevention MMWR Morb Mortal Wkly Rep 2002; 51:1.

82. Banerjee SN, Emori TG, Culver DH, et al. Saccular trends in nosocomial primary bloodstream infections in the United States, 1980–1989. Am J Med 1991; 91:86S.

83. Eng RH, Bishburg E, Smith SM, et al. Staphylococcus aureus bacteremia during therapy. J Infect Dis 1987; 155:1331.

84. Fowler VG, Li J, Corey GR, et al. Role of echocardiography and evaluation of patients with Staphylococcus aureus bacteremia: experience in 103 patients. J Am Coll Cardiol 1997; 30:1072.

85. Ringberg H, Thoren A, Lilja B. Metastatic complications of Staphylococcus aureus septicemia: to seek is to find. Infection 2000; 28:132.

86. Durack DT, Beeson PB. Protective role of complement in experimental Escherichia coli endocarditis. Infect Immun 1977; 16:213.

87. Yersin B, Glauser M-P, Guze L, et al. Escherichia coli endocarditis in rats: roles of serum bactericidal activity and duration of catheter placement. Infect Immun 1988; 56:1273.

87a. Fridel JM, Stehlik J, Desai M, Granato JE. Infective endocarditis after oral body piercing. Cardiol Rev 2003; 11:252.

88. Scheld WM, Thomas JH, Sande MA. Influence of preformed antibody on experimental Streptococcal sanguis endocarditis. Infect Immun 1979; 25:71.

89. Van de Rijn I. Analysis of cross-protection between serotypes and passively transferred immune globulin in experimental nutritionally variant streptococcal endocarditis. Infect Immun 1988; 56:117.

90. Scheld WM, Calderone RA, Brodeur JP, et al. Influence of preformed antibody on the pathogenesis of experimental Candida albicans endocarditis. Infect Immun 1983; 40:950.

91. Sieling, Van de Rijin I. Evaluation of the immune response in protection against experimental Streptococcus defectivus endocarditis. J Lab Clin Med 1991; 117:402.

92. Greenberg DP, Ward JI, Bayer AS. Influence of Staphylococcus aureus antibody on experimental endocarditis in rabbits. Infect Immun 1987; 55:3030.

93. Adler SW II, Selinger DS, Reed WP. Effect of immunization on the genesis of pneumococcal endocarditis in rabbits. Infect Immun 1981; 34:55.

94. Scheld WM, Thomas JH, Sande MA. Influence of preformed antibody on experimental Streptococcus sanguis endocarditis. Infect Immun 1979; 25:71.

95. Patti JM, Allen BL, McGavin MJ, Hook M. MSCRAMM-mediated adherence of microorganisms to host tissues. Ann Rev Microbiol 1994; 48:585.

96. Gould K, Ramirez-Ronda CH, Holmes RK, et al. Adherence of bacteria to heart valves in vitro. J Clin Invest 1975; 56:1364.

97. Parker MT, Ball LC. Streptococci and aerococci associated with systemic infection in man. J Med Microbiol 1976; 9:275.

98. Ramirez-Ronda CH. Adherence of glucan-positive and glucan-negative streptococci strains to normal and damaged heart valves. J Clin Invest 1978; 62:805.

99. Dall L, Barnes WG, Lane JW, et al. Enzymatic modifications of glycocalyx in the treatment of experimental endocarditis due to viridans streptococci. J Infect Dis 1987; 156:736.

100. Lowrance JH, Baddout LM, Simpson WA. The role of fibronectin in the rat model of endocarditis caused by *Streptococcus sanguis*. J Clin Invest 1990; 86:7.

101. Viscount HB, Munro CL, Burnette-Curley D, et al. Immunization with Fim A protects against *Streptococcus parasanguis* endocarditis in rats. Infect Immun 1997; 65:994.

102. Manning JE, Geyelin AJ, Ansmits LM, et al. A comparative study of the aggregation of human, rat and rabbit platelets by members of the *Streptococcus sanguis* group. J Med Microbiol 1994; 41:10.

103. Jenkinson HF. Cell surface protein receptors in oral streptococci. FEMS Microbiol Lett 1994; 121:133.

104. Becker RC, Dibello PM, Lucas FV. Bacterial tissue tropism: an in vitro model for infective endocarditis. Cardiovasc Res 1979; 21:813.

105. Lowy FD. *Staphylococcus aureus* infections. N Engl J Med 1998; 339:520.

106. Cheung AL, Koomey JM, Butler CA, et al. Regulation of exoprotein expression in *Staphylococcus aureus* by a locus (sar) distinct from agr. Proc Natl Acad Sci USA 1992; 89:6462.

107. Que YA. Pathogenesis of Staphylococcal Endovascular Infections. Ph.D. Thesis. University of Lausanne, 2001.

108. Yeaman MR, Sullam PM, Ramos M, et al. Characterization of *Staphylococcus aureus*—platelet binding by quantitative flow cytometric analysis. J Infect Dis 1992; 166:65.

109. Herrmann M, Suchard SJ, Boxer LA, et al. Thrombospondin binds to *Staphylococcus aureus* and promotes staphylococcal adherence to surfaces. Infect Immun 1991; 59:279.

110. Bayer AS, Sullam PM, Ramos M, et al. *Staphylococcus aureus* induces platelet aggregation via a fibrinogen-dependent mechanism which is independent of principal platelet glycoprotein IIb/IIIa fibrinogen-binding domains. Infect Immun 1995; 63:3634.

111. Southwick FS, Durack DT. Chemotherapy of experimental streptococcal endocarditis. III. Failure of a bacteriostatic agent (tetracycline) in prophylaxis. J Clin Pathol 1975; 27:261.

112. Malinverni R, Overholser C, Bille J. Antibiotic prophylaxis of experimental endocarditis after dental extractions. Circulation 1988; 77:183.

113. Lowry FD, Chang DS, Neuhaus EG et al. Effect of penicillin on the adherence of *Streptococcus sanguis* in vitro and in the rabbit model of endocarditis. J Clin Invest 1983; 71:668.

114. Glauser MP, Bernard JP, Moreillon P, et al. Successful single-dose amoxicillin prophylaxis against experimental streptococcal endocarditis: evidence for two mechanisms of protection. J Infect Dis 1983; 147:568.

115. Kitten T, Munro CL, Wang A, et al. Vaccination with Fim A from *Streptococcus parasanguis* protects rats from endocarditis caused by other viridans streptoccoci. Infect Immun 2002; 70:422.

116. McCormick JK, Tripp TJ, Dunny GM, et al. Formation of vegetations during infective endocarditis excludes binding of bacterial specific host antibodies to *Enteroccocus faecalis*. J Infect Dis 2002; 185:994.

117. Vignes S, Fantin B, Elbim C, et al. Critical influence of timing of administration of granulocyte-stimulating factor on antibacterial effect in experimental endocarditis due to *Pseudomonas aeruginosa*. Antimicrob Agent Chemother 1995; 39:2702.

118. Camerer E, Kolsto AB, Prydz H. Cell biology of tissue factor, the principal initiator of blood coagulation. Thromb Res 1996; 81:1.

119. Durack DT. Experimental bacterial endocarditis. IV. Structure and evolution of very early lesions. J Pathol 1975; 115:81.

120. Bansci MJ, Thompson J, Bertina RM. Stimulation of monocyte tissue factor expression in an in vitro model of bacterial endocarditis. Infect Immun 1994; 62:5669.

121. Bansci MJ, Veltrop MH, Bertina RM, Thompson J. Role of phagocytosis in activation of the coagulation system in *S. sanguis* endocarditis. Infect Immun 1996; 64:5166.

122. Bansci MJ, Veltrop MH, Bertina RM, Thompson J. Role of monocytes and bacteria in *Staphylococcus epidermidis* endocarditis. Infect Immun 1998; 68:4818.

123. Veltrop MH, Beekhuizen H, Thompson J. Bacterial species—and strain dependent-induction of tissue factor in human vascular endothelial cells. Infect Immun 1999; 67:6130.

124. Herzberg MC, Britzenhofe KL, Clawson CC. Aggregation of human platelets and adherence of *Streptrococcus sanguis*. Infect Immun 1983; 39:1457.

125. Dankert J, Van den Werff J, Zaat SAJ, et al. Involvement of bactericidal factors from thrombin-stimulated platelets in clearance of adherent viridans streptococci in experimental infective endocarditis. Infect Immun 1995; 63:663.

126. Koo SP, Bayer AS, Kagan BL, Yeaman MR. Membrane permeabilization by thrombin-induced platelet microbicidal protein 1 is modulated by transmembrane voltage polarity and magnitude. Infect Immun 1999; 67:2475.

127. Fowler VG Jr., McIntyre LM, Yeaan MR, et al. In vitro resistance to thrombin-m induced platelet microbicidal protein in isolates of *Staphylococcus aureus* from endocarditis patients correlates with an intravascular device source. J Infect Dis 2000; 182:1251.

128. Kupferwasser LI, Yeaman MR, Shapiro SM, et al. Acetylysalicylic acid reduces vegetation bacterial density, hematogenous bacterial dissemination and frequency of embolic events in experimental *Staphylococcus aureus* endocarditis through antiplatelet and antibacterial effects. Circulation 1999; 99:2791.

129. Thompson J, Euidernik F, Lemkes H, et al. Effect of warfarin on the induction and course of experimental endocarditis. Infect Immun 1976; 14:1284.

130. Johnson CE, Dewar HA, Aherne WA. Fibrinolytic therapy in subacute bacterial endocarditis. An experimental study. Cardiovasc Res 1982; 14:482.
131. Libman E, Friedberg CK. Subacute Bacterial Endocarditis. Oxford: Oxford University Press, 1941.
132. Arnett EC, Roberts WC. Acute infective endocarditis: a clinicopathological analysis of 137 necropsy patients. Curr Probl Cardio 1976; 1(7):3.
133. Durack DT, Beeson PB. Experimental endocarditis. I Colonization of a sterile vegetation. Br J Exp Pathol 1982; 53:44.
134. Sinha B, Francois P, Que YA, et al. Heterologously expressed *Staphylococcus aureus* fibronectin-binding proteins are sufficient for invasion of host cells. Infect Immun 2000; 69:6871.
135. Novick RP, Muir TW. Virulence gene regulation by peptides in staphylococci and other gram-positive bacteria. Curr Opin Microbiol 1999; 2:40.
136. Durack DT, Petersdorf RG. Chemotherapy of experimental streptococcal endocarditis. I Comparison of commonly recommended prophylactic regimens. J Clin Invest 1973; 52:592.
137. Karchmer AW. Infective Endocarditis. In: Zips DP, Libby P, Bonow R, Braunwald E, eds. Braunwald's Heart Disease. 7th ed. Philadelphia: Elseiver, 2005:1633.
138. Weinstein L, Brusch JL. Pathology. In: Weinstein L, Brusch JL. Infective Endocarditis. New York: the Oxford University Press, 1995:123.
139. Cates JE, Christie RV. Subacute bacterial endocarditis. A review of 442 patients treated in 14 centres appointed by the Penicillin Trials Committee of the Medical Research Council. Q J Med 1951; 20:93.
140. Volger WR, Dorney ER. Bacterial endocarditis in congenital heart disease. Am Heart J 1962; 64:198.
141. Mansur AJ, Grinberg M, Lamos de Luz P, Bellotti G. The complications of infective endocarditis. A reppraisal in the 1980s. Arch Intern Med 1992; 152:2428 .
142. Kerr A Jr. Subacute Bacterial Endocarditis. Springfield, IL: Charles C Thomas, 1955.
143. Menzies CJG. Coronary embolism with infarction in bacterial endocarditis. Br Heart J 1961; 23:464.
144. Zinmet I. Nervous system complications in bacterial endocarditis. Am J Med 1969; 47:493.
145. Salgado AV, Furlan AJ, Keys TF, et al. Neurologic complications of endocarditis: a 12 year experience. Neurology 1989; 39:173.
146. Cabell CH, Pond KK, Peterson GE, et al. The risk of stroke and death in patients with aortic and mitral valve endocarditis. Heart J 2001; 142:75.
147. Greenlee J, Mandell G. Neurological manifestations of infective endocarditis: a review. Stroke 1983; 4 :958.
148. Tunkel AR, Kaye D. Neurologic complications of infective endocarditis. Neurol Clin 1993; 11:419.
149. Bullock R, Van Dellen JR, Van den Heever CM. Intracranial mycotic aneurysms: a review of 9 cases. S Afr Med J 1961; 60:970.
150. Cordeiro A, Costa H, Laghena F. Immunologic phase of subacute bacterial endocarditis. A new concept and general considerations. Editorial. Am J Cardiol 1965; 16:477.
151. Phair J, Clarke J. Immunology of infective endocarditis. Prog Cardiovasc Dis 1979; 22:137.
152. Messner R, Laxdal T, Quie P, et al. Rheumatoid factors in subacute bacterial endocarditis. Bacterium, duration of disease or genetic predisposition. Ann Intern Med 1968; 68:746.
153. Williams R Jr., Kunbel H. Rheumatoid factors and their disappearance following therapy in patients with subacute bacterial endocarditis. Arthritis Rheum 1962; 5:126.
154. Carson D, Bayer A, Eisenberg R, et al. IgM rheumatoid factor in subacute bacterial endocarditis: relationship to IgG rheumatoid factor and circulatory complexes. Clin Exp Immunol 1970; 31:100.
155. Sheagren JN, Tuazon CU, Griffin C, et al. Rheumatoid factor in acute bacterial endocarditis. Arthritis Rheum 1976; 19:887.
156. Williams R. Rheumatoid factors in subacute bacterial endocarditis and other infectious diseases. Scand J Rheum 1988; 75 (suppl):300.

157. Bayer AS, Theofilopoulos AN, Tillman DB, et al. Use of circulating immune complex levels in the serodifferentiation of endocarditic and non endocarditic septicemias. Am J Med 1979; 66:58.
158. Gutman RA, Striker GE, Gilliland BC, et al. The immune complex glomerulonephritis of bacterial endocarditis. Medicine 1972; 51:1.
159. Libman E. Characterization of various forms of endocarditis. JAMA 1923; 80:813.
160. Alpert JS, Krous HF, Dalen JE, et al. Pathogenesis of Osler's nodes. Ann Intern Med 1976; 85:471.
161. Silverberg HHM. Roth spots. Mt Sinai J Med 1977; 37:77.
162. Kerr A Jr., Tan J. Biopsies of the Janeway lesion of infective endocarditis. J Cutan Pathol 1979; 6:24.
163. Churchill M, Geraci J, Hunder G. Musculoskeletal manifestations of bacterial endocarditis. Ann of Intern Med 1977; 87:754.

6

Clinical Manifestations of Native Valve Endocarditis

John L. Brusch
Harvard Medical School and Department of Medicine and Infectious Disease Service, Cambridge Health Alliance, Cambridge, Massachusetts, U.S.A.

INTRODUCTION

Although all types of infective endocarditis (IE) share a common pathogenesis, nonbacterial thrombotic endocarditis (NBTE) (Chapter 5), there are marked differences in their manifestations. Nowhere is this difference as striking than that between subacute and acute (IE) of native valves. The former disease is an indolent process that is marked by fever, fatigue, and anorexia. It is a wasting disease that may go on for longer than a one year if untreated. Acute IE follows an extremely aggressive course with intractable heart failure leading to death in a few days (1,2).

The sharp distinction between these two clinical extremes has become blurred. The failure to recognize underlying endocarditis as the cause of recurrent fevers can lead to inadequate courses of antibiotics aimed at less serious infections. These can suppress but not eradicate the valvular infection. This situation may be termed muted IE. Muted IE probably most commonly occurs in the setting of the healthcare-associated IE (HCIE) (3). Such empirical use of antibiotics may convert the clinical picture of a *Staphylococcus aureus* IE to resemble that of *Streptococcus viridans*.

CAUSATIVE ORGANISMS OF NATIVE VALVE INFECTIVE ENDOCARDITIS

In adults who were not intravenous drug abusers (IVDA), *S. aureus* is responsible for approximately 40% of cases while the oral streptococci cause 31%. The nonoral streptococci (*Streptococcus bovis, Streptococcus agalactiae, Streptococcus pneumoniae, Streptococcus pyogenes*, and *Abiotrophia* spp.) account for 10% of the cases. Enterococci produce <10% of cases. Eighty percent of enterococci are *Streptococcus faecalis* or gram-negative aerobes isolated in <10%. Fungi are recovered in <1%. *Streptococcus viridans* remains the classic organism of subacute disease. *Staphylococcus aureus* is the predominant pathogen of acute IE.

In IVDA IE, *S. aureus* is responsible for 70% of isolates. Polymicrobial IE and gram-negative anaerobic IE each account for 10% of the cases (Chapters 1–3, 7) (4).

SIGNS, SYMPTOMS, AND COMPLICATIONS OF SUBACUTE INFECTIVE ENDOCARDITIS

When the clinical manifestations of IE are presented, it is most important to specify that the data pertain either to acute or subacute disease or both. Too many series fail to do so. An additional criticism is that referral bias has marked influence on the results from a given hospital. Simply, the uncomplicated cases currently remain in the community. Tertiary-care hospitals care for those that require acute cardiac surgery.

The rate of death in these facilities is two to three times greater (5). The complication rate of IE is approximately the same in both subacute and acute diseases. However, the development of complications occurs at a much greater pace in the latter variety. Almost 60% of patients suffer at least one complication; 26% develop two; 8% demonstrate three or more, and 6% have more than six complications (6).

Incubation/Prodromal Period of Subacute Infective Endocarditis

The incubation time for IE is defined as the interval between the performance of the procedure that gives rise to the inciting transient bacteremia and the onset of clinical disease (7). In the case of streptococcal IE, in 80% of individuals, the incubation period was one week and symptoms appear within two weeks for 85% of the patients. Rarely was the incubation period more than four weeks. However, the diagnosis of IE was made in only 16% of cases during this time. The average interval between the onset of bacteremia and the diagnosis of valvular infection was six weeks. Several factors underly this significant delay in diagnosis. Among these are: (*i*) the nonspecific nature of the signs and symptoms of the early stages of subacute IE; (*ii*) patients infrequently seek medical attention during this time because of the mildness of their symptoms; (*iii*) failure of physicians to even consider the diagnosis of IE until weeks or months go by; and (*iv*) and the stage of muted IE brought about by the poorly reasoned administration of antibiotics (1). From their study of these important time periods, Starkebaum et al. (7) concluded that in those valvular infections caused by medical interventions, signs and symptoms of disease usually appear within two weeks (1). They suggested that people at risk for development of IE be instructed to report any symptoms consistent with IE for two weeks postprocedure. Symptoms that develop after this time frame are unlikely to be related to the intervention and should not be considered to represent failure of antibiotic prophylaxis.

More recent data supports and expands Starkebaum's findings to include cases of acute IE (8). This series studied 683 cases of IE. Twenty-five percent of the cases were hospitalized within 10 days of the development of symptoms. About 36.5% of the individuals received antibiotics prior to hospitalization. Symptoms were prolonged before diagnosis when an antibiotic was given (58.8 vs. 44.8 days); there were detectable vegetations by echocardiogram (53.5 vs. 38.8 days) and in cases prior to 1990 (54.2 vs. 42.3). Prosthetic valve IE had the shortest delay in diagnosis (26.8 days). However, 26.5% of cases of prosthetic valve IE were not detected for >30 days. As would be expected, *S. aureus* were the pathogens most isolated among patients with symptoms of 10 days or less. Streptococcal species were the most frequent cause of disease >20 days. Mortality was inversely proportional to the duration of the symptoms. Those with disease <10 days before diagnosis had a mortality rate of 36.1% as opposed to the overall rate of 25.6%. These striking figures demonstrate, in a quantified manner, the major clinical differences between subacute and acute IE.

The early symptoms of subacute disease are quite nonspecific and often masquerade as more common diseases of the elderly such as polymyalgia rheumatica or urinary tract infections. When outpatient antibiotic therapy is started empirically for treatment of fever in the aged patient, blood cultures are often not obtained. As the pathogens of subacute IE are sensitive to many antimicrobial agents, the favorable clinical response reinforces the correctness of misdiagnosis in the clinician's mind. A week or two after the antibiotic is stopped, fever returns.

TABLE 1　Noncardiac Signs and Symptoms of Early Subacute
Infective Endocarditis

Low-grade fever[a]
Presence of pre-existent murmur[a]
Influenza-like syndrome with myalgias
Hemoptysis with pleuritic pain (right-sided endocarditis)
Syndrome of fever and arthritis suggesting rheumatic fever, Lyme disease, polymyalgia rheumatica, and other rheumatologic disorders
Typhoid-like syndrome with fever, dulled sensorium, and headache
Facial rash resembling systemic lupus erythematosus
Biliary tract symptoms of fever and right upper quadrant abdominal pain
Early satiety and vomiting resembling gastric carcinoma
Right lower quadrant pain and nausea mimicking acute appendicitis

[a]May be absent in 3% to 15% of patients.

Pretreatment with the same antibiotic is often instituted with the justification that the initial course was just not long enough. This can continue over several cycles. The greater the time before the correct diagnosis is made, the higher the risk that it may be a permanent valvular damage. The initial symptoms of untreated disease or symptoms of muted IE are quite nonspecific (Table 1) There is little indication that there is an infection of the heart or of any other organ. The most common of these are low-grade fever, fatigue, and weight loss as a result of anorexia. Fever may be absent in up to 15% of patients. In 1885, Osler wrote "it is well recognized that fever is not an invariable accompaniment of endocarditis" (9). This dictum remains true in the present day (10). Patients may be afebrile on presentation and remain so throughout the course of the infection. Body temperature must be assessed in relationship to the patient's age. Older patients often have a lower basal temperature than younger. As subacute disease is now a disease of the elderly, the apparently normal temperature may well represent a bona fide fever. When their temperatures are closely monitored, spikes in temperature may become apparent, although still remaining below 98.6°F. Concurrent congestive heart failure or renal failure may contribute to the blunted febrile response (11). Chills are not common in subacute IE patients except in those whom salicylates or nonsteroidal anti-inflammatory drugs (NSAIDs) are used. As the effect of the antipyretic wears off, rigors develop as part of the process in raising the core temperature in response to endogenous pyrogen.

The absence of a murmur is quite unusual in subacute IE and may indicate the presence of mural endocarditis (1,12). Patients have been encountered in whom a murmur has never been heard either before or after their development of valvular infection. One such patient was a 36-year-old man who developed persistently low-grade fevers. On several physical examinations, no murmurs were audible. He suffered an occlusion of the right middle cerebral artery. At that time, blood cultures grew out *S. viridans*. With appropriate therapy, he recovered completely. No murmurs were detected by auscultation of echocardiography during his hospitalization or for 15 years of follow-up. Many of the murmurs heard during IE are not hemodynamically significant, but no murmurs should be considered innocent in an elderly patient with unexplained fever. Only about 17% of pre-existing murmurs change characteristics during subacute valvular infection.

Splenomegaly was present in most patients in the preantibiotic era. It is currently present in about 30%. Its presence is directly correlated with the duration the of disease. There is no difference in its incidence between IE of native and prosthetic valves. Splenic enlargement is unusual in acute IE. Splenic complications include: infarcts (1%) (see the following) and splenic artery aneurysms. Splenic abscesses are seen primarily in acute disease. Splenomegaly may persist long after the valvular infection has been cured (13–16).

Libman et al. (17,18) described several presentations of early IE that mimic a number of extracardiac infections. Among these are: (*i*) prominent myalgias resembling that of influenza; (*ii*) fever and arthritis suggesting rheumatic fever; (*iii*) a dulled sensorium suggesting typhoid fever; (*iv*) pain in right upper quadrant of the abdomen mimicking biliary tract infection; (*v*) vomiting and postprandial indigestion resembling carcinoma of the stomach; (*vi*) the signs and symptoms of acute appendicitis; and (*vii*) erythema of the nose and cheeks similar to the rash of systemic lupus erythematosus.

Intracardiac Complications of Subacute Infective Endocarditis

Complications of subacute IE develop weeks or months after the beginning of the disease. These may be owing to one of three major processes: embolic phenomenon, inexorable valvular destruction, and immunological mechanisms. Heart failure occurs in 15% to 65% of cases. This rate is lower in the setting of congenital heart disease (25%). The rate of congestive heart failure does not differ between subacute and acute IE, only the time span. Cardiac decompensation usually becomes evident within six months after the onset of subacute disease. It may delay its appearance up to one year after microbiological cure has been achieved. In an acute process, congestive heart failure may appear within a few days of presentation (1). It is the most common cause of death in all types of IE and the most frequent indication for surgery. In subacute disease, it is caused primarily by progressive destruction of the valve leaflets. Eighty percent of cases of congestive heart failure are because of development of aortic insufficiency (19). The force of the regurgitant aortic jet on the mitral valve contributes to the ventricular failure by perforating a valvular cusp or rupturing a papillary muscle or chordae tendineae of the mitral valve (20). Occasionally, bits of the valvular thrombus may embolize into the ostia of the coronary arteries. Rarely do the vegetations become large enough to physically obstruct the orifice of the valve (21). Myocarditis may initiate or exacerbate cardiac failure (22) in subacute disease; it is most frequently caused by deposition of immune complexes in the walls of the coronary arteries which leads to their occlusion. Bracht-Wachter bodies, collections of lymphocytes and polymorphonuclear leukocytes in the myocardium, are the pathological hallmarks of this type of myocarditis.

Pericarditis is rarely seen in patients with subacute IE. It is immunologically mediated as compared with the more common pericarditis of acute infection. The latter usually represents direct extension of infection into the pericardial space (23).

The other intracardiac complications of IE will be discussed in the acute IE section.

Neurological Complications of Subacute Infective Endocarditis

Traditionally, it has been estimated that 25% to 35% of patients suffer some type of neurologic complication during IE. By far, the most common of these is stroke (24). A more recent series of 700 cases reported a lower incidence of stroke rate, 18% of cases of mitral valve IE and 10% of cases of aortic valve IE (25). Stroke was the presenting symptom in over 50% of these cases. Embolic ischemic strokes were more common than hemorrhagic ones by a ratio of 3 to 1. Quite similar results were generated in a series from Finland (26). The middle cerebral artery is involved most frequently (27). In this study, embolic stroke was the presenting symptom in >75% of the individuals. There is no connection between the neurological complications of IE and the age and sex of the patient and the type of underlying heart disease. The death rate of valvular infection increases markedly in the setting of a neurological insult. It increases approximately fourfold (from 6–24% to 22–92%) (28). One reason why mortality is greater in patients with stroke is the high rate of concurrent congestive heart failure.

Until two decades ago, streptococci were the most common pathogens involved in IE-associated neurological disorders (29). This role has been played by *S. aureus* (28). The embolic infarcts of subacute disease may be microscopic or macroscopic. Approximately 11% of stroke patients demonstrate multiple punctate lesions. In cases of subacute IE, brain infarcts occur within two to four weeks or as late as one to three months after the onset of the disease. In acute IE with its more aggressive pathogens, brain infarcts occur within the first two weeks of the disease (see later) and 18% of patients with mitral valve IE suffered stroke as compared with 10% of patients with aortic valve IE (25). The rate of cerebral embolization is greater in those patients who exhibit large friable vegetations. More than 50% of patients with cerebral emboli have evidence of embolization to other organs.

It appears that anticoagulation increases the risk of embolization. Pruitt et al. (30) demonstrated that more than 23% of cerebral hemorrhage occurred in the 3% of patients given anticoagulants; 50% of these developed a cerebral hematoma. Appropriate antibiotic reduces by twofold the recurrence of stroke within two weeks of their initiation (31,32).

Cerebral mycotic aneurysms complicate 2% to 10% of cases of IE. This may be a low figure. The true incidence of the cerebral mycotic aneurysms is probably significantly underestimated as they may remain clinically silent. In subacute disease, they most likely result from to the infected microemboli of the vasa vasorum. These then trigger an inflammatory response, which weakens the adventitia and muscular layers of the vessel. Deposition of immune complexes on the wall of the artery may also play a role in the pathogenesis of mycotic aneurysm (33). *Streptococcus viridans* is more involved in mycotic aneurysms of IE than is *S. aureus*. However, those produced by the latter organism rupture at a far greater rate. Most remain asymptomatic throughout the patient's lifespan. Others may not declare themselves until years after bacteriological cure has been achieved. About 17.7 % of aneurysms are multiple and may develop at different stages of IE (34). Single or multiple aneurysms are located peripherally to the first bifurcation of a major intracranial artery near the surface of the brain. The most feared consequence of these is rupture. Although, that can occur at any time, the mean time between the onset of valvular infection and rupture of these mycotic aneurysms is 18 days. Some series (35) put into question the long-held belief that cerebral mycotic aneurysms provide no pre-event warning of their presence. Severe headaches and visual field defects, usually homonymous hemianopsia, may occur early enough to provide adequate time to perform imaging studies to verify their existence. A useful screening test is a computed tomography (CT) scan, which often identifies secondary signs of mycotic aneurysms. These include peri-aneurysmal inflammation due to small leak in the structure. Bleeding into an ischemic infarct, and not the rupture of a mycotic aneurysm, is the most common cause of IE-associated intracerebral hemorrhage (36).

TABLE 2 Neurological Manifestations of Infective Endocarditis[a]

Toxic manifestations
Headache, decreased concentration, insomnia, drowsiness, vertigo, and irritability
Psychiatric disorders
Neuroses, psychoses, confusion, disorientation, emotional instability, delirium,
auditory visual disturbances, apathy, and altered personality
Stroke
Aphonia, hemi-di-para-or quadriplegia, stupor, and coma
Meningoencephalitis
Involvement of the cranial nerves
Visual disturbances and cranial nerve sensory impairment
Dyskinesia
Tremor, ataxia, parkinsonism, seizures, chorea, hemifacial dyskinesia, hiccups,
and myoclonus
Spinal cord or small nerves involvement
Girdle pain, weakness, paraplegia, paresis, sensory disturbances, myalgia,
and peripheral neuropathy.

[a]Although most of these categories are more commonly seen in subacute disease, many may be present in acute disease (see text).
Source: From Ref. 38.

Embolic abscesses complicate 1% of subacute and 4% of acute cases of valvular infection. They are almost invariably silent during life (30). Most often, they are less than 1 cm in diameter. Encephalomalacia and endarteritis are caused by infectious vasculitis of the cerebral arteries. Petechial lesions of the brain are found usually in the white matter adjacent to the lateral ventricles and the gray matter proximate to the aqueduct and corpus callosum (30).

Ocular complications of IE include embolic retinal artery occlusion, retinal and conjunctival hemorrhages, papilledema, iridocyclitis, panophthalmitis, nystagmus, and conjugate deviation of the third cranial nerves (37). Emboli to a retinal artery lead to ipsilateral blindness, retinal infarction, and retinopathy. Prepapillary embolic abscess are unusual (38).

Cerebrospinal fluid is abnormal in 72% of all cases of IE (30). In subacute IE, the chemical and microscopic profile of cerebrospinal fluid resembles that of aseptic meningitis except that gross blood is present in about 15% of the patients.

In his seminal article, Ziment classified the multiple neurological complications of IE according to six major etiologies: (*i*) toxic manifestations, (*ii*) psychiatric disorders, (*iii*) stroke, (*iv*) meningoencephalitis, (*v*) cranial nerve involvement, (*vi*) dyskinesia, and (*vii*) spinal cord or small nerve involvement (Table 2) (39).

Non-Nervous System Emboli and Mycotic Aneurysms of Subacute Infective Endocarditis

Although in the antibiotic era the incidence of arterial embolization has decreased from 70–97% to 15–35% of cases, it remains the second most common complication of both subacute and acute IE. This reduction is primarily due to the effectiveness of antibiotic administration on reducing the risk of embolization. The rate of embolization is reduced from 13/1000 patient days to <1.2/1000 patient days after two weeks of antimicrobial administration (40). Table 3 presents the risk factors for arterial embolization (1,27,41–47).

The spleen, kidneys, and coronary arteries are the most common non-neurologic organs involved. The skin, bones, and joints are less affected. Of the

TABLE 3   Risk Factors for Embolization in Infective Endocarditis

The size of vegetations[a]
Significant mobility of the vegetation[a]
Location-mitral valve is greater than aortic valve (25% vs. 10%). The anterior leaflet of the
  mitral valve has the highest incidence of embolization (37%)
Organisms that are associated with giant vegetations (*Candida* spp., *Aspergillus* spp.,
  Staphylococcus aureus, Group B streptococci)
Patient age between 20 and 40 years
Vegetations that can be visualized by both TEE and TTE
Presence of a hypercoagulable state, such as the presence of antiphospholipid antibodies

[a]Degree of significance is greater for the time period after initiation of antibiotic therapy.
Abbreviations: TEE, transesophageal echocardiogram; TTE, transthoracic echocardiogram.
Source: From Refs. 1, 26, 40–46.

peripheral arteries, embolization occurs most frequently in the legs (45%), carotid arteries (23%), and arms (14%) (48). It is unusual for subacute disease to be complicated by embolization of a large artery. The effects of the generally larger emboli of acute disease are more readily apparent than those of the smaller ones of subacute IE. However, studies based on both clinical and postmortem data indicate that the rate of embolization is essentially identical for both forms of IE. It is important to keep in mind that the emboli of subacute IE usually produce a sterile infarct both because of the small number of organisms contained within the embolus and their minimally invasive nature.

Emboli frequently involve the spleen (44%) but are often clinically silent. Those of subacute disease usually cause sterile infarcts and seldom suppurate (49) unless infected by a bloodstream infection (BSI) unrelated to the valvular infection (27). The infarcted spleen may produce symptoms of left upper quadrant abdominal pain with radiation to the shoulder. A small left pleural effusion may be present. Examination may detect a splenic rub. In the past, macroembolic infarction of the kidney occurred in 50% of patients, currently much less frequently so. Patients may develop flank pain and hematuria (49,50). Embolization to the coronary arteries may produce small and multiple myocardial infarctions which seldom produce electrocardiographic changes. Congestive heart failure may result, especially when the infarction occurs in the vicinity of the aortic valve (51,52). Although they may occur in both types of IE, they more often result in a myocardial abscess in the acute form.

The incidence of noncerebral mycotic aneurysms is approximately 2.5%. Their true incidence is unknown as most remain asymptomatic. Their pathogenesis is discussed previously and in Chapter 5. The most common sites are the vessels of the limbs, especially those of the legs (20–30%), and the superior mesenteric artery (10–20%). Emboli or mycotic aneurysms of the mesenteric arteries may produce acute abdominal pain, melena, or ileus. Less frequently involved are the splenic arteries and the coronary arteries (1). In the preantibiotic era, 23% of cases of IE were found to have a mycotic aneurysm of the descending aorta; currently 6% (53).

Renal Complications of Subacute Infective Endocarditis
Presently, the most common causes of renal dysfunction in IE are congestive heart failure and untoward reactions to antimicrobial therapy (54,55). The renal lesions associated with antibiotics include: interstitial nephritis, toxic nephropathy, and

TABLE 4   Timing of the Renal Complications of Subacute Infective Endocarditis

Process	Time frame
Antibiotic-related interstitial nephritis	Usually occurs after 10 days of therapy
Antibiotic-related acute tubular necrosis	Occurs after at least 5 days of therapy
Diffuse and focal glomerulonephritis	Noted prior to institution of antibiotic therapy

acute tubular necrosis (Table 4). The development of interstitial nephritis (10%) is most Fosinophiluria frequently associated with the penicillins, quinolones, and cephalosporins; that of acute tubular necrosis with the aminoglycosides (56,57). Eosinophilia and eosinophiluria may occur in interstitial nephritis. A preponderance of white blood cells and white blood cell casts distinguishes antibiotic-associated interstitial nephritis from glomerulonephritis. The latter condition is marked by red cell casts and hematuria. The urinanalysis of drug-induced acute tubular necrosis reveals muddy brown granular casts, renal epithelial cells, and epithelial casts.

The second most common lesion of the kidney is focal embolic glomerulonephritis (58). It occurs in 17% to 80% of untreated cases and 15% of treated ones. Only 7% of cases of acute IE develop this lesion. It is marked by a localized proliferation of endothelial and mesangial cells. Neutrophils and red cells infiltrate this area. Fibrinoid necrosis with crescent formation develops (59). A diffuse glomerulonephritis may develop in 30% to 60% of untreated individuals compared with 10% of those treated (59–61). It is caused by deposition of immune complexes, not emboli onto the basement membrane. These findings often resolve on appropriate treatment of the valvular infection. Coagulase-negative staphylococcal IE can produce a membranoproliferative glomerulonephritis. Macroemboli to the kidney rarely occur presently. Cortical necrosis may be a consequence of disseminated intravascular coagulation.

Musculoskeletal Complications of Subacute Infective Endocarditis
Approximately, 40% of patients develop musculoskeletal complaints during the course of their infection. The vast majority are seen in subacute IE. The majority of these symptoms appear prior to the diagnosis of IE being made (Table 5) (62,63). The prominence of musculoskeletal symptoms at an early stage can avert the clinicians attention away from the heart and to a variety of rheumatological diseases (rheumatoid arthritis, Reiters syndrome, and Lyme disease) as the cause of the patient's complaints. This is especially likely when there is a positive rheumatoid

TABLE 5   Musculoskeletal Manifestations of Infective Endocarditis

Symptom	Number of cases developed before diagnosis	Number of cases developed after diagnosis
Arthralgias	30	2
Arthritis	22	4
Low back pain	19	—
Leg myalgias	11	11
Disc space infection	5	5
Nail clubbing	4	4
Hypertrophic osteoarthropathy	1	1
Achilles tendinitis	—	1
Avascular necrosis	—	1

factor as part of the disease process (Chapter 5). Acute synovitis most frequently affects the ankle, knee, wrist, sternoclavicular joint, low back pain, elbow metatarsophalangeal, and metacarpophalangeal joints. Joint fluid is sterile except in those few cases owing to *S. aureus*. Myalgias and arthralgias are the most prominent symptoms. This process is typically monoarticular or oligoarticular and asymmetrical. In recent years, low back pain has become a more frequent presenting symptom. Spondylodiscitis has been increasingly reported as a possible explanation. In a recent series, spondylodiscitis was present in 15% of cases of IE. At the time of the diagnosis of this articular infection, IE was not suspected in 71% of these cases involved the lumbar area. Group D enterococci, coagulase-negative staphylococci, and *Streptococcal* spp. were the most commonly identified organisms. Because of this association, valvular infection needs to be ruled out in all cases of spondylodiscitis (64). Other potential causes of low back pain in IE include: (*i*) emboli to the vertebral blood vessels; (*ii*) aseptic necrosis of an intervertebral disc; (*iii*) vertebral osteomyelitis; and (*iv*) deposition of immune complexes in the disc space. Spondylodiscitis appears to be the most plausible explanation. Whatever may be their origin, low back pain dramatically resolves after 7 to 10 days of appropriate antibiotic therapy. Table 6 summarizes the musculoskeletal manifestations of IE.

Classical Peripheral Manifestations of Subacute Infective Endocarditis
The peripheral lesions of subacute IE are considered to be Osler nodes, petichae, subungual hemorrhages, Janeway lesions, clubbing, and Roth spots. In the pre-antibiotic era, one or more of these were present in up to 85% of the patients. Currently, 19% to 40% of patients exhibit any of these manifestations of subacute IE (13,17,24,65–68). Most of these are produced by immunological mechanisms that are driven by prolonged untreated infection (Chapter 5). Petechiae, with pale centers, are more significant than those with yellow ones. They are usually located in the eyelids, on the dorsum of the hands and feet, the chest and abdominal walls, the oral pharyngeal mucosa, and soft palate. Petechiae are also found in: (*i*) a variety of hematological disorders; (*ii*) scurvy; (*iii*) Libman-Sacks disease; (*iv*) renal failure; (*v*) various viral infections; (*vi*) atrial myxoma; (*vii*) marantic endocarditis; and (*viii*) various types of uncomplicated bacteremias. Fatty microemboli produce contralateral petechiae in 50% of patients who undergo cardiopulmonary bypass.

Subungual hemorrhages are quite uncommon in patients with IE. It is most commonly seen in individuals whose hands are traumatized in the workplace (typists; carpenters are also part of the physical findings of trichinosis). The two chief characteristics of a significant splinter hemorrhage is its linearity and its failure to reach the distal edge of the nail. They number from 1 to 10 and may involve the toenails.

Osler nodes are small, elevated, tender nodules that vary in color from red to purple. They are located in the pulp spaces of the terminal phalanges of the fingers, on the backs of the toes, soles of the feet, and on the thenar and hypothenar areas of the hands. They are present on the sides of the fingers. Their appearance is often heralded by pain. They may be evident for only a few hours or last for four to five days; they do not frequently necrose. Most often, they are the product of the immunological phenomenon of subacute IE. However, they may appear during the course of acute valvular infection. In this setting, they are caused by septic emboli. Osler node-like lesions may be seen in marantic endocarditis, systemic lupus erythematosus, chronic gonococcemia, and cannulation of the radial artery. Since described by Osler, its incidence has fallen from 70% to 10% of cases.

Janeway lesions are painless, erythematosus macules with irregular margins. They range in size from 1 to 4 mm. They are most often are found on the thenar and hypothenar eminences of the hands and soles of the feet. Less frequently, they are located on the tips of the fingers and plantar surfaces of the toes. Rarely, they may present as a diffuse, macular, erythematous rash over the trunk and extremities which blanches on pressure. It appears that most are caused by septic emboli.

Clubbing of the fingers and toes occurs now in only 10% of the patients. It usually resolves with antibiotic therapy. Other ocular findings are associated with IE. Roth spots are circular or flame-shaped hemorrhages that appear in the retina, near the optic disk, and sometimes in the sclera. They presently occur in less than 5% of the cases. Litten' sign represents a cotton wool exudate (a perivascular collection of lymphocytes in the nerve layer of the retina) that is sometimes surrounded by hemorrhage. There are also boat-shaped retinal hemorrhages that are caused by returned showers of petechiae. Optic neuritis is an uncommon complication of IE.

Bacteria-Free Stage of Subacute Infective Endocarditis

In 1913, Libman recognized as a syndrome cases of valvular infections distinctive for persistently sterile blood cultures in which diagnosis was delayed for months (69). Its distinctive features included severe congestive heart failure, arthralgias especially of the thighs, and massive edema of the legs. Fever is usually absent except during periods of recurrent embolization. New murmurs do not appear; in fact, pre-existing ones may disappear. Renal failure is a cause of death in at least one-third of the patients. Profound anemia is common. It may represent the renal failure or the ongoing chronic disease. Massive splenomegaly occurs and may be the most obvious physical finding. Surprisingly for the setting of a prolonged inflammatory course, Osler nodes and petechiae are seldom present. Purpura occurs in the early stages of the syndrome. There is significant sternal tenderness. Brown pigmentation involving the face and dorsum of the hands, should alert the clinician. Multiple aneurysms are common. These involve the sinus of Valsalva, femoral and iliac arteries, and septum membranaceum. The criteria for making the diagnosis of the stage of subacute IE are: (*i*) the absence of any obvious clinical signs or symptoms suggesting the presence of valvular infection; (*ii*) persistently sterile cultures of blood; (*iii*) the presence of organisms within the valvular vegetations; (*iv*) renal failure; (*v*) severe anemia; (*vi*) recurrent embolic disease; (*vii*) striking brown pigmentation of the face; (*viii*) massive splenomegaly; and (*ix*) the absence of fever (9).

Because of improved diagnostic methods and the availability of effective antibiotics, for all intents and purposes the bacteria-free stage of IE does not occur in the developed world. Its disappearance is because of both the accuracy of current diagnostics and the availability of effective antimicrobial agents. It serves as a dramatic demonstration of how lowly pathogenic organisms, if left unchecked, can be fatal simply by continuous and prolonged stimulation of the patient's own immune system (Chapter 5).

SIGNS, SYMPTOMS, AND COMPLICATIONS
OF ACUTE INFECTIVE ENDOCARDITIS

Incubation /Prodromal Period of Acute Infective Endocarditis

Acute IE starts abruptly and proceeds aggressively. The patient notices sudden onset of high-grade fever and chills. There is usually no previous history of valvular disease. The duration of symptoms of acute staphylococcal IE is generally <10 days prior to diagnosis. This is because of the intensity and rapidly progressive symptoms. This period is longer when antibiotics are given before diagnosis of valvular infection (8). In great part, this is owing to the slowing down of the progression of the valvular infection by the antimicrobial agents (muted IE).

Intracardiac Complications of Acute Infective Endocarditis

Table 6 lists the life-threatening intracardiac complications of acute IE. Congestive heart failure occurs in 30% to 40% of patients with acute IE. It is the most common cause of both death and cardiac surgery in IE (43). As in the case of subacute disease, the cardiac failure of acute IE is most commonly caused by valvular insufficiency, especially that of the aortic valve. The valvular leaflets primarily suffered from the destructive process of infection. Classically, the vegetations are found on the closure line of the leaflets of the atrial surface of the mitral or tricuspid valves or on the ventricular surface of the aortic valve. The infectious process may produce fenestration cord tearing of the valvular leaflets, detachment of the valve from the supporting annulus, and rupture of the chordae tendineae or the papillary muscles. Less often, cardiac failure is the result of myocardial damage provoked by emboli to the coronary artery (70) or myocarditis. Rarely, it may be because of an intracardiac fistula produced by a paravalvular abscess (PVA) (see later). The hemodynamic profile of acutely developing aortic insufficiency is significantly different than that of chronic regurgitation (71). The mean pulse and left ventricular end-diastolic pressure in stroke volume are markedly reduced in those individuals with rapid onset of dysfunction as compared to those with chronic insufficiency. Because ventricular pressures of late diastole are greater than those in the left atrium, the mitral valve prematurely closes. This early closure of the mitral valve may be heralded by the appearance of an Austin-Flint murmur. Such patients have severe volume overload of the ventricle and so are candidates for early valvular replacement. The initial presentation of congestive failure may be very subtle, such as the development of resting tachycardia. This finding may be directly attributed to the presence of fever (72). Patients may appear quite stable early in the course of IE and then suffer a sudden onset of pulmonary edema (Chapter 15).

Extension of the valvular infection beyond the leaflets into the annulus or myocardium is termed PVA. Approximately 35% of patients with acute IE develop this complication (73,74). Not surprisingly, because of its extensive repertoire of virulence factors [Chapter 2, *S. aureus* is not only the most common pathogen found

TABLE 6 Intracardiac Complications of Acute Infective Endocarditis

Refractory heart failure
Myocardial and septal abscesses
Paravalvular abscesses
Valvular leaflet destruction
Infection of intracardiac devices and sewing patches
Papillary muscle ruptures
Obstruction of prosthetic valves
Suppurative pericarditis
Loosening of prosthetic valves from sewing ring
Intracardiac fistulas

Source: From Ref. 23.

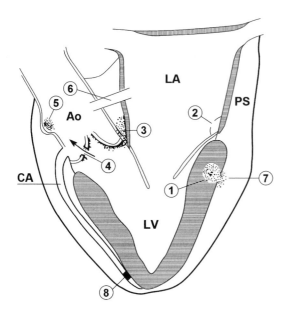

FIGURE 1 Intracardiac complications of native valve infective endocarditis. *Keys:* 1, myocardial/septal abscesses; 2, ruptured papillary muscle; 3, paravalvular abscess; 4, destruction of valvular leaflets; 5, mycotic aneurysm of the sinus of valsalva; 6, aortic/cardiac fistula; 7, suppurarative pericarditis; 8, septic/sterile coronary artery embolus. *Abbreviations:* LA, left atrium; AO, aorta; LV, left ventricle; PS, pericardial space; CA, coronary artery.

in PVA but also the most deadly (75)], PVA is more common in patients with aortic valve disease (41%) as compared with mitral valve IE (6%). Intravenous drug abusers also are at a greater risk of developing PVA. PVA develops frequently in patients with prosthetic valve IE with mechanical prosthetic valves more involved than the bioprosthetic ones (76). However, the size of the vegetation does not seem to be correlated with the risk of extension of valvular infection. In a series of 23 patients who died of acute IE, Arnett and Roberts determined that a PVA of the aortic valve is not related to age or sex, the condition of the valve before the development of IE, or to the antibiotics administered. Because of its critical location situated between the left atrium left, ventricle, and aorta and adjacent to the conduction system (Fig. 1), they can produce several significant deleterious effects. These include: (*i*) conduction abnormalities, (*ii*) fistula formation, (*iii*) persistent infection, (*iv*) exacerbation of congestive heart failure, and (*v*) increased rates of systemic embolization (77).

Roberts and Somerville were among the first to recognize the effect of PVA on intracardiac conduction as determined by the appearance of a prolonged P-R interval or by the presence of A-V dissociation, left bundle branch block during the course of IE. (78). Actually, most of these patients had infected aneurysms of the septum. Twenty-two percent of these patients died suddenly. Conduction abnormalities are most frequent when the PVA lies between the right and the noncoronary cusp of the aortic valve. This area overlies the proximal ventricular conduction system. Interference with normal conduction either may be reversible if caused by an inflammatory response around the conduction fibers, or permanent if there is direct damage to them (21,75). Septal abscesses that arise from a mitral valve PVA usually are situated at the lower end of the interventricular septum. Their existence should be considered when there is a gradual increase in the P-R and Q-T intervals combined with a left bundle branch block. An abscess of the upper septum produces much less specific EKG changes and these occur later in the course of IE. Serial EKGs may detect ventricular tachycardia (79). The surgical removal of an

TABLE 7 Conduction Abnormalities in 20 Patients with Acute Infective Endocarditis

Conduction abnormality	Number of patients
First-degree AV block	9
Isolated	5
+ Left bundle branch block	3
+ Left anterior hemiblock	1
Second-degree AV block	3
Isolated	2
+ Incomplete right bundle branch block	1
Third degree AV block	4
Isolated	2
+ Left bundle branch block	1
+ Right bundle branch block	1
Isolated left bundle branch block	1
Isolated right bundle branch block	2
Left posterior hemiblock	1

Abbreviation: AV, atrioventricular.
Source: From Ref. 80.

abscess from this location usually necessitates the placement of a pacemaker. Table 7 presents the various conduction abnormalities seen in acute IE (80).

The sensitivity of EKGs for detecting the presence of a PVA is low. In a recent prospective series, 36 of 137 patients with IE of a native valve developed dysfunction of the conducting system (81). Eight of the 15 patients with PVA by echocardiography had an infranodal on their EKGs. The significantly higher death rate of patients with infranodal block than those without (41% vs. 15%) mandates a sensitive and specific method for their detection. Transesophageal echocardiography (TEE) has become the diagnostic standard. It has superceded transthoracic echocardiography (TTE), which fails to detect up to 50% of PVA that are detected by TEE (82). The sensitivity of the TEE modality was 87% versus 28% for TTE. Both TEE and TTE were highly specific (95% and 99%, respectively). The positive and negative predictive values of TEE were 91% and 92%, respectively. The TEE signs of PVA include: (*i*) interventricular septal perivalvular densities >14 mm; (*ii*) anterior or posterior aortic root thickness >9 mm; (*iii*) abnormal rocking motion of prosthetic valves; and (*iv*) sinus of Valsalva aneurysms (21) (Chapter 13). It is challenging for TEE to differentiate PVA from postoperative changes in patients with prosthetic heart valves. Occasionally, uninfected prosthetic valves may demonstrate small paravalvular leaks.

Paravalvular abscess is a significant cause of refractory fevers during acute IE. The mortality rate of unoperated upon PVA ranges between 38% and 75% (21,75). In one series, the overall death rate was 38% (75). Those who died lived an average of 43 days after surgery. Fifty-seven percent of those with significant valvular and paravalvular regurgitation died. Persistent infection was the most common cause of death (56%). It is recommended that all patients with PVA received surgery unless there are contraindications (Chapter 15).

Intracardiac fistulas (incidence of 1.6%) may result from myocardial abscesses or PVA (83). These most commonly develop when PVA burrows into the aorta, the pulmonary arteries, or the sinuses of Valsalva (84). Transesophageal echocardiography provides the only noninvasive way of diagnosing this complication.

The pericarditis of acute IE may be multifactorial in origin (23). Organisms may be deposited into the pericardial space during the course of a bacteremia.

Other infectious causes are: (*i*) rupture of a myocardial abscess into the pericardial space and (*ii*) extension of PVA of the aortic valve to the wedge of pericardium situated between the root of the aorta and the pulmonary arteries. Noninfectious causes include: (*i*) uremia secondary to the renal failure of IE and (*ii*) flare-up of rheumatic fever. Whatever may be the cause, IE-associated pericarditis seldom is painful. It does not produce hemodynamically significant tamponade.

Myocarditis is more frequently seen in subacute disease. When it occurs during acute IE, it may be a result of embolic occlusion of a coronary artery or of toxic injury to the myocardium by bacterial toxins or by direct invasion of the pathogen (1).

Extracardiac Complications of Acute Infective Endocarditis

Table 8 presents the extracardiac complications of acute IE.

Neurological Complications of Acute Infective Endocarditis

Cerebral abscess and stroke are the most common neurological complications of acute IE. Embolic infarcts seem to occur at the same rate as in subacute disease. Cerebral abscesses and purulent meningitis are more common in acute IE (28). Hemorrhagic strokes in acute IE are particularly devastating. Unlike their role in subacute disease, strokes rarely are the presenting symptom of acute valvular infection. The cerebral abscesses of staphylococcal IE may be single or multiple. Unlike the meningeal emboli of *S. viridans* that can lead to aseptic meningitis, those of *S. aureus* produce one typical of bacterial meningitis. In one report, 31% of *S. aureus* meningitis was associated with IE (85).

Non-Neurological Emboli and Mycotic Aneurysms of Acute Infective Endocarditis

In order of importance of complications of acute IE, septic emboli are secondary only to the intracardiac catastrophes discussed previously. Suppurative foci are the inevitable result wherever the emboli of acute IE, especially that because of *S. aureus*, are deposited. Clinical clues to their presence are: (*i*) initial defervescence after the initiation of treatment; (*ii*) recurrent febrile episodes during or after discontinuation of treatment; (*iii*) failure to respond at all to appropriate antibiotics; and (*iv*) the persistence of bacteremia during therapy. The metastatic suppurative complication most closely associated with IE is the splenic abscess (86,87). There usually is no pain or splenic enlargement. The mortality rate of this infection approaches 100% in those who do not undergo a splenectomy. Although, percutaneous drainage is curative for most types of abscesses, it is less effective in the case of those of the spleen.

TABLE 8 Extracardiac Complications of Acute Infective Endocarditis

Stroke
Spinal cord embolus
Splenic abscess
Mycotic aneurysm of the brain
Cerebral abscess
Non-neurological systemic septic emboli

Certainly, a disease of medical progress is the high rate of infection of prosthetic joints during the bacteremia of valvular infection (88). In one series, 34% of patients with *S. aureus* endocarditis developed infection of the prosthetic joint. The joint infection may not become clinically apparent when the patient is receiving antibiotics for treatment of the IE. They often become manifest after cure of IE has been achieved. Because the prosthetic joint is usually not a source of bacteremia, it is not recommended that the joint be removed during treatment of the valve infection. Eventually, the joint should be removed if definite signs of infection develop such as fistula formation or loosening of its components. Occasionally vertebral osteomyelitis may be seen in *S. aureus* IE.

Mycotic aneurysms are not frequently seen in acute IE (see earlier).

Renal Complications of Acute Infective Endocarditis

The kidney may be involved in 40% to 50% of *S. aureus* IE. The most common pathological findings are: (*i*) renal infarction (31%); (*ii*) acute glomerulonephritis (26%); (*iii*) interstitial nephritis (10%); and (*iv*) acute cortical necrosis (10%). These changes are because of septic emboli and vasculitis and are not mediated by immunological phenomena as are the renal changes of subacute IE (61,89).

Musculoskeletal Complications of Acute Infective Endocarditis

Osteomyelitis (usually vertebral) is not a common feature of acute IE. *Staphylococcus aureus* is its most common cause. Septic arthritis is seen in a small percentage of patients. Infective endocarditis should be considered as its source: (*i*) if joint infection appears abruptly in the joints of the axial skeleton; (*ii*) when multiple joints are involved; and (*iii*) when organisms, closely associated with IE, are retrieved from the joint space (90).

Classic Peripheral Manifestations of Acute Infective Endocarditis

As discussed before, most of the peripheral manifestations of valvular infection are part of the syndrome of subacute IE. Osler nodes and Janeway lesions, in certain cases, may be associated with acute staphylococcal infections.

Right-Sided Infective Endocarditis

Approximately, 5% of cases of native valve IE involve the right side of the heart. Rarely does the pulmonic valve become infected (91,92). Patients with isolated pulmonic valve IE present with hypertension and interstitial pulmonary infiltrates. Infective endocarditis occurs 28 times less frequently in pulmonic stenosis than in aortic stenosis. It occurs twice as often in those with pulmonic stenosis than in patients with normal valves (93). Most of the cases of right-sided IE involve the tricuspid valve and are acute in nature with *S. aureus*, fungi, and gram-negative aerobes as the pathogens most commonly involved. One most commonly associates right-sided infection with IVDA IE [Chapter 7 (94)]. However, there are other causes of right-sided valvular infection. Among these are congenital defects, septic abortion, skin infection, and infections of the respiratory or genitourinary tract. Understandably, pulmonary complications predominate. Embolic phenomenon to the lungs occurs early in the course of the disease. These occur more frequently when there are predominant left or right shunts, defects in the intraventricular septum, or presence of patent ductus arteriosus (95). Emboli involve the systemic circulation as the course of IE progresses. Symptoms include: embolic pneumonia, pleurisy, and hemoptysis. In the case of tricuspid valve IE, a murmur may be absent in 80% of the cases. In the setting of congenital heart disease or valvular regurgitation, the thrombus is located downstream of the orifice through which an elevated pressure gradient propels the blood at high velocity. The smaller the intraventricular septal defect is, the more likely a vegetation/infection will occur because of the larger pressure gradient generated (96). Under these circumstances, the vegetations are located surrounding the opening in the right septal wall and at the point of impact of the jet stream on the ventricular endocardium. Ostium secundum atrial septal defects are rarely involved in IE because the low-pressure gradients between the two atria do not promote the development of NBTE.

When emboli result from infection with poorly pathogenic organisms such as *S. viridans*, the resultant pulmonary infarcts are sterile. Those owing to *S. aureus* are almost always infected and may develop into micro- or macropulmonary abscesses. Pneumonia, arterial thrombosis, and septic arteritis of the branches of pulmonary artery are other complications of septic emboli. If left unchecked, the sterile emboli of organisms like *S. viridans* may lead to repeated episodes of pulmonary infarction complicated by pneumonia, hepatosplenomegaly, jaundice, and progressive renal failure. The underlying valvular infection may be cryptic because these patients are often afebrile and right-sided murmurs are absent or difficult to hear. In addition, blood cultures often are sterile.

Relapse, Recurrence, and Mortality of Native Valve Infective Endocarditis

Early relapse of IE is defined as return of clinical disease combined with positive blood cultures during antibiotic therapy or three months after its completion (1,97). The longer the time between the onset of the disease in its relapse, the greater the chance for the blood cultures to be sterile. The bacteria, recovered from the initial infection and the relapse, may be the same or different. Early relapses may be associated with several factors: (*i*) ineffective antibiotic; (*ii*) improper dosing regimen; (*iii*) too short a duration of therapy; (*iv*) presence of a tolerant organism; (*v*) superinfection with another microorganism, bacterial or fungal; (*vi*) secondary bacteremia from an infected intravenous catheter or from suppurative thrombophlebitis; (*vii*) development of resistance by the initially infecting organism; (*viii*) presence of perivalvular abscess other than myocardial abscesses or intracardiac fistulas; and (*ix*) development of cell wall-deficient organisms (microbial persisters) promoted by the use of antibiotics that inhibit cell wall synthesis. The rate of relapse of *S. viridans* native valve IE is <2%. For enterococcal IE, the corresponding number ranges from 8% to 20%. *Staphylococcus aureus*, gram-negative aerobes, and fungal IE have a much higher rate of failure (97).

Extracardiac staphylococcal abscesses may mimic the phenomenon of early relapse. Abscesses of the spleen are the ones most likely to do this (23,87). The abscessed spleen is neither enlarged nor tender. It may or may not produce a bacteremia. A splenic abscess should always be ruled out by CT scan, before cardiac surgery is performed to treat a "failure" of antimicrobials or relapse of valvular infection.

Late relapse is defined as the return of signs and symptoms of the original valvular infection three to six months after treatment has been completed. As with early relapse, the organism may or may not be the same one that caused the original infection. Fungal infections have been implicated in producing late relapses.

It is proposed that fungal growth is enhanced by the prolonged use of broad-spectrum antibiotics employed to treat the initial bacterial valvular infection. A relapse of fungal is associated with failure to sterilize the core of a large thrombus and the tendency of the fungus to spread into the areas of myocardium proximate to the infected valve.

The overall rate of recurrent endocarditis ranges from 1% to 10% (99) with much higher rates in certain groups (see later). Organisms have been detected in surgical specimens more than 10 months after the patients had achieved clinical cure (100). This is comparable with an 8.5% rate of persistent endocardial infection (101). Recurrence occurs in almost 10% of patients with subacute IE (102). About 2.5% of these patients suffered a third attack of IE. Some series show an overall recurrence rate of greater than 30% (103). Intravenous drug abusers IE is the most likely to recur with a rate >48%. Mokotoff (104) described a remarkable patient who dramatically demonstrated this feature. The individual was an IVDA who experienced seven episodes of IE over 9.5 years. Five of these were because of *S. aureus* and one of *Entercoccal* spp. The last attack was culture negative. The final conclusion by these investigators was that the recurrences were because of inadequate treatment. Baddour identified three major characteristics that increase the risk of recurrence (105). These included an underlying cardiac disorder, periodontal disease, and a variety of surgical procedures such as placement of prosthetic valves and grafts in patients with congenital defects. Congestive heart failure and dual invasion of both mitral and aortic valves occur more commonly in recurrent infection than during an initial episode of IE. In a series of 420 patients with IE who were cared for in a tertiary-care teaching hospital, there was an overall recurrence rate of 11.4%. Mean follow-up of the patients was 6.1 years. There were two recurrences in 0.5% of cases, three in 0.2%, and five recurrences in 0.2% (106). Risk factors for recurrent IE were advanced age and male sex. The overall mortality rate was 12.3%. Recurrent IE was the factor that most highly correlated with death (risk ratio of 2.06). The authors of this study concluded that the long-term, event-free post-treatment of IE of patients was currently lower than previously thought.

Another study established a risk classification for death owing to complicated left-sided native valve endocarditis (Table 9) (107). The authors found that all cause mortality rate was 25% at six months after the onset of IE. They identified five baseline characteristics that are independently associated with death within six months. These included: (*i*) abnormal mental status; (*ii*) moderate to severe congestive heart

TABLE 9 Charlson Comorbidity Scale

One-point value category	Diabetes with end-organ damage
Myocardial infarction	Any type of tumor
Congestive heart care	Leukemia
Peripheral vascular disease	Lymphoma
Cerebrovascular disease	Three-point value category
Connective tissue disease	Moderate-to-severe liver disease
Ulcer disease	Six-point value category
Mild liver disease	Metastatic solid tumor
Diabetes	AIDS
Two-point value category	
Hemiplegia	
Moderate to severe renal disease	

Source: From Ref. 107.

failure; (*iii*) non-*S. viridans* etiology; (*iv*) more than two comorbidities (Table 9); and (*v*) medical therapy alone without valvular surgery. Cases of IE could be risk stratified into four prognostic categories that were derived from these five characteristics. Six-month mortality ranged from 7% in prognostic group 1 to 69% in prognostic group 4. A significant feature of this risk classification is the importance given to the underlying comorbidities. The importance of these, in determining outcomes of IE, is often overshadowed by the underlying heart disease and the pathogenic potential of the infecting organism.

Case Study 1 ■ The patient is an 85-year-old woman who was brought to the emergency room by her family because of the rapid onset of symptoms consistent with delirium. Her neighbors had contacted the patient's daughter to alert her that her mother was wandering throughout the neighborhood looking for her home. Her type II diabetes mellitus and essential hypertension have been under good control. She lives alone and does her own activities of daily living. She requires some help with changing the beds but does all her home-line work except for mowing the grass. Over the preceding three months, the patient had been several times to see her primary care physician for increasing arthritic symptoms, which were more consistent with myalgias. She had received two courses of oral antibiotics to cover hospital bronchitis and urinary tract infection without much symptomatic effect. No cultures were obtained prior to starting these agents. Ten days prior to being brought to the emergency room, her doctor drew some additional blood work. Among this group of tests was a sedimentation rate. Its value was 120. Because of the symptoms of myalgia, elevated sedimentation rate, and normal white count, her doctor prescribed low-dose prednisone (10 mg daily) for the presumptive diagnosis of polymyalgia rheumatica. She started to improve symptomatically until her change in mental status.

On physical examination, the patient looked younger than her stated age. Her temperature was 100.2°F; blood pressure was 115/80 sitting and standing with an apical pulse of 88 and regular. Skin was normal for her age. She showed signs of mild gingivitis. There was no adenopathy. On chest exam, there were a few scattered crackles. A 2/6 early systolic murmur was present in the aortic area with a "wiff" of regurgitation. Abdominal exam revealed no hepatosplenomegaly of masses. Neurological exam was normal without any focal deficits peripherally or centrally. No neck stiffness was present. Her primary care physician related that there was no change in the patient's systolic murmur.

Hemoglobin, hematocrit, and white blood cell count were all within normal limits. Liver function tests, serum calcium, and electrolytes were within normal limits. There was evidence of senile emphysema on the chest X-ray along with calcification of the aortic valve. EKG showed nonspecific S-T segment changes. Computed tomography scan of the brain was read to be normal. Because of her low-grade fever and her neuropsychiatric symptoms, a lumbar puncture was performed. The cerebrospinal fluid glucose was 60 and serum glucose was 150. There were 33 cells, 31 lymphocytes, and two polymorphonuclear leukocytes. The diagnosis of aseptic meningitis was made. She was started on acyclovir, pending the results of a spinal fluid Herpes simplex PCR test.

Her prednisone was begun to be tapered because of the possibility that this medication may have contributed to her mental status changes. On the second hospital day, the PCR test came back negative. The cerebrospinal fluid was sterile. Acyclovir was discontinued. On the third hospital day on a prednisone dosage of 5 mg, her temperature increased to 101.2°F. Shortly thereafter, she became short of breath with an increase in her respiratory rate. On physical examination, there was clear-cut evidence of congestive heart failure. Her murmur seemed somewhat more harsh with more prominent findings of aortic regurgitation on auscultation and echocardiogram was performed which showed an 8-mm vegetation on the aortic valve.

Three sets of blood cultures that were drawn in the emergency room became positive for *S. viridans* on the following day.

Discussion: This is a classic case history for subacute IE. This is currently a disease primarily of the elderly. Previously abnormal valves, usually not hemodynamically dysfunctional, are the sites of infection. The murmur usually does not change from baseline. Most often, there is no cause, evident, of the infecting bacteremia. Only approximately 10% of cases can be linked to dental procedures or to other interventions. Most likely, the *S. viridans* originated from her gingivitis. Presenting symptoms are nonspecific and often musculoskeletal in nature. They are less frequent but not less important highly neurological changes that are brought about by subacute disease. She did have aseptic meningitis, not viral in origin, but due to sterile emboli to the central nervous system.

Case Study 2 ■ A 27-year-old man is brought to the emergency room with a 104°F fever and shaking chills. His only significant past medical history was the onset of juvenile diabetes at the age of 10. His diabetes is under excellent control. He leads a full and vigorous life. Three days before admission, he was playing ice hockey and was checked against the boards. He continued playing despite increasing pain in his thigh. At the end of the game, he went directly home and took a warm bath. The next morning he noticed a large bruise and hematoma at the point of contact. He went to work. As the day progressed, he felt "flu-like" with fever and chills. When he went home, he took his temperature. It was 101°F. He took some over-the-counter cold medication. Although he felt better when he woke up, he was unable to go to work. He continued taking the cold medication until the day of admission when he developed severe rigors and acute onset of shortness of breath. A friend drove him to the emergency room.

On physical examination, his temperature was 104°F. His blood pressure was 90/60 and the heart rate was regular at 120. He was shaking uncontrollably. Because of severe dyspnea, he acted almost combatively to the staff and did not allow them to do much of an examination initially. For a brief time, the caregiver felt that he may have been in withdrawal or had developed malignant hyperthermia from some unknown antipsychotic. When an oxygen saturation of 82% on room air was obtained, he was placed on a rebreathing mask. With his dyspnea improved, he was more co-operative. At that point, it was appreciated that he had rales two-thirds the way up his chest fields. In addition, there was a 4/6 systolic ejection murmur in the aortic area as well as a 2/6 diastolic regurgitant murmur with a summation gallop. Chest X-ray showed signs of pulmonary edema. There was a small hematoma on his left thigh.

The diagnosis of acute bacterial IE was made. Antibiotics were begun. He was taken to surgery within eight hours. A large PVA was drained. The aortic valve was replaced. Three sets of blood cultures, obtained in the emergency room, and tissue obtained by operation grew out methicillin-resistant *S. aureus* (MRSA). After a stormy postoperative course, he made a complete recovery.

Discussion: His presentation is very typical of acute staphylococcal valvular infection. Its course is rapidly progressive with severe valvular destruction leading to congestive heart failure. There was no evident portal of entry. This is often the case in staphylococcal bacteremia/IE. It is postulated that the staphylococci penetrate the skin through microscopic rents. Damage to the microcirculation by pressure trauma (being checked against the boards) prevents migration of polymorphonuclear leukocytes. This interference with the migration of the leukocytes allows local proliferation of the staphylococcus and entry into the circulation. The fact that he is diabetic indicates that there was pre-existing impairment of his microcirculation. In addition, the high rate of MRSA in the community makes it imperative to empirically cover for this organism.

Case Study 3 ■ A 42-year-old fisherman was taken to the emergency room because of fever and acute shortness of breath. His health was always excellent. About 10 days prior to his admission, he stuck his finger with a metal piece of the fishing net. The next day, he noticed that this finger had become red and swollen and painful. He applied bacitracin ointment and soaked it. Over the day, the digit grew more painful. He developed fever and chills. At the end of this day, he went to the emergency room. A diagnosis of cellulitis and the flu was made. Except for the swollen finger, the physical examination was normal. It was noted that no murmur was heard. He was started on cephalexin for five days. No cultures were obtained. He began to feel better. He defervesced and his finger improved. His temperature never fully went away. His symptoms started to return within 36 hours of finishing the prescribed course of antibiotic. Again, he went to the emergency room. He was given another five days of cephalexin. He initially started to feel better but after a few days he became more febrile. Gradually, he noted the onset of dyspnea on exertion.

For the third time, he returned to the emergency room. There, it was noted that his temperature was 103.8°F. He was in severe congestive heart failure with the heart sounds hardly audible. An emergency echocardiogram revealed severe aortic regurgitation. An EKG indicated that he was in third-degree heart block. He was transferred to a tertiary-care center. Within four hours, he was operated upon. In addition to a destroyed valve, there was found a large PVA tracking well into the myocardium and into the septum. The valve was replaced and the areas were drained as well as possible. He died four hours after the completion of surgery. Blood cultures and operatively obtained cultures grew out *S. aureus*.

Discussion: This clearly is a case of acute staphylococcal IE with extensive intracardiac complications of PVA leading to disruption of the conducting system. It also is a form of "muted" endocarditis. Although caused by a very virulent organism, symptoms of his valvular infection were suppressed for several days with a relatively mild orally administered antibiotic. However, during this time, the infection was given an opportunity to spread and produce the deadly intracardiac complications. By the time the correct diagnosis was realized, the patient was beyond medical help.

REFERENCES

1   Weinstein L, Brusch JL. Clinical manifestations of native valve endocarditis. In: Weinstein L, Brusch JL, eds. Infective Endocarditis. New York: Oxford University Press, 1996:165.
2. Brusch JL. Infective endocarditis. E-medicine 2006.
3. Gouello JP, Asfar P, Brenet O, et al. Nosocomial endocarditis in the intensive care unit: an analysis of 22 cases. Crit Care Med 2000; 28:377.
4. Moreillon P, Yok-Ai Q. Infective endocarditis. Lancet 2004; 363:139.
5. Verheul HA, van den Brink RB, van Vreeland T, et al. The effects of changes in management of active infective endocarditis on outcome in a 25-year period. Am J Cardiol 1993; 72:682.
6. Mansur AJ, Grinburg M, da Luz PL, Bellotti G. The complications of infective endocarditis. A reappraisal in the 1980s. Arch Intern Med 1992; 152:2428.
7. Starkebaum M, Durack D, Beeson P. The "incubation period" of subacute bacterial endocarditis. Yale J Biol Med 1977; 50:49.
8. Sarli Issa V, Fabri J Jr, Pomerantzeff PM, et al. Duration of symptoms in patients with infective endocarditis. Intern J Cardiol 2003; 89:63.
9. Osler W. Malignant endocarditis. Lancet 1885; 1:415.
10. Nager F. Changing clinical spectrum of infective endocarditis. In: Horstkotte D, Bodnar B, eds. Infective Endocarditis. London: ICR Publishers, 1991:25.
11. Terpenning MS, Buggy BP, Kauffman CA. Infective endocarditis: clinical features in young and elderly patients. Am J Med 1987; 83:626.
12. Pankey GA. Subacute bacterial endocarditis at University of Minnesota Hospitals, 1939–1959. Ann Intern Med 1961; 55:550.

13. Lerner PI, Weinstein L. Infective endocarditis in the antibiotic era. N Engl J Med 1966; 274:199.
14. Pelletier LL, Petersdorf RG. Infective endocarditis: a review of 125 cases from the University of Washington Hospitals. 1963–1972. Medicine (Baltimore) 1977; 72:90.
15. Weinstein L, Rubin RH. Infective endocarditis—1973. Prog Cardiovasc 1973; 16:239.
16. Weinstein L. Infected prosthetic valves: a diagnostic and therapeutic dilemma. N Engl J Med 1972; 286:1100.
17. Libman E, Friedberg CK. Subacute Bacterial Endocarditis. Oxford: Oxford University Press, 1948.
18. Libman E, Celler HL. The etiology of subacute infective endocarditis. Am J Med Sci 1910; 140:516.
19. Mills J, Utley J, Abbott J. Heart failure in infective endocarditis: predisposing factors, course and treatment. Chest 1974; 66:151.
20. Gonzales-Lavin L, Lise M, Ross D. The importance of the "jet lesion" in bacterial endocarditis involving the left heart: surgical considerations. J Thorac Cardiovasc Surg 1970; 59:185.
21. Sexton DJ, Spelman D. Current practices and guidelines: assessment and management of complications in infective endocarditis. Cardiol Clin 2003; 21:27.
22. Perry EL, Fleming RG, Edwards JE. Myocardial lesions in subacute bacterial endocarditis. Ann Intern Med 1952; 36:126.
23. Weinstein L. Life-threatening infective endocarditis. Arch Intern Med 1986; 46:953.
24. Garvey GJ, Neu HC. Infective endocarditis-an evolving disease. A review of endocarditis at the Columbia-Presbyterian, 1968–1973. Medicine (Baltimore) 1978; 57:105.
25. Anderson DJ, Goldstein LB, Wilkinson WE, et al. Stroke location, characterization, severity and outcome in mitral versus aortic valve endocarditis. Neurology 2003; 61:1341.
26. Heiro M, Nikskelainen J, Engblom E, et al. Neurologic manifestation of infective endocarditis. A 17-year experience in a teaching hospital in Finland. Arch Intern Med 2000; 160:2781.
27. Weinstein L, Schlesinger JJ. Pathoanatomic, pathophysiologic and clinical correlation in endocarditis (first of two parts).N Eng J Med 1974; 291:832.
28. Venezio FR, Weaterfielder GO, Cook FV, et al. Infective endocarditis in a community hospital. Arch Intern Med 1982; 142:789.
29. Salgado AV, Furlan AJ, Keys TF, et al. Neurologic complications of endocarditis: a 12-year experience. Neurology 1989; 39:173.
30. Pruitt AA, Rubin RH, Karchmer AW, et al. Neurologic complications of bacterial endocarditis. Medicine 1978; 57:329.
31. Hart Evasani, Foster JW, Luther MF, Kanter MC. Stroke in infective endocarditis. Stroke 1990; 21:695.
32. Vuile C, Nidorf M, Weyman AE, et al. Natural history of vegetations during successful medical treatment of endocarditis. Am Heart J 1994; 128:1200.
33. Molinari GF, Smith L, Goldstein MN, et al. Pathogenesis of cerebral mycotic aneurysms. Neurology 1974; 23:325.
34. Bohmfalk GL, Story JL, Wissinger JP, et al. Bacterial intracranial aneurysms. J Neurosurg 1978; 48:369.
35. Wilson WR, Lie JT, Houser OW, et al. The management of patients with mycotic aneurysm. Curr Clin Top Infect Dis 1981; 2:51.
36. Masuda J, Yutani C,Waki R, et al. Histopathologic analysis of the mechanisms of intracranial hemorrhage complicating infective endocarditis. Stroke 1992; 23:843.
37. Rubin RH, King MA, Mark EJ. Case 7-2003: a 43 year old man with fever, rapid loss of vision in the left eye and cardiac findings. N Engl J Med 2003; 348:834.
38. Manor RS, Mendel I, Savir H. Precapillary metastatic abscess in a case of subacute bacterial endocarditis. Ophthalmologica 1975; 170:22.
39. Ziment I. Nervous system complications in bacterial endocarditis. Am J Med 1969; 47:593.
40. Steckelberg JM, Murphy JG, Ballard B, et al. Emboli in infective endocarditis: the prognostic value of echocardiography. Ann Intern Med 1991; 114:635.
41. Sanfillipo AJ, Picard MH, Newell JB, et al. Echocardiographic assessment of patients with infectious endocarditis: prediction of risk for complications. J Am Coll Cardiol 1991; 18:1191.

42. Di Salvo G, Habib G, Pergola V, et al. Echocardiography predicts embolic events in infective endocarditis. J Am Coll Cardiol 2001; 37:1069.
43. Bayer AS, Bolger AF, Taubert KA, et al. Diagnosis and management of infective endocarditis and its complications. Circulation 1998; 98:2936.
44. Fowler VG Jr, Sanders LL, Kong LK, et al. Infective endocarditis due to *Staphylococcus aureus*: 59 prospectively identify cases with follow-up. Clin Infect Dis 1999; 28:106.
45. Rohmann S, Erbel R, Gorge G, et al. Clinical relevance of education location by transesophageal echocardiography in infective endocarditis. Eur Heart J 1992; 13:446.
46. Thuny F, DiSalvo G, Belliard O, et al. Risk of embolism and death in infective endocarditis: prognostic value of echocardiography: a prospective multicenter study. Circulation 2005; 112:69–75.
47. Kupferwasser LI, Hafner G, Mohr-Kahaly S, et al. The presence of infection-related antiphospholipid antibodies in infective endocarditis determines a major risk factor for embolic events. J Am Coll Cardiol 1999; 33:1365.
48. Elliott JP, Smith RF. Peripheral embolization. In: Magilligan DJ, Quinn EL, eds. Endocarditis: Medical and Surgical Management. New York: Marcel Dekker, 1986:165.
49. Baehe G. Renal complications of endocarditis. Trans Am Assoc Phys 1931; 46:87.
50. Glassock RJ, Cohen AG. Secondary glomerular disease. In: Brenner BM, Rector FC, eds. The Kidney. Philadelphia: Saunders, 1981:1536.
51. Pfeiffer JM, Lipton MJ, Oury JH, et al. Acute coronary embolus complicating bacterial endocarditis: operative treatment. Am J Cardiol 1976; 37:920.
52. Menzies CJG. Coronary embolus with infarction in bacterial endocarditis. Br Heart J 1961; 23:464.
53. Trevasani MF, Ricci MA, Michaels RM, et al. Multiple mesenteric aneurysms complicating subacute bacterial endocarditis. Arch Surg 1987; 122:823.
54. Feinstein E, Eknoyan G, Lister B. Renal complications of bacterial endocarditis. Am J Nephrol 1985; 5:457.
55. Weinstein L. "Modern" infective endocarditis. JAMA 1975; 223:260.
56. Neilson EG. Pathogenesis and therapy of interstitial nephritis. Kidney Int 1989; 35:1257.
57. Moore R, Smith C, Lipsky J, et al. Risk factors for nephrotoxicity in patients treated with aminoglycosides. Ann Intern Med 1989; 100:352.
58. Morel-Maroger L, Sraer JD, Herreman G, et al. Kidney in subacute endocarditis: pathological and immunofluorescence findings. Arch Pathol 1993; 26:689.
59. Kauffman RH, Thompson J Valentjn RM, et al. The clinical implications and the pathogenic significance of circulating immune complexes in infective endocarditis. Am J Med 1981; 71:17.
60. Bell ET. Glomerular lesions associated with endocarditis. Am J Pathol 1932; 6:639.
61. Majumdar A, Chowdhary S, Ferreira MA, et al. Renal pathological findings in infective endocarditis. Nephrol Dial Transplant 2000; 15:1782.
62. Churchill M, Geraci J, Hunder G. Musculoskeletal manifestations of bacterial endocarditis. Ann Intern Med 1977; 87:755.
63. Thomas P, Allal J, Bontoux D. Rheumatological manifestations of bacterial endocarditis. Ann Rheum Dis 1989; 93:716.
64. Le Moal G, Robolot F, Paccalin M, et al. Clinical and laboratory characteristics of infective endocarditis when associated with spondylodiscitis. Eur J Clin Microbiol Infect Dis 202; 21:671.
65. Willerson JT, Moellering RC Jr, Buckley MJ, et al. Conjunctival petechiae after open-heart surgery. N Engl J Med 1971; 24:539.
66. Kilpatrick ZM, Greenberg PA, Sanford JP. Splinter hemorrhages—their clinical significance. Arch Intern Med 1965; 115:730.
67. Kerr A, Tan JS. Biopsies of the Janeway lesion of infective endocarditis. J Cutan Pathol 1979; 6:124.
68. Doherty WB, Trubeck M. Significant hemorrhagic retinal lesions in bacterial endocarditis (Roth's spots). JAMA 1931; 97:308.
69. Libman E. The clinical features of cases of subacute bacterial endocarditis that have spontaneously become bacteria-free. Am J Med Sci 1913; 126:625.
70. Millaire A, Van Belle E, de Grotte P, et al. Obstruction of the left main coronary ostium due to an aortic vegetation: survival after early surgery. Clin Infect Dis 1996; 22:192.

71. Mann T, McLaurin L, Grossman W, et al. Assessing the hemodynamic severity of acute regurgitation due to infective endocarditis. N Engl J Med 1975; 293:108.
72. Mills J, Utley J, Abbott J. Heart failure in infective endocarditis: predisposing factors, course and treatment. Chest 1974; 66:151.
73. Graupner C, Vilacosta I, San Roman J, et al. Periannular extension of infective endocarditis. J Am Coll Cardiol 2002; 39:1204.
74. Arnett EN, Roberts WC. Valve ring abscess in active infective endocarditis: frequency, location, clues to clinical diagnosis from the study of 95 necropsy patients. Circulation 1976; 54:140.
75. Cosmi JE, Tunick PA, Kronzon I. Mortality in patients with paravalvular abscess diagnosed by transesophageal echocardiography. J Am Soc Echocardiogr 2004; 17:21.
76. Lytle BW. Surgical treatment of prosthetic valve endocarditis. Semin Thorac Cardiovas Surg 1995; 7:13.
77. Omari B, Nelson RJ, Shapiro S, et al. Predictive risk factors for periannular extension of native valve endocarditis. Clinical and echocardiographic analyses. Chest 1989; 96:1273.
78. Roberts NK, Somerville J. Pathological significance of electrocardiographic changes in aortic valve endocarditis. Br Heart J 1969; 31:395.
79. Ryon DS, Pastor BH, Myerson RM. Absence of the myocardium. Am J Med Sci 1966; 251:698.
80. DiNubile MJ, Calderwood SB, Steinhaus DM, et al. Cardiac conduction abnormalities complicating native valve active infective endocarditis. Am J Cardiol 1986; 58:1215.
81. Meine TJ, Nettles RE, Anderson TJ, et al. Cardiac conduction abnormalities in endocarditis defined by the Duke criteria. Am Heart J 2001; 142:280.
82. Daniel WG, Mugge A, Martin RP, et al. Improvement in the diagnosis of abscesses associated with endocarditis by transesophageal echocardiography. N Engl J Med 1991; 324:795.
83. Anguera I, Miro JM, Vilacosta I, et al. Aorto-cavitary fistulous tract formation in infective endocarditis: clinical and echocardiographic features of 76 cases and risk factors for mortality. Eur Heart J 2005; 26:288.
84. Ebringer A, Goldstein G, Sloman G. Fistula between aorta and atrium due to bacterial endocarditis. Br Heart J 1969; 31:133.
85. Schlesinger LS, Ross SC, Schaberg DR. *Staphylococcus aureus* meningitis: a broad-based epidemiologic study. Medicine (Baltimore) 1987; 66:148.
86. Chun CH, Raff MJ, Contreras L, et al. Splenic abscess. Medicine (Baltimore) 1980; 59:50.
87. Robinson SL, Saxe JM, Lucas CE, et al. Splenic abscess associated with endocarditis. Surgery 1992; 112:781.
88. Murdock DR, Roberts SA, Fowler VG Jr, et al. Infection of orthopedic prostheses after *Staphylococcus aureus* bacteremia. Clin Infect Dis 2001; 32:647.
89. Neugarten J, Baldwin DS. Glomerulonephritis in bacterial endocarditis. Am J Med 1984; 77:297.
90. Speechly-Dick ME, Swanton RH. Osteomyelitis and infective endocarditis. Postgrad Med J 1994; 70:885.
91. Pandis I, Kotler M, Mintz G. Right heart endocarditis: clinical and echocardiographic features. Am Heart J 1989; 107:759.
92. Hamza N, Ortiz J, Bonomo RA. Isolated pulmonic valve infective endocarditis: a persistent challenge. Infection 2004; 32:170.
92a. Bain R, Edward J, Scheiffen C. Right-sided bacterial endocarditis and endarteritis: clinical and pathologic study. Am J Med 1958; 29:9.
93. Matthew J, Addai T, Anand A, et al. Clinical features, site of involvement, bacteriologic findings and outcome of infective endocarditis in intravenous drug users. Arch Intern Med 1995; 155:1641.
94. Gersony WM, Hayes CJ, Driscoll DJ, et al. Bacterial endocarditis in patients with aortic stenosis, pulmonary stenosis and ventricular septal defect. Circulation 1993; 87(suppl I):121.
95. Altschule MD. Subacute bacterial endocarditis of the right heart. Med Sci 1964; 15:50.
96. Rodbard S. Blood velocity and endocarditis. Circulation 1963; 27:18.

97. Mylonakis E, Calderwood SB. Infective endocarditis in adults. N Engl J Med 2001; 345:1318.
98. Ooi LL, Leong SS. Splenic abscesses from 1987 to 1995. Am J Surg 1997; 174:87.
99. Garvey GJ, Neu HC. Infective endocarditis: an evolving disease. Medicine 1978; 57:105.
100. Cordeiro A, Pimental C. Novas fisionomias da endocardite subaguda. Ref Medica Angola 1961; 13:5.
101. Morgan WL, Bland EF. Bacterial endocarditis in the antibiotic era. Circulation 1959; 19:753.
102. Pankey GA. Subacute bacterial endocarditis at the University of Minnesota hospitals. Am Heart J 1962; 64:583.
103. Welton DE, Young JB, Gentry WO, et al. Recurrent infective endocarditis: analysis of predisposing factors and clinical features. Am J Med 1979; 66:932.
104. Mokotoff D, Young JB, Welton DE, et al. Recurrent infective endocarditis in a drug addict. Multiple separate episodes in nine years. Chest 1979; 76:592.
105. Baddour L. Twelve year review of recurrent native valve infective endocarditis: a disease of the modern antibiotic era. Rev Infect Dis 1988; 10:1163.
106. Mansur AJ, Dal Bo CM, Fukushima JT, et al. Relapses, recurrences, valve replacements and mortality during the long-term follow-up after infective endocarditis. Am Heart J 2001; 141:78.
107. Hasbun R, Holenarasipur VR, Barakat LA, et al. Complicated left-sided native valve endocarditis in adults: risk classification for mortality. JAMA 2003; 289:1933.

7 Endocarditis in Intravenous Drug Abusers

John L. Brusch
Harvard Medical School and Department of Medicine and Infectious Disease Service, Cambridge Health Alliance, Cambridge, Massachusetts, U.S.A.

INTRODUCTION

In any discussion of intravenous drug abuser infective endocarditis (IVDA IE), it is important to keep in mind that this form of valvular infection closely resembles the other types of IE, especially healthcare-associated infective endocarditis (HCIE). At first glance, to make such an association appears a bit outlandish. However, on closer inspection, it becomes more apparent that the pathogenesis of IVDA IE does parallel that of HCIE. Both forms are usually the consequence of some intravascular intervention albeit that of the IVDA is one that occurs without protocols or much of an attempt at sterile technique. The involved organisms are very much the same. Intravenous drug abuser IE and its growing association with HIV infection bridges the gap between native valve endocarditis and the immunosuppressed patient.

EPIDEMIOLOGY

In the United States, the incidence of valvular infection in IVDA ranges from 2% to 5% per year with 1.5 to 2 cases per 1000 years of intravenous drug abuse (1,2). These figures may underestimate the true problem because of the erratic use of medical care by these individuals (3). In addition, there may be actual spontaneous cures and "street-treated" right-sided IVDA IE (see later). Both of these possibilities would interfere with a valid assessment of the rate of acquisition of IVDA IE. Prior to 1950, IE had not been documented as a complication of injection drug use (4). Between 1950 and 1970, there were only 72 cases of IVDA IE reported in the literature (5). Levine estimated that 60% of hospitalizations of IVDA are because of infectious causes, 5% to 20% of which are IE (6). Five to ten percent of all deaths of IVDA are because of valvular infection (7). Of all injectable substances, intravenous cocaine puts the IVDA at greatest risk of developing IE (8), and hence those who use cocaine are at the greatest risk. The IVDA are at a significantly higher risk than individuals with underlying rheumatic heart disease or with prosthetic valves in place. The prevalence of IVDA IE depends on the specific population studied. This is an urban-focused disease. In the 1980s, the use of intravenous drugs was responsible for 40% of cases of IE in San Francisco but only 1% of those were reported in Olmsted County, Minnesota (9). Median age of IVDA ranges between 30 and 40 years (10). Males are affected three times more often than females (11). This does not hold for all organisms such as *Streptococcus pyogenes*. The reason for this imbalance between the sexes has not been established. There may be intrinsic differences in host defenses and injection techniques between men and women. Both the shorter duration of illicit drug use and a lesser rate of self-medication with antibiotics by females may preserve the normal flora of their skin and prevent overgrowth of *S. aureus* and *Pseudomonas aeruginosa* (12,13).

The relative incidence of IE of IVDA, infected with HIV, is 2.6 to 4.0 higher than in those who are not (14–16). The prevalence of HIV-1, among IVDA, varies from 40% to 90% (7). HIV-positive IVDA with CD4 counts >350 had an increased risk of 2.31 (range 0.61–8.8) of developing IE. Those with a CD4 count <350 had an 8.31-fold risk of developing valvular infections (range 1.2–56) (14). Female IVDA have an increased risk of developing valvular infections. There is a direct correlation with risk of developing the IE and the increasing frequency of illicit drug injections (16). There is some evidence that the development of IE, among HIV-positive IVDA, is decreasing because of needle-exchange programs (17). This may not be true for the United States. Non-IVDA HIV patients appear to have no increased risk of developing IE (18).

In 1977, Watanakunakorn published that the valvular involvement in IVDA IE was: the tricuspid valve, alone or with another valve, was infected in 52.2% of cases; the aortic valve was involved in 18.5%; the mitral valve in 10% to 18%, and the aortic and mitral valves in 12.5% (19). More recent series show the same type of distribution. The tricuspid valve is involved in greater than 50% of the cases, in some series up to 70%. The aortic valve is affected in 25% and the mitral valve in 20%, mixed lesions (combined infection of right- and left-sided valves) in 5% to 10% (20,21). There is increasing clinical evidence that left-sided disease may become more common in IVDA IE (22). This may be due, in part, to improved diagnostic methods. The pulmonic valve is seldom infected.

An autopsy-based study of patients, dying of their first attack of endocarditis, documented a higher rate of left-sided infection than appreciated by the clinical series shown before (23). This series documented that the right heart was infected in 30% of these cases; mixed cases were present in 13% and the mitral or aortic valve was infected in 41% (Table 1). These results support the clinical impression that left-sided IVDA valvular infection has a much poorer outcome than the right-sided (10).

TABLE 1 Autopsy Findings of the Location of Valvular Vegetations, Resulting from the First Episode of Infective Endocarditis in 80 Intravenous Drug Abusers

Location	Number of patients
Right-sided single valve	
Tricuspid valve	23
Pulmonic valve	1
Mixed right- and left-sided valves	
Tricuspid + mitral valves	8
Tricuspid + aortic valves	4
Pulmonic + mitral valves	1
Pulmonic + aortic valves	0
Left-sided single valve	
Mitral valve	15
Aortic valve	18
Two left-sided valves	
Aortic and mitral valves	10

Source: From Ref. 23.

PATHOGENESIS OF INTRAVENOUS DRUG ABUSER INFECTIVE ENDOCARDITIS

Is important to note that, at most, 30% of IVDA IE have underlying valvular disease (15). Most often, the predisposing valvular pathology is left-sided but the majority of the clinical disease (as opposed to autopsy data) involves the tricuspid valve. Until fairly recently, this distinctive feature has posed a significant challenge to fully comprehending the pathogenesis of IVDA IE. The common denominator of all of the varieties of IE is the lesion of nonbacterial thrombotic endocarditis (NBTE)—the sterile platelet/fibrin thrombus (Chapter 6). Many mechanisms have been invoked to explain the origin of the NBTE of IVDA IE. The particulate matter, which is contained within injectable illicit drugs, over time, may cause cumulative damage to the tricuspid valve (24). In support of this possibility is the detection of talc embedded within the tricuspid valves of IVDA (1,2). Much of the infected particulate matter is small enough to cross the pulmonary capillaries into the arterial circulation and ultimately damage the mitral or aortic valves (10). Intravenous drug abusers may have evidence of damage to the tricuspid valve on examination by transthoracic echocardiography (TTE) (24). Repeated injections of foreign proteins may induce NBTE by a variety of immunological mechanisms (25). In rats, stress has been shown to induce the formation of the NBTE (26,27). These may resolve spontaneously when the stressful situation is removed. One could theorize that the addict's overwhelming drive to acquire drugs is the human counterpart to this model. The ability of cocaine to stimulate the sympathetic nervous system may amplify these effects of stress. There may be increased expression of matrix molecules on the endothelium of the tricuspid valve (28) However, it was not possible to reproduce tricuspid IE in rabbits by injecting street heroin into them over several weeks followed by a very high concentration of *S. aureus* administered intravenously (29).

In the final analysis, the most important factor in the pathogenesis of IVDA IE is the pathogenic mechanisms of the most commonly associated organisms, *S. aureus* (Chapter 2). These bacteria can infect normal endothelial cells (endotheliosis) (30). The presence of fibronectin on the valvular surface can promote this invasion (31). Binding of *S. aureus* to fibronectin, by means of its vascular cell adhesion (VCA) molecules starts the process of endothelial uptake of the staphylococci. In summary, there are several possible, noninfectious triggers of NBTE production. *S. aureus* does not require a preformed fibrin platelet thrombus but will readily take advantage of one if already present.

Usually infection does not extend beyond the valvular cusps. Paravalvular abscess and perforation of the leaflets are quite unusual. Absence of aggressive infection is consistent with the more favorable clinical course of IVDA IE than other types of IE (32).

ORGANISMS OF INTRAVENOUS DRUG ABUSER INFECTIVE ENDOCARDITIS

The profile of infecting organisms in IVDA IE has remained substantially the same since first described by Hussey and Katz in 1950 (4). *S. aureus* infected the tricuspid valve of seven of their eight patients; *P. aeruginosa* was recovered from the aortic valve of the remaining patient. This constancy of the prominence of *S. aureus* is due primarily to the fact that this organism is commonly found in the patient's own mucocutaneous flora. This was originally documented by Tuazon and Sheagran in 1975 (33). They observed that in almost 100% of cases of IVDA IE, a single strain of *S. aureus* was recovered from the blood as well as from the oropharynx, nasopharynx, and skin. When the organism colonizes the pharynx, it is then able to be transferred to the skin. From there, it may penetrate into the bloodstream during the process of injection. Addiction to heroin increases the carriage of *S. aureus* by at least threefold. Upon withdrawing from heroin, the oropharyngeal carriage of *S. aureus* drops back close to that of the nonaddict.

There are clearly temporal and geographic trends in the types of organisms that cause IVDA IE. Because of this, the distribution of non-*S. aureus* pathogens is quite time- and site-specific. During the 1970s, *P. aeruginosa* was the most common cause in Chicago and Detroit. *Serratia* played the same role in San Francisco (34,35). Both have been supplanted by *S. aureus*. More current data from Spain indicates a lower percentage of both entercoccal and nonentercoccal streptococci than recorded in the United States (7). These past and present trends most likely reflect local patterns of contamination of injection paraphernalia, the drugs themselves, or techniques of injection. *Pseudomonas aeruginosa* lives in mixtures of pentazocaine and/or tripelennamine (36). Lemon juice that is used to prepare a "brown heroin" may be contaminated by *Candida albicans* (37). Some addicts lick their needles prior to injection for good luck. In many respects, right-sided IVDA IE is quite distinct from other types of valvular infection including even left-sided IVDA IE. With some exceptions, the profile of organisms producing left-sided IVDA IE is quite similar to that of nondrug abuser-associated valvular infections. Nonentercoccal streptococcal species and enterococci are recovered in cases of left-sided IVDA and non-IVDA IE in approximately the same numbers. These pathogens infect, almost exclusively, abnormal valves. *Streptococcus viridans* accounts for less than 5% of cases currently as opposed to 40% 30 years ago (2). Group A streptococci had been reported in up to 25% of cases of IVDA IE (6). Now it is seldom seen. Fungal infection, most commonly *Candida parapsilosis*, is closely associated with IVDA IE. It usually produces left-sided disease. Other *Candida* species found in IVDA IE are *C. tropicalis, C. guilleromondi, C. kruisei,* and *C. stellatoidea* (38,39). Less frequently isolated organisms include: *Hemophilus influenzae, Neisseria* spp., *Pseudomonas* spp., *Erysipelothrix, Gemella morbillorum, Clostridial* spp., *Corynebacteria, Citrobacter* spp., and *Eikenella corrodens* (40–44). This last organism may produce skin abscesses in those who use a mixture of pentazocaine and tripelennamine (T's and blues).

Staphylococcus aureus produces approximately 50% of overall cases of IVDA IE but >70% of right-sided disease. Forty percent of these are methicillin-resistant *S. aureus* (MRSA). Currently in the United States, it appears that fungal and gram-negative aerobes are quite unusual causative pathogens (45–47). When they affect the left side, they do so not more often than in non-IVDA. Why this differential distribution exists is not known. Table 2 summarizes the microbiology of right-sided IVDA IE.

Five to nine percent of IVDA IE are polymicrobial. Usually there are no more than two organisms, but valvular infection with eight has been reported. *Staphylococcus aureus* is almost inevitably retrieved. Other common isolates of polymicrobial IVDA IE are constituents of the patient's mouth flora. This may be related to their habit of licking the needle before insertion (48). Other frequently involved pathogens are *P. aeruginosa, Hemophilus,* and *Candida* spp. (1,39).

TABLE 2 Microbiology of Right-Sided Intravenous Drug
Abuser Infective Endocarditis Currently in the United States

Organism	Percentage of cases
Staphylococcus aureus	70
Entercoccal spp.	2
Non-Entercoccal streptococci	8
Fungal	2
Gram-negative aerobes	5
Polymicrobial	9

Source: From Refs. 43, 45.

CLINICAL MANIFESTATIONS OF INTRAVENOUS DRUG ABUSER INFECTIVE ENDOCARDITIS

The presenting manifestations of IVDA IE were determined not only by the causative organism but by the valves involved. Left-sided IVDA IE presents in a very similar fashion to non-IVDA IE of native valves (Chapter 6) (13). A significant consequences of mitral or aortic valve infection with *P. aeruginosa* is a high incidence of neurological insult (see later) and persistence of bacteremia despite the use of appropriate antibiotics (9). Pseudomonas may involve both ventricles simultaneously. Left-sided IVDA IE, as a result of *S. aureus* and less commonly due to *Streptococcus* spp., is also complicated by a high rate of arterial embolization to the renal and cerebral arteries (2). Murmurs are usually present (49). The incidence of peripheral stigmata of IE may be slightly less than that of other types of IE (10,50). More commonly seen are splinter hemorrhages (10%) and conjunctival petechiae (50%) (51).

Infection of the tricuspid valve by *S. aureus* leads to a high rate of septic embolization early on in the course of disease. This process overwhelmingly involves the lungs (3,10,15,48). Right-sided IVDA IE may present in a noncardiac manner in 25% to 50% of the individuals. The majority of these patients acutely develop cough, pleuritic pain, and hemoptysis. In 50% to 95%, septic pulmonary emboli underlie these symptoms. Thirteen percent develop empyema (Table 3). There is little systemic embolization compared with the left-sided disease. On presentation, only 5% of individuals with right-sided disease have a murmur. A murmur will later develop in half of these patients. In all cases of IVDA IE, murmurs are present in 35% of the cases (6). Right-sided IVDA, even when because of *S. aureus*, rarely leads to congestive heart failure. This may be because of the rarity of the perforation of valvular leaflets and paravalvular abscess in this type of IE (32).

Significant abdominal pain may occur in those with abdominal abscesses, splenic infarcts, or ischemic colitis (51). A splenic abscess may lead to persistent bacteremia. Neurological involvement in IVDA IE is quite similar to non-IVDA IE. There are two distinctive central nervous system features of IVDA gram-negative valvular infections. Panopthalmitis occurs in 10% of the patients and there is a high rate of cerebral mycotic aneurysms (52). Toxic encephalopathy is present in 30%. The infecting organism often can be grown out of the cerebrospinal fluid.

Ten to twenty percent of cases of IVDA IE, as a result of *S. aureus*, are complicated by septic arthritis. In subacute left-sided IVDA IE, arthralgias, which are the result of deposition of immune complexes in the synovium, are common (53).

TABLE 3 Signs and Symptoms of Right- and Left-Sided Intravenous
Drug Abuser Infective Endocarditis

Signs or symptoms	Right-sided (%)	Left-sided (%)
Pleuropulmonary complaints	80	35
Systemic complaints	25	50
Congestive heart failure	—	35–50
Fever >38°C	97	98
Murmur	5	80
Vegetations	38	58

Concurrent infection with HIV does not significantly alter the clinical presentation of IVDA IE. HIV fraction is not associated with a lower degree of fever even in patients with a CD4 count of <200 (54). Table 3 summarizes the signs and symptoms of right- and left-sided IVDA IE.

DIAGNOSIS OF INTRAVENOUS DRUG ABUSER INFECTIVE ENDOCARDITIS

There are multiple disease processes, both infectious and noninfectious, which produce fever in the IVDA. In those patients with concurrent HIV infection, the list of possible pathogens markedly increases. It is almost impossible to diagnose accurately valvular infection in febrile addicts on the basis of degree of temperature and physical examination. Only 33% of the diagnoses of IVDA IE made in the emergency room are correct (12,55,56). The aspect of the clinical history that is most highly correlated with the presence of IVDA IE is the individual's use of heroin (8). It is stated that the diagnosis of right-sided IVDA is challenging in those patients who have neither a murmur nor any signs of systemic embolization. Physical examination, especially in right-sided disease, is usually unremarkable. The murmur and other physical signs of tricuspid regurgitation (large V-waves or pulsatile liver) are present in only 33% of the cases (57). However, because of the high rate of valvular infection in IVDA, IE must be highly suspected in any addict with a temperature >38°C. Murmurs, congestive heart failure, and systemic embolization are present as frequently as they are in non-IVDA IE of native valves (2). Table 4 presents laboratory findings in febrile IVDA with and without valvular infection (55).

The classic chest radiographic signs of right-sided IVDA IE are multiple or solitary pulmonary infiltrates that result from septic emboli. These appear eventually in 87% of the patients (58). They may either cavitate or be complicated by

TABLE 4 Temperature and Laboratory Values in Febrile Intravenous Drug
Abusers With and Without Infective Endocarditis

Test	Endocarditis patients	Nonendocarditis patients
Median temperature	39.2°C	38.2°C
Leukocyte count	11,000/mL	8000/mL
Sedimentation rate	48 mm/hr	60 mm/hr

Source: From Ref. 55.

empyema in up to 75% of cases (3,48). *S. aureus* is responsible for 90% of these radiographic findings with *P. aeruginosa* accounting for 5% (48).

The principle method for diagnosing IVDA IE is, as it is for all types of valvular infections, the blood culture (see Chapter 12). Bacteremia lasting >30 minutes (continuous bacteremia) is the primary diagnostic criteria of IE (2,59). Continuous bacteremia is the hallmark of an endovascular infection. Three sets of blood cultures should be obtained by separate venipunctures. The interval between each is determined by the clinical situation. If the clinical presentation is subacute, then 24 hours is desirable. If it is acute in presentation, antibiotic therapy needs to be instituted rapidly (see later). In this situation, the blood cultures should be drawn within 30 minutes (60). Performing a venipuncture at the exact site of a previous illicit injection should be avoided because of the possibility of rupturing an underlying mycotic aneurysm (2).

Five percent of blood cultures in IVDA IE are truly negative. Most likely, many more are falsely so because of the preadmission use of street-obtained antibiotics, which are self-administered. Anecdotally, this number may be much greater. Such a practice can suppress the growth of many organisms including *S. aureus*. Persistently sterile cultures, which are obtained over several days after the self-administration of antibiotics, has ceased should lead to the reconsideration of the diagnosis of IE (61). It is important to emphasize that the presence of septic emboli by chest X ray and positive blood cultures may also be produced by septic thrombophlebitis (48). Probably, the best way of differentiating these two diseases is by demonstrating valvular thrombi by echocardiography.

Whenever there is a chest infiltrate in the patient with HIV-IVDA IE, Pneumocystic jirovecci must be considered in the differential diagnosis. The Duke criteria for diagnosing endocarditis have been shown to be valid in IVDA IE (62,63). Transthoracic echocardiography may demonstrate tricuspid vegetations in up to 80% cases of IVDA IE. Transesophageal echocardiography (TEE) has somewhat a higher sensitivity (64,65). In most cases of IVDA IE, echocardiography is not required as a primary diagnostic tool as it would not provide any means of monitoring the development of complications of the valvular infection (paravalvular abscess or valvular insufficiency). Usually, TTE is sufficient. TEE is most helpful to the clinician in the evaluation of two types of patients. First, those patients who have a high likelihood of infection but who have persistently negative blood cultures because of either fastidious organisms or the recent use of antibiotics. The other category of patients are those who have positive blood cultures for a well-established endocarditis pathogen but who have no other radiological or clinical evidence consistent with the diagnosis of IVDA IE (2,60).

A prominent noninfectious cause of fever in IVDA is the entity labeled cotton fever (61,66). Cotton fever is described as the sudden onset of fever, chills, and dyspnea developing shortly after injection of the illicit drug. These typically disappear within a few hours. It is thought to be caused by pyrogens present in the injectable substance. At times however, it may be caused by actual bacterial contamination.

TREATMENT OF INTRAVENOUS DRUG ABUSER INFECTIVE ENDOCARDITIS

This section will cover the treatment of right-sided IVDA IE and not left-sided disease, as therapy of the latter is basically the same as that of native or prosthetic valve IE (Chapter 14).

Patients who are medically stable, who have low-grade fever, and who present with no definite evidence of IE upon admission to hospital do not require emergent therapy unless a prosthetic valve is present. Twenty percent of these defervesce within a few hours after the hospitalization (12). None of this subgroup of patients ever ends up having the diagnosis of valvular infection. In the case of individuals who have taken antibiotics prior to hospitalization and who are medically stable, blood cultures are obtained at presentation. If these are sterile, they should be repeated over a period of days while suppressive effect of the antibiotic disappears. The length of time this would take depends on the antibiotic, clearance from the vegetations, and nature of the infecting organism. If during this time of watchful waiting, the patient deteriorates or develops signs or symptoms of IE (pleuritic pain or embolic changes on the chest X ray) or the blood cultures exhibit growth, antibiotic therapy should be begun immediately (61).

More often than not, treatment must be initiated immediately because of the unstable nature of the patient. There are four major factors to be taken into consideration when making this initial therapeutic decision: (*i*) the location of the valvular infection, right- or left-sided, (*ii*) the HIV status of the patient, (*iii*) the nature of the bacterial flora of the local IVDA community, and (*iv*) the type of drug injected (Table 5) (67).

Oxacillin or nafcillin are the antibiotics of choice for treating methicillin-sensitive *S. aureus* (MSSA) of native valves of either ventricle (68,69). For treatment of patients with a history of minor reactions to penicillins (e.g., typical macular drug rash), cefazolin is almost as efficacious as the antistaphylococcal penicillins. Vancomycin has been the antibiotic of choice for patients who have significant allergies to penicillins. However, vancomycin is not the therapeutic equivalent of the penicillinase-resistant penicillins in the treatment of MSSA. Small and Chambers documented a failure rate of 35% in 13 cases of MSSA IE treated with appropriate doses of the drug (70). There were cases of right-sided endocarditis in this series. Another study demonstrated that 70% of cases of MSSA bacteremia that were treated with vancomycin were relapses (71). There are several causes for failure of vancomycins in treating MSSA. Their bactericidal action is less pronounced than the penicillinase-resistant penicillins (71). They diffuse poorly into valvular vegetations (72) and they are cleared more readily by the kidney in IVDA (73). Vancomycin should be used in only those patients who are significantly allergic to beta-lactams.

An alternative antibiotic to vancomycin would be the oxazolidinone, linezolid. Outcomes for this agent have been shown to be superior to those of vancomycin against

TABLE 5 Factors and Their Rationale that Are Important in Choosing Empiric Antibiotic Therapy in Intravenous Drug Abuser Infective Endocarditis

Factors	Rationale
Location of the valvular infection	Right-sided disease is almost always currently caused by *Staphylococcus aureus*
HIV status	HIV-positive IVDA have a significantly higher rate of right-sided disease due to *S. aureus*
Nature of local IVDA flora	Prevalence of methicillin-resistant *S. aureus* and *Pseudomonas aeruginosa*
Type of drug injected	Pentazocaine use is associated with *P. aeruginosa*; use of brown heroin, dissolved in lemon juice, associated with *Candida*

Abbreviation: IVDA, intravenous drug abuser.

many types of infections caused by both MSSA and MRSA (74,75). There have been treatment failures of MRSA IE. These seem to be related to subtherapeutic levels of the antibiotic in serum (76). Other favorable aspects of linezolid are its excellent gastrointestinal absorption that helps facilitate transition to oral therapy and its lack of dosing adjustment in renal failure. It does have important hematological toxicities (myelosuppression, thrombocytopenia, and anemia); being a monoamine oxidase inhibitor, it potentially causes peripheral and optic neuropathy (77,78). The author has had a good deal of favorable experience with this antibiotic in the treatment of IE. In fact, it often is my empiric choice for treatment of *S. aureus* IE while awaiting sensitivities. The treatment successes of the bacteriostatic linezolid seem to defy the important therapeutic principles that bactericidal antibiotics are necessary for cure of valvular infections. Chapter 14 presents a more thorough discussion of the role of linezolid. In treatment of MSSA IE, there are few other alternatives. There is little clinical experience with quinupristin–dalofopristin to recommend its use in therapy of IE (79).

Korzeniowski first showed that a combination of penicillinase-resistant penicillin (nafcillin) and an aminoglycoside (gentamicin) resulted in a more rapid defervescence and decreases in both the white blood cell count and in the duration of bacteremia in MSSA IE (80). This pairing did not improve the ultimate cure rates. However, because of its favorable effects, it has been recommended to combine gentamicin in the first three to five days of treatment with the beta-lactam (68).

The aforementioned favorable effects of the addition of gentamicin was one of the justifications for evaluating a short-course (two weeks) treatment of *S. aureus* right-sided IVDA IE with nafcillin and tobramycin (81). In the original study of Chambers, the cure rate was 94%. This has been substantiated in six other studies between 1993 and 2001 (7). These additional studies investigated the addition of aminoglycosides to other beta-lactam drugs and vancomycin.

Combinations of beta-lactams and aminoglycosides produced quite favorable results (at least 90% cure rate). The failure rate of vancomycin and aminoglycosides ranged from 40% to 67%.

Short-term therapy is not appropriate for any type of MSSA left-sided valvular infection, either IVDA- or non-IVDA-related. This is due in part to the inherent differences in their outcomes. Mortality rates of left-sided disease range from 25% to 30%. Comparable rates for right-sided MSSA IVDA IE are 2% to 5% (7). This favorable prognosis for right-sided disease was first established in the experimental rabbit model of Freedman (82) (Chapter 6). In addition, there is evidence that the combination of nafcillin and gentamicin sterilizes the vegetations of *S. aureus* in half the time of nafcillin when used singly (83). There is recent evidence that it is not necessary to combine the beta-lactam with an aminoglycoside to successfully treat right-sided MSSA by the short- course method (84). Because of its synergistic effect with beta-lactams (85), many in this field (7), including this author, would advise adding the aminoglycoside for the first five days of therapy. Table 6 summarizes the contraindications for the use of a two-week course of therapy of MSSA right-sided IVDA IE (86,87).

Oral therapy is desirable for many reasons including difficulty in obtaining intravenous access in IVDA and misuse of the intravenous line by IVDA as a route of administering their own recreational drugs. The combination of ciprofloxacin and rifampin, given orally, has been used successfully in treating MSSA right-sided IE. Changing sensitivity patterns and the documented risk of developing resistance to rifampin during therapy have made this regimen a less attractive possibility for either definitive or transition therapy (88,89). Linezolid has real potential to be a

TABLE 6   Contraindications for Two-Week Therapy of Right-Sided Intravenous
Drug Abuser Infective Endocarditis

Inadequate initial clinical and/or bacteriological response to initial antibiotic therapy
Complicated valvular infection[a]
Use of nonpenicillinase-resistant penicillins
Immunosuppressed patient

[a]Presence of large vegetations (>2 cm in diameter); congestive heart failure; septic metastatic
 infection or significant organ failure.
Source: From Refs. 85, 86.

TABLE 7   Antibiotic Regimens for Treatment of Methicillin-Sensitive *Staphylococcus aureus*
Right-Sided, Native Valve Infective Endocarditis in Intravenous Drug Abusers

Type of valvular involvement	Dosage regimen
Uncomplicated	Nafcillin/oxacillin 2 g every 4 hrs intravenously (IV) for 2 weeks + gentamicin 1 mg/kg every 8 hrs IV/IM for 5 days[a]
Complicated disease[b]	Nafcillin/oxacillin 2 g every 4 hrs IV for 4–6 weeks + gentamicin 1 mg/kg every 8 hrs IV/IM for 5 days[a]

[a]Assuming normal renal function.
[b]See definition of complicated in Table 6.

viable oral antibiotic in treatment of MSSA right-sided IVDA IE (see earlier). Table 7
presents alternative treatment regimens for treatment of MSSA right-sided IE.

The treatment of MSSA left-sided IVDA IE and MRSA IVDA IE and IVDA
IE of prosthetic valves will be presented in Chapter 12. *Pseudomonas aeruginosa* is
the primary gram-negative involved in IVDA IE. For several reasons, coverage of
Pseudomonas does not need to be included in the empiric antibiotic regimen. It is
infrequently encountered. Above-average doses of gentamicin are required to achieve
therapeutic levels in serum of IVDA suffering from IE. Because of its relatively indolent clinical course, delay in treating this pathogen does not appear to adversely
affect the outcome (90). Fungal IVDA IE is primarily a surgical disease. Prolonged
treatment with antifungal is indicated after excision of the infected valve (1,13,39).

RECURRENCE OF INTRAVENOUS DRUG ABUSER
INFECTIVE ENDOCARDITIS

Intravenous drug abuser IE has the highest recurrent rate of any type of valvular
infection (1,91) ranging up to 40%. This is due primarily to the continued use of intravenous drugs in this population. This reality has tremendous importance in deciding
whether a patient is a surgical candidate or not (see the following section).

SURGICAL THERAPY OF INTRAVENOUS DRUG
ABUSER INFECTIVE ENDOCARDITIS

The current discussion will be focused on right-sided infections. The indications for
surgery in left-sided and prosthetic valve IVDA IE are similar to those for other
types of valvular infection and will be discussed in Chapter 15. Drug abuse should
not be considered with an absolute contraindication to cardiac surgery of the patient
who no longer uses illicit drugs and is competent and responsible to adhere to

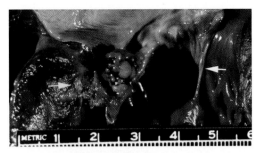

FIGURE 4.2 Vegetations along the mitral valve. The anterior leaflet of the mitral valve shows large polypoid vegetations owing to *Staphylococcus aureus* infection. Note the predominant involvement of the atrial surface of the leaflet. The valve was distorted by rheumatic valvular disease as evidenced by the thickened and shortened chordae tendinae (*white arrow*). Calcification of the mitral annulus is present (*outline arrow*).

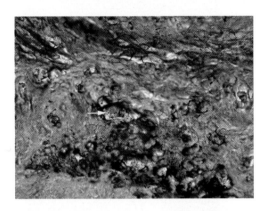

FIGURE 4.9 Silver impregnation (Warthin–Starry) in case of *Coxiella burnetti.* Warthin–Starry stain demonstrates small intracellular organisms that proved to be *Coxiella burnetti* by polymerase chain reaction assay.

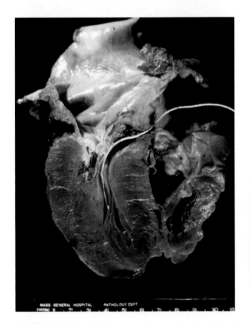

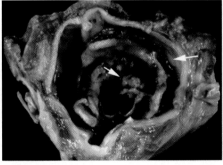

FIGURE 4.11 Fistulous tract complicating mitral valve endocarditis. Extension of infection from a vegetation of the mitral valve led to fistula formation between the left ventricle and right atrium. The patient died from acute right ventricular failure owing to a large left to right shunt. A small thread illustrates the fistula.

FIGURE 4.12 Infective endocarditis of a bioprosthetic valve. An aortic bioprosthesis shows vegetations bridging the cusps (*small arrow*) and involvement of the sewing ring that led to paravalvular insufficiency (*long arrow*).

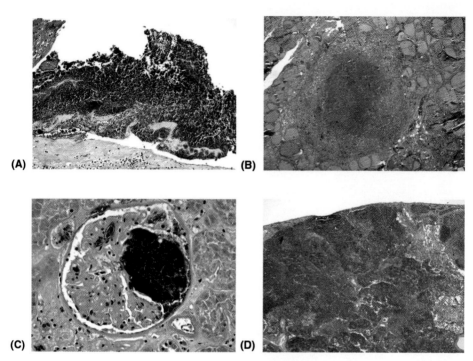

FIGURE 4.15 Tricuspid endocarditis in a patient with a patent foramen ovale. (**A**) Intravenous drug user with HIV-1 infection developed *Staphylococcus aureus* endocarditis of the tricuspid valve. At autopsy, infected lesions were found in (**B**) thyroid, (**C**) kidney, and (**D**) lung.

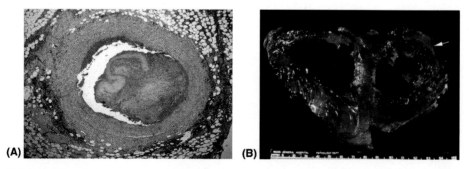

FIGURE 4.19 Coronary artery embolus from vegetation of aortic valve. (**A**) An infected embolus is seen in the circumflex artery. (**B**) The heart at autopsy shows an acute myocardial infarction of the lateral wall of the left ventricle caused by the embolus.

(A)   **(B)**

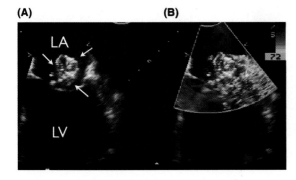

FIGURE 13.5 (**A**) Mitral valve vegetation. The large vegetation (*arrow*) involving the mitral valve is seen on a systolic frame of transesophageal echocardiography. (**B**) Color Doppler imaging reveals moderate mitral regurgitation. *Abbreviations*: LA, left atrium; LV, left ventricle.

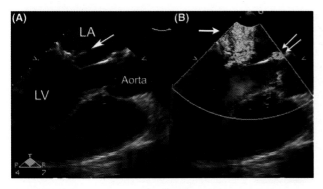

FIGURE 13.14   A transesophageal long axis view of a patient with dehiscence of a mitral annular ring (**A**, B mode image; **B**, Color Doppler). A linear echodensity arises from the posterior portion of the ring consistent with a torn suture (**A**: *arrow*). The posterior portion of the mitral valve ring is dehisced with severe mitral regurgitation (**B**: *single arrow*). A fistulous channel is identified in the intervalvular fibrosa between the aorta and the left atrium (**B**: *double arrow*) with a moderate amount of shunt by color Doppler. *Abbreviations*: LA, left atrium; LV, left ventricle.

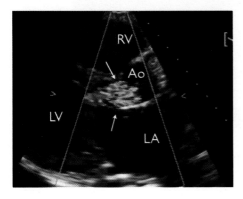

FIGURE 13.17 A transthoracic parasternal long axis view demonstrating severe aortic insufficiency (*arrows*) owing to acute infective endocarditis of the native aortic valve. *Abbreviations*: Ao, aorta; LA, left atrium; LV, left ventricle; RV, right ventricle.

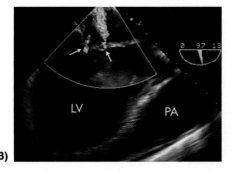

(B)

FIGURE 13.18 A transesophageal endocardiographic long axis view illustrating aneurysms of the mitral valve leaflets due to acute infective endocarditis in (**B**) two separate jets of mitral regurgitation as seen on color. *Abbrevaitions*: LA, left atrium; LV, left ventricle; PA, pulmonary artery.

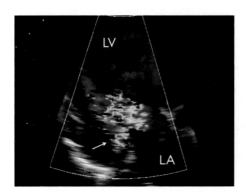

FIGURE 13.22 A transthoracic apical three-chamber view with color illustrating color flow into the pseudoaneurysm (*arrow*). *Abbreviations*: LA, left atrium; LV, left ventricle.

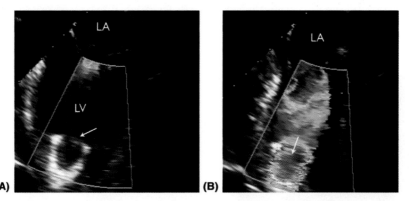

(A)   **(B)**

FIGURE 13.27 (**A**) Transeophageal long axis view of the left ventricle demonstrating an inflow left ventricular-assist devices cannula at the left ventricular apex (*arrow*). (**B**) Transesophageal long axis view of the left ventricle demonstrating unobstructed flow into the left ventricular-assist devices cannula on color Doppler (*arrow*). *Abbreviations:* LA, left atrium; LV, left ventricle.

appropriate treatment regimens. In a carefully selected population of IVDA, surgery improves overall survival (92,93). The major indications for surgery in IVDA IE are: (*i*) infection due to fungi, (*ii*) persistent or recurrent bacteremia exceeding seven days of appropriate therapy, (*iii*) tricuspid vegetations >2 cm, (*iv*) recurrent pulmonary emboli, and (*v*) right-sided failure (2,7,94). The most important prognostic indicator for surgery in tricuspid IVDA IE is the size of the vegetation. There were no deaths in patients with vegetations <1 cm. Three percent of those with vegetations of 1.1 to 2 cm died and 33% with vegetations >2 cm succumbed (95).

Because of the risk of continued drug use and its complications, tricuspid valvulectomy without prosthetic replacement is the most frequently employed surgical technique (96). Removal of the infected valve is curative. Most patients remained hemodynamically normal, however bothersome the symptoms of tricuspid regurgitation might be. Prior to cardiac surgery, a splenic abscess must be ruled out as it can closely mimic resistant valvular infection (Chapter 6).

Case Study ■ A 32-year-old male IVDA IE was admitted to the hospital for evaluation of a fever of 103.2°F. Three sets of blood cultures grow out MSSA. Chest X-ray showed a pattern consistent with septic pulmonary emboli. Transthoracic echocardiography demonstrated vegetation of 2.1 cm in diameter. He refused an HIV test. The patient was placed on ciprofloxacin 750 mg b.i.d. and rifampin 300 mg b.i.d. and discharged home on the second hospital day. The patient failed to keep his appointment in medical clinic. Two weeks after discharge, the patient was readmitted because of recurrent fever and chills. Three sets of blood cultures were positive for MSSA that was now resistant to rifampin. He was started on six weeks of therapy with 12 g of nafcillin daily. For the first five days of treatment, gentamicin was added. He defervesced and was doing well overall. The patient had a constant stream of visitors. Into the final week of therapy, he developed shaking chills and fever to 104°F. All blood cultures grew out *C. albicans*. Repeat TTE revealed a massive tricuspid vegetation >3 cm in diameter. One day later, the patient suffered a massive cerebral embolus. He developed Cheyne-Stokes respirations and was placed on a ventilator. Three days later, the ventilator was removed after being declared brain dead by hospital protocol. On clearing out his belongings, drug injection paraphernalia was discovered along with a supply of brown heroin.

This case illustrates the challenges in caring for the IVDA IE. On medical grounds alone, the patient was most likely not an oral treatment candidate because of the size of the vegetation. Compliance is always a concern in treating the drug abusing patient in a nonsupervised setting. Noncompliance is a major factor for the development of antibiotic resistance during treatment. Unless there is no other alternative, I generally avoid using outpatient oral antibiotic regimens in the treatment of IVDA IE. In no other area of infectious diseases is the behavior of the patient so important in the final outcome as in IVDA IE. Presumably, one of the patient's friends brought in the heroin, which led to the fungal superinfection. As discussed previously, the lemon juice used to prepare the brown heroin may be contaminated with *C. albicans*. Consideration must be given to markedly restricting visitors to IVDA patients in whom intravenous lines are present. Tragedies, such as this case, make one consider such restrictive measures.

REFERENCES

1. Sande MA, Lee BL, Mills J, Chambers HF. Endocarditis in intravenous drug users. In: Kaye D, ed. Infective Endocarditis. New York: Raven Press, 1992:345.
2. Weinstein L, Brusch JL. Endocarditis in intravenous drug abusers. In: Weinstein L, Brusch J Laus, eds. Infective Endocarditis. New York: Oxford University Press, 1996:194.

3. Reisberg B. Infective endocarditis in the narcotic addict. Prog Cardiovasc Dis 1979; 22:193.
4. Hussey H, Katz S. Infections resulting from narcotic addiction. Am J Med 1950; 9:186.
5. Ramsey RG, Gunnar RM, Tobin JR, Jr. Endocarditis in the drug addict. Am J Cardiol 1970; 25:608.
6. Levine D, Crane L, Servos M. Bacteremia in narcotic addicts and the Detroit Medical Center II. Infective endocarditis: a prospective study. Rev Infect Dis 1986; 8:374.
7. Miro JM, del Rio A, Mestres CA. Infective endocarditis in intravenous drug abusers and HIV-1 infected patients. Infect Dis Clin NA 2002; 16:273.
8. Chambers HF, Morris DL, Tauber MG, Modin G. Cocaine use and the risk of endocarditis in intravenous drug abusers. Ann Intern Med 1987; 106:833.
9. Steckelberg JM, Melton LJ, Listrup DM, et al. Influence of referral bias on the apparent clinical spectrum of infective endocarditis. Am J Med 1990; 88:582.
10. Mathew J, Addai T, Anand A, et al. Clinical features, site of involvement, bacteriologic findings and outcome of infective endocarditis in intravenous drug users. Arch Intern Med 1995; 155:1641.
11. Simberkoff MS. Narcotic-associated infective endocarditis. In: Kaplan EL, Taranta AV, eds. Infective Endocarditis. Dallas: American Heart Association, 1977:46.
12. Levine D. Infectious endocarditis in intravenous drug abusers. In: Levine D, Sobel J, eds. Infections in Intravenous Drug Abusers. New York: Oxford University Press, 1991:258.
13. Niebel J. Infective endocarditis in immune compromised patients. In: Horstkotte D, Bodnar E, eds. Current Heart Valve Disease: Infective Endocarditis. London: ICR Publishers, 1991:156.
14. Manoff SB, Vlahov D, Herskowitz A, et al. Human immunodeficiency virus infection in infective endocarditis among injecting drug users. Epidemiology 1996; 7:566.
15. Miro JM, Engemann JJ, Cabell CH, et al. Intravenous drug use and infective endocarditis: report from the ICE investigators. Sixth International Symposium on Modern Concepts Endocarditis and Cardiovascular Infections, Sitges, Barcelona, Spain, June, 2001.
16. Wilson LE, Thomas DL, Astemborski J, et al. Prospective study of infective endocarditis among injection drug users. J Infect Dis 2002; 25:1761.
17. Currie PF, Sutherland GR, Jacob AJ, et al. A review of endocarditis in acquired immuno-deficiency syndrome and human immunodeficiency virus infection. Eur Heart J 1995; 16(suppl B):15.
18. Losa JE, Miro JM, Cruceta A, et al. Infective endocarditis in HIV-infected patients with-out active IV drug addiction: review of 24 episodes (abstract #562) thirty fifth Annual Meeting of the Infectious Diseases Society of America (IDSA) San Francisco (CA) 1997. Clin Infect Dis 1997; 25:459.
19. Watanakunakorn C. Changing epidemiology and newer aspects of infective endocardi-tis. Adv Intern Med 1977; 22:21.
20. Niebel J, Held E. Endokarditis bei Drogenabhangigen. Fortschr der Antimikr und Antineopl. Chemotherapie1987; 6:781.
21. Eichacker PQ, Miller K, Robbins M. Echocardiographic evaluation of heart valves in IV drug abusers without a previous history of endocarditis. Rev Infect Dis 1988; 10:1163.
22. Graves MK, Soto L. Left-sided endocarditis in parenteral drug abusers: recent experience at a large community hospital. South Med J 1992; 85:387.
23. Dressler FA, Roberts WC. Infective endocarditis in opiate addicts: analysis of 80 cases studied at necropsy. Am J Cardiol 1989; 63:1240.
24. Pons-Llado G, Carreras F, Borras X, et al. Findings on Doppler echocardiography in asymptomatic intravenous heroin users. Am J Cardiol 1992; 69:238.
25. McGeown MG. Bacterial endocarditis: an experimental study of healing. J Path Bacteriol 1954; 67:179.
26. Angrist AA, Oka M, Nakao K, et al. Studies in experimental endocarditis. I production of alveolar lesions by mechanisms not involving infection or sensitivity factors. Am J Pathol 1960; 36:181.
27. Highman B, Atland PD. Infective exposure and acclimazation to: on susceptibility of rats to bacterial endocarditis. Proc Soc Exp Biol Med 1962; 110:663.

28. Miro JM, del Rio A, Mestres CA. Infective endocarditis and cardiac surgery in intravenous drug abusers and HIV-1 infected patients. Cardiol Clin 2003; 21:200.
29. Frontera JA, Gradon JD. Right-side endocarditis in injection drug users: review of proposed mechanisms of pathogenesis. Clin Infect Dis 2002; 30:374.
30. Que YA. Pathogenesis of staphylococcal endovascular infections. Ph.D. thesis, University of Lausanne, 2001.
31. Greene C, McDevitt D, Francois P, et al. Adhesion properties of mutants of *Staphylococcus aureus* defective in fibronectin-binding proteins in studies in the expression of fnb genes. Mol Microbiol 1995; 17:1143.
32. Roberts WC, Buchbinder NA. Right-sided valvular infective endocarditis: a clinicopathologic study of twelve necropsy patients. Amer J Med 1972; 53:7.
33. Tuazon CU, Sheagran JN. Staphylococcal endocarditis in parenteral drug abusers: source of the organism. Ann Intern Med 1975; 82:790.
34. Reyes MP, Palutke WA, Wylin RF. Pseudomonas endocarditis in the Detroit Medical Center 1969–1972. Medicine 1973; 52:173.
35. Mills J, Drew D. *Serratia marcescens* endocarditis: a regional illness associated with intravenous drug abuse. Ann of Intern Med 1976; 84:29.
36. Shekar R, Rice TW, Ziedert CH, et al. Outbreak of endocarditis caused by *Pseudomonas aeruginosa* serotype 011 among pentazocine and tripelemmamine abusers in Chicago. J Infect Dis 1985; 151:203.
37. Bisbe J, Miro JM, Latorre X, et al. Disseminated candidiasis in addicts who use brown heroin: report of 83 cases and review. Clin Infect Dis 1992; 15:910.
38. Weens J, Jr. *Candida parapsilosis* pathogenicity: clinical manifestations and antimicrobial susceptibility. Clin Infect Dis 1992; 14:756.
39. Rubenstein E, Noiega E, Simberkoff MS, et al. Fungal endocarditis: analysis of 24 cases and review of the literature. Medicine 1975; 54:331.
40. Dreyer NP, Fields BN. Heroin-associated infective endocarditis. A report of 28 cases. Ann Intern Med 1973; 78:69.
41. Pollack S, Mogatder A, Lange M. *Neisseria subflava* endocarditis case report and review of the literature. Am J Med 1984; 76:752.
42. Thornhill-Joynes M, Li MW, Canawati HN, et al. *Neisseria sicca* endocarditis in intravenous drug abusers. West J Med 1985; 22:255.
43. Yi VL, Rumans LW, Wing EJ, et al. *Pseudomonas maltophilia* causing heroin-associated infective endocarditis. Arch Intern Med 1978; 138:1667.
44. Brooks GF, O'Donoghue JM, Rissing JP. *Eikenella corrodens*, a recently recognized pathogen: infection in medical-surgical patients and in association with methylphenidate abuse. Medicine 1974; 53:325.
45. Watanakunakorn C, Burkert T. Infective endocarditis at a large community teaching hospital, 1980–1990. A review of 210 episodes. Medicine 1993; 72:90.
46. Sandre RM, Shafran SD. Infective endocarditis: review of 35 cases over 9 years. Clin Infect Dis 1996; 22:276.
47. Bouza E, Mensalves A, Munoz P, et al. Infective endocarditis—a prospective study the end of the 20th century: new predisposing conditions, new etiologic agents and still a high mortality. Medicine 2001; 80:298.
48. Cheubin CE, Sapira JD. The medical complications of drug addiction and the medical assessment of the intravenous drug users. Ann Intern Med 1993; 119:1017.
49. Brown PD, Levine D. Infective endocarditis in the injection drug user. Infect Dis Clin NA 2002; 16:645.
50. Joseph WL, Fletcher HS, Giordano JM, et al. Pulmonary and cardiovascular implications of drug addiction. Ann Thorac Surg 1973; 69:1148.
51. Chambers H, Mills J. Endocarditis associated with intravenous drug abusers: In Sande J, Kaye D, eds. Contemporary Issues Infectious Disease. Vol. 2. Endocarditis. New York: Churchill Livingstone, 1984:186.
52. Cohen PS, Maguire JH, Weinstein L. Infective endocarditis caused by Gram-negative bacteria: a review of the literature 1945–1977. Prog Cardiovasc Dis 1980; 22:205.
53. Chadrasekar P, Narule A. Bone and joint infections in intravenous drug abusers. Rev Infect Dis 1969; 8:909.

54. Robinson DJ, Lazo MC, Davis T, Kufera JA. Infective endocarditis in intravenous drug users: does HIV status alter the presenting temperature and white blood cell count? J Emerg Med 2000; 19:5.

55. Marantz PR, Linzer M, Feiner CJ, et al. Inability to predict diagnosis in febrile intravenous drug abusers. Ann Intern Med 1987; 106:823.

56. Chambers HF, Korzeniowski OM, Sande MA, et al. *Staphylococcus aureus* endocarditis: clinical manifestations in addicts and nonaddicts. Medicine (Baltimore) 1983; 62:170.

57. Thadepalli H, Francis CK. Diagnostic clues in metastatic lesions of endocarditis in addicts. West J Med 1978; 128:1.

58. Sklaver AR, Hoffman TA, Greenman RL. Staphylococcal endocarditis in addicts. South Med J 1978; 71:638.

59. Bayer AS, Bolger AF, Taubert KA, et al. Diagnosis and management of infective endocarditis and its complications. Circulation 1998; 98:2936.

60. Weinstein L, Brusch JL. Diagnosis. In: Weinstein L, Brusch J Laus, eds. Infective Endocarditis. New York: Oxford University Press, 1996:236.

61. Pazin GJ, Saul S, Thompson ME. Blood culture positivity. Suppression by outpatient antibiotic therapy in patients with bacterial endocarditis. Arch Intern Med 1982; 142:263.

62. Durack DT, Lukes AS, Bright DK. Duke Endocarditis Service. New criteria for diagnosis of infective endocarditis: utilization of specific echocardiographic findings. Am J Med 1994; 26:200.

63. Palepu A, Cheung SS, Montessori V, et al. Factors other than the Duke criteria associated with infective endocarditis among injection drug users. Clin Invest Med 2002; 25:118.

64. Manolis AS, Melita H. Echocardiographic and clinical correlates of drug addicts with infective endocarditis. Implications of vegetation size. Arch Burn Med 1988; 148:2461.

65. San Roman JA, Vilacosta I, Zamorano JL, et al. Transesophageal echocardiography right-sided endocarditis. J Am Coll Cardiol 1993; 21:1226.

66. Ferguson R, Feeney C, Chiruigi L. *Enterobacter agglomerans*-associated cotton fever. Arch Intern Med 1993; 153:381.

67. Pulvirenti JJ, Kerns E, Benson C, et al. Infective endocarditis in injection drug users: importance of human immunodeficiency virus serostatus and degree of immunosuppression. Clin Infect Dis 1996; 22:40.

68. Wilson WR, Karchmer AW, Dajani AS, et al. Antibiotic treatment of adults with infective endocarditis due to streptococci, enterococci, staphylococci and HACEK microorganisms. JAMA 1995; 274:1706.

69. Working Party of the British Society for Antimicrobial Chemotherapy. Antibiotic treatment of streptococcal, entercoccal and staphylococcal endocarditis. Heart 1998; 79:207.

70. Small PM, Chambers HF. Vancomycin for *Staphylococcus aureus* endocarditis in intravenous drug abusers. Antimicrob Agent Chemother 1998; 34:1227.

71. Harstein AL, Mulligan ME, Morthland VH, et al. Recurrent *Staphylococcus aureus* bacteremia. J Clin Microb 1991; 30:670.

72. Cremieux AC, Maziere B, Vallois JM, et al. Evaluation of antibiotic diffusion into cardiac vegetations by quantitative autoradiography. J Infect Dis 1989; 159:938.

73. Rybak MJ, Albrecht LM, Berman JR, et al. Vancomycin pharmacokinetic in burn patients and intravenous drug abusers. Antimicrob Agent Chemother 1990; 34:792.

74. Moise PA, Forrest A, Birmingham MC, Schentag JJ. The efficacy and safety of linezolid as treatment for *Staphylococcus aureus* infections in compassionate use patients who are tolerant of, or who have failed to respond to vancomycin. J Antimicrob Chemother 2002; 50:1017.

75. Sperber S, Levine JF, Gross PA. Persistent MRSA bacteremia in a patient with low linezolid levels. Clin Infect Dis 2003; 36:675.

76. Ruiz ME, Guerrero IC, Tuazon CU. Endocarditis caused by methicillin-resistant *Staphylococcus aureus*. Treatment failure with linezolid. Clinical Infect Dis 2002; 35:1018.

77. Moellering RC, Jr. Linezolid: the first oxazolidinone antimicrobial. Ann Intern Med 2003; 138:135.

78. Gerson SL, Kaplan SL, Bruss JB, et al. Hematologic effects of linezolid: summary of clinical experience. Antimicrob Agent Chemother 2002; 46:2723.

79. Vouillamoz J, Entenza JM, Ferger C, et al. Quinpristin-dalfopristin combined with beta-lactams for treatment of experimental endocarditis due to *Staphylococcus aureus* constitutively resistant to macrolide-lincosamide-streptogramin B antibiotics. Antimicrob Agent Chemother 2000; 24:1789.
80. Korzeniowski O, Sande MA. The National Collaborative Endocarditis Study Group. Combination antimicrobial therapy for *Staphylococcus aureus* in patients addicted to parenteral drugs and in non addicts: a prospective study. Ann Intern Med 1982; 27:496.
81. Chambers HF, Miller T, Newman MD. Right-sided *Staphylococcus aureus* endocarditis in intravenous drug abusers: two-week combination therapy. Ann Intern Med 1988; 109:619.
82. Garrison PK, Freedman LR. Experimental endocarditis I. Staphylococcal endocarditis in rabbits resulting from placement of polyethylene catheter in a right-sided heart. Yale J Biol Med 1978; 42:394.
83. Sande MA, Courtney KB. Nafcillin-gentamicin synergism in experimental staphylococcal endocarditis. J Lab Clin Med 1976; 88:118.
84. Ribera E, Gomez V, Cortes E, et al. Effectiveness of cloxacillin with or without gentamicin in short-term therapy for right-sided *Staphylococcus aureus* endocarditis: a randomized, controlled trial. Ann Intern Med 1996; 125:969.
85. Rubinstein E, Carbon C. The Endocarditis Working Group of the International Society of Chemotherapy. Staphylococcal endocarditis—recommendations for therapy. Clin Microbiol Infect 1998; 4:S27.
86. Chambers HF. Short-course combination and oral therapies for Staphylococcus endocarditis. Infect Dis Clin NA 1993; 7:69.
87. DiNubile MJ. Short-course antibiotic therapy for right-sided endocarditis caused by *Staphylococcus aureus* in injection drug users. Ann Intern Med 1994; 121:873.
88. Heldman AW, Hartert TV, Ray SC, et al. Oral antibiotic treatment of right-sided staphylococcal endocarditis in injection drug users: prospective randomized comparison with parenteral therapy. Am J Med 1996; 101:68.
89. Tebas P, Ruiz M, Roman F, et al. Early resistance to rifampin and ciprofloxacin in the treatment of right-sided *Staphylococcus aureus* endocarditis. J Infect Dis 1991; 163:204.
90. Reyes MP, EL-Khatib MR, Brown WJ, et al. Synergy between carbenicillin and an aminoglycoside (gentamicin or tobramycin) against *Pseudomonas aeruginosa* isolated from patients with endocarditis and sensitivity of isolates to normal human serum. J Infect Dis 1979; 140:192.
91. Welton DE, Young JB, Gentry WO, et al. Recurrent infective endocarditis: analysis of predisposing factors and clinical features. Am J Med 1979; 66:932.
92. Matthew J, Abreo G, Namburi K, et al. Results of surgical treatment for infective endocarditis in intravenous drug users. Chest 1995; 108:73.
93. Arbulu A, Holmes RJ, Asfaw I. Surgical treatment of intractable right sided endocarditis in drug addicts: 25 years experience. J Heart Valve Dis 1993; 2:129.
94. Alsip SG, Blackstone EH, Kirklin J, et al. Indications for cardiac surgery in patients with active infective endocarditis. Am J Med 1985; 78(suppl 6B):138.
95. Hecht SR, Berger M. Right sided endocarditis in intravenous drug users. Prognostic features in 102 episodes. Ann Intern Med 1992; 117:560.
96. Arbulu A, Holmes RJ, Asfaw I. Tricuspid valve colectomy without replacement. Twenty years experience. J Thorac Cardiovasc Surg 1991; 102:917.

8   Prosthetic Valve Endocarditis

John L. Brusch
Harvard Medical School and Department of Medicine and Infectious Disease Service, Cambridge Health Alliance, Cambridge, Massachusetts, U.S.A.

COMMENT AND BACKGROUND

This author will continue the tradition of devoting a chapter to the discussion of prosthetic valve infective endocarditis (PVE) although infection of all the intravascular devices is quite similar in epidemiology, pathogenesis, and even treatment. With the exception of vascular catheters, prosthetic heart valves were the first intravascular devices. In 1960, Starr and Edwards (1) and Harkness (2) performed the first successful implantation of prosthetic aortic and mitral valves. Wallace et al. (3) performed the first valve replacement to treat a case of refractory *Klebsiella*-infective endocarditis (IE). Despite appropriate antibiotic therapy, blood cultures had remained positive for over one month. Along with the persistent fever, intractable cardiac failure developed due to progressive aortic insufficiency. The surgeons removed the infected valve and replaced it with Starr Edwards prosthesis. The patient recovered completely and remained free of disease. The attending surgeons concluded that the presence of active infection was not a contraindication to surgical replacement of an infected valve. Indeed, it may be the only therapeutic option when antimicrobial therapy fails. In his review of the infectious aspects of prosthetic valves, Weinstein concluded that the cardiac surgeon truly wields a double-edged scalpel (4) that both cures valvular infection and is responsible for inducing it.

EPIDEMIOLOGY

Sixty thousand prosthetic valves are implanted yearly in the United States (5). Sixty percent of these are mechanical valves. The rest are bioprosthetic devices that are either heterografts, made up of porcine or bovine tissues; or homografts, preserved human aortic valves; or pulmonary autografts. Currently, PVE account for 2% to 30% of all cases of IE (6–8) with an incidence of 0.94 cases per 100,000 population in a large urban area. The incidence of PVE in recipients varies with respect to the type of patients studied and the type of prosthetic valve infected. It ranges from 0.65 to 2.16 events per 100 patient years (9). The valve is at a highest risk of being infected within the first three months after its implantation (10). It remains at this high level for three months and then starts to decline to a fairly constant rate of 0.4% yearly. At the end of 12 months, 1% to 3.1% are infected; at the 60-month mark, 3.0% to 5.7% (11–16); after 180 months, 17% of the prosthetic valves are infected (17). These figures are certainly less than that recorded in the early days of prosthetic valve surgery in which there was approximately a 10% incidence of PVE within the first year (18). Antibiotic prophylaxis is the major reason for the rates of infection to typically decline from those of the 1960s. Greater numbers of prosthetic valves were implanted during the 1990s. Unfortunately, the rate of infection outstripped that of placement (50% vs. 31%) despite appropriately administered prophylaxis (19).

Most likely, this disproportionate increase is due to acquisition of infection not in the operating room but in a variety of patient-care units and their device-associated bacteremias. The long-term increase in PVE reflects the rise in healthcare-associated bacteremias (20) (see later).

Older data supported the concept that mitral bioprosthetic valves were more likely to be infected than their mechanical counterparts because of the greater mechanical stress applied to valves in the mitral position (21). Currently, it appears that the location has no correlation with the risk for infection (11–13,22). This decrease in risk may be because of advances in valve design. However, a prosthetic valve of any type that is implanted because of inactive or active native valve endocarditis (NVE) has a greater potential to be infected (11,14,15). Patients who receive more than one valve and those with longer "pump time" are at greater risk of developing PVE (11,12). These factors may simply reflect the seriousness of the underlying disease.

There is no overall difference between the incidence of infection of mechanical and bioprosthetic valves. Both, however, do have their own distinctive temporal pattern of developing endocarditis. Within the first six months of implantation, mechanical prostheses have a higher rate of PVE than bioprosthetic ones (11,12). Through the fifth year anniversary, there was no significant difference between the rates of mechanical (5%) and bioprosthetic valvular infections (6.3%) (13). After this point, PVE occurs much more frequently in bioprosthetic devices. This appears because of the "wear and tear" on the bioprosthetic's leaflets (11).

PATHOGENESIS OF PROSTHETIC VALVE ENDOCARDITIS

Prosthetic valve endocarditis is unique among the endocarditites by having a timeline characterizing not only when certain types of valves are likely to be infected but also by what organisms. PVE that is clinically manifest within 60 days of valvular surgery is termed early PVE. Those cases that are evident past 12 months are considered as late PVE. Intermediate PVE occurs between 2 and 12 months after implantation (9). To understand what underlies this timeline, it is necessary to understand the pathogenesis of PVE. The common denominator behind all types of IE is the sterile platelet/fibrin thrombus or nonbacterial thrombotic endocarditis [NBTE (23)] (Chapter 5). NBTE palms are native valves because of damage to the valve leaflets, hypercoagulable states, or various hemodynamic factors (24). After a prosthetic valve is implanted, it undergoes a process called conditioning. The first stage is a nonspecific reaction that varies with the particular shape of the implanted material as well as the physicochemical composition of the prosthesis. Various body fluids, especially blood (fibronectin and fibrinogen) and tissue proteins, as well as cells bind to the prosthetic material. These protein components may either promote or interfere with staphylococcal attachment to the valve (25,26). In general, they promote the adherence of *Staphylococcus aureus* but interfere with that of coagulase-negative staphylococci (CoNS). The second phase of conditioning is the deposition of fibrin/platelet thrombi (NBTE) at the interface of the native cardiac tissue and the sewing cuff that has not yet been endothelialized (27). Until it is endothelialized at approximately 60 days after placement, the sewing cuff remains susceptible to the deposition of platelets and fibrin. At about the 60-day mark, the annulus and sewing cuff become encased in endothelial cells. However, these layering cells do not function normally in preventing localized thrombus formation. Because of this, the cuff remains susceptible to infection throughout the life of the valve albeit at a lower frequency than earlier. The anchoring sutures, themselves, serve as a conduit for the organisms to invade the adjacent cardiac tissues. This process may result in the formation of paravalvular leaks and ring abscesses (10,28).

The details of bacterial adherence have been addressed earlier in detail [Chapters 2, 3, and 5 (29)]. The sewing cuffs of bioprosthetic valves are equally prone to becoming infected. In addition, their leaflets are vulnerable to infection in a manner quite similar to that of the native valves (30,31). Over a period of many years the blood flow through the valve damages the surface of the leaflets of bioprosthetic valves. This roughening of the surfaces leads to the deposition of microthrombi (NBTE) to which circulating bacteria may eventually adhere, as well as calcification of the leaflets. From the infected thrombi, bacteria may invade the cusps of the valves despite their being pretreated with glutaraldehyde. This chemical partially protects porcine valvular leaflets and bovine pericardial tissue from infection (32,33). The enlarging thrombus, by further disturbing the smooth rheology of blood flow, contributes to the growth of either an infected thrombus or NBTE. It is important to emphasize that bioprosthetic valve IE is not strictly limited to the cusps. The nonendothelialized sewing ring of this type of valve is probably equally infected as that of the mechanical valves (34). As time goes on, bioprosthetic valves are at increasing risk of developing endocarditis (11) because of the continued degeneration of the valvular leaflets.

The source of infecting organisms varies according to what part of the timeline one refers to. In almost all cases of early PVE and many intermediate PVE, the bacteria are nosocomial or healthcare facility-related. The microorganisms of early PVE have been recovered from the surgical field and the cardiopulmonary bypass equipment (35,36). Seventy-five percent of cardiopulmonary bypass equipment was found to be contaminated by the organisms that cause early PVE (CoNS, streptococci, gram-negative aerobes, diphtheroids, and fungi) (see later) (37). The ambient air is a major source of bacterial contamination. The concentration of organisms in the air of the operating suite appears to be directly related to the amount of personnel present. Seventy-one percent of cultures of the valve and its bed, obtained just before closure of the sternal wound, have been positive. Most early PVE has been because of infection secondary to intravenous lines, including pacer wires, and wound infections (14,38). Water, which is contaminated by species of *Legionella* (*L. pneumophilia* and *L. dumoffi*), has been documented by means of restrictive DNA analysis as the source of early *Legionella* PVE (39). Personnel are seldom the direct source of valvular infection except in that they may contribute to contamination of the operating room air. It has been documented that a cardiac surgeon, who was colonized by CoNS, was the source of an outbreak of PVE (40) with his particular staphylococcal strain. Rarely is the prosthetic valve, itself, a cause of infection. In the 1980s, contamination during their manufacture of porcine valves by *Mycobacterium chelonei* was well documented (41).

Late cases of PVE, and some intermediate ones, usually are because of many of the same underlying factors and organisms that cause NVE (42). It is important to remember that PVE is five times more frequent in patients whose prosthetic valve was inserted during active infection (43). This situation, in which the prosthesis was placed because of an infected native valve, is called secondary PVE. When PVE develops in a valve that replaced a noninfected one, it is termed primary PVE (44). Often the infecting organism is different than the original. At least 50% of the patients with intermediate or late-onset PVE have nonhealthcare-associated bloodstream infections (HCBSI) as the source of the invading organisms. These non-HCBSI are because of a variety of infections that are acquired in the community including urinary tract infections, soft-tissue infections, and pneumonias (44).

A particular type of late PVE is that caused by HCBSI, which is an increasing challenge since 16% developed clinically apparent PVE within 28 days (range, 7–170 days) of the bacteremia (45). A similar risk (11%) is seen arising from noso-comial fungemias in which PVE developed after 26 to 690 days (46). As the conse-quences of PVE are so catastrophic, all reasonable efforts must be made to first limit those devices and interventions that are at high risk of producing bacteremia in those patients with prosthetic valves in place. In addition, the bacteremia must be regarded as the potentially representing infection of that valve. Unfortunately, even expeditious administration of appropriate antibiotics often fails to protect the valve (45).

PATHOLOGY OF PROSTHETIC VALVE ENDOCARDITIS

Prosthetic valve endocarditis of mechanical valves usually penetrates into the annulus and underlying myocardium (Fig. 1). This invasion of the myocardium from aortic PVE can burrow into the pericardial space causing pericarditis. It also can lead to second- or third-degree block by injuring the conducting system because of either an inflammatory or destructive process involving the various bundles. These complications occur primarily in aortic valve PVE. Dehiscence of the sewing sutures results in paravalvular regurgitation. Vegetations may partially block the valve opening. This occurs much more commonly in PVE of the mitral valve (44,47–49). Table 1 presents these complications of mechanical PVE.

From the initial studies of porcine valves, tissue PVE was considered to be primarily an infection of the leaflets (50). Only 6% of the cases were noted to have invasion of the paravalvular tissues. The collagen of the cusps of the infected valves was found to be damaged. Similar to the microscopic findings of NVE there was significant infiltration by bacteria and inflammatory cells. These histological changes lead to a high rate of valvular stenosis. Magilligan (34) first documented a higher rate of paravalvular infection in PVE (13%). Currently, it is felt that myocardial involvement PVE is almost identical for both mechanical and bioprosthetic valves (51). More recent studies demonstrate that paravalvular spread involves between

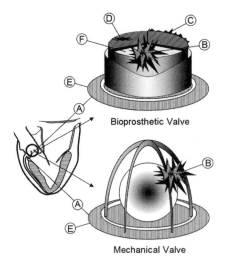

Bioprosthetic Valve

Mechanical Valve

FIGURE 1   Intracardiac complications of prosthetic valve infective endocarditis. Complications of mechanical and bioprosthetic valve infective endo-carditis: (A) paravalvular extension of sewing ring infection; paravalvular abscess; valvular dehiscence; septal abscess; pericardial abscess; intracardiac fis-tulas. (B) Infected vegetations blocking the valvular orifice: outlet obstruction; valvular incompetence; (E) sewing ring; (F) bioprosthetic valve orifice. Complications of bioprosthetic infective endocarditis. (C) leaflet destruction; (D) leaflet perforation; (E) sewing ring.

TABLE 1 Complications of Mechanical Prosthetic Valve Infective Endocarditis

Complication	Percentage of cases[a]
Invasion of annulus	42–85
Dehiscence of valve	64–82
Obstruction of valve	4–19
Pericarditis	2–5
Myocardial abscess	14–32

[a]Lower values obtained from clinical series with a significant amount of nonautopsy cases.

TABLE 2 Complications of Infective Endocarditis of Bioprosthetic Valves

Complication	Percentage of cases
Invasion of annulus/myocardial abscess	25–80
Dehiscence of valves	42
Obstruction/stenosis	33
Perforation of cusps	43

50% and 80% of tissue PVE (10,52,53). An important difference between the pathology of mechanical and bioprosthetic valve endocarditis is that paravalvular infection spread of mechanical PVE occurs commonly in both early and late types of diseases whereas that of tissue valve infections occur much more frequently during the first year of valvular implantation (79%) than after (31%) (54). The aortic location is also associated with a higher rate of paravalvular involvement. During active infection, valvular stenosis can result from large vegetation. Delayed stenosis, up to 98 months after microbiological cure, is because of the stiffening of the leaflets secondary to the rearrangement of collagen that is produced by infection (34,53). The complications of tissue PVE are summarized in Table 2.

MICROBIOLOGY OF PROSTHETIC VALVE ENDOCARDITIS

A wide variety of microorganisms, *Mycoplasma* spp., *Legionella* spp., *trophynema whippeli*, have been documented to cause PVE (10). However, the microbiology of PVE reflects primarily its site of acquisition (Table 3). Therefore, in reality just a few types produce the majority of the cases. Early and intermediate PVE is dominated by CoNS, usually *S. epidermidis*. In early-stage disease, these organisms can be quite locally destructive. Such behavior is not commonly attributed to CoNS. As discussed previously, the presence of these pathogens is because of perioperative contamination or device-related HCBSI (55–58). The fact that the incidence of CoNS, PVE remains essentially the first year of implantation supports the notion that all of these were acquired perioperatively. Eighty-five percent of CoNS which are isolated during the first year of implantation are primarily *S. epidermidis* that are methicillin-resistant. Methicillin-resistant CoNS posses the resistant genotype but often do not express the phenotype. This heteroresistance poses a challenge in identifying methicillin-resistant examples. After one year, 50% of CoNS are *S. epidermidis* and only 30% are methicillin-resistant. This pattern of resistance is a significant factor on the empiric choice of antibiotics in treating PVE (see later) (59). Likewise, the incidence of *S. aureus* PVE remains essentially constant through the first year, probably for the same reasons

TABLE 3 Microbiology of Prosthetic Valve Infective Endocarditis

	Percentage of cases		
Organisms	Early PVE	Intermediate PVE	Late PVE
CoNS[a]	33–45	32	11–12
Staphylococcus aureus	22	12	18–20
Streptococcal spp.[b]	0–2	9	25–31
Entercoccal spp.	7–8	12	7–11
HACEK organisms	0	0	1.5–6
Other gram-negatives	13	3	6
Diphtheroids (*Corynebacterium jekium*)	6	0	3
Candida spp.	8	12	1
Other bacteria	0	0	3
Polymicrobial	0	0	1.5
Culture negative	5–27	6	7–8

[a]Usually *Staphylococcus epidermidis*.
[b]*Streptococcus viridans*, *Streptococcus bovis*, and *Abiotrophia* spp.
Abbreviations: CoNS, coagulase-negative staphylococci; PVE, prosthetic valve infective endocarditis
Source: From Refs. 55–58.

that apply to CoNS. The organisms that produce late PVE resemble those that infect native valves with the exception of a high rate of CoNS involvement.

In the early days of prosthetic valve surgery, gram-negative aerobes (coliforms) were often isolated in early PVE (9). Because of improved surgical procedures, they are currently seldom isolated. Members of the HACEK group now play a significant role in late PVE (60).

Corynebacteria spp. are occasionally isolated from cases of PVE. Most common of these are members of the J-K, which cause early PVE (61). They are difficult to grow in culture because of their fastidious nutritional requirements. These organisms are quite resistant to many antibiotics, especially the cephalosporins. Vancomycin appears to be the agent most consistently active against them (62).

In endemic areas, *Coxiella burnetti* is a major cause of PVE. Currently, prosthetic valve infections constitute 69% of all cases of Q fever IE (63). Fungal PVE is being more frequently encountered. This is probably because of the increase in immunosuppressed patients' intravenous drug abusers (IVDA) and greater numbers of intravascular devices. *Candida albicans*, *Candida* spp., and *Aspergillus* spp. are the most common fungi isolated from cases of PVE. *Histoplasma capsulatum* and *Cryptococcus neoformans* are less frequently involved in cases of PVE. Fungal PVE became manifest from eight days to 3.4 years after implantation. In only 35% of the patients was there a source documented. The chief predisposing factors were intravascular catheters and a preceding bacterial IE. *Candida* spp. produce 32% to 67% of fungal IE, and 50% of cases of fungal IE involve prosthetic valves. Forty-one percent of cases of candidal IE are produced by nonalbicans species. This holds true for PVE as well. *Candida stellatoidea* is a common cause of candidal PVE but unusually isolated from other types of candidal infections (64–68). Candida has been demonstrated to be able to adhere to the NBTE that would result from surgical damage to the endocardium/myocardium (Chapter 3) (69). *Candida* spp. have been documented to superinfect cases of bacterial PVE. This would be presumably due to an increase in fungemia brought about by the prolonged usage of wide-spectrum antibiotics.

Culture-negative infection occurs uniformly through the three stages of PVE. It was formerly felt that this type of IE did not occur until after six months of

TABLE 4 Time Line for Development of Prosthetic Valve Infective Endocarditis

Time in months[a]	0 ___ 2 ___	6 ___	12 ___		
Pathological changes	(1) (2) (3)		(4)	(5)	(6)
Organisms	(A)		(A + B)	(B)	

(1) First stage of conditioning (see text).
(2) Second stage of conditioning (see text).
(3) Endotheliozation of the sewing cuff begins.
(4) Endotheliozation of the sewing cuff is completed.
(5) Nonbacterial thrombotic endocarditis formation occurs.
(6) Degeneration of bioprosthetic valve cusps begins.
(A) Pathogens of early PVE.
(B) Pathogens of late PVE.

[a]All times are approximate.
Abbreviation: PVE, prosthetic valve infective endocarditis.

implantation. Table 4 correlates the time line of pathological changes in PVE with the microorganisms that predominate in each phase.

CLINICAL MANIFESTATIONS OF PROSTHETIC VALVE ENDOCARDITIS

Overall, the signs and symptoms of PVE are quite similar to those of NVE with several notable exceptions (9,49,59,70). The presence of PVE that begins within a few weeks of valve implantation may be obscured by more common surgical complications such as pneumonia or wound infections. This masking effect of PVE by other more obvious infections continues to be a challenge to the clinician throughout the life of that valve. Early PVE, as a result of *S. aureus,* may present as septic shock due to the complications of overwhelming paravalvular extension (valve incompetence, conduction disturbances, and septic emboli) (71). The central nervous system appears to be targeted by the emboli of early *S. aureus* PVE (72), especially within the first three days (73). However, this septic picture may occur at any stage of PVE when it is caused by *S. aureus* or *Streptococcus pyogenes* (28). There appears to be a lower rate of the central nervous system emboli (10%) in early PVE caused by other organisms. Because PVE usually is superimposed upon an already dysfunctional heart, congestive failure develops earlier and is more severe than in NVE (74). Heart failure occurs in 30% to 100% of patients. Dehiscence of the sewing ring may be caused in mechanical and tissue valves. Destruction of the bioprosthetic leaflets may produce congestive failure at any time depending on the virulence of the pathogen. Paravalvular spread of infection leads to abnormalities of the conducting system, myocarditis, or pericarditis (9). Ten percent of mechanical PVE is complicated by thrombosis significant enough to impede ventricular outflow. Forty percent of cases are complicated by clinically significant arterial emboli. Among the most important of these are the embolic infarcts and hemorrhages of the central nervous system (75). Murmurs of valvular regurgitation develop in 50% of the cases. They occur early in those caused by *S. aureus,* later in those due to *Streptococcus viridans* (76). It is important to recognize that paravalvular leaks, because of mechanical causes, develop immediately after valve surgery in 1% of the patients (77).

Late PVE may follow a subacute or almost chronic course with the classic peripheral stigmata of valvular infection. Both the skin and eye manifestations of PVE are increasing in frequency. Janeway lesions, Osler nodes, and Roth spots are documented in 20% of the patients (78). Hepatosplenomegaly occurs in 3%

TABLE 5 Clinical Manifestations of Prosthetic Valve Infective Endocarditis

Symptom/sign	Early PVE (%)	Intermediate–late PVE (%)
Fever	95–100	97–100
Septic shock	31	9
Congestive heart failure	36–100	30–44
New or changing murmur	47–70	40–63
Hepatosplenomegaly	20–36	15–42
Central nervous system emboli	11	28
Other emboli	5–30	10–40
Petechiae	30–60	40–50
Dermal signs[a]	5–14	15–28
Anemia	75–89	72–75
Leukocytosis	40–78	30–51
Hematuria	—	65

[a]Osler's nodes, Janeway lesions, Roth spots.
Abbreviation: PVE, prosthetic valve infective endocarditis.
Source: From Refs. 70, 79–81.

of the patients with PVE, especially those infected with *S. viridans*. The presence of hematuria is a frequent but neglected sign of PVE (Table 5).

DIAGNOSIS OF PROSTHETIC VALVE ENDOCARDITIS

The major clinical factors that raise the possibility of PVE in a given patient are the presence of fever and valvular dysfunction—either a paravalvular leak or thrombus. Because prosthetic valves are continuously at significant risk of being infected from even a transient bacteremia, the threshold for instituting an evaluation is low. As discussed previously, the presenting symptoms of PVE may be masked by those of a more mundane infection. Conversely, many extracardiac infections can produce many of the same symptoms of PVE. Arguably, of all the types of IE, the Duke criteria may inhibit their value in the diagnosis of PVE for all of the aforementioned reasons. As it is the case for all types of IE, blood cultures remain the mainstay of diagnosis (Chapter 12). The hallmark of a valvular infection is the presence of a continuous bacteremia. The modified Duke criteria define a significant continuous bacteremia as a recognized endocarditis pathogen retrieved from at least two sets of blood cultures drawn more than 12 hours apart or by three sets drawn at least one hour apart (82). There are challenges to the interpretation of the results of blood cultures obtained during the work-up of PVE.

The bacteremia of PVE actually may not be continuous in up to 10% of the patients (83). One explanation for this discontinuity is that the primary lesion may be an abscess of the sewing cuff that is not in direct communication with the intravascular space. In that case, more than the usual amount of blood cultures should be drawn to confirm reproducibility of the organism as well as making use of echocardiography and the Dukes modified criteria (see later). Unfortunately, bona fide causes of PVE, such as CoNS and diphtheroids but especially CoNS, are also well-known contaminants of blood cultures. This situation also causes more than the usual amount of blood cultures to be drawn as well as determining that the intermittent bacteremia is secondary to a single strain of CoNS by one of a number of molecular techniques (84). The analysis of positive blood cultures for organisms which are highly associated with IE (enterococci, HACEK organisms), is difficult as these are rarely contaminants. *Streptococcus viridans* or *S. aureus* may be contaminants. If one set of blood cultures is positive for one of these two, it is very hard to decide its significance. The addage "one set of blood cultures is worse than none at all" remains quite diagnostic true (the author, unpublished). The high rate of embolization in PVE may provide a surrogate for blood cultures, an embolized vegetation. Culture and microscopic examination may be very rewarding. Not all bacteremias represent PVE. The more common nonendocarditis causes of bacteremia, in the setting of cardiac surgery, are mediastinal infections or infected vascular catheters. Factors which favor uncomplicated bacteremia include: (*i*) bacteremia within 25 days of surgery; (*ii*) a proven or strongly suspected noncardiac source; (*iii*) failure to develop a new murmur; and (*iv*) gram-negative bacteremias (85). In general, false-negative blood cultures in IE are usually because of the recent use of antibiotics (86). This may be especially true for PVE, as perioperatively there are so many noncardiac infections which require antimicrobial therapy. In addition, there is always the fastidious organism to be considered. Non-*Candida* fungi are seldom grown out of blood cultures. Culture and histological examination of fungal emboli may yield the diagnosis (87). Polymerase chain reaction (PCR) analysis and similar techniques hold great promise for minimizing the amount of false-negative cultures.

At times because of the discussed diagnostic challenges, imaging techniques are employed to corroborate the diagnosis of PVE. Cinefluoroscopy was considered the procedure of choice for diagnosing valvular dysfunction such as abnormal excursions of the valvular cage or of the occluder component. This technique does not distinguish infectious from noninfectious causes of valvular abnormalities (88).

Echocardiography has taken over as the imaging technique of choice for both diagnosing and managing PVE. It can determine the degree of heart failure by estimating left ventricular end-diastolic volume and the premature closing of the mitral valve. Doppler modification of echocardiography provides useful estimates of the degree of valvular regurgitation (89,90).

Overall, transesophageal echocardiography (TEE) is superior to transthoracic echocardiography (TTE). TEE has a sensitivity of diagnosing PVE of 82% to 96% as compared with 17% to 36% for TTE (91). High-resolution multiplane transducers that allow continuous-wave and pulse-wave Doppler and color flow imaging have become the echocardiographic standard (92). A prospective comparison between TTE and TEE, used in patients with prosthetic valves, indicated that both agreed in 55% of the cases. TEE reclassified the results of TTE in 34%. Ten of 34 patients were reassigned to definitely having PVE (93).

Transthoracic echocardiography yields better images of the ventricular surfaces of mitral and aortic valves. TEE is superior to TTE in imaging the atrial surfaces of the mitral and tricuspid valves and aortic prosthetic valves as well as being able to detect paravalvular abscesses, paraprosthetic leaks, fistulae, and perforated bioprosthetic valve leaflets (94,95).

Transesophageal echocardiography has a positive predictive value for PVE of 89% and a negative one of 86% to 94%. In those cases in which there is a high suspicion of PVE but no definite echocardiographic or microbiological proof, repeating the echocardiographic studies in one week can often clarify the situation (96). The results of echocardiography should never constitute the sole basis of diagnosing PVE.

TREATMENT OF PROSTHETIC VALVE ENDOCARDITIS

To achieve the best of the therapeutic outcomes, the clinician must be attentive to three major areas when treating PVE: the choice of antibiotics, evaluating the necessity of and timing of surgical intervention, and issues of anticoagulation.

PRINCIPLES OF ANTIBIOTIC THERAPY OF PROSTHETIC VALVE ENDOCARDITIS

As with any type of valvular infection, it is mandatory to retrieve the causative organism in order to know its antibiotic sensitivity pattern. One can withhold antibiotic therapy until these values are available unless the patient is septic or hemodynamically unstable. If one or both of these states are present, antimicrobial therapy is begun on an empiric basis aimed at the most likely pathogens. If the patient has recently been put on an oral antibiotic regimen because of misdiagnosis, it is best to wait until the blood cultures become positive and then start specifically targeted therapy (see next). It may take up to seven days off antibiotics for cultures to become positive. The duration of antibiotic therapy is at least six weeks. This prolonged course is dictated by the difficulty in treating infections of prosthetic material (97).

The antibiotic regimens used in the treatment of PVE are generally the same as those administered to cases of NVE (98). The major exceptions to this are found in the approach to treating staphylococcal PVE. When prosthetic material is involved, staphylococci isolates should be considered to belong to one of the two groups on the basis of their sensitivity patterns and not whether they are coagulase-positive or -negative: (*i*) methicillin-sensitive *S. aureus* (MSSA) and (*ii*) methicillin-resistant *S. aureus* (MRSA) and methicillin-resistant CoNS (99). The treatment of PVE caused by nonstaphylococcal microorganisms will be presented in Chapter 14. A semisynthetic penicillin is the core component of the antibiotic regimen for MSSA. For those with mild reactions to the penicillins, a first-generation cephalosporin may be substituted. In those who have had severe reactions, vancomycin is employed. Vancomycin also plays the key treatment role in MRSA PVE (Table 6). What is unique about eradicating staphylococci from prosthetic material is the need for triple therapy (100,101). Rifampin is the unique part of this combination. It has a special ability to eradicate staphylococci that are inherent to prosthetic material. This is because of the fact that it is the only compound with bactericidal activity against CoNS that are residing within a layer of the biofilm (59,98,102–104). Its efficacy in the treatment of MSSA or MRSA PVE is less well understood (99). In part, it may be its ability to promote the intracellular killing of *S. aureus* that underlines its observed efficacy. However, its use in NVE can be controversial because of its ability

TABLE 6 Treatment of Staphylococcal Prosthetic Valve Endocarditis

Organism	Antibiotic regimen[a]
MSSA	Oxacillin 2 g intravenously (IV) every 4 hrs for at least 6 wk or nafcillin 3 g IV every 4 hrs for at least 6 wk[b] or cefazolin 1.5 g every 6 hrs for at least 6 wk[c] or vancomycin 1 g IV every 12 hrs for at least 6 wk[d,e] + rifampin 300 mg PO every 8 hrs for at least 6 wk + gentamicin 1 mg/kg IV every 8 hrs for 2 wk[f]
MRSA	Vancomycin 1 g IV every 12 hrs for at least 6 wk[d,e] + rifampin 300 mg PO every 8 hrs for at least 6 wk + gentamicin 1 mg/kg IV every 8 hrs for 2 wk[f]

[a]Assuming normal renal function.
[b]Larger doses than for oxacillin required because of larger volume of distribution.
[c]To be used in patients with minor allergies to beta-lactam antibiotics.
[d]Can be used in patients with significant allergies to beta-lactam antibiotics.
[e]Consider use of linezolid (see text).
[f]Seek alternatives to gentamicin if the organism is resistant to gentamicin (see text).
Abbreviations: MRSA, methicillin-resistant staphylococci; MSSA, methicillin-sensitive staphylococci; PVE, prosthetic valve infective endocarditis.

to antagonize the actions of several antibiotics (105). The need for a triple antibiotic combination was demonstrated in the study that compared the effectiveness in treating CoNS PVE of vancomycin and rifampin versus vancomycin and rifampin given for six weeks plus gentamicin for the first two weeks of therapy (106,107). Thirty-three percent of those treated with only vancomycin and rifampin developed resistant organisms. The addition of gentamicin for the first two weeks prevented this development. Each constituent has a particular role. Vancomycin or the penicillinase-resistant beta-lactam is the primary agent. The rifampin augments the antibacterial effect of the glycopeptide or beta-lactam in the "hostile" environment of implantable material as well as having a potent antistaphylococcal effect. For the best possible result, it is necessary that the targeted organism be sensitive to all three agents. Whenever possible, initiation of rifampin should wait until it is ascertained that the staphylococcus is sensitive to the other two antibiotics. If resistance is present to one of them, then it needs to be replaced by a compound which is effective in vitro. Isolates of CoNS are becoming resistant to gentamicin. Another aminoglycoside should be used if demonstrated to be effective. In the case of the pathogen demonstrating pan-resistance to the aminoglycosides, a quinolone whose effectiveness has been documented may be substituted (108). If the bacteria are resistant to aminoglycosides and quinolones treatment should be initiated with nafcillin/vancomycin plus rifampin (98). When immediate therapy is necessary, the empiric treatment of PVE would consist of vancomycin, gentamicin, and rifampin while awaiting full identification of the organism.

For several reasons, the "weak link" of the therapeutic team is vancomycin. After decades of use, there is still uncertainty regarding the value of vancomycin serum levels as well as the desired levels to be achieved for the successful treatment of infections (109). Against the high concentrations of *S. aureus* that are found in the infected vegetations, vancomycin is dynamically less bactericidal than the semisynthetic penicillinase-resistant penicillins. This fact correlates clinically with the experience that vancomycin treatment of *S. aureus* right-sided IE is associated with a high rate of failure (40%) (110). Although the addition of the aminoglycoside can potentiate the effect of vancomycin, it is also associated with a higher risk of nephrotoxicity. Because of its poor penetration of the fibrin/platelet thrombus, many clinicians will aim for a vancomycin trough of 15 to 20 µg/mL. There is no specific evidence that trough levels >15 µg/mL achieve any greater benefit in outcomes. In treating IE, the recent guidelines (98) advocate vancomycin troughs between 10 and 15 µg/mL. This necessitates vancomycin therapeutic drug monitoring in IE. Trimethoprim/sulfamethoxazole has been used successfully in treating MRSA NVE in IVDA (111). There is no adequate data relevant to the use of this drug in non-IVDA NVE and certainly not for treating PVE. Desensitization of the patient with MSSA IE who is highly allergic to the penicillins has been recommended (112). However, this is carried out with some real risk especially, when it is performed by individuals with no prior experience in desensitizing patients.

Some of the newer antibiotics may provide reasonable alternatives to vancomycin. Quinupristin/dalfopristin (113) and linezolid (114) are the most promising clinically available candidates. There is no large published series documenting the effect of either drugs in the treatment of NVE or PVE. There are case reports supporting the efficacy of quinupristin/dalfopristin in the treatment of complicated MRSA PVE (115). There is somewhat more experience with the use of linezolid in IE. Besides experimental models, there are reports of a few cases. Both types of sources provide mixed evidence (116–120). In their case report of two patients with PVE successfully treated with linezolid, one set of investigators concluded that linezolid "challenges the conventional wisdom that bactericidal synergy is required for the effective treatment of most cases of IE due to gram-positive organisms" (121). It appeared that combining gentamicin and vancomycin did not achieve synergy with linezolid. There is some experimental evidence that treatment failures are related to subtherapeutic levels of the antibiotic (122). A desirable feature of the drug is that it is extremely well absorbed orally. Indeed, there is experience treating NVE with orally administered linezolid (123). The author has a good deal of experience in using linezolid in the treatment of NVE. Its major negative aspect is the development of significant side-effects, hematological and neurological, during its prolonged usage, and not microbiological failures. Certainly, it is premature to recommend linezolid as standard therapy in the treatment of PVE. However, its use should be considered in special circumstances, especially when patients have lost intravenous access. Table 6 summarizes the treatment of staphylococcal PVE.

Fungal PVE requires a surgical approach except perhaps in cases caused by *Histoplasma capsulatum* (65,77). Early valve replacement is dictated by the risk of major emboli and paravalvular invasion. The role of antifungal agents is purely ancillary. Isolates of *C. albicans*, within a prosthetic valve-associated biofilm, become progressively more resistant to amphotericin and fluconazole (124).

SURGICAL TREATMENT OF PROSTHETIC VALVE ENDOCARDITIS

Indications for surgical intervention in PVE are well established (65,77,125). Table 7 summarizes the indications for surgery in PVE. Overall, approximately 30% of patients with PVE do not require surgery. Sixty-five percent presenting with significant renal failure early in the course of PVE is a strong indication for surgery (51).

TABLE 7   Indications for Surgery in Prosthetic Valve Endocarditis

Major indications
  Progressive congestive heart failure refractory to medical therapy
  Fungal PVE (excluding *Histoplasma capsulatum*)
  Persistent sepsis >72 hrs despite antimicrobial therapy
  Recurrent septic thromboemboli
  Indicators of paravalvular extension of infection (atrioventricular block,
    conduction disturbances, and myocardial abscesses)
  Other indicators of paravalvular extension (rupture of sinus of valsalva,
    intracardiac fistulas, pericarditis, and aortic aneurysm)
  Significant perivalvular dehisence
  "Kissing" infection of the anterior mitral valve leaflets with infection of the aortic valve
  Persistent bacteremia due to PVE after 7–10 days of appropriate antibiotic therapy
  Relapse after appropriate therapy.
Lesser indications
  Compensated congestive heart failure
  Nonstreptococcal PVE
  Single episode of thromboembolism
  Vegetations detected on echocardiography
  Small perivalvular dehiscence
  Early (<60 days) PVE
  Multiply resistant organisms such as *Pseudomonas aeruginosa* and *Entercocci*
    for which there is no bactericidal regimen
  Staphylococcus aureus PVE without obvious paravalvular extension

Abbreviation: PVE, prosthetic valve infective endocarditis.

Repeat surgery for mechanical or infectious causes ranges from 18% to 26% (54,126,127). Five-year survival rates following surgical intervention for PVE vary from 54% to 82%. Overall, there is little difference in mortality between surgical and nonsurgical patients. However, in-hospital rates of death were reduced significantly by surgery. If intraoperative cultures are positive for the infecting bacteria, an additional six weeks of antibiotic therapy is required (101). When the patient is identified as being a candidate for surgery, there is nothing to be gained by preoperatively administering antibiotics "to clean up" the field. Extended antibiotic administration before surgery neither sterilizes the valve base nor improves outcome (126). The indications for surgery are the same for mechanical and tissue prosthetic valves (128). When seriously complicated PVE requires advanced surgical techniques such as aortic ventriculoplasty and reconstruction of the annulus, preoperative antibiotic therapy for 10 to 14 days is mandatory (129). The major determinants of outcome are timing of the onset of infection after implantation and the presence of intracardiac complications (130). Survival was 60% in patients with intermediate early PVE as compared with 44% in those with early disease. Patients with fungal PVE should be considered for lifelong suppressive therapy with fluconazole (65).

ANTICOAGULATION IN PROSTHETIC VALVE ENDOCARDITIS

Wilson reported on the effect of continuing anticoagulation during treatment of PVE. Thirty percent of patients in whom anticoagulation was stopped suffered significant neurological complications (130). These results have been confirmed (131). However, other studies indicate that cerebrovascular events occurred more commonly in those receiving coumadin (28). The author's approach to this problem is to discontinue anticoagulation for 48 to 72 hours if a cerebrovascular event takes place during the treatment of PVE. When the bleeding is stabilized, anticoagulation may be resumed with all things being equal. This decision must be made on an individual basis. Heparin is used to resume coagulation because it is rapidly reversed if further complications occur. When thrombotic disease develops in other areas than the heart (i.e., venous thrombosis of the legs), appropriate anticoagulation is indicated. In such a case, placement of a vena cava umbrella may be an alternative.

PROPHYLAXIS OF PROSTHETIC VALVE ENDOCARDITIS

Prevention of the development of PVE will be discussed in Chapter 16.

REFERENCES

1. Starr A, Edwards ML. Mitral replacement: clinical experience with a ball valve prosthesis. Ann Surg 1960; 154:726.
2. Harkness JE, Soroff M, Taylor MC. Prostheses in aortic insufficiency. J Thorac Cardiovasc Surg 1960; 40:744.
3. Wallace AG, Young WG Jr, Osterhout J. Treatment of acute bacterial endocarditis by valve excision and replacement. Circulation 1965; 31:450.
4. Weinstein L. The double-edged scalpel. Editorial. N Engl J Med 1968; 279:775.
5. Vongpatanasin W, Hillis LD, Lange RA. Prosthetic heart valves. N Engl J Med 1996; 335:407.
6. Sidhu P, O'Kane H, Ali N, et al. Mechanical or bioprosthetic valves in the elderly: a 20-year comparison. Ann Thorac Surg 2001; 71(suppl):257.
7. Varstela E. Personal follow-up of 100 aortic valve replacement patients for 1081 patients years. Ann Chir Gynaecol 1998; 87:205.

8. Hoen H, Alla F, Selton-Suty C, et al. Changing profile of infective endocarditis: results of a 1 year survey in France. JAMA 2002; 288:75.
9. Weinstein L, Brusch JL. Prosthetic valve endocarditis. In: Weinstein L, Brusch JL, eds. Infective Endocarditis. New York: Oxford University Press, 1996:210.
10. Karchmer AW, Longworth DL. Infections of intracardiac devices. Infect Dis Clin NA 2002; 16:477.
11. Calderwood SB, Swinski LA, Waternaux CM, et al. Risk factors for the development of prosthetic valve endocarditis. Circulation 1985; 72:31.
12. Ivert T, Dismukes W, Cobbs G, et al. Prosthetic valve endocarditis. Circulation 1984; 69:223.
13. Rutledge RR, Leim BJ, Applebaumb RE. Actuarial analysis of the risk prosthetic valve endocarditis in 1598 patients with mechanical and bioprosthetic valves. Arch Surg 1985; 120:469.
14. Agnihorti AK, McGiffin DC, Galbraith EJ, O'Brien MF. Surgery for acquired heart disease. J Thorac Cardiovasc Surg 1995; 110:1708.
15. Arvay A, Lengel M. Incidence and risk factors of prosthetic valve endocarditis. Eur J Cardiothorac Surg 1988; 2:340.
16. Glower DD, Landofolo KP, Cheruvu S, et al. Determinants of 15-year outcome with 1119 standard Carpentier-Edwards porcine valves. Ann Thorac Surg 1998; 66:S44.
17. Hammermeister KE, Sethi G, Henderson WG, et al. Outcomes 15 years after valve replacement with a mechanical versus a bioprosthetic final report of the Veterans Affairs randomized trial. J Am Coll Cardiol 2002; 36:1152.
18. Geraci JE, Dale AJD, McGoon DC. Bacterial endocarditis following cardiac operation. Wis Med J 1963; 62:302.
19. Talkington CM, Thompson JE. Prevention and management of infective prostheses. Surg Clin NA 1982; 62:515.
20. Gouello JP, Asfar P, Brenet O, et al. Nosocomial endocarditis in intensive care units: an analysis of 22 cases. Crit Care Med 2002; 28:377.
21. Broom ND. Fatigue-induced damage in glutaraldehyde-preserved heart valve tissue. J Thoracic Cardiovasc Surg 1978; 76:202.
22. Grover FL, Cohen DJ, Oprian C, et al. Determinants of the occurrence of and survival from prosthetic valve endocarditis. J Thorac Cardiovasc Surg 1994; 108:207.
23. Weinstein L, Schlesinger JJ. Pathoanatomic, pathophysiologic and clinical correlations in endocarditis (second of two parts). N Engl J Med 1974; 291:1122.
24. Weinstein L, Schlesinger JJ. Pathoanatomic, pathophysiologic and clinical correlations in endocarditis (first of two parts). N Engl J Med 1974; 291:832.
25. Gristina AG. Biomaterial-centered infection: microbial adhesion versus tissue integration. Science 1987; 237:1588.
26. Vaudaux P, Francois P, Lew DP, Waldvogel FA. Host factors predisposing to and influencing therapy of foreign body infections. In: Waldvogel FA, Bisno AL, eds. Infections Associated with Indwelling Medical Devices. 3rd ed. Washington DC: ASM Press, 2000:1.
27. Chen SC, Sorrell TC, Dwyer DE. Endocarditis associated with prosthetic cardiac valves. Med J Aust 1990; 152:458.
28. Karchmer AW, Dismukes WE, Buckley MJ, et al. Late prosthetic valve endocarditis: clinical features influencing therapy. Am J Med 1978; 64:199.
29. Gotz F, Georg P. Colonization of medical devices by coagulase-negative staphylococci. In: Waldvogel FA, Bisno AL, eds. Infections Associated with Indwelling Medical Devices. 3rd ed. Washington DC: ASM Press, 2000:55
30. Zussa C, Galloni MR, Zattera CF. Endocarditis in patients with bioprostheses: pathology and clinical correlations. Intern J Cardiol 1984; 6:719.
31. Sabbah HN, Hamid MS, Stein PD. Mechanical stresses on closed cusps of porcine bioprosthetic valves: correlation with sites of calcification. Ann Thorac Surg 1986; 22:93.
32. Lakler JB, Khaja F, Magilligan DJ, et al. Porcine valves. Long-term (60–89 months) follow-up. Circulation 1980; 62:313.
33. Camilleri JP, Pornin B, Carpentier A. Structural changes in glutaraldehyde-treated porcine bioprosthetic valves. Arch Pathol Lab Med 1982; 106:490
34. Magilligan DJ. Bioprosthetic valve endocarditis. In: Magilligan DJ Jr, Quinn EL. eds. Endocarditis-Medical and Surgical Management. New York: Marcel Dekker, 1986:253.

35. Blakemore WS, McGarrity RJ, Thurer HW, et al. Infection by airborne bacteria with cardiopulmonary bypass. Surgery 1971; 70:830.
36. Block PC, DeSanctis RW, Weinberg AN, et al. Prosthetic valve endocarditis. J Thorac Cardiovasc Surg 1978; 60:540.
37. Kluge RM, Calia FM, McLaughlin JS, et al. Sources of contamination in open-heart surgery. JAMA 1974; 230:1415.
38. Freeman R, King D. Analysis of results of catheter tip cultures in open-heart surgery patients. Thorax 1975; 30:26.
39. Tompkins LS, Roessler BJ, Redd SC, et al. Legionella prosthetic valve endocarditis. N Engl J Med 1988; 318:530.
40. Van den Broek PJ, Lampe AS, Berbee GAM. Epidemic of prosthetic valve endocarditis caused by *Staphylococcus epidermidis*. Brit Med J 1985; 291:949.
41. Wallace RJ Jr., Musser JM, Huss SI. Diversity sources of rapidly growing mycobacteria associated with infections following cardiac surgery. J Infect Dis 1989; 159:708.
42. Hortkotte D, Rosin H, Friedreichs W, et al. Contribution for choosing the optimal prophylaxis of bacterial endocarditis. Eur Heart J 1987; 8(suppl):379.
43. Cowgill LD, Addonizio VP, Hopeman AR, et al. Prosthetic valve endocarditis. Curr Probl Cardiol 1986; 11:617.
44. Ismail MB, Hananachi F, Abid Z, et al. Prosthetic valve endodocarditis: a survey. Brit Heart J 1987; 58:72.
45. Fang G, Keys TF, Gentry LO, et al. Prosthetic valve endocarditis resulting from nosocomial bacteremia. A prospective, multicenter study. Ann Intern Med 1993; 11(9):560.
46. Nasser RM, Melgar GR, Longworth DL, Gordon SM. Incidence in risk for developing fungal prosthetic valve endocarditis after nosocomial candidemia. Am J Med 1997; 103:25.
47. Rose AG. Prosthetic valve endocarditis: a clinicopathological study of 31 cases. S Afr Med J 1986; 6:441.
48. Anderson DJ, Bulkley BH, Hutchins GM. A clinicopathological study of prosthetic valve endocarditis in 22 patients: morphologic basis for diagnosis and therapy. Am Heart J 1977; 94:325.
49. Arnett EN, Roberts WC. Prosthetic valve endocarditis: clinicopathologic analysis of 22 necropsy patients with comparison of observations in 74 necropsy patients with active infective endocarditis involving natural left-sided cardiac valves. Am J Cardiol 1976; 38:281–291.
50. Ferrans VJ, Boyce ME, Billingham TL, et al. Infection of glutaraldehyde-preserved porcine valve heterografts. Am J Cardiol 1979; 43:1123.
51. Cortina JM, Martinelli J, Artiz V, et al. Surgical treatment of active prosthetic valve endocarditis. Results in 66 patients. Thorac Cardiovasc Surg 1987; 35:209.
52. Fernicola DJ, Roberts WC. Frequency of ring abscess and cuspal infection in active infective endocarditis involving bioprosthetic valves. Am J Cardiol 1993; 72:314.
53. Sett SS, Hudon MPJ, Jaimeson WRE, Chow AW. Prosthetic valve endocarditis: experience with porcine bioprostheses. J Thorac Cardiovasc Surg 1993; 105:428.
54. Lytle BW, Priest PC, Taylor FD, et al. Surgery for acquired heart disease: surgical treatment of prosthetic valve endocarditis. J Thorac Cardiovasc Surg 1996; 111:198.
55. Watankunakorn C, Burkert T. Infective endocarditis in a large community teaching hospital, 1988–1990. A review of 210 episodes. Medicine 1993; 72:90.
56. Sandre RM, Shafran SD. Infective endocarditis: review of 135 cases over 9 years. Clin Infect Dis 1996; 22:276.
57. Bouza E, Menasalves A, Munoz P, et al. Infective endocarditis—a prospective study at the end of the twentieth century: new predisposing conditions, new etiologic agents, and still a high mortality. Medicine 2001; 80:298.
58. Archer GL, Vishniavsky N, Stiver HG. Plasmid pattern analysis of *Staphylococcus epidermidis* isolates from patients with prosthetic valve endocarditis. Infect Immun 1982; 35:627.
59. Karchmer AW, Archer GL, Dismukes WE. *Staphylococcus epidermidis* causing prosthetic valve endocarditis: microbiologic and clinical observations as guides to therapy. Ann Intern Med 1983; 98:447.

60. Karchmer AW, Swartz MN. Infective endocarditis in patients with prosthetic heart valves. In: Kaplan EL, Taranta AV, eds. Infective Endocarditis. American Heart Association Symposium Monograph No 52. Dallas: American Heart Association, 1977:58.

61. Meyer DJ, Gerding DN. Favorable prognosis of patients with prosthetic valve endocarditis caused by gram-negative bacilli of the HACEK group. Am J Med 1988; 85:104.

62. Murray BE, Karchmer AW, Moellering RC. Diphtheroid prosthetic valve endocarditis: a study of clinical features and infecting organisms. Am J Med 1988; 69:838.

63. Raoult D, Tissot-Dupont H, Foucault C, et al. Q-fever 1985-1998: clinical and epidemiologic features of 1,383 infections. Medicine (Baltimore) 2000; 79:109.

64. Edwards JE. Candida species. In: Mandell GL, Bennett JE, Dolin R, eds. Principles and Practice of Infectious Diseases. 6th ed. Philadelphia: Elseiver, Livingston, 2005:2938.

65. Melgar GR, Nasser RM, Gordon SM, et al. Fungal prosthetic valve endocarditis in 16 patients: an 11-year experience in a tertiary care hospital. Medicine 1997; 76:94.

66. Aslam PA, Gourley R, Eastridge CE. Aspergillus endocarditis after aortic valve replacement. Int Surg 1970; 53:91.

67. Kaygusuz I, Mulazimoglu L, Cerikcioglu N, et al. An unusual native tricuspid valve endocarditis caused by *Candida colliculosa*. Microbiol Infect 2003; 9:319.

68. Ellis M. Fungal endocarditis. J Infect 1997; 35:99.

69. Calderone RA, Scheld WM. Role of fibronectin in the pathogenesis of candidal infections. Rev Infect Dis 1987; 9(suppl 4):S400.

70. Karchmer AW. In: Mandell GL, Bennett JE, Dolin R, eds. Principles and Practice of Infectious Diseases. 5th ed. Philadelphia: Elseiver Livingston, 2000:903.

71. Wilson WR, Jaumin GK, Danielson ER, et al. Prosthetic valve endocarditis. Ann Intern Med 1975; 82:751.

72. Keys TF. Early-onset prosthetic valve endocarditis. Cleve Clin J Med 1993; 60:455.

73. Wolff M, Witchitz S, Chastang C, et al. Prosthetic valve endocarditis in the ICU: prognosis factors of overall survival in a series of 122 cases and consequences for treatment decisions. Chest 1995; 108:688.

74. Leport C, Vilde JL, Bricaire A, et al. Fifty cases of late prosthetic valve endocarditis: improvement in prognosis over 15 year period. Br Heart J 1987; 58:66.

75. Chen SC, Sorrell TC, Dwyer DE, et al. Endocarditis associated with prosthetic cardiac valves. Med J Aust 1990; 152:458.

76. Quenzer RW, Edwards LD, Levin S. A comparative study of 48 post valves and 24 prosthetic valve endocarditis cases. Am Heart J 1976; 92:18.

77. Horstkotte D. Prosthetic valve endocarditis. In: Horstkotte D, Bodnar E, eds. Current Issues in Heart Valve Disease: Infective Endocarditis. London: ICR Publishers, 1991:238.

78. Horstkotte D. Prosthetic valve endocarditis. In: Horstkotte D, Bodnar E, eds. Current Issues in Heart Valve Disease: Infective Endocarditis London: ICR Publishers, 1991:242.

79. Burckhardt D, Stultz P, Follath F, et al. Prosthetic valve endocarditis: conservative therapy and indications for reoperation. In: Horstkotte D, Bodnar E, eds. Current Issues in Heart Valve Disease: Infective Endocarditis London: ICR Publishers, 1991:262.

80. Mausur H, Johnson WD. Prosthetic valve endocarditis. J Thorac Cardiovasc Surg 1980; 80:31.

81. Dismukes WE, Karchmer AW, Buckley M, et al. Prosthetic valve endocarditis: analysis of 38 cases. Circulation 1973; 48(2):365–377.

82. Li JS, Sexton DJ, Mick N, et al. Proposed modifications to the Duke criteria for the diagnosis of infective endocarditis. Clin Infect Dis 2000; 30:633.

83. Heimberger T, Duma R. Infections of prosthetic heart valves and cardiac pacemakers. Infect Dis Clin N A 1989:228.

84. Archer GL, Karchmer AW, Vishnaivsky N, et al. Plasmid-pattern analysis differentiation of infecting from non-infecting *Staphylococcus epidermidis*. J Infect Dis 1984; 149:913.

85. Parker FB, Grenier-Hayes C, Tomar RH. Bacteremia following prosthetic valve replacement. Ann Surg 1983; 197:147.

86. Hoen B, Selton-Suty C, Lacassin F, et al. Infective endocarditis in patients with negative blood cultures: analysis of 88 cases from a one-year nationwide survey in France. Clin Infect Dis 1985; 20:501.

87. Melgar GR, Nasser SM, Gordon BW, et al. Fungal prosthetic valve endocarditis in 16 patients. An 11 year experience in a tertiary care hospital. Medicine 1997; 76:94.
88. Sands MJ, Lachman AS, O'Reilly DJ. Diagnostic value of cinefluoroscopy in the evaluation of prosthetic heart valve dysfunction. Am Heart J 1982; 104:622.
89. Mann T, McLaurin L, Grossman W, et al. Assessing the hemodynamic severity of acute aortic regurgitation due to infective endocarditis. N Engl J Med 1975; 293:108.
90. McFadden M, Gonzalez-Lavin L, Remington JS. Limited reliability of the "negative" two-dimensional echocardiogram in the evaluation of infectious vegetative endocarditis: Diagnostic and surgical implications. J Cardiovasc Surg 1985, 26:59.
91. Daniel WG, Mugge A, Grote J, et al. Comparison of transthoracic and transesophageal echocardiography for detection of abnormalities of prosthetic and bioprosthetic valves in the mitral and aortic positions. Am J Cardiol 1993; 71:210.
92. Cheitlin MD, Armstrong WF, Aurigemma GP, et al. ACC/AHA/ASE 2003 guideline for the clinical application of echocardiography: summary article: a Report of the American College of Cardiology/American Heart Association Task Force on Practice Guidelines (ACC/AHA/ASE Committee to Update the 1997 Guidelines for the Clinical Application of Echocardiography). Circulation 2003; 108:1146.
93. Roe MT, Abramson MA, Li J, et al. Clinical information determines the impacted transesophageal echocardiography in the diagnosis of infective endocarditis by the Duke criteria. Am Heart J 2000; 139:945.
94. Daniel WG, Mugge A, Martin RP, et al. Improvement in the diagnosis of abscesses associated with endocarditis by transesophageal echocardiography. N Engl J Med 1991; 324:795.
95. Sochowski RA, Chan KL. Implication of negative results on a monoplane transesophageal echocardiographic study in patients with suspected infective endocarditis. J Am Coll Cardiol 1993; 21:216.
96. Morguet AJ, Werner GS, Andreas S, Kreuzer H. Diagnostic value of transesophageal compared with transthoracic echocardiography in suspected prosthetic valve endocarditis. Herz 1995; 20:390.
97. Baddour LM, Wilson WR Infections of prosthetic valves and other cardiovascular devices In: Mandell GL, Bennett JE, Dolin R, eds. Principles and Practice of Infectious Diseases. 6th ed. Philadelphia: Elsevier, Livingston, 2005:2938.
98. Karchmer AW. Infections of prosthetic heart valves. In: Waldvogel FA, Bisno KL, eds. Infections Associated with Indwelling Medical Devices. Washington D.C.: American Society for Microbiology, 2000:145.
99. Wilson WR, Karchmer AW, Bisno AL, et al. Treatment of adults with infective endocarditis due to viridans streptococci, enterococci, other streptococci, staphylococci and Hacek microrganisms. JAMA 1995; 274:1706.
100. Baddour LM, Wilson WR, Bayer AS, et al. Infective endocarditis: diagnosis, antimicrobial therapy and management of complications: a statement for healthcare professionals from the Committee on Rheumatic Fever, Endocarditis and Kawasaki disease, Council on Cardiovascular Disease in the Young and the Council on Cardiology Stroke and Cardiovascular Surgery and Anesthesia, American Heart Association—executive summary: Endorsed By Infectious Diseases Society of America. Circulation 2005; 111:3167.
101. Horstkotte D, Follath F, Gutschik E, et al. Guidelines on prevention, diagnosis and treatment of infective endocarditis, executive summary; The Task Force on Infective Endocarditis of the European Society of Cardiology. Eur Heart J 2004; 25:267.
102. Drinkovic D, Morris AJ, Pottumarthy S, et al. Bacteriologic outcome of combination versus single-agent treatment for staphylococcal endocarditis. J Antimicrob Chemother 2003; 52:820.
103. Kosba WD, Kaye KL, Shapiro T, et al. Therapy for experimental endocarditis due to *Staphylococcus epidermidis*. Rev Infect Dis 1983; 5(suppl 3):S533.
104. Lucet JC, Hermann M, Vaudaux P, et al. Treatment of experimental foreign body infection caused by methicillin-resistant *Staphylococcus aureus*. Antimicrob Agents Chemother 1990; 34:2312.
105. Bayer AS, Lam K. Efficacy of vancomycin plus rifampin in experiment from the aortic valve for an endocarditis due to methicillin-resistant *Staphylococcus aureus*: in vitro–in vivo correlations. J Infect Dis 1985; 151:157.

106. Archer GL, Johnson JL, Vasquez GJ, et al. Efficacy of antibiotic combinations including rifampin against methicillin-resistant *Staphylococcus epidermidis*. Rev Infect Dis 1983; 5(suppl):S538.
107. Karchmer AW. Treatment of prosthetic valve endocarditis. In: Sande MA, Root R, eds. Endocarditis. New York: Churchill Livingstone, 1985:163.
108. Chuard C, Herrmann M, Roehner P, et al. The treatment of experimental foreign body infection caused by methicillin-resistant *Staphylococcus aureus*. Antimicrob Agents Chemother 1990; 34:2312.
109. Saunders AJ. Vancomycin administration and monitoring reappraisal. J Antimicrob Chemother 1995; 36:279.
110. Small PM, Chambers HF. Vancomycin for *Staphylococcus aureus* endocarditis in intravenous drug users. Antimicrob Agent Chemother 1990; 34:1227.
111. Markowitz N, Saramolatz L, Pohlod D, et al. Comparative efficacy and toxicity of trimethoprim-sulfamethoxazole versus vancomycin for therapy of serious *S. aureus* infections (638). Abstracts of the 25th Interscience Conference on Antimicrobial Agents and Chemotherapy, American Society for Microbiology, October 1983.
112. Bayer AS. Infective endocarditis. Clin Infect Dis 1993; 17:313.
113. Bouanchaud DH. In-vitro and in-vivo antibacterial activity of quinupristin/dalfopristin. J Antimicrob Chemother 1997; 39(suppl A):15.
114. Bain KT, Wiibrodt ET. Linezolid for the treatment of resistant gram-positive cocci. Ann Pharmacother 2001; 35:566.
115. Mohan SS, Mc Dermott BP, Cunha BA. Methicillin-receptor *Staphylococcus aureus* prosthetic aortic valve endocarditis with paravalvular abscess treated with daptomycin. Heart Lung 2005; 34:69.
116. La Plante KL, Rybak MJ. Impact of high inoculum *Staphylococcus aureus* on the activities of nafcillin, vancomycin, linezolid and daptomycin, alone and in combination with gentamicin, in vivo and in vitro pharmacodynamic model. Antimicrob Agent Chemother 2004; 48:2665.
117. Chiang FY, Climo M. Efficacy of the linezolid alone or in combination with vancomycin for treat. Treatment failure of experimental endocarditis due to methicillin-resistant *Staphylococcus aureus*. Antimicrob Agent Chemother 2003; 47:3002.
118. Leung KT, Tong MK, Siu YP, et al. The bend of vancomycin-intermediate *Staphylococcus aureus* endocarditis with linezolid. Scand J Infect Dis 2004; 36:483.
119. Asseray JC, Batard E, Le Mabecque V, et al. In fetal efficacy of linezolid in combination with gentamicin for the treatment of experimental endocarditis due to methicillin-resistant *Staphylococcus aureus*. Intern J Antimicrob Ag 2004; 4:393.
120. Marchandin CP, Macia JC, Jonquet O. Treatment failure of methicillin-resistant *Staphylococcus aureus* endocarditis with linezolid. Scand J Infect Dis 2005; 37:946.
121. Wareham DW, Abbas H, Karcher AM, Das SS. Treatment of prosthetic valve infective endocarditis due to multi-resistant Gram-positive bacteria with linezolid. J Infect 2006; 52:300.
122. Dailey CF, Dileto-Fang CL, Buchanan LV, et al. Efficacy in the treatment of experimental endocarditis caused by methicillin-resistant *Staphylococcus aureus*. Antimicrob Agent Chemother 2001; 45:2304.
123. Nathani N, Iles P, Elliott TS. Successful treatment of MRSA native valve endocarditis with oral linezolid therapy. J Infect 2005; 51:e213.
124. Mateus C, Crow SA, Ahearn DG, Jr. Adherence of Candida have against silicone induces immediate enhanced tolerance to fluconazole. Antimicrob Agent Chemother 2004; 48:3358.
125. Bonow RV, Carabello B, de Leon AC, et al. Guidelines for management of patients with valvular heart disease: executive summary. A report of the American College of Cardiology/American Heart Association Task Force on Practice Guidelines (Committe on Management of Patients with Valvular Heart Disease). Circulation 1998; 98:1949.
126. Baumgartner WA, Miller DC, Reitz BA, et al. Surgical treatment of prosthetic valve endocarditis. Ann Thorac Surg 1983; 35:87.
127. Jault F, Gandjbakch I, Chastre C, et al. Prosthetic valve endocarditis with ring abscesses. Surgical management and long-term results. J Thorac Cardiovasc Surg 1993; 105:1106.

128. Calderwood SB, Swinski LA, Karchmer AW, et al. Prosthetic valve endocarditis: analysis of factors affecting outcome of therapy. J Thorac Cardiovasc Surg 1986; 92:776.

129. Ketosugbo AD, Basu S, Greengart A, et al. Aortventriculoplasty in the management of an infected Cabrol graft. Ann Thorac Surg 1992; 6:106.

130. Grover FL, Cohen DJ, Oprian C. Participants in the Department of Veterans Affairs Cooperative Study on Valvular Heart Disease. Determinants of the occurrence and survival from prosthetic valve endocarditis. J Thorac Cardiovasc Surg 1994; 108:207.

130. Wilson W, Geraci J, Danielson G. Anticoagulant therapy and central nervous system complications in patients with prosthetic valve endocarditis. Circulation 1978; 57:1004.

131. Carpenter J, McAllister C. U.S. Army Collaborative Group: anticoagulation in prosthetic valve endocarditis. South Med J 1983; 76:1372.

9 Infective Endocarditis of Intracardiac Devices

John L. Brusch
Harvard Medical School and Department of Medicine and Infectious Disease Service, Cambridge Health Alliance, Cambridge, Massachusetts, U.S.A.

EPIDEMIOLOGY OF PACEMAKER INFECTIVE ENDOCARDITIS

By the year 2000, there were approximately 200,000 implantable cardiac defibrillators and 3.5 million permanent pacemakers throughout the world (1). It is estimated that 400,000 intracardiac defibrillators (ICDs) are placed in the United States each year (2). This has increased by more than 600% in the 1990s. The insertion of left ventricular-assist devices (LVAD) is also growing. Through the 1990s, implantation of intracardiac devices of all types increased by 42%. However, total device infections went up by 124%. The rate of device-related infective endocarditis (IE) remained fairly constant (0.5% of insertions) (3). This alarming increase in infections may be due to the disproportionate rise in placement of ICDs (4,4a) and their infectious complications. As with prosthetic valves, intracardiac devices are a double-edged sword. They prolong and improve the quality of life while always posing significant infectious risks to the patient.

The permanent pacemaker was first employed in 1960 (5) and so has been studied the longest of any of these devices. Despite this experience, a valid incidence of pacemaker infections is not available. This is due, in great part, to the various types of pacemaker infections with a ride range of clinical presentations. Infections of the modern transvenous pacemaker system may be divided into three major types: (*i*) pulse generator pocket infections; (*ii*) infection of epicardial electrodes; and (*iii*) pacemaker infective endocarditis (PIE). PIE is defined by the finding of positive blood cultures in a febrile patient with no other detectable sources of the bloodstream infection (BSI). PIE represents infection of the pacemaker leads, usually the intracardiac portions (6,7). Pacemaker system infections (PSI) may be characterized early (<2 months after placement) and late (>2 months after placement). The incidence of pacemaker infections is currently about 5%. Prior to 1980, this figure approached 12%. This decrease most likely is due to the routine administration of prophylactic antibiotics aimed at staphylococci (8).

Because the transvenous pacemaker is a contiguous system, understanding of the pathogenesis of PIE depends on recognizing the vulnerability of the individual components to infection. Over the years, PSI/PIE have been associated with a variety of risk factors including: diabetes, various types of immunosuppressive states, malignancies, increasing age, treatment with anticoagulant corticosteroids, and the degree of experience of the interventionist (Table 1) (2). Of greatest importance appears to be any type of manipulation of the pacemaker system (9). The most common of these interventions appears to be battery replacement. The complication rate, associated with initial implantation of pacemakers, is 1.4%. That of subsequent interventions is 6.5%. Of this, 67% of the complications are infectious in nature (10). There is no difference between the rates of PSIs of single- and dual-chamber

TABLE 1 Risk Factors for Development of Pacemaker System Infective Endocarditis

Risk factor	Comments
Manipulation of the pacemaker system	Most significant and well-established risk factor
Diabetes mellitus	Conflicting supportive evidence
Prior temporary transvenous pacer	2.9% developed pocket infections vs. 0.4% of those without a temporary pacer
Inexperienced interventionist	History of doing <100 procedures
Presence of a hematoma in the pacemaker pocket	Protects infecting bacteria from host defenses
Coumadin usage	Promotes hematoma formation
Various immunosuppressive states	Not well characterized
Increasing age of the patient	Not well characterized

Source: From Refs. 3, 10, 12–15.

pacemakers suggesting that the number of leads does not increase the risk of infection (10,11). About 33.3% of cases of PIE occur within three to six months of an intervention in a pacemaker system. About 66.6% of cases of PIE become clinically apparent far beyond this time span. The average delay in development of symptoms of valvular infection is 25 months (6,12).

PATHOGENESIS OF PACEMAKER INFECTIVE ENDOCARDITIS

The pathogenesis of PIE is quite similar to that of prosthetic valve endocarditis (PVE; Chapter 8). Implanted foreign material is "conditioned" by the deposition of blood-derived protein complexes (fibrinogen, fibronectin), laminin, and collagen. These promote bacterial adherence to the implanted device (16,17) by means of adherence factors of staphylococci (Chapter 2). In addition, both *Staphylococcus aureus* and coagulase-negative staphylococci (CoNS) adhere to these devices by means of *biofilm*. This structure is a colony of microorganisms enmeshed in a polysaccharide matrix (slime) (18–20). The slime layer protects the pathogen from administered antibiotics as well as from the host's leukocytes (21). Within hours of their placement, conditioning of the generator box, the transvenous leads, and epicardial electrodes commences. In approximately one week, the segments of the leads and electrodes, which abut the walls of the veins, vena cava, and right atrium, are engulfed by connective tissue. At the points of contact with the walls of these blood vessels, there is continued deposition of collagen. Eventually, the leads and electrodes become firmly anchored to the great vessels and right atrium. For several months after implantation, the fibrotic cocoon provides a favorable surface for the adherence of circulating organisms. Later, this encasement becomes endothelialized and much less susceptible to infection by BSI (22,23). Therefore, pacemaker leads are dissimilar to prosthetic valves in that they are relatively resistant to being infected by BSIs with *Streptococcus viridans*, other streptococci, and gram-negatives. An exception to this is *S. aureus*, which can infect the leads at any time after placement (24). The infection rate of the leads, during a *S. aureus* BSI occurring any time after implantation, ranges from 33% to 50%. The negative side of this endothelialized fibrotic sheath is a high rate of thrombotic venous obstruction. Usually, it is a partial blockage (23). Pacemaker system infections with CoNS do resemble that of PVE in that the pacemaker pocket becomes contaminated during the procedure. The rate of colonization varies from 37% to 48%. Less than 5% of these contaminated sites give rise to PSI (25). Analogous to PVE, strains of CoNS have been documented to cause PSI/PVE up to 29 months after implantation.

Breakdown of the skin, which overlies the pacemaker pocket, may lead to infection of the deeper components of the system. This erosion is usually due to the pressure effect of the underlying components on the vascular supply of the dermis. Unusually, it may be secondary to an occult, smoldering pocket infection (25). Breakdown of the skin becomes a more significant cause of PSI that occurs after 24 months of implantation (3,6,26,27). Seventy-nine percent of PSI at this point is produced by erosions of the overlying skin. Infections in this subcutaneous area can migrate down the leads and result in valvular infection. Interoperative contamination is the usual source for infection of the epicardial electrodes. It is less likely that are they affected by infection that has spread from an infected pacer pocket. Infection of the epicardial electrodes by BSI, after they are enveloped by endothelial cells, is unusual, except in the setting of *S. aureus* bacteremia. As presented, an infected epicardial electrode or intracardiac results in a right-sided endocarditis.

MICROBIOLOGY OF PACEMAKER INFECTIVE ENDOCARDITIS

S. aureus and CoNS dominate the microbiology of PIE (85% of cases) (1,6,8,26). In most series, there is a higher proportion of *S. aureus* in early infections and of CoNS in late infections (25,28). This distribution of staphylococci is the reverse of that seen in PVE. The prominence of CoNS in late disease may be attributed to the importance to the contribution of the skin flora to infecting the ulcerated pacemaker pocket seen in late disease. In addition, many of these late CoNS infections delay presentations of intraoperative contamination. The remaining 15% to 20% of cases are caused by gram-negative organisms (coliforms, *Serratia*, and *Pseudomonas* spp.). Enterococci and atypical mycobacteria have also been isolated from cases of PSI/PIE. Fungal infection of the pacemaker system is quite unusual (29). There is increasing evidence that PSI/PIE may be due to multiple organisms (30,31). Klug et al. compared the results of culturing blood and the extravascular and intravascular portions of pacemaker leads. In 12.3% of the cases, cultures of the leads showed no growth. Infection was caused by multiple organisms in 25% of the patients. Most of these were examples of skin flora. *S. aureus* is found in 66% of the cases; while CoNS was responsible for 29.5%. Approximately 50% of the organisms obtained in one set of blood cultures were also retrieved from cultures of leads. Despite the high rate of lead cultures, less than 20% of cases of PSI had more than two positive blood cultures. Whatever the clinical features, whether they indicate pocket or intravascular lead involvement, both extra- and intravascular segments of the leads were infected. The results of this series strongly support DaCosta's proposal that most cases of PSI arise from intraoperative contamination by local skin flora for both early and late disease (25). These findings also may have significant diagnostic and therapeutic implications.

CLINICAL PRESENTATION OF PACEMAKER
INFECTIVE ENDOCARDITIS

Pacemaker system infections clinically may be present as a localized infectious process of the generator pocket, or as a bacteremia in a febrile patient, or as right-sided IE. Many studies of the clinical presentation of infections of permanent pacemakers do not adequately separate the symptoms of pocket infections from those deeper in the system. In general, PIE itself presents with more systemic signs and symptoms than do the more superficial processes (1,3,6,12,32,33).

However, the absence of fever does not preclude the presence of BSI. In one series, 80% of patients with infections of implantable devices were afebrile in the face of a rate of bacteremia of 33% (33). Table 2 presents a profile of the manifestations of implantable medical devices (pacemakers and ICDs) that is based on the study by Chua et al. (1). This data clearly dominated the infections of the generator pocket. Based on the epidemiological data (3), approximately 90% of the cases, represented in Table 2, were non-PIE ones.

Early pacemaker pocket infections most often manifest themselves as typical wound infections (1). On occasions patients may have systemic symptoms of fever and chills with associated BSI. In late infections, signs of erosion of the overlying skin predominate. Surprisingly, there may be a low rate of constitutional signs and symptoms.

Infection of the intravascular leads have a higher rate of fever and bacteremia, especially when the epicardial electrodes are involved. Septic pulmonary emboli occur even in the absence of endocarditis, albeit at a lower frequency (34).

Pacemaker infective endocarditis is usually subacute in nature, although a septic picture is not rare. Fever (84–100%) and chills (75–84%) are much more commonly seen than in other types of PSI (Table 2). Forty-five percent of cases of PIE had abnormalities on chest X ray, which were consistent with pneumonia, abscess, or emboli (6,12,35). Septic pulmonary emboli complicate approximately 30% to 45% of the cases. Less than 10% of the patients with emboli had no clinical signs and symptoms as such (12). *S. aureus* is the organism most commonly isolated from patients who are present with bacteremia and vegetations. Vegetations >10 mm in diameter are more commonly associated with pulmonary emboli (36). Emboli, because of PIE, are much less likely to completely obstruct the pulmonary arteries and those arising from deep venous thrombosis of the lower extremities. This is because it is a type of emboli much more friable than the latter that tends to break apart as it wedges into the arterial circulation. Both tricuspid regurgitation (25%) and functional stenosis may occur (3,37). The former may be because of direct

TABLE 2 Clinical Signs and Symptoms of Infections of Implantable Cardiac Devices[a]

Category	Percentage of cases
Pocket-related	
Pain and redness	55
Drainage	42
Erosion	32
Total cases of BSI	33
Symptomatic BSI	20
Signs	
Fever	19
Sepsis	12
Tachycardia	8
Symptoms	
Chills	22
Malaise	21
Anorexia	12

[a]Implantable pacemakers and cardioverter defibrillators.
Abbreviation: BSI, bloodstream infections.
Source: From Ref. 1.

valvular involvement or increased right-sided pressures due to massive embolization. The latter is caused by obstructing vegetation.

Pacemaker system infections may occur with or without concurrent valvular
infection. Conversely, the pacemaker system may be unaffected by active IE. Duval
et al. described these two groups on the basis of clinical history and echocardiography
(transesophageal method) (35). The first was made up of patients who had detectable
heart valve and intracardiac lead involvement. These patients had undergone multiple
reimplantations of their devices. The last procedure occurred less than one year (ranging from one month to eight years) from the onset of symptoms; 70% were because
of staphylococci. The second group had evidence of valvular infection without demonstrable involvement of the pacemaker lead. Reimplantations were quite infrequent.
In these patients, the average time between the last procedure and the development of
symptoms was 2.2 years. Staphylococci were responsible for 42% of the cases; streptococci and enterococci for 50%. Gram-negatives accounted for the remaining 8%.

DIAGNOSIS OF PACEMAKER INFECTIVE ENDOCARDITIS

The diagnosis of PIE should be strongly considered in any bacteremic and/or febrile
patient, with a permanent transvenous pacemaker whose source of these symptoms
is not established. Clearly, the presence of pocket erosion or pulmonary emboli
dictates a vigorous approach in diagnosing PIE. The standard Duke criteria (38)
are quite insensitive for diagnosing PIE with a sensitivity of 16% for acute PIE and
59.3% for chronic PIE (6). By adding the findings of an infected pacemaker pocket
and pulmonary emboli as major criteria, Klug et al. were able to increase the sensitivity of the Duke criteria for acute and chronic PIE to 87.5% and 85.2%, respectively.
Echocardiography is a key component of the criteria. Transthoracic echocardiography
(TTE) is relatively insensitive in diagnosing lead or tricuspid valve involvement
(20–43%) (3,6,29). Transesophageal echocardiography (TEE) is the much superior
technique (91–96%). Several other studies have yielded almost identical results
(12,29). As is the case with the vegetations of native valves, the predictive value for
PIE of vegetations on pacemaker leads is unknown (39).

The differential diagnosis of PIE should include: septic pelvic thrombophlebitis,
septic jugular thrombophlebitis, and thromboembolic disease of the low extremities.

TREATMENT OF PACEMAKER INFECTIVE ENDOCARDITIS

There is very little solid evidence pointing the way to the best possible therapy of PSI
especially PIE. In general, the approach should be the employment of appropriate antibiotics in conjunction with the removal of the entire system. Eggimann and Waldvogel
present a strong case. There are many challenges in treating these infections (40–54).

REFERENCES

1. Chua JD, Wilkoff BL, Lee I, et al. Diagnosis and management of infections involving
   implantable electrophysiologic cardiac devices. Ann Intern Med 2002; 133:604.
2. Cabell CH, Heidenreich PA, Chu VH, et al. Increasing rates of cardiac device infections
   among Medicare beneficiaries. Am Heart J 2004; 147.
3. Arber N, Pras E, Copperman Y, et al. Pacemaker endocarditis. Report of 44 cases and
   review of the literature. Medicine (Baltimore) 1994; 73:299.
4. Hlatky MA, Saynina O, McDonald K, et al. Utilization and outcome of the implantable
   cardioverter defibrillator, 1987 to 1995. Am Heart J 2002; 144:397.

4a.   Gordon RJ, Quagliarello B, Lowry FD. Ventricular assist device-related infections the Lancet: Infections Diseases 2006; 626.
 5.   Chardack WM, Gage AA, Greatbach W. Correction of complete heart block by a self contained subcutaneously implanted pacemaker. J Thorac Cardiovasc Surg 1961; 42:814.
 6.   Klug D, Lacroix D, Savoye C, et al. Systemic infection related to endocarditis on pacemaker leads: clinical presentation and management. Circulation 1997; 95:2098.
 7.   Choo MH, Holmes DR Jr, Gersh JD, et al. Permanent pacemaker infections: characterization and management. Am J Cardiology 1981; 48:559.
 8.   Eggimann P, Waldvogel F. Pacemaker and defibrillator infections. In: Waldvogel FA, Bisno AL, eds. Infections Associated with Indwelling Medical Devices. Washington D.C.: ASM Press, 2000:247.
 9.   Hildick-Smith DJ, Lowe MD, Newell PM, et al. Ventricular pacemaker upgrade: experience, complications and recommendations. Heart 1998; 79:383.
10.   Harcome AA, Newell PF, Ludman TE, et al. The complications following permanent pacemaker implantation or elective unit replacement. Heart 1998; 80:240.
11.   Victor F, DePlace C, Camus H, et al. Pacemaker lead infection: echocardiographic features, management and outcome. Heart 1999; 81:82.
12.   Cacoub P, LePrince P, Nataf P, et al. Pacemaker infective endocarditis. Am J Cardiol 1998; 82:480.
13.   Bluhm GL. Pacemaker infections. 2-year follow-up of antibiotic prophylaxis. Scand Thorac Cardiovasc Surg 1985; 19:231.
14.   Matsuura Y, Yamashina H, Higo M, Fujii T. Analysis of complications permanent transvenous implantable cardiac pacemaker related to operative and post operative management in 717 consecutive patients. Hiroshima J Med Sci 39:131.
15.   Mounsey JP, Griffith MJ, Tynan M, et al. Antibiotic prophylaxis in permanent pacemaker implantation: a prospective randomized trial. Br Heart J 1994; 72:339.
16.   Passerini L, Lam K, Costerton JW, King EG. Biofilms on indwelling vascular catheters. Crit Care Med 1992; 20:665.
17.   Peters GE, Saborowski F, Locci R, Pulverer G. Investigations on staphylococcal infection of transvenous endocardial pacemaker electrodes. Am Heart J 1984; 108:359.
18.   Baddour LM, Sullam PM, Bayer AS. Pathogenesis of infective endocarditis. In: Sussman M, ed. Molecular Medical Microbiology. London: Academic Press, 2002:999.
19.   Donlan RM. Biofilm formation. A clinically relevant microbiological process. Clin Infect Dis 2001; 33:1387.
20.   Moreillion Que YA, Bayer AS. Pathogenesis of streptococcal and staphylococcal endocarditis. Infect Dis Clin NA 2002; 16:297.
21.   Lew DP, Pittet D, Waldvogel FA, Mayhall G. Infections that complicate the insertion of prosthetic devices. In: Mayhall G, ed. Hospital Epidemiology and Infection Control. Baltimore: Williams and Wilkins, 1996:731.
22.   Cox JN. Pathology of cardiac pacemakers and central catheters. Curr Top Pathol 1994; 86:199.
23.   Spittell PC, Hayes DL. Venous complications after insertion of a transvenous pacemaker. Mayo Clin Proc 1992; 67:258.
24.   Chamais AL, Peterson GE, Cabell CH, et al. *Staphylococcus aureus* bacteremia in patients with permanent pacemakers or implantable cardioverter-defibrillators. Circulation 2001; 104:1029.
25.   DaCosta A, Lacroix D, Savoye C, et al. Role of the preaxillary flora in pacemaker infections: a prospective study. Circulation 1998; 97:1791.
26.   Lewis AB, Hayes DL, Holmes PR Jr, et al. Update in infections involving permanent pacemakers. Characterization and management. J Thorac Cardiovasc Surg 1985; 89:758.
27.   Camus C, Leport C, Raffi F, et al. Sustained bacteremia in the 26 patients with a permanent endocardial pacemaker: assessment of wire removal. Clin Infect Dis 1993; 17:46.
28.   Bluhm G. Pacemaker infections. A clinical study with special reference to prophylactic use of some as isoxazolyl penicillins. Acta Med Scand Suppl 1985; 699:1.
29.   Victor F, DePlace C, Camus H, et al. Pacemaker lead infections: echocardiographic features, management and outcome. Heart 1999; 81:82.
30.   Brook I, Frazier EH. Role of anaerobic and anaerobic bacteria in pacemaker infections. Clin Infect Dis 1997; 24:1010.

31. Klug D, Wallet F, Kacet S, Courcol RJ. Detailed bacteriologic tests to identify the origin of transvenous pacing system infections indicate a high prevalence of multiple organisms. Am Heart J 2005; 149:322.

32. Spratt KA, Blumberg EA, Wood CA, et al. Infections of implantable cardioverter defibrillators approach to management. Clin Infect Dis 1993; 17:679.

33. Kearney RA, Eisen HJ, Wolf JE. Nonvalvular infections of the cardiovascular system. Ann Intern Med 1994; 121:219.

34. Wilhelm MJ, Schmid JC, Hammel S, et al. Cardiac pacemaker infection: surgical management with and without extracorporeal circulation. Ann Thorac Surg 1997; 64:1707.

35. Robbins MJ, Frater RWM, Soeiro R, et al. Influence of vegetation size on clinical outcome of right-sided infective endocarditis. Am J Med 1986; 80:165.

35. Duval X, Selton-Suty C, Alla F, et al. Endocarditis in patients with a permanent pacemaker: a 1-year epidemiological survey on infective endocarditis due to valvular and/or pacemaker infection. Clin Infect Dis 2004; 39:68.

36. Robbins MJ, Frater RWM, Soeiro R, et al. Influence of vegetation size on the clinical outcome of right-sided infective endocarditis. Am J Med 1986; 80:165.

37. Unger P, Clevenbergh P, Crasset V, et al. Pacemaker-related endocarditis inducing tricuspid stenosis. Am Heart J 1997; 133:605.

38. Durack DT, Lukes AS, Bright DK. New criteria for diagnosis of infective endocarditis: utilization of specific echocardiographic findings. Am J Med 1994; 96:200.

39. Vilacosta I, Sarria J, San Roman J, et al. Usefulness of transechocardiography for diagnosis of infected transvenous pacer permanent pacemakers. Circulation 1994; 89:2684.

40. Eggimann P, Pittet D. Central line sepsis in intensive care units: overview and updates. Opin Anesth Crit Care 1999; 10:14.

41. Wilson WR, Karchmer AW, Dajani AS. Antibiotic treatment of adults with infective endocarditis due to streptococci, enterococci, staphylococci and Hacek microorganisms. JAMA 1995; 274:1706.

42. del Rio A, Anguera I, Miro JM, et al. Surgical treatment of pacemaker and defibrillator lead endocarditis: the impact of electrode lead extraction on outcome. Chest 2003; 124:1451.

43. Meier-Ewert HK, Gray ME, John RM. Endocardial pacemaker or defibrillator leads with infective vegetations: a single-center experience and consequences of transvenous extraction. Amer Heart J 2003; 146:203.

44. Bracke FA, Meijer A, vanGelder LM. Pacemaker lead complications: when is extraction appropriate and what can we learned from published data? Heart 2001; 85:254.

45. Manolis AS, Manounis J, Chiladakis J, et al. In percutaneous extraction of pacemaker leads with a novel (vascoextor) pacing lead removal system. Am J Cardiol 1998; 81:935.

46. Wilkoff BL, Byrd CL, Love CJ, et al. Pacemaker lead extraction with the laser sheath: results of the pacing lead extraction with the excimer sheath (PLEXES) Trial. J Am Cardiol 1999; 33:1671.

47. Wade J, Cobbs C. Infections in cardiac pacemakers. In: Remington J, Swartz M, eds. Current Topics in Infectious Diseases. New York: McGraw-Hill, 1988:9, 44.

48. Baddour LM and the Infectious Diseases Society America—Emerging Infectious Network. Long-term suppressive antimicrobial therapy for intravascular device-related infections. Am J Med Sci 2001; 322:209.

49. Kron J, Herre J, Renfroe EG, et al. Lead and device-related complications in the antiarrhythmics versus implantable defibrillators trial. Am Heart J 2001; 121:92.

50. Samuels LE, Samuels FL, Kaufman MS, et al. Management of infected implantable cardiac defibrillators. Ann Thorac Surg 1997; 64:1702.

51. Al-Khatib SM, Lucas FL, Jollis JG, et al. Relation between patients' outcomes and the volumes of cardioverter-defibrillator implantation procedures performed by physicians treating Medicare beneficiaries. J Am Coll Cardiol 2005; 46:1536.

52. Rose EA, Geligns AC, Moskowitz AJ, et al. Long-term use of a left ventricular assist device for end-stage heart failure. N Engl J Med 2001; 345:1435.

53. Vilchez RA, McEllistrem MC, Harrison LH, et al. Relapsing bacteremia in patients with ventricular assist device: an emerging complication of extended circulatory support.

54. deJonge KC, Laube HR, Dohmen PM, et al. Diagnosis and management of left ventricular assist device valve-endocarditis: LVAD valve replacement. Ann Thorac Surg 2001; 70:1404.

Nosocomial and Health Care-Associated Infective Endocarditis (Iatrogenic Infective Endocarditis)

John L. Brusch
Harvard Medical School and Department of Medicine and Infectious Disease Service, Cambridge Health Alliance, Cambridge, Massachusetts, U.S.A.

INTRODUCTION

Prosthetic valve infective endocarditis (PVE) and infective endocarditis of intra-cardiac devices have already been presented (Chapters 8 and 9). For many reasons, they could rightfully be labeled examples of iatrogenic infective endocarditis (IIE). IIE represents the negative consequences of medicine's invasive efforts to treat a variety of diseases. This chapter focuses on the more common types of IIE, those due to a variety of intravascular catheters, and the profound impact they have had on the epidemiology and microbiology of IE as a whole. The characteristics of IE, acquired in various healthcare venues, will be compared with that acquired in the community (nonhealthcare-connected IE). Valvular infections of intravenous (IV) drug abusers will not be included in this analysis as this topic has been discussed in Chapter 7.

EPIDEMIOLOGY

Since the mid 1960s, there has been a marked change in the epidemiological pat-terns of IE. It has been marked by a significant "graying" of the IE population. Excluding patients with IV drug abuser endocarditis (IVDA IE), 55% of patients are above 60 years of age. Rheumatic heart disease underlies only 15% of the cases; whereas 30% are associated with mitral valve prolapse and 20% have one or more prosthetic valves in place; 50% of the elderly with valvular infection have underly-ing calcific aortic stenosis. The most significant change has been the increase in cases of acute IE to the point that they now outnumber subacute ones. *Staphylococcus aureus* has become the premier pathogen of IE due in great part to its involvement in infections of various types of intravascular devices (central IV, hemodialysis cath-eters, tunneled lines) [Chapter 1, (1)]. These devices are increasingly employed in the outpatient setting as well as in the hospital. In the past, 67% of bloodstream infections (BSI) were acquired in the hospital setting (2). Currently, BSI arise almost equally from the community and from the hospital (3). From 1990 to 1993, 20% of *S. aureus* BSI developing outside the hospital were related to intravascular devices. Ten years earlier, this was not the situation (4). In the past, *S. aureus* IE was more highly associated with the nonintravascular catheter-related BSI (CR-BSI). *S. aureus* is secondary only to coagulase-negative staphylococci (CoNS) in causing nosoco-mial BSI. Methicillin-resistant *S. aureus* (MRSA) is involved in approximately 50% of the cases. Sixty percent of individuals are intermittent carriers of either MRSA or of methicillin-sensitive *S. aureus* (MSSA). Because these devices are the major risk fac-tors for the development of staphylococcal and other types of nosocomial BSI and nosocomial infective endocarditis (NIE), this chapter focuses primarily on their role in producing nosocomial valvular infections. Bloodstream infections, associated with intravascular lines, have increased by more than 100% while those produced by urinary tract infections, pneumonias, and wound infections have not. The risk of nosocomial BSI due to intravascular catheters is only exceeded by the traumatic procedures of tonsillectomy, transurethral resection of the prostate, dental extractions, and suction abortion. Other risk factors for staphylococcal BSI include cancer and diabetes, use of corticosteroids, IVDA, alcoholism, and renal failure.

Up to 78% of *S. aureus* bacteremia in the United States (200,000 cases per year), occurring in either the community or in a healthcare facility, are associated with intravascular catheters (5). In the past, those individuals, who developed a *S. aureus* BSI in the hospital (nosocomial BSI), which was caused by a removable focus (intravascular catheter), were felt to be at much lower risk of developing metastatic infections including IE (6,7). These changes emphasize the blurring of the once sharp distinctions between the nature of BSI/IE acquired within the hospital and in the community. The following paragraphs discuss in detail the three major sites of acquisition of valvular infections.

In 1970, investigators at the Boston City Hospital described an increase in IE, due to organisms not previously highly associated with valvular infection, during the period 1935–1955 (8). *S. aureus*, gram-negative, enterococci and *Staphylococcus epidermidis* were the chief examples of this group. The investigators concluded that these changes of this initial phase of NIE were brought about by the availability of antibiotics and were primarily nosocomial in nature. In a 1981 study, which compared cases of IE that developed both within and without the hospital, von Reyn defined NIE as a valvular infection that presented itself after 48 hours of hospitalization or up to four weeks following a procedure performed in the hospital (9). Friedland compared patients with community-acquired IE to those with NIE (10). Individuals belonging to the latter group were generally older, more likely to be female, with a greater degree of valvular abnormalities, and with more bacteremic episodes due to invasive procedures. Nosocomial infective endocarditis was found to have a mortality rate greater than 40% as compared with 11% of the community cases. Probably, the most important conclusion of this study was that "nosocomial endocarditis occurs in the definable population of hospitalized patients and is potentially preventable." In the 1960s and 1970s, NIE affected women more than men. Community-acquired IE had the opposite gender distribution (11). Currently, males seem to dominate in both types of IE except in community-acquired PVE (12).

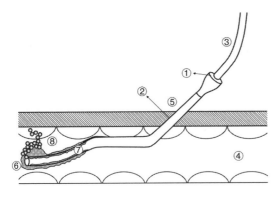

FIGURE 1 Sources of infection and proliferation of established infection of intravascular catheters. 1, colonized hub; 2, colonized skin; 3, contaminated infusate; 4, endothelial cells; 5, exit tunnel; 6, external fibrin sleeve/thrombus, 7, internal fibrin sleeve/thrombus; 8, dispersion of *S. aureus* from the infected catheter sheath.

The second phase of NIE can be considered to have begun in the 1970s with the implantation of the first of the intracardiac devices, prosthetic valves. Early PVE is by definition nosocomial [Chapter 8 (13,14)]. The first case of early PVE was reported in 1961. Presently, PVE is responsible for 9% to 15% of all cases of IE. Nineteen percent of late PVE is nosocomially acquired. Nearly 17% to 45% of individuals with NIE have prosthetic valves in place. These statistics regarding infection of prosthetic valves have remained fairly constant over the last two decades. For further discussion of PVE, see Chapter 8.

In 1976, Watanakunakorn and Baird reported the first series of NIE associated with intravascular catheters (15). The dramatic effect that intravascular devices had on the incidence of NIE, especially that of native valves, was not realized until the 1990s. In the 1980s, NIE constituted less than 4% of all cases of IE of native valves (NVE). In the early 1990s, NIE caused 9.3% of all noncardiac surgery-related IE (16). At the end of the 20th century, it was responsible for 7.5% to 31% of cases of NVE (12,17,18) in tertiary care hospitals. The concurrent rate in community hospitals for NIE of native valves runs between 14% and 25% (19). Giamrellou (13) speculates that these rates will increase for both types of facilities because of: (*i*) the increase in BSI; (*ii*) greater numbers of immunocompromised patients; (*iii*) greater numbers of more severely ill patients who are admitted to intensive care units; and (*iv*) the increased numbers of older and more frail patients who are living longer because of a variety of intracardiac devices. Fifty percent of patients with NIE are >60 years of age as compared with 21% of cases acquired outside of healthcare institutions (10).

Nearly, 23% to 70% of cases of NIE of native valves have predisposing valvular pathology (12,16,20). These may vary between series. They include rheumatic heart disease, degenerative valvular disease, prior attacks of IE, hypertrophic cardiomyopathy, and previously implanted prosthetic valves (21). More than 80% affect the left side of the heart. Fifty percent of the cases involve the mitral valve; the aortic valve in 11%; both of these valves in 11%; the tricuspid in 11%; and mural endocarditis in 7% (12). Right-sided NIE is usually the result of pacemaker/internal cardiac debrillators-associated IE (Chapter 9). Generally, the mitral position is the most commonly infected valve in late PVE. There is no difference in predisposing conditions between NIE and valvular infection arising outside the hospital.

Bloodstream infections are the most common underlying events in most cases of IIE, whatever the type (16,18). Infections of intravascular devices are the source of up to 60% of hospital-associated BSI. The number of nosocomial BSI has increased by more than 100% in the last 20 years. The rate of nonintravascular device-related BSI, such as that caused by pneumonia or pyelonephritis, has remained essentially the same. The contribution of the various types of intravascular lines to cases of device-related NIE is as follows: (*i*) peripheral intravenous catheters (6–22.7%); (*ii*) central intravenous catheters (9.1–48%); (*iii*) Swan–Ganz catheters (2–9%) (13,16,18,22). Most of these catheters will have been in place for 3.25 days before giving rise to the causative BSI. Sixty-eight percent of them are present for 5 to 10 days. There is a significant and independent association between hemodialysis catheters, infected with *S. aureus* and valvular infections with this pathogen (23). Thirty percent of NIE are due to BSI that arise from the urinary tract. This is especially important as regards enterococcal NIE (24). A variety of other types of infections contribute to the causative BSI including skin and soft-tissue infections (24). The source of the BSI could not be determined in up to 17% of cases of NIE. Table 1 presents the sources of infection for NIE.

TABLE 1   Sources of Blood Stream Infections in Cases of Native Valve
Nosocomial Infective Endocarditis

Source	Percent of cases of NIE	Comments
IVC		
Peripheral IVC	6–22.7%	
Central IVC[a]	9.1–48%	
Swan–Ganz catheters	2–9%	
Hemodialysis catheters	—	Highly associated with S. aureus NIE
GU tract infections or procedures	20–30%	
No definable source	17%	

[a]Most are peripherally inserted.
Abbreviations: BSI, bloodstream infections; GU, genitourinary tract; IVC, intravenous catheters; NIE, nosocomial infective endocarditis.
Source: From Refs. 13, 16–18.

MICROBIOLOGY OF NOSOCOMIAL INFECTIVE ENDOCARDITIS

The predominance of staphylococci (both coagulase-negative and -positive) in producing NIE reflects their frequent colonization of the skin of hospitalized patients Table 2. Exactly 77.4% of NIE are because of these isolates as compared with 39.4% of IE that develops outside of the hospital (18). Presently, *S. aureus* produces 55% of all cases of NIE. Ninety-one percent of these are associated with intravascular lines. Enterococci (*Streptococcus faecalis*) are the second most common pathogens isolated from cases of NIE (5–30%) (24). These usually originate from the urinary tract. About 8% of enterococcal BSI are complicated by NIE, usually in the elderly and those with severe vascular disease. Ten percent of the cases of NIE are caused by CoNS (25,26). Despite their frequency, gram-negative bacteremias seldom produce valvular infection (3–7% of cases of IE) (17). This is probably due to their decreased ability, as compared with the gram-positives, to adhere to the cardiac endothelium. Of all the gram-negatives, *Pseudomonas aeruginosa* possesses the greatest ability to invade normal endothelial cells. Bloodstream infections as a result of *P. aeruginosa* are almost twice as likely to cause IE among IVDA in the community than it does in hospitalized non-IVDA (27). Hemodialysis and cardiac surgery appear to be additional risk factors for *P. aeruginosa* NIE (13).

TABLE 2   Microbiology of Nosocomial Infective Endocarditis

Organism	Percentage of cases
Staphylococcus aureus	55
CoNS	10
Enterococci	16
Streptococcal spp.	7
Gram-negatives	5
Fungal	4
Culture negative	3

Abbreviation: CoNS, Coagulase-negative staphylococci.
Source: From Ref. 26.

Polymicrobial endocarditis has become more frequent over the last 10 to 20 years. It is most commonly observed in IVDA and cardiac surgery patients. The most frequent combination is that of *P. aeruginosa* and *S. faecalis*.

There has been a significant increase in fungal IE over the last 10 years (17). Fungi currently account for 5% of cases of NIE. This rise parallels that of candidal BSI (1200% in the 1990s). Most of these are caused by *Candida albicans* (28,29). Twenty-eight percent of fungal IE is produced by nonalbicans spp. (30). *Candida parapsiliosis* has become especially important because of the following abilities: (*i*) to survive not only on the skin but in infused glucose solutions; (*ii*) to adhere to the synthetic materials that make up the various types of intravascular devices because of its ability to make slime; (*iii*) to its propensity to colonize intravascular pressure-monitoring systems. It has a mortality of 36% to 50% (31,32). There is a close association between *C. parapsilosis* NIE and cardiac surgery (44% of cases). Major systemic emboli are common (44%).

There are specific associations between the microbial nature of a CR-BSI and specific types of patients (29). *S. aureus* is the primary cause of device-related BSI in patients with AIDS and dialysis catheters while *P. aeruginosa* is the most frequently retrieved from those with extensive burns (32a). Translocation of organisms due to chemotherapy produced gut mucosal breakdown is the most likely cause of gram-negative BSI in patients with a variety of neoplastic processes. Noncoliform pathogens (*Serratia marcesens, Acinetobacter* spp., and *Pseudomonas* spp.) predominate in hemodialysis patients (32b, 32c).

CLINICAL MANIFESTATIONS, DIAGNOSIS, AND THERAPY
OF NOSOCOMIAL INFECTIVE ENDOCARDITIS
Health Care-Associated Bloodstream Infections

Of the 200,000 cases of nosocomial BSI produced by *S. aureus*, approximately 25% of these result in IE/noncardiac metastatic infections (1). Realization that at least 50% of staphylococcal bacteremia acquired in the hospital or in the community arose from infected vascular catheters has prompted the reclassification of BSI. More and more seriously ill patients are cared for outside the hospital, in nursing homes, rehabilitation facilities, and in their homes receiving various therapies that require an intravascular catheter. The complications of these devices, including infectious ones, are similar whatever the location. This makes sense as the clinical characteristics of the patients and the treatments that they receive are essentially the same whatever the venue of care. Friedman et al. have crafted the term "healthcare-associated bloodstream infections" (HCBSI) to describe BSIs occurring in this type of patient (33,34). As an example, these authors cite the study that described 91% of *S. aureus* BSI in HIV-positive patients as community-acquired despite the fact that 78% of these individuals had an indwelling intravascular catheter (35). Table 3 presents the criteria for diagnosing an HCBSI. A community-acquired BSI is one that does not meet the definition of an HCBSI. Friedman et al. emphasize the fact that patients with HCBSI share many characteristics with those of the classically described nosocomial BSI. Both have a similar rate of BSIs resulting from intravascular devices and from the gastrointestinal tract. *S. aureus* is the most frequently identified pathogen. However, to Fowler et al., the differences between community-acquired BSI and HCBSI are of more significance. In community-acquired BSI, there was a higher frequency of underlying urinary tract infections than in nosocomial or HCBSIs. *Escherichia coli* and *Streptococcus pneumoniae* were more commonly

TABLE 3 Definition of Health Care-Associated Bloodstream Infection

A positive blood culture from a patient obtained within 48 hours of admission to a hospital and any one of the following conditions:
1. Received intravenous home therapy or specialized nursing care, including wound care, by a healthcare agency or by individuals within 30 days of the BSI.
2. Attended a hospital or dialysis clinic or received intravenous chemotherapy within 30 days of the BSI.
3. Was hospitalized in an acute care hospital for at least two days within 90 days of the BSI.

Abbreviation: BSI, bloodstream infection.

isolated from community-acquired BSIs. However, 20% of cases of MRSA IE occur in individuals who do not meet the criteria of a HCBSI (1). These isolates have the exotoxin genes (Panton—Valentine leukocidinn genes) that are characteristic of community-acquired MRSA. Patients with healthcare-acquired IE (HCIE) are more likely to be diabetic, to be on hemodialysis, to have experience with an intravascular device, to have MRSA, and to have persistent BSI with *S. aureus* healthcare-associated IE. Table 4 contrasts the properties of HCBSI with that of BSI arising from the community. The concept of HCBSI has major implications for diagnosis, therapy, and prevention. Being aware of the concept of HCBSI should alert the clinician to the possibility that the BSI, which fits the criteria for a healthcare-acquired one, may have the same complications as that from an intensive care unit (ICU) of a tertiary care hospital.

Pathogenesis of Iatrogenic Infective Endocarditis

All types of IE follow the same pathogenic pathway. First, the organisms arrive at the valve's surface by means of nosocomially derived or spontaneous bacteremia. Then, the bacteria attach themselves in large enough numbers to initiate invasion of the valve. The common denominator of both adherence and invasion is the sterile platelet-fibrin thrombus or nonbacterial thrombotic endocarditis (NBTE). The typical bacteria of subacute IE (*Streptococcus viridans*) depend on the presence of a preformed thrombus as their target for valvular invasion (Chapter 4). Those of acute IE, such as *S. aureus*, are able to initiate thrombus formation on undamaged

TABLE 4 Characteristics of Nosocomial Infective Endocarditis Bloodstream Infection/ Health Care-Associated Bloodstream Infections and Community Bloodstream Infection

NIE BSI/HCBSI	Community BSI
Organisms	*Escherichia coli,*
Staphylococcus aureus, CoNS,	*S. pneumoniae*
Enterococci, Candida spp.	
MRSA 46.1%/29.8%	19.9%
Mortality 37%/29%	16%
Source	
Intravascular devices 52%/42%	0
Urinary tract 17%/18%	46%
Pneumonia 16%/16%	27%
Gastrointestinal tract 13%/17%	4%

Abbreviations: BSI, bloodstream infections; CoNS, coagulase-negative staphylococci; HCBSI, health care-associated bloodstream infections; MRSA, methicillin-resistant *S. aureus*.
Source: From Refs. 1, 13, 33.

endocardium. Fibronectin bridging promotes uptake of *S. aureus* by endothelial cells. These cells then produce tissue factor activity and cytokines that initiate both thrombus formation and extension of the inflammation. Eventually, the endothelial cells are lysed by the *S. aureus* within them. *S. faecalis*, and probably the nutritionally variant streptococci, also promote the production of fibronectin by the endothelium (36).

The pathogenesis of intravascular catheter infections is similar to the aforementioned processes. Bacterial adherence to these devices is dependent on the response of the host to the presence of the foreign body, properties of the organism itself, and position of the catheter. Within a few days of its insertion, a sleeve of fibrin and fibronectin is deposited along with platelets, albumin, and fibrinogen (Chapter 8). *S. aureus* and *Candida* isolates preferentially adhere to the fibrin component, whereas CoNS attaches to fibronectin. CoNS also attaches avidly to the host biofilm by its glycoccalyx. Slime is utilized by both bacteria and fungi not only for adherence but also as a shield against the various chemotherapeutic agents employed against them (37–40). Within the exglycocalyx, bacteria are able to resist up to 1000 times the minimal bactericidal concentration of most antibiotics. The "community" of slime also shields the pathogens from the host's antibodies and phagocytes. *S. aureus* and *Candida* isolates attach more efficiently to catheters made of polyvinylchloride than to those made of teflon. Foreign materials have a significant negative effect on the host's defense system, in particular neutrophil function and concentration of complement (37).

The processes by which intracardiac devices, such as implanted cardioverter-defibrillators and permanent pacemakers, become infected is quite similar to that described previously. These devices are more likely to be the point of origin of staphylococcal BSI within one year of their placement. After this, bacteremia with *S. aureus* is more likely to originate from infected tissue that then proceeds to seed the intracardiac device (Chapter 9).

Not all intravascular catheters have the same potential to produce BSI. Bacteremias in the range of 80% to 90%, owing to intravascular devices, are related to central venous catheters. The noncuffed central venous catheter is the worst offender (with rates of BSI ranging from 4% to 14%). Peripherally inserted central venous catheters (PICCs) have a much lower rate of infection (1.2%). Swan-Ganz lines have a risk of approximately 2%. Cuffed central catheters (Hickman, Broviac) and subcutaneous central venous ports (Infusaport, Port-a-Cath) have the lowest rate of all. Because of the extended period of time that they remain, they do have the highest total risk of infection (Table 5). Lines placed in the subclavian area have a much lower risk than those inserted in the internal jugular. Femoral lines are the most likely to become infected (41–43). Catheter infections are directly related to its thrombotic potential (44,45). Silicone elastomers and polyurethrane devices are less thrombogenic than polyvinylchloride ones. Most intravascular catheters are currently polyurethrane in composition. No matter what their composition or location, the longer they are in use, the greater the risk of BSI. Prior to four days of placement, there is very little risk of CR-BSI for any type of device.

The pathogens, which produce CRBSI, contaminate the infusion system at one of four possible sites (37,46): (*i*) the site of insertion; (*ii*) the catheter's hub; (*iii*) contamination of the infusate itself; and (*iv*) infection of the device's fibrin sheath by a bacteremia arising from a distant source. For catheters that are in place for <15 days, the skin flora is the most common source of infection. Increasingly, the skin of patients is becoming colonized by antimicrobial-resistant *S. aureus*, *Enterococcal* spp.,

TABLE 5 Assessment of Risk and Rates of Bloodstream Infections Produced by Intravascular Catheters

Types of vascular catheters	Risks of BSI per catheter (%)	Rates of catheter BSI/1000 catheter days
Standard CVC	3.3	2.3
Antibiotic-coated CVC	0.2	0.2
PICC	1.2	0.4
Hemodialysis catheters	—	2.8
Tunneled and cuffed CVC	20.9	1.2
Swan–Ganz CVC	1.9	5.5

Abbreviations: BSI, bloodstream infections; CVC, central venous catheter; PICC, peripherally inserted central venous catheter.
Source: From Refs. 41–43.

gram-negatives, and *Candida* spp. Identifiable risk factors for the presence of these pathogens include: age, chronic disease, severity of illness, interinstitutional patient transfer especially from nursing homes, extended hospitalizations, transplant and gastrointestinal surgeries, exposure to antibiotics especially cephalosporins, and the presence of intravascular catheters (47). Local applications of disinfectant compounds can lower the degree of colonization and the risk of infection of the insertion site. A silver impregnated cuff or Dacron cuff sheath is able to interfere with the migration and colonization of the cuff of the catheter (48–51). Infection of the intracutaneous tract that leads to bacterial migration all the way from the insertion point to the tip of the catheter is the most common source of CRBSI within the first seven to nine days of after insertion. This process results in extraluminal infections. Later on (mean 23.4–26.5 days), contamination of the catheter hub becomes the major source of CRBSI. The pathogens transiently colonize the hands of healthcare providers. Contamination of the hub results from various types of manipulations of the device's port/ports. The organisms produce intraluminal infection as they migrate down the inner wall of the catheter. In the case of long-term catheters (mean 109 days), the concentration of microorganisms within the biofilm of the inner wall of the catheter is twice that found on the exterior surface.

Shortly after their insertion, the extraluminal wall of most intravascular catheters become coated with fibrin (52). This sheath of fibrin/thrombin is at risk of being seeded by a transient bacteremia that originated from a distant site (53). This scenario probably occurs quite infrequently. Over time, this sleeve is "transformed into a cellular/collagen tunnel covered by endothelium" (54). In addition, thrombi may form at the point of insertion within 24 hours of placement. After the 24-hour mark, thrombi develop at the tip of the catheter. The infusion itself appears to be behind the formation of this clot (55). These thrombi are also at risk to be infected during a transient BSI.

Unusually, the infused solution itself may be the source of HCBSI/IE. Any type of solution or compound may become contaminated during its manufacture or preparation (intrinsic contamination). These include blood products (platelets, albumin) and any type of IV solution [total parenteral nutrition (TPN) formula, lipid emulsions, crystalloid solutions, and multidose drug vials] (56–58). This type of BSI is most commonly produced by gram-negative aerobes (*Enterobacter*, *Serratia*, and *Pseudomonas* species). Platelet packets have become tainted with *Salmonella* spp., *Yersinia*, and other gram-negatives when they have been stored at room temperature in order to extend the period of their viability. Even vacutainer tubes, povidione–iodine, and other disinfectants have been contaminated during their manufacture. The risk of intrinsic contamination has significantly become lessened with implantation of stricter quality controls. Preparation of total parenteral nutrition solutions in the pharmacy still poses a significant risk of internal contamination (45).

Fifty percent of BSIs associated with arterial catheters are because of infection of the infusate solutions, such as those that are used in external pressure-monitoring devices, hemodialysis-related materials, crystalloid solutions, lipid emulsions, blood products, and hyperalimentation solutions which have been documented to have become contaminated during the time of their administration (extrinsic contamination). One to two percent of IV administered solutions are so tainted (59,60). Representative organisms of a patient's normal skin flora are usually unable to grow in most infusates. Gram-negatives such as *Pseudomonas* spp., *S. marcescens*, and *Enterobacter* spp. can multiply in normal saline. The rate of BSI markedly increases when the concentrations of the organisms is >1000 colony-forming units per milliliter of the fluid. At this concentration, there is no visible turbidity that could serve as a warning of possible contamination. TPN infusates are able to support the growth of many pathogens, especially *Candida* spp. (61,62). Many types of bacteria and fungi, especially *Malassezia furfur*, may flourish in lipid emulsions (63,64). Once infection is established in an infusion system, it will persist until all the hardware of that system is changed (60).

The risk of contamination is directly related to the length of time that the IV apparatus is in place (65). A more significant factor is the degree of manipulation by healthcare personnel (i.e., drawing blood from the line). Arterial catheters have a high rate of CRBSI (>1%). Half of these are secondary to contaminated saline. This is attributable to the stagnant nature of the fluid as these devices are used to obtain hemodynamic measurements so as not to infuse solutions. They are also subjected to a great deal of manipulation as these measurements are being conducted. The pathogens implicated are those gram-negatives that can flourish in normal saline (66,67).

Clinical Manifestations of Iatrogenic Infective Endocarditis

Although the signs and symptoms of NIE and how they differ from community-acquired valvular infection were well-described by 1988, knowledge of them and appreciaton of how they differ from those of community-acquired valvular infection are not widespread. This lack of familiarity is a significant factor in the failure to expeditiously diagnose IIE (18). Most of the data concerning the clinical aspects of IIE are based on studies of NIE. Because they share so many characteristics, it is reasonable for this portion of the discussion to place NIE and HCIE under the common heading of IIE (1).

IIE differs from the community form of the disease in that it presents itself less often with fever, chills, and leukocytosis (55% vs. 25% and 82% vs. 61%, respectively). There is a lower rate of hepatosplenomegaly, embolic, dermatological manifestations of IE (Osler nodes and Janeway lesions) in cases of IIE. These observations may be explained, in part, by the older age of patients with IIE. Hypotension, pulmonary edema, and other manifestations of the sepsis syndrome do occur more frequently in IIE (53% vs. 23% and 27% vs. 9%, respectively). Only 40.6% of the patients with community-acquired IE have a defined source for the inciting bacteremia IE. The muted response of the older patient with IIE leads to a high rate of delay in diagnosis in this group. It has been felt that underlying valve abnormalities are more common in IIE. More recent evidence suggests that healthy native valves are becoming more frequently involved. As with many aspects of IE, the frequency of previous abnormalities is dependent on the population studied (12,13,18,21,22). Where rheumatic fever is widespread, rheumatic valvulitis is a major predisposing abnormality. Likewise, those institutions that perform cardiac surgery will see a higher rate of PVE.

The hallmarks of fungal IIE are failure to make a timely, correct diagnosis in 82% of the cases, delay in hospitalization (32 ± 39 days), and a high rate of macro-embolization (13,68). The brain, kidneys, extremities, and coronary arteries are the major targets (45% of cases). Significant neurological insults (seizures, hemiplegia, facial palsies, and confusion) are seen in 26% of the patients. Similar to the situation in bacterial IIE, there is a low rate of splenomegaly and embolic dermal manifestations.

Diagnosis of Iatrogenic Infective Endocarditis

The purpose of this section is to discuss the means of making an expeditious diagnosis of IIE. The reader should refer to other chapters for discussions of the diagnosis of specific types of IE. The diagnostic approach to IIE should focus on four major areas: (*i*) Is a BSI present? (*ii*) If so, what is its source? (*iii*) If the source is an infected intravascular catheter, what is the best form of treatment? and (*iv*) Has it produced IE of one or more valves.

The major criteria for diagnosing any type of IE is the documentation of a continuous bacteremia Chapter 12. This has been defined as two separate blood cultures growing out of organisms that are associated with IE in the absence of a primary focus; or blood cultures, persistently positive for any microorganism, drawn >12 hours apart; or at least three out of four sets positive for any microorganism drawn over at least one hour (69). The diagnosis of NIE may be quite challenging for many reasons. Forty percent of NIE were not recognized until the end stages of the patient's life or even only upon autopsy. The manifestations of acute IE may resemble noninfectious processes, such as vasculitis or drug reactions. The presence of fever and a sudden decline may be attributed to another source, such as bacteria in a Foley catheter or a possible infiltrate on the chest X ray. Because of a precipitous clinical deterioration in the patient, antibiotic therapy is often empirically instituted before the patient is adequately assessed. This should primarily be by the appropriate drawing of blood cultures (discussed earlier).

Not less than three nor more than five blood cultures should be drawn. As the bacteremia of IE is continuous, the interval between draws is not critical as long as blood is obtained through different venipunctures. Blood cultures should be drawn through intravascular lines only for the purpose of diagnosing CR-BSI (70–72) these catheters that are frequently colonized with skin flora. A CR-BSI is defined as at least one positive blood culture drawn from a peripheral vein of the patient with a central catheter in place within 48 hours of the positive blood cultures. Contamination of the infusate must always be excluded in the process of diagnosing a CR infection. The presence of a gram-negative BSI is highly suggestive of the infusion system being the source. The presence of line infection is documented by either culturing the tip of the catheter by the roll-plate method or blood may be drawn simultaneously through the line and a vein. The former method has the marked disadvantage that the catheter must be removed and only its external surface is cultured. In the latter approach, a ratio of the colony counts obtained from the catheter to those collected from a peripheral vein of 10/1 is diagnostic of line-related BSI. Growth from blood cultures, obtained through the central venous catheter, which occurs more than two hours earlier than that obtained from a peripheral vein, is also indicative of a CR-BSI (73). Criteria have been established for determining whether a blood culture is truly positive. Those with a positive predictive value are: retrieval organisms that are strongly correlated with IE, a short incubation period, multiple cultures positive for the same organism, and high degree of acuity of illness (74).

Multiple courses of empirically administered antibiotics often mute the progression of the infected platelet fibrin thrombus and is probably the chief cause of false-negative blood cultures in NIE. For this type of patient, indirect diagnostic methods must be realized. The most useful of these is echocardiography (Chapter 13). This technique not only visualizes the valvular vegetations of IE but also the complications of infection, such as myocardial abscesses, valvular insufficiency, and congestive heart failure. The sensitivity of transthoracic echocardiography (TTE) is approximately 60% to 70%. In at least 15% of the patients, small vegetations are not able to be visualized by TTE because of pulmonary changes due to chronic obstructive pulmonary disease or aging. Transesophageal echocardiography (TEE) was developed because of the inability to visualize the right-sided lesions of IVDA as well as to compensate for the distortion of the transducer beam by mechanical prosthetic valves. Seventy-five percent of PVE can be detected by TEE as opposed to 35% by TTE. The overall sensitivity of TEE is higher (83–100%). TEE can detect smaller vegetations (<8 mm) and is more useful in detecting perivalvular and myocardial abscesses (75,76). Echocardiography has a role in predicting the risk of embolization (77). It is important to remember that only approximately 50% of vegetations, which are visualized by either type of echocardiography, are actually infected (78). Additionally, 10% to 20% of cases of IE at any one time do not have any demonstrable vegetation by TTE. One series indicates that a negative TEE effectively rules out IE. In this author's opinion, the evidence remains inadequate to support this conclusion in clinical practice. Conversely, a recent study demonstrated that 23% of patients with staphylococcal BSI associated with intravascular catheters and negative TTEs had evidence of IE by TEE (79). Without culturing actual valvular tissue, it is impossible to say whether these vegetations were not or were infected. However, because of the high association between staphylococcal BSI and endocardial infection, echocardiography should be performed in all these cases. Clearly, TEE is the preferred methodology in cases of prosthetic PVE and perhaps IVDA. Otherwise, TTE should be the initial approach due to its lower rate of complications (IE has resulted from the endoscopic component of TEE). If this study is negative, then a TEE should be performed.

The documentation of *S. aureus* bacteriuria, in the absence of a history of urinary tract abnormalities, is an important clue to the existence of either bacteremia or IE with a *S. aureus*. Most cases of *S. aureus* bacteriuria are because of instrumentation (80). Twenty-seven percent of the cases of *S. aureus* BSI have been documented to have concurrent bacteriuria (81,82). In the setting of *S. aureus* BSI, the presence of hematuria often represents staphylococcal IE. The hematuria may be caused by embolic renal infarction or immunologically mediated glomerulonephritis. Hematuria usually results with appropriate antibiotic therapy.

Abnormalities of cardiac conduction are present in 10% of the patients (83). These blocks may be secondary to myocarditis or more likely to the development of septal abscesses. It is recommended that electrocardiography be performed every

72 hours during the initial two weeks of antibiotic therapy to monitor the development of a septal abscess.

Treatment of Iatrogenic Infective Endocarditis

In this author's opinion, the major challenge of treatment of *S. aureus* CR-BSI is not selecting the agents to be used but rather how long to treat. With ever-increasing rates of CR-BSI, the most important is to determine the appropriate length of therapy. It should be as short as possible in order to avoid the medical complications of prolonged antibiotic administration as well as the overwhelming economic consequences.

One approach to reaching a solution is to classify *S. aureus* BSI into simple, uncomplicated, continuous, and complicated (IE/metastatic infection). Simple BSI has been described as a bacteremia that is not associated with vegetations underlying valvular abnormalities on TEE negative blood cultures obtained two to four days after initiation of enzymatic therapy; and a removable focus of infection and resolution of clinical symptoms within 72 hours of the start of antibiotic therapy (84). Some authorities contend that seven days of IV antibiotics are adequate in this setting. Given the fact that *S. aureus* has the overwhelming capability of infecting normal valves, this author cannot endorse such a short course of therapy when treating *S. aureus.*

Uncomplicated bacteremia is defined as underlying valvular abnormalities without any vegetations demonstrable by TEE; a positive blood culture obtained two to four days after the beginning of therapy; a nonremovable source of infection; and persistent signs of infection after 72 hours of effective antibiotic therapy. Fourteen days of therapy of uncomplicated BSI are felt by many to be adequate. This view is a consensus statement that is based on limited evidence. The fact that Fernandez-Guerrero documented that 53% of his patients with proven NIE exhibited relapsing/breakthrough bacteremia that persists for >72 hours after the start of antibiotic therapy or catheter removal (16). This should make one cautious about using an abbreviated antibiotic course.

One of the premier challenges in the field of IE is whether a continuous *S. aureus* bacteremia, in the presence of an intravascular line, represents valvular infection. The essential characteristic of IE is the presence of a continuous BSI. However, an infected intravascular catheter may mimic an infected valve by producing a continuous BSI. This is understandable as an infected catheter, like an infected heart valve, sits in the vascular space with an attached infected thrombus. Although there is no direct evidence to support this concept, it is reasonable to speculate that *S. aureus* may disperse from the infected fibrin sleeve of intravascular catheter and infect the adjacent endothelium (endotheliosis) (85,86). Under such conditions, CR-BSI may become perpetuated. Infectious disease specialists often utilize longer courses of antibiotics in this situation. These resulted, in some series, in higher cure rates and lower relapse rate (87,88). Therefore, at this time, this author favors treatment of a continuous CR-BSI for at least four weeks. Clearly, more studies need to be undertaken to provide adequate evidence to settle these questions. It is essential that infected, short-term, non-tunneled intravascular catheters be removed. Cure rates are as low as 20% with antibiotic therapy alone and without prompt catheter removal (89). Long-term catheters (Broviac or Hickman) do not need to be automatically removed except in the presence of proven IE, infection of the vascular, septic thrombophlebitis, or infection with pathogens

TABLE 6 Management of Noncontinuous, Short-Term Catheter-Related Bacteremia Due to *Staphylococcus aureus*

Prompt removal of the catheter
Institution of appropriate antibiotic therapy
Follow-up surveillance blood cultures within 48 hours
If the follow-up blood cultures are negative and
The TEE shows no signs of infective endocarditis
There is no evidence of metastatic infection, then two weeks of antibiotic therapy would be appropriate
If follow-up blood cultures are positive and the TEE shows signs of infective endocarditis, then four weeks of intravenous antibiotic therapy is appropriate
If follow-up blood cultures are positive and the TEE shows no signs of infective endocarditis, further imaging studies should be performed to rule out other sources of bacteremia

TEE, transesophageal echocardiography.
Source: From Refs. 79, 88.

such as *Corynebacterium* of JK, *Pseudomonas* spp., fungal species, or *Mycobacterium* spp. Intraluminal infusions of antibiotics have at least a 30% success rate against sensitive organisms (90). The use of thrombolytic agents to dissolve the fibrin sheath of the catheter most likely improves (91) the effect of the infused antibiotic (90). Table 6 presents an approach to the management of noncontinuous, short-term CR-BSI as a result of *S. aureus*.

Discussion of the antimicrobial therapy of all types of IE has been presented in detail elsewhere in this text. Some key points in the therapy of *S. aureus* BSI are presented here. Because of the development of HCBSI, the clinician should initiate antibiotic therapy as if that patient were hospitalized. In addition, MRSA has become endemic in many communities (33). Therefore, vancomycin may be the drug of empiric choice. It is significantly less effective against MSSA than the beta-lactams. It is associated with a high rate of failure (35%) and relapse (at least 40%) (88) because of its high protein binding and reduced bactericidal properties combined with its relatively poor penetration into the vegetations (92,93). Linezolid may be a better alternative. However, resistance to this antibiotic has already been reported (94). Strong consideration should be given to the addition of gentamicin for two weeks to either vancomycin or the antistaphylococcal beta-lactams. These combinations have not been proven to lessen mortality, but do produce both a more rapid clearing of the BSI and a more rapid defervescence (95).

Outcomes of Iatrogenic Infective Endocarditis

Fifty years ago, more than 80% of the patients with NIE died (96). This value has decreased from 35% to 56% overall (97). *S. aureus* IIE has mortality rates of up to 75% compared with 20% for cases of *S. aureus* NVE developing in the community (16). Mortality of CR *S. aureus* NIE is related to age >60 years, development of heart failure, infection of prosthetic valves, arterial embolization, and need of emergency surgery (13).

In fungal endocarditis, individuals treated with antifungal agents and cardiac surgery have a significantly greater survival rate at one year than those receiving medical therapy alone (55% vs. 36%) (30). Nosocomial infective endocarditis caused by *Candida* spp. has more favorable outcomes than cases due to *Aspergillus* spp.

TABLE 7 Evidence-Based Measures to Prevent Catheter-Related Bloodstream Infections

Insertion site and duration of catheterization
Subclavian site preferred over femoral or internal jugular (101).
Despite the fact that the rate of CR-BSI increases with longer periods of catheterization, routine changing over a guide wire or placement of a new site does not decrease this rate (102).
Precautions taken during insertion of catheter
Use of maximum sterile techniques during insertion (103).
Preparation of the skin-chlorhexidine is preferred over povidone–iodine[a] (104).
Prophylactic heparin during insertion may well have an effect on CR-BSI ability to reduce catheter thrombosis[a] (105).
Equipment type and dressings
Type of intravascular catheter minocycline-/rifampin-impregnated catheters are significantly better than chlorhexidine-/silver sulfadiazine-impregnated ones in preventing CR-BSI (12-fold CR-BSI risk reduction). The superiority may be because of the fact that the former catheter has both intraluminal and extraluminal coatings as compared with the latter which has only extraluminal coating (106).
CR-BSI may occur more frequently in multiluminal catheters[a] (107).
Transparent dressings may be associated with a greater risk of CR-BSI[a]. Gauze dressings should always be used when there is bloody drainage from the insertion site (108).

[a]Evidence does not reach statistical significance.
Abbreviation: CR-BSI, catheter-related bloodstream infections.
Source: From Refs. 99, 100.

Prophylaxis Against Catheter-Related Bloodstream Infections

In the case of NIE, prophylaxis takes a somewhat different form than the classic tenets for prophylaxis of IE. The key to the prevention of IIE is the reduction of infection of intravascular devices. Preventive measures focus on several major areas: (*i*) choice of insertion site and duration of catheterization; (*ii*) preventive measures during catheter insertion; and (*iii*) devices and dressings. In a study of ICU patients, adherence to evidence-based infection control guidelines was almost abolished CR-BSI (98).

There is good evidence that the following lessen the risk of catheter infection: formal training in insertion and care of catheters; use of sterile barriers during placement; use of chlorhexidine instead of povidone–iodine for cutaneous antisepsis; use of a chlorhexidine-impregnated dressing or application of a topical anti-infective ointment wound to the insertion site. The use of catheters with anti-infective properties may also be effective. Their use should be currently restricted to those patients most at risk of developing CR-BSI (catheters to be in position for more than five days). One should avoid insertion of intravascular catheters in the internal jugular and femoral veins. Exchanging catheters over a guide wire should be discouraged as the new catheter may be placed through a contaminated tract or positioned in proximity to an infected thrombus or area of endotheliosis (99,100,110). Table 7 presents an approach in preventing CR-BSI.

Case Study ■ A 75-year-old man was admitted to the ICU because of respiratory failure secondary to *Klebsiella pneumonia*, which necessitated that he be placed on the ventilator. He initially responded to IV ceftriaxone to which the organism is susceptible. He was making progress weaning until day 5 when he developed clinical sepsis with a temperature of 103°F and worsening hypoxia. A portable chest X ray indicated a left lower lobe infiltrate. He was aggressively treated with fluids. The antibiotic regimen was changed to vancomycin and gentamicin. Within 24 hours, he was hemodynamically stable with marked improvement in his temperature. A sputum culture caused the growth of *P. aeruginosa*. Blood cultures were not drawn. Vancomycin and gentamicin were discontinued after five days and ceftazadime was begun. He was treated for a total of 10 days. Five days after completion of antibiotics, he again slipped into a septic course. At the same time, another patient in the unit was "crashing." Because the urine in the Foley bag looked "dirty," the covering resident ordered ciprofloxacin to be given intravenously. The urine was cultured. Again, no blood cultures were obtained. Methicillin-sensitive *S. aureus*, which is sensitive to ciprofloxacin, grows out of the urine. The Foley catheter was changed and the patient received a total of 10 days of cipro-floxacin. Because, overall, he was making little progress weaning, peripherally inserted central catheter was replaced by a guide wire. After being off antibiotics for seven days, the patient again became febrile and hypotensive. Ciprofloxacin was restarted. He clinically did not respond and began to go into congestive heart failure. The cardiology consult heard a new early diastolic murmur. Echocardiogram was performed at the bedside, which revealed a large vegetation of an aortic valve leaflet associated with a perforated cusp. The patient then became bradycardiac. The EKG revealed a third-degree heart block. The patient's heart failure worsened. The patient then became unresponsive. The family at this point refused emergency cardiac surgery and expressed their wish for comfort measures only. Postmortem examination revealed a large paravalvular abscess tracking into the interventricular septum.

Comments ■ This is a common scenario for NIE. Without blood culture results, a patient's deterioration in the ICU is attributed to many possibilities but not to IIE. In this setting, the most obvious possible cause of sepsis is often not the real one. Only 25% of infiltrates seen by portable chest X-ray of ventilated patients represent pneumonia (110). "Dirty" urine does not always represent the cause of systemic infection. The fact that this man grew out S. aureus from the urine should have raised the possibility that a BSI was the underlying cause. There is almost no circumstance under which the patient is too ill to allow at least two sets of blood cultures to be drawn before the institution of empiric therapy.

REFERENCES

1. Fowler VG, Miro JM, Hoen B, et al. *Staphylococcus aureus* endocarditis: a consequence of medical progress. JAMA 2005; 293:3012.
2. Weinstein MP, Towns ML, Quartey SM, et al. The clinical significance of positive blood cultures in the 1990s: a prospective comprehensive evaluation of the microbiology, epidemiology and outcome of bacteremia and fungemia in adults. Clin Infect Dis 1997; 24:584.
3. Weinstein MP, Reller LB, Murphy JR, Lichtenstein KA. The clinical significance of positive blood cultures: a comprehensive analysis of 500 episodes of bacteremia and fungemia in adults I. Laboratory and epidemiological observations. Rev Infect Dis 1983; 5:35.
4. Steinberg JP, Clark CC, Hackman BO. Nosocomial and community acquired *Staphylococcus aureus* bacteremias from 1980 to 1993: impact of intravascular devices and methicillin resistance. Clin Infect Dis 1996; 23:255.
5. Thompson RL. Staphylococcal infective endocarditis. Mayo Clin Proc 1982; 57:106.
6. Nolan CM, Beaty HN. *Staphylococcus aureus* bacteremia. Am J Med 1976; 60:495.
7. Iannini PB, Crossley K. Therapy of *Staphylococcus aureus* bacteremia associated with a removable focus of infection. Ann Intern Med 1975; 84:558.
8. Finland M, Barnes MW. Changing etiology of bacterial endocarditis in the antibacterial era. Experiences at the Boston City Hospital 1933–1955. Ann Intern Med 1970; 72:341.
9. VonReyn CF, Levy B Arbeit R. Infective endocarditis: an analysis based on strict case definitions. Ann Intern Med 1981; 94 (Part 1):505.
10. Friedland G, von Reyn CF, Levy B. Nosocomial endocarditis. Infect Control 1984; 15:193.
11. Weinstein L, Rubin LH. Infective endocarditis. Prog Cardiovasc Dis 1973; 16:239.
12. Martin-Davila P, Fortun J, Navas E, et al. Nosocomial endocarditis in a tertiary hospital. An increasing trend in native valve cases. Chest 2005; 128:772.
13. Giamarellou H. Nosocomial cardiac infections. J Hosp Infect 2002; 50:91.

14. Block PC, DeSanctis RW, Weinberg AN, et al. Prosthetic valve endocarditis. J Thorac Cardiovasc Surg 1970; 60:540.
15. Watanakunakorn C, Baird IM. *Staphylococcus aureus* bacteremia and endocarditis associated with a removable infected intravenous device. Am J Med 1977; 63:253.
16. Fernandez-Guerrero ML, Verdejo C, Azofra J, Gorgolas M. Hospital-acquired infectious endocarditis not associated with cardiac surgery. An emerging problem. Clin Infect Dis 1995; 20:16.
17. Gilleece A, Fenelon L. Nosocomial infective endocarditis. J Hosp Infect 2000; 46:83.
18. Terpenning MS, Buggy B, Kauffman CA. Hospital-acquired infective endocarditis. Arch Intern Med 1988; 148:1601.
19. Kazanjian PH. Infective endocarditis: review of 60 cases treated in community hospitals. Infect Dis Practice 1993; 2:41.
20. Lamas CC, Ekyn SJ. Hospital acquired native valve endocarditis: analysis of 22 cases presenting over 11 years. Heart 1998; 79:442.
21. Haddad SH, Arabi YM, Ziad MA, AL-Shimemeri AA. Nosocomial infective endocarditis in critically ill patients: a report of three cases and review of the literature. Intern J Infect Dis 2004; 8:210.
22. Chen S, Dwyer D, Sorrell TA. A comparison of hospital and community-acquired infective endocarditis. Am J Cardiol 1992; 70:1449.
23. Petti CA, Fowler VG Jr. *Staphylococcus aureus* bacteremia and endocarditis. Infect Dis Clin NA 2002; 16:413.
24. Fernandez-Guerrero ML, Herrero L, BellverM, et al. Nosocomial enterococcal endocarditis: a serious hazard for hospitalized patients with enterococcal bacteraemia. J Intern Med 2002; 252:510.
25. Gilleece A, Fenelon L. Increasing incidence of coagulase negative staphylococcal endocarditis. J Infect 1998; 36:A22.
26. Karchmer AW. Infective endocarditis. In: Zipes DP, Libby P, Bonow R, Braunwald E, eds. Braunwald's Heart Disease: A textbook of Cardiovascular Medicine. Chap. 58. 7th ed. Philadelphia: Elseiver, Saunders, 2005:1633.
27. Finklestein R, Boulos M, to a Markivicz. Hospital-acquired *Pseudomonas aeruginosa* endocarditis. J Hosp Infect 1991; 18:161.
28. Pittet D, Wenzel R. Nosocomial bloodstream infections. Secular trends in rates, mortality and contribution to hospital deaths. Arch Intern Med 1995; 155:1117.
29. Wisplinghoff H, Bischoff T, Tallent SM, et al. Nosocomial bloodstream infections in US hospitals: analysis of 24,179 cases from a prospective nationwide surveillance study. Clin Infect Dis 2004; 39:309.
30. Ellis ME, AL-AbdelyH, Sandridge A, et al. Fungal endocarditis: evidence in world literature, 1965–1995. CID 2001; 32:50.
31. Weems JJ Jr. *Candida parapsilosis*: epidemiology, pathgogenicity, clinical manifestations and antimicrobial susceptibility. CID 1992; 14:756.
32. Hawser SP, Douglas LJ. Biofilm formation by *Candida* species on the surface of catheter material in vitro. Infect Immun 1994; 62:915.
32a. Goetz AM, Squier C, Wagener MM, et al. Nosocomial infections in the human immuno-deficiency virus-infected patient: a two-year survey. Am J Infect Control 1994; 23:334.
32b. Weinke A, Schiller R, Fehrenbach FJ, et al. Association between *Staphylococcus aureus* nasopharyngeal colonization and septicemia in patients infected with human immuno-deficiency virus. Eur J Clin Microbiol Infect Dis 1992; 11:985.
32c. Do AN, Ray BJ, Banerjee SN, et al. Bloodstream infection associated with needleless devices use and the importance of infection control practiced in the home health care setting. J Infect Dis 1999; 179:442.
33. Friedman ND, Kaye KS, Stout JE, et al. Health care-associated bloodstream infections in adults: a reason to change the accepted definition of community-acquired infections. Ann Intern Med 2002; 137:791.
34. Gaynes R. Health care-associated bloodstream infections: a change in thinking. Ann Intern Med 2002; 137:850.
35. Senthilkumar A, Kumar S, Sheagren JN. Increased incidence of *Staphylococcus aureus* bacteremia in hospitalized patients with acquired immunodeficiency syndrome. Clin Infect Dis 2001; 33:1412.

36. Moreillon P, Que YA, Bayer AS. Pathogenesis of streptococcal and staphylococcal endocarditis. Infect Dis Clin NA 2002; 16:297.
37. Vaudaux P, Francois P, Lew DP, Waldvogel FA. Host factors predisposing to and influencing therapy of foreign body infections. In: Waldvogel FA, Bisno AL, eds. Infections Associated with Indwelling Medicasl Devices. 3rd ed. Washington, D.C.: ASM Press, 2000:1.
38. Donlan RM. Role of biofilms in antimicrobial resistance. ASAIO J 2000; 46:S47.
39. Stewart PS, Costerton JW. Antibiotic resistance of bacteria in biofilms. Lancet 2001; 358:135.
40. Watnick P, Kolter R. Biofilm, city of microbes. J Bacteriol 2000; 182:2675.
41. Kluger D, Maki D. The relative risk of intravascular device-related bloodstream infections with different types of intravascular devices in adults: a meta-analysis of 206 published studies (abstract). Infect Control Hosp Epidemiol 2000; 21:95.
42. Maki DG. Infections caused by intravascular devices used for infusion therapy: pathogenesis, prevention and management. In: Bisno AL, Waldvogel FA, eds. Infections Associated with Indwelling Medical Devices. 2nd ed. Washington, D.C.: ASM Publishers, 1994:155.
43. Brusch JL. Infective endocarditis in critical care. In: Cunha B, ed. Infectious Diseases in Critical Care Medicine. New York: Marcel Dekker, 1998:387.
44. Linder L, Curelaru I, Gustavsson B, et al. Material thrombogenicity in central venous catheterization: a comparison between soft, antibrachial catheters of silicone elastomer and polyurethrane. J Parenter Nutr 1984; 8:399.
45. Beekman S, Henderson DK. Infections caused by percutaneous intravascular devices. In: Mandell GL, Bennett JE, Dolin R, eds. Principles and Practice of Infectious Diseases. Chap. 300. 6th ed. Philadelphia: Elseiver, Churchill Livingstone, 2005:3347.
46. Durack DT. Prevention of infective endocarditis. N Engl J Med 1995; 332:38.
47. Safdar N, Maki DG. The commonality of risk factors for nosocomial colonization and infection with antimicrobial-resistant *Staphylococcus aureus*, enterococcus, gram-negative bacilli, *Clostridium difficile* and *Candida*. Ann Intern Med 2002; 136:834.
48. Maki DG, Cobb L, Gurman JK, et al. Unattachable silver impregnated cuff for prevention of infection with central venous catheters. A prospective randomized multicenter trial. Am J Med 1988; 80:307.
49. Sitges-Serra A, Linares J, Garau J. Catheter sepsis: the clue is the hub. Surgery 1985; 97:355.
50. Raad I, Costerton JW, Sabharwar U, et al. Central venous catheters (CVC) studied by quantitative cultures and scanning electron microscopy (SEM): the importance of luminal colonization. In: Programs and Astracts of the 31st Interscience Conference on Antimicrobial Agents and Chemotherapy. Washington, D.C.: ASM, 1991, Abstract 450.
51. Chaiyakunapruk N, Veenstra DL, Lipsky BA, et al. Chlorhexidine compared with povidone-iodine solution for vascular catheter-site care: a meta-analysis. Ann Intern Med 2002; 136:792.
52. Bozzetti F. Central venous catheter sepsis. Surg Gynecol Obstet 1985; 161:293.
53. Sheth NK, Franson TR, Rose HD. Colonization of bacteria on polyvinyl chloride and teflon intravascular catheters in hospitalized patients. J Clin Microbiol 1983; 18:1061.
54. Sheretz RJ. Pathogenesis of vascular catheter infection. In: Bisno AL, Waldvogel FA, eds. Infections Associated with Indwelling Medical Devices. 3rd ed. Washington, D.C.: ASM Publishers, 2000:111.
55. Everitt NJD, Krupowicz DW, Evans JA, McMahon MJ. Ultrasonographic investigation of the pathogenesis of infusion thrombophlebitis. Br J Surg 1997; 84:642.
56. Maki DG. Nosocomial bacteremia: an epidemiologic overview. Am J Med 1981; 70:719.
57. Maki DJ. Infections caused by intravascular devices used for infusion, pathogenesis, prevention and management. In: Bisno AL, Waldvogel FA, eds. Infections Associated with Indwelling Medical Devices. 2nd ed. Washington, D.C.: ASM Publishers, 1994:155.
58. Bucholz DH, Yound VM, Fredman NR, et al. Bacterial proliferation in platelet products stored at room temperature. Transfusion induced *Enterobacter* sepsis. N Engl J Med 1971; 285:429.
59. Maki DG. Infections due to infusion therapy. In: Bennett JL, Brackman PS, eds. Hospital Infections. Boston: Little Brown, 1992:849.
60. Snydman DR, Reidy MD, Perry LK, Martin WJ. Safety of changing intravenous (IV) administration sets at longer than 48 hour intervals. Infect Control 1987; 8:113.

61. Goldmann D, Martin W, Worthington J. Growth of bacteria and fungi in total parenteral nutrition solutions. Am J Surg 1973; 126:314.
62. Maki DJ. Growth properties of microorganisms in infusion fluid and method of detection. In: Philips I, ed. Microbiologic Hazards of Intravenous Therapy. Lancaster, England: MTP Press, 1973:13.
63. Jarvis W, Highsmith A. Bacterial growth and endotoxin production in lipid emulsions. J Clin Microbiol 1984; 19:17.
64. Dankner W, Spector S, Fierer J. Malassezia fungemia in neonates and adults: complication of hyperalimentation. Rev Infect Dis 1987; 9:743.
65. Raadl I, Bodey GP. Infectious complications of indwelling vascular catheters. Clin Infect Dis 1992; 15:197.
66. Maki DG, Hassemer CH. Endemic rate of fluid contamination related septicemia in arterial pressure monitoring. Am J Med 1981; 70:733.
67. Saint S, Matthay MA. Risk reduction in the intensive care unit. Am J Med 1998; 105:515.
68. Ellis ME, Al-Abdely H, Sandridge A, et al. Fungal endocarditis evidence in world literature, 1965–1995. CID 2001; 32:50–62.
69. Durack DT, reading and Lukes BS, Bright DK. Duke Endocarditis Service. New criteria for diagnosis of the infective endocarditis: utilization of specific echocardiographic findings. Am J Med 1994; 96:200.
70. Collignon PG, Sone NO, Pearson I, et al. Is surface quantitative culture of central venous catheter tips useful in the diagnosis of catheter associated bacteremia? J Clin Microbiol 1986; 24:532.
71. Miller M, Casey J. Infective endocarditis: new diagnostic techniques. Am Heart J 1978; 96:123.
72. Bryant JK, Strand CL. Reliability of blood cultures collected from intravascular catheters versus venipuncture. Am J Clin Pathol 1987; 88:113.
73. O'Grady NP, Alexander M, Dellinger EP, et al. Guidelines for the prevention of intravascular catheter-related infections. Centers for Disease Control and Prevention. MMWR—Morb Mortal Wkly Rep 2002; 51:1.
74. Bates D, Lee TH. Rapid classification of positive blood cultures: prospective validation of a multivariate algorithm. JAMA 1992; 267:1962.
75. Mortara L, Bayer A. *Staphylococcus aureus* bacteremia and endocarditis: new diagnostic and therapeutic concept. Infect Dis Clin NA 1993; 7:53.
76. Shivley BK, Gurule FT, Roldan CA, et al. Diagnostic value of transesophageal compared with transthoracic echocardiography in infective endocarditis. J Am Coll Cardiol 1991; 18:391.
77. Mugge A, Daniel WG, Frank G, et al. Echocardiography in infective endocarditis: reassessment of prognostic implications of vegetation size determined by the transthoracic and transesophageal approach. J Am Coll Cardiol 1989; 14:631.
78. Lowry RW, Zogbhi WA, Baker WB, et al. Clinical impact of transesophageal echocardiography in the diagnosis and management of infective endocarditis. Am J Cardiol 1994; 73:1089.
79. Fowler VG, Li J, Corey GR, et al. Roles of echocardiography in evaluation of patients with *Staphylococcus aureus* bacteremia: experience in 103 patients. J Am Coll Cardiol 1997; 30:1072.
80. Demuth P, Gerding D, Crossley K. *Staphylococcus aureus* bacteria. Arch Intern Med 1979; 139:78.
81. Lee B, Crossley K. The association between *Staphylococcus aureus* bacteremia and bacteriuria. Am J Med 1978; 65:303.
82. Kim AI, Adal KA, Schmitt SK. *Staphylococcus aureus* bacteremia: using echocardiography to guide length of therapy. Cleveland Clin J Med 2003; 20:517.
83. Arnette N, Roberts SI. Valve ring abscesses in active infective endocarditis. Circulation 1976; 54:140.
84. Fowler V, Sanders L, Sexton D, et al. Outcome of *Staphylococcus aureus* bacteremia according to compliance recommendations of infectious diseases specialists: experience with 244 patients. Clin Infect Dis 1998; 27:478.
85. Gristina AG. Biomaterial-sensitive detection: microbial adhesion versus tissue integration. Science 1987; 237:1588.

86. Tompkins DC, Blackwell LJ, Hatcher VB, et al. *Staphylococcus aureus* proteins that bind to human endothelial cells. Infect Immun 1992; 60:965.
87. Lundbery J, Nettleman M, Costigan M, et al. *Staphylococcus aureus* bacteremia: the cost-effectiveness of long-term therapy associated with infectious diseases consultation. Clin Perform Qual Health Care 1988; 6:9.
88. Fowler VG, Sanders LL, Li Kuo Kong R, et al. Infective endocarditis due to *Staphylococcus aureus*: 59 prospectively identified cases with follow-up. CID 1999; 28:106.
89. Dudale DC, Ramsey PG. *Staphylococcus aureus* bacteremia in patients with Hickman catheters. Am J Med 1990; 89:137.
90. Press OW, Ramsey PG, Larson EB, et al. Hickman catheter infections in patients with malignancies. Medicine 1984; 63:189.
91. Ascher DP, Shoupe BA, Maybee D, et al. Persistent catheter-related bacteremia: clearance with antibiotics and urokinase. J Pediatr Surg 1993; 28:628.
92. Small P, Chambers HF. Vancomycin for *Staphylococcus aureus* endocarditis in intravenous drug abusers. Antimicrob Agent Chemother 1990; 34:1227.
93. Levine DP, Fromm BS, Reddy BR. Slow response to vancomycin or vancomycin plus rifampin in methicillin-resistant *Staphylococcus aureus* endocarditis. Ann Intern Med 1991; 115:674.
94. Norrby R. Linezolid—a review of the first oxazolidinone. Expert Opin Pharmacother 2001; 2:293.
95. Korzeniowski O, Sande MA. Combination antimicrobial therapy for *Staphylococcus aureus* endocarditis in patients addicted to parenteral drugs and nonaddicts. Ann Intern Med 1982; 97:496.
96. Guze L, Pearce M. Hospital-acquired bacterial endocarditis. Archiv Intern Med 1963; 112:56.
97. Benn M, Hagelskjaer LH, Tvede M. Infective endocarditis, 1984 through 1993: a clinical and microbiology survey. J Intern Med 1997; 242:15.
98. Berenholtz SM, Pronovost PJ, Lipsett PA, et al. Eliminating catheter-related bloodstream infections in the intensive unit. Crit Care Med 2004; 32:2014.
99. Cepkova M, Matthay MA. Reducing risk in the ICU: vascular catheter-related infections. Infect Med 2006; 23:141.
100. Centers for Disease Control and Prevention. Guidelines for the prevention of intravascular catheter-related infections. MMWR—Morbid Mortal Wkly Rep 2002; 51 (RR-10):1.
101. Merrer J, DeJonghe B, Golliot F, et al. Complications of femoral and subclavian venous catheterization in critically ill patients: a randomized controlled trial. JAMA 2001; 286:700.
102. Eyer S, Brummitt C, Crossley K, et al. Catheter-related sepsis: prospective, randomized study of three methods of long-term catheter maintenance. Crit Care Med 1990; 18:1073.
103. Raad II, Hohn DC, Gilbreath BJ, et al. Prevention of central venous catheter-related infections by using maximal sterile area of cautions during insertion. Infect Control Hosp Epidemiol 1994; 15:231.
104. Cobett S, LeBlanc A. IV site infection: a prospective, randomized clinical trial comparing the efficacy of three methods of skin antisepsis. CINA: Official J Can Intraven Nurses Assoc 1999; 15:48.
105. Randolph AG, Cook DJ, Gonzalez CA, et al. Benefit of heparin in central venous and pulmonary artery catheters: a meta-analysis of randomized controlled trials. Chest 1998; 113:165.
106. Darouchie RO, Berger DH, Khadori N, et al. Comparison of antimicrobial impregnation with tunneling of long-term central venous catheters: a randomized controlled trial. Ann Surg 2005; 242:193.
107. Hanna HA, Raad II, Hackett B, et al. Clinical investigations in critical care. Antibiotic-impregnated catheters associated with significant decrease in nosocomial and multidrug-resistant bacteremias in critically ill patients. Chest 2003; 124:1.
108. Yeung C, May J, Hughes R. Infection rate for single lumen versus triple lumen subclavian catheters. Infect Control Hosp Epidemiol 1988; 9:154.
109. Hoffmann KK, Weber DJ, Samsa GP, et al. Transparent polyurethane film as an intravenous catheter dressing. A meta-analysis of the infection risks. JAMA 1992; 267:2072.
110. Meduri GU, Maudlin GL, Wunderink RG, et al. Causes of fever and pulmonary densities with clinical manifestations of ventilator associated pneumonia. Chest 1994; 106:221.

11 Infective Endocarditis of Immunocompromised Patients

John L. Brusch
Harvard Medical School and Department of Medicine and Infectious Disease Service, Cambridge Health Alliance, Cambridge, Massachusetts, U.S.A.

GENERAL PRINCIPLES

The numbers of immunosuppressed individuals have risen markedly over the last 25 years. These patients belong to several varied categories of immunosuppression including those with AIDS, organ transplant recipients, and increasingly aggressive therapy for hematologic and solid malignancies. In addition, there are those patients with less dramatic degrees of immunosuppression who are also at increased risk of developing infective endocarditis (IE). Among these are the elderly, patients with chronic liver disease, those with chronic renal failure, and alcoholics (1). Overall, the most common categories of patients with immunosuppressive IE (ISIE) are intravenous drug abusers (IVDA) with AIDS and those with healthcare-associated IE (HCIE) and nosocomial IE (NIE). Both of these categories are closely associated with catheter-related bloodstream infections (CR-BSI) (Chapter 10) (2). The author has placed both of these in the category of iatrogenic IE (IIE). A less frequent factor leading to ISIE is the infection of an underlying, sterile valvular thrombus, such as that seen in marantic endocarditis or the sterile platelet/fibrin thrombus of systemic lupus erythematosus (Libman–Sachs endocarditis). Many of the clinical manifestations of these sterile vegetations resembled by closely those of IE, especially fever-elevated sedimentation rate and signs and symptoms of meningoencephalitis. Approximately, 4% of these vegetations become infected (3,4). When secondarily infected, these behave as any other infected vegetation. Renal failure [Blood Urea Nitrogen (BUN) >60 mg/100m mL], prednisone doses of >20 mg/day, and treatment with cyclophosphamide increase the risk of infection in both diseases (Chapter 12) (5).

Infection of any type occurs when the pathogen is able to overwhelm the host's defenses. Immunosuppression facilitates development of infection. The concept of net immunosuppression (NIS) semiquantitatively estimates both the risk of developing and type of infection in the immunocompromised (6). The NIS has several components: (*i*) dose, duration, and sequence of immunosuppressive agents; (*ii*) damage to the mucosal and dermal barriers; (*iii*) neutropenia; (*iv*) metabolic abnormalities (diabetes, renal failure, and malnutrition) and presence of immunomodulating viruses (cytomegalovirus, Epstein-Barr virus, hepatitis B virus, and HIV).

The aspects of NIS most pertinent to the development of IE are the breakdown of the mucosal barriers, neutropenia, and the presence of the immunomodulating viruses. All of these promote the development of BSI that is necessary for the development of IE. The most important of these is damage to the mucosa of the gastrointestinal tract, including the oropharynx, and to the skin. Bloodstream infections arise when there are breaks in the integrity of the skin and mucus membranes that are is combined with a decrease in local immunity usually because of neutropenia. Disturbances in the normal flora of the intestinal tract or skin can lead to overgrowth of both gram-positive and gram-negative organisms (7). The normal skin flora may be altered by several factors including antibiotics (ciprofloxacin) that are actively secreted by the sweat glands (8). Radiation may cause necrosis of the hair follicles that may become a permanent focus of infection. Inserting an intravascular catheter percutaneously induces the secretion of fibronectin that facilitates the adherence of *Staphylococcus aureus* to the device.

Equally important in the development of ISIE is injury to the gastrointestinal mucosa produced by both chemotherapy and radiation. Transmigration of the bowel flora is markedly increased and results in BSI capable of infecting native valves, prosthetic valve, or one of several intracardiac devices. Absorption of nutrients and medications, including the quinolones, are significantly decreased by these therapeutic modalities (9). The availability of hemopoietic and granulocyte colony-stimulating factors allows the use of high doses of radiation and chemotherapy with resultant more pronounced cytotoxic effects. Disturbances in intestinal motility lead to overgrowth of *Candida* spp., *Streptococcus viridans*, and various types of gram-negatives, which in turn promote entry of these microorganisms into the blood (10). Various types of antibiotics lead to the mucosal damage by promoting the overgrowth of *Pseudomonas aeruginosa*, *Stenotrophomonas mucilginosus*, and *Capnocytophaga* spp. (11,12). The penicillins, cephalosporins, rifampin, and clindamycin demonstrate the greatest effect on the normal bowel flora. The quinolones and trimethoprim sulfamethoxazole exhibit the least. Fungemia, especially Candidemis may also be the result of disruption of the normal bowel flora with concurrent mucosal damage. Other contributors to candidemia/candidal IE are: (*i*) prolonged use of antibiotics and corticosteroids, which can lead to primary fungal valvular involvement or superinfection of bacterial IE; (*ii*) gynecological/genitourinary procedures; (*iii*) extensive burns and oral surgery (1,13). The true frequency of *Candida* valvular infection is difficult to establish as candidal involvement of other organ systems may obscure the valvular infection (14).

Aspergillus spp. are the second most common cause of fungal ISIE. The most common examples are *A. fumigatus* and *A. flavus*. The rate of *Aspergillus* infections in the immunosuppressed is rapidly rising. This may be because of the success of *Candida* prophylaxis by fluconazole (1,15). Neutropenia is a major risk factor for acquiring deep-seated *Aspergillus* infection. Whether this holds true for valvular IE has not been determined.

One of the most intensively studied areas of ISIE has been the effects of the AIDS virus on the clinical course of IE. The association between HIV infection and IVDA IE has already been discussed in Chapter 8. There is a very high prevalence of concurrent HIV infection and IVDA IE (40–90%) (16,17). However, the rate of endocarditis among non-IVDA HIV-positive patients is very low at 0.3% (18). This figure represents 2% of all cases of non-IVDA IE. In one series (19), most patients were men (95%) due to the high rate of homosexuality (45%) and hemophilia (14%). The median range of CD4 cell counts was 31.9% of cases, which involved prosthetic valves. Forty-one percent of cases were acquired in healthcare institutions. Most cases were left-sided. What is quite distinctive for this group of patients is the profile of the infecting organisms (Table 1). Although the number in this series is small (22 cases), it is the largest series of non-IVDA HIV-associated IE. The distribution of pathogens seems quite valid. It represents a combination of organisms that are associated with HIV immunodeficiency (*Salmonella* spp. and *Streptococcus pneumoniae*) to those that are typically associated with IE (viridans streptococci) and those

TABLE 1 Organisms that Have Been Involved in Nonintravenous Drug Abuser HIV-Associated Infective Endocarditis

Organism	Percentage of cases
Salmonella spp.	23
Enterococcus faecalis	18
Other organisms (*Listeria, Bartonella quintana,* *Coxiella burnetii*)	14
Viridans streptococci	9
Streptococcus pneumoniae	9
Candida spp.	9
Other fungi	9

that are caused by catheter-related BSI (CR-BSI) (*S. aureus*). There was no evidence that clinical presentation was different from that of patients who were HIV-negative; 18% of patients eventually required cardiac surgery. This is a lower rate than that observed for the non-HIV-associated IE (16). Interestingly, cardiac surgery and extracorporeal circulation did not impact on the immune status of the patient. Eighteen percent of patients died during hospitalization, which is comparable with that of the general population with IE. On the basis of this limited data, it appears that infection with HIV by itself does not increase the risk of developing IE or the overall prognosis of valvular infection. Abraham et al. (20) provided another type of data to support this conclusion. This group compared the frequency of IE, diagnosed by echocardiographic criteria, in bacteremic patients with or without HIV infection. Fourteen percent of HIV-positive patients were IVDA; 15% of HIV-negative individuals were IVDA. Almost half of each group had *S. aureus* BSI. BSI, with any organism, resulted in IE in 12% of the HIV-positive patients and 42% in HIV-negative patients. This held true for the group with *S. aureus* BSI as well. In summary, severe immunosuppression (CD4 count <200) markedly worsens prognosis of HIV-positive, IVDA IE (21), but probably has little effect on the outcome of non-IVDA HIV IE.

INFECTIVE ENDOCARDITIS IN THE ELDERLY

As presented in Chapter 1, IE has become a disease of the elderly. Overall, more than 50% of the patients are older than 60 years. Much of this is because of the fact that the underlying valvular abnormalities are primarily "wear and tear" degeneration as well as the proliferation of intravascular devices. However, the effects of aging on the immune system may play a role in this "graying" of IE. It appears that as one gets older, there is "a state of immune dysregulation and not of immune deficiency" (22). There is decreased ability to generate naive lymphocytes as one gets older. There is no effect on the production of monocytes and neutrophils nor is their functioning impaired. It has long been realized that there is a decrease in antibody responsiveness to antigenic stimuli. Total antibody production is not affected because of the rise in autoantibodies. In summary, there is little evidence that, by itself, aging significantly affects the immune system. More important are the mucosal and skin changes that occur as one grows older. There is a significant rise in streptococcal BSI, which originates from the mouth, as people keep their teeth longer with the inevitable attendant gingivitis (23).

The frequency and mortality of BSI is increased in the geriatric population. There is less of a systemic response of the aged host. Many patients never mount a significant fever or white count. The symptoms may be quite nonspecific such as fatigue, disordered thinking, or musculoskeletal complaints mimicking polymyalgia rheumatica (24–27). On physical examination, there is a decrease in the incidence of splenomegaly and the integumentary signs of IE. The febrile response is muted. The murmurs that are heard are misleading in that they have been noted to be present and unchanged for long periods of time and are not hemodynamically significant. This is the classic presentation of calcific degenerative valvular disease. Appreciable numbers of cases are misdiagnosed at their presentation (67%) (28).

Among the elderly, it appears that there is a disproportionately increased number of *Enterococcus faecalis* and *Streptococcus bovis*. The former source is chronic prostatitis; the latter arises from colonic abnormalities such as neoplasms and polyps (29). Otherwise, the spectrum of pathogens is similar to that of younger patients.

Because of other cardiac problems such as coronary artery disease, surgery should probably be considered earlier in the course of congestive heart failure that is a consequence of significant aortic regurgitation. In many patients, the risk of inadequately treated heart failure significantly outweighs the morbidity and mortality of the operation (30).

Many elderly "fall through the cracks" of the official recommendations for prophylaxis. Even though most cases of IE in this group are due to calcific valvular disease, such lesions are put in a lower risk category (31). Aging as well as placement of dentures or implantations or antibiotic use may alter the oral flora to one of *S. aureus*, lactobacilli, yeasts, or other organisms (32). The most effective prophylaxis against IE is to establish good oral hygiene (33). These principles will be discussed in more detail in Chapter 16.

INFECTIVE ENDOCARDITIS IN END-STAGE RENAL DISEASE AND DIALYSIS

Infections of various types are second only to current artery disease as the most common cause of death in patients on dialysis (34). Uremia has a significant effect on the host's defense systems (35). Table 2 lists the most significant deficiencies. In addition, dialysis is a "double-edged sword" as regards the immune system of the patient with chronic renal failure. The implantation of various types of intravascular catheters, both temporary and permanent, provides a significant risk factor for BSI. The dialyzer membrane itself may produce a significant leukopenia owing to its ability to activate complement (36). Diagnosis of infection is made more difficult in uremic/dialyzed individuals because of the blunting of the febrile response to the decreased production of endogenous pyrogen and decreased skin-test

TABLE 2   Immune Deficiencies that Contribute to Infection in Uremia

Abnormal white cell function
Impaired phagocytosis
Circulating inhibitors of chemotaxis
Increased intracellular calcium
Leukopenia caused by complement activation
Decreased B- and T-cell functions
Decreased natural killer cell function
Decreased endogenous pyrogen

Source: From Ref. 34.

TABLE 3 Contributing Factors to Infection in Uremia

Factor	Comments
Low albumin	—
Excess iron stores	Stimulates bacterial growth
Metabolic acidosis	Decreases neutrophil function
Intravascular catheter placement	Most important source of bloodstream infections

Source: From Refs. 3, 4.

reactivity to various antigens (37). Table 3 presents factors that contribute to the development of infection, including IE, in uremic/dialyzed patients.

These factors are present no matter what the cause of renal failure in a given patient. Diabetes mellitus currently is the most common cause of renal failure in the United States. Diabetes does not directly affect the immune system, but does indirectly by producing renal failure, which in turn leads to deficiencies noted in Table 2. Diabetes does increase the morbidity and mortality of IE (31% vs. 15%). Diabetic patients exhibit heart failure more frequently than nondiabetic ones [69% vs. 38% (38,39)]. Diabetic patients with IE were older than nondiabetics with valvular infections.

Another factor predisposing to IE in renal failure patients is an anatomical one. Patients with renal failure have greater rates of mitral annular calcification and aortic valve calcification. These also occur at a younger age in these patients as compared with individuals with normal renal function. Aortic valve calcification more frequently evolves into aortic stenosis than does aortic calcifications of patients without renal failure. Both aortic and mitral valvular calcifications and aortic stenosis serve as prime predisposing factors for the development of IE (40). These ectopic deposits are the results of the typical alterations in calcium and phosphate levels in renal failure. They usually develop after five years of hemodialysis.

Intravascular catheters are the major cause of BSI in patients with renal failure (41). The rate of BSI has been determined to be 1.6–7.7 BSI/1000 catheter days with temporary and noncuffed dialysis catheters and 0.2–0.5 BSI/1000 catheter days with tunneled and cuffed catheters (34). Synthetic vascular grafts have much higher rates of BSI than do arteriovenous fistulas (42). It has been held that the rate of BSI was significantly lower with tunneled and cuffed catheters (0.2–0.5 BSI/1000 catheter days). Follow-up studies did not support this concept and documented the BSI rate of 3.9/1000 catheter days with these types of devices. This difference in results may be due to the fact that the subjects of the later studies did not receive any special type of catheter care and presumably have a higher rate of luminal infection than those receiving special care (43). Risk factors for CR-BSI include: increased length of use, diabetes mellitus, iron overload, and previous CR-BSI (44). Access-associated infections spread to many areas of the body, including the heart in at least 25% of the cases (range of 3–50%) (41,45). This rate has been on the rise, in part due to the increased placement of cuffed catheters (46).

Staphylococcus aureus causes over 50% of vascular access infections. Only about 10% of these isolates are methicillin-resistant, but their involvement should be expected to grow considerably. The remainder is produced chiefly by *Enterococci* spp. and gram-negative bacilli (47). Because of the increased use of vancomycin in these patients, the isolation of vancomycin-resistant enterococci (VRE) is on the increase (48).

Both prevention and treatment of infection of these access catheters is quite similar to other intravascular catheters. Antibiotic-coated hemodialysis catheters appear to prevent access-related infections. In one study, catheters impregnated with minocycline and rifampin were inserted in the femoral veins (49). Both the treated devices and control devices were in place for a mean of eight days. Eleven percent of the untreated catheters became infected, none of the treated ones. This is especially impressive in light of the fact that they were inserted in the groin. Minocycline and rifampin-US with treated catheters were quite effective against enterococcus and methicillin-resistant *S. aureus* (MRSA). Patients who undergo hemodialysis have increased rates of long-term nasopharyngeal carriage of *S. aureus* (50), which acts as the source for staphylococcal intravascular catheter infection. Elimination of carriage of this organism lessens the risk of dialysis-associated infections. Administration of this ointment to the nasal mucosa twice daily for five days lowers access infections without inducing resistance of *S. aureus* to this compound (51). For a more thorough discussion of intravascular access, see Chapter 10.

The results of a large retrospective review from 1991 to 1999 indicates that the rate of *S. aureus* BSI in end-stage renal disease ranges from 5.7% to 27.4% per year (50). Two to five percent of patients receiving chronic dialysis develop IE (52,53). Mean length of hospitalization for each case was 22.9 ± 19.3 days with mean Medicare paid costs of $\$29,306 \pm 28,276$. In the recent series of hemodialysis-associated IE, the mean age of the patients was approximately 54 years (54–57). The causative bacteremia is overwhelmingly associated with hemodialysis access devices (approximately 65% of the cases). The most common types are the dual lumen-tunneled catheter and the synthetic arteriovenous grafts. However, arteriovenous fistulas have a high rate of involvement (approximately 35% of cases). Most cases of hemodialysis-associated IE occur between one and five years of initiating dialysis. This may be related to the time required for calcification of the valves to develop. Aortic and mitral valves are most commonly infected. Subclavian catheters more often produce right-sided disease.

Minnaganti and Cunha (34) emphasize the need to a have a high degree of awareness about the possibility of hemodialysis-associated IE. Often, common clues to the presence of infection, such as an elevated white count of fever, are suppressed in renal failure. Conversely, various forms of renal disease can produce many of the features of valvular infections. These include hematuria, anemia, pericarditis, and leukocytosis. As is true for all types of IE, blood cultures remain the mainstay of diagnosis. They are positive in 90% to 94% of the cases. Echocardiography is sometimes required in those with culture negative disease that is primarily because of the administration of antibiotics prior to the drawing of the blood cultures.

Successful treatment depends mainly on the timely administration of appropriate antibiotics. Unless it responds to infused antimicrobial agents, the infected access site must be removed (Chapter 10). On establishing the diagnosis of access-associated IE, serious consideration must be given to switching the patient to peritoneal dialysis until the valvular infection is cleared. A small series that employed this approach in the treatment of *S. aureus* IE demonstrated that the in-hospital mortality was 8.3% in those switched to peritoneal dialysis and 55.5% in those who continued to receive hemodialysis (58).

In 1977–1991, long-term survival rates of dialysis patients who were hospitalized for IE at one, two, and five years were 45.9%, 33.3%, 24.3%, and 14.7%, respectively. In 1992–1996, the long-term survival rates at one, two, and three years were 38.4%, 25.3%, and 18.3%, respectively. The most important independent predictors of survival from IE are, age, end-stage renal disease due to diabetes, and cerebrovascular disease (59). The one- and two-year survival of these patients is essentially the same as that of dialysis patients who have suffered an acute myocardial infarction (60). Nonrenal failure/hemodialysis patients with IE overall survival rates of 71% and 60% for *S. aureus* have been reported for the period of 1984–1993 (61,62). The cause or causes of this increased mortality have not been well-defined.

Infective endocarditis is quite unusual in renal transplant patients (63). The interval between the transplant of the kidney and the onset of valvular infection is 3.5 years. *Staphylococcus aureus* and fungi were the most common organisms isolated, 22% of cases apiece. Other organisms included *S. viridans, Corynebacteria, Nocardia,* and *Erysipelothrix.* Dermal manifestations were not present. Overall mortality was 50%.

INFECTIVE ENDOCARDITIS IN CIRRHOSIS

Infective endocarditis is an unusual complication of cirrhosis (64). There are numerous immunological abnormalities in these patients. These include impaired defects in complement and immunoglobulins and dysfunction of macrophages in neutrophils as well as the reticuloendothelial system. The significance of these defects in the pathogenesis of cirrhotic-associated IE is not clear. Most likely, they all contribute to prolonged BSI, which allows a greater opportunity for valvular infection. In alcoholic cirrhotics, *S. pneumoniae* and *Escherichia coli* are the most common pathogens (65). In the Far East, where the etiology of liver disease may well be different, the most common organisms found were *S. aureus, S. viridans, Streptococcus sanguis, Pseudomonas* spp., and *Enterococcus faecalis* (66). The many of the staphylococci were MRSA. The mortality rate was high due to the complications of septic emboli and mycotic aneurysms.

INFECTIVE ENDOCARDITIS IN CANCER

Infective endocarditis is quite uncommon in patients suffering from all types of cancer. A major diagnostic and therapeutic challenge is distinguishing culture-negative IE from truly sterile platelet fibrin thrombi (nonbacterial thrombotic endocarditis, marantic endocarditis). This topic recently has been thoroughly reviewed (67). Fifty-eight percent had positive blood cultures 69% of patients with positive blood cultures had a central venous catheter in place: whereas only 26% of culture-negative endocarditis had these lines in place. *Staphylococcus aureus* and coagulase-negative staphylococci were the most common pathogens. Clearly, culture-positive IE in cancer patients frequently represents IIE. In those with negative blood cultures, emboli to the central nervous system and coronary arteries occurred much more frequently than in those with positive blood cultures (37% vs. 12% and 21% vs. 0%). Because both these types of embolic events are seen in nonbacterial thrombotic endocarditis (NBTE), one has to question whether many of these cases represent paraneoplastic sterile fibrin/platelet thrombi and not infected vegetations. Without pathologic examination of the thrombus, one cannot really distinguish between the two (68). Table 4 presents the possible causes of sterile blood cultures in cancer patients.

TABLE 4   Causes of Negative Blood Cultures in Patients with Cancer

Increased use of antibiotics in cancer patients for prophylaxis and empirical treatment
Increased susceptibility of an immunosuppressed host to small infecting inoculum
Infections as a result of fastidious organisms which are difficult to culture

Case Study ■ A 73-year-old woman was admitted to the hospital for evaluation and treatment of the sudden onset of right hemiparesis. A computed tomography (CT) scan revealed a cerebral infarct in the distribution of the left middle cerebral artery. An MRA confirmed the finding of a large thrombus in this vessel. Because there was no abnormality of the carotid arteries on MRA, a transthoracic echocardiogram (TTE) was performed. The study showed a large thrombus on a leaflet of the aortic valve. The woman had been in good health until two months prior to her admission. At that time, she developed symptoms of mild depression that were associated with an 8-lb weight loss. Two days before her admission, she was started on levaquin 500 mg daily for treatment of a urinary tract infection that was characterized by urgency and a temperature of 100.4°F. Blood cultures were withdrawn, but all remained sterile. Her low-grade fever persisted. Because of the findings of the echocardiogram and the persistence of fever, the patient was started on ampicillin and gentamicin for treatment of culture-negative IE. The levaquin was discontinued. Her fever failed to resolve. On the seventh day, the patient suffered a massive as a right-sided stroke. A repeat echocardiogram demonstrated an enlarging vegetation. At this point, it was felt that the valvular finding was more consistent with marantic endocarditis. In an effort to locate the primary neoplasm, a CT scan of the abdomen was performed. This study demonstrated a large cancer in the pancreas. In compliance with the family's wishes, all medical care was withdrawn. She died three days later.

Comments ■ This case demonstrates the difficulty in distinguishing NBTE from an infected vegetation. In an older individual who develops involuntary weight loss and depression, the possibility of an underlying neoplasm, especially pancreatic, must be considered. The development of a neoplastic-associated embolic stroke is a very bad prognostic feature. At times, this situation may be controlled with heparin.

REFERENCES

1. Brusch JL. Cardiac infections in the immunosuppressed patients. Infect Dis Clin NA 2001; 15:613.
2. Brusch JL. Infective endocarditis in critical care. In: Cunha B, ed. Infectious Diseases in Critical Care Medicine. 1st ed. New York: Marcel Decker, 1998:387.
3. Harris ED Jr. Rheumatoid arthritis: the clinical spectrum. In: Kelly WN, Harris ED, Ruddy S, et al., eds. Textbook of Rheumatology. Philadelphia: WB Saunders, 1985:915.
4. Rothfield N. Clinical features of systemic lupus erythematosus. In: Kelly WN, Harris ED, Ruddy S, et al., eds. Textbook of Rheumatology. Philadelphia: WB Saunders, 1985:1870.
5. Payan D. Evaluation and management of patients with collagen vascular disease. In: Rubin RH, Young LS, eds. Clinical Approach to Infection in the Compromised Host. 3rd ed. New York and London: Plenum Medical Book Company, 1994:581.
6. Rubin RH. Infection in the organ transplant recipient. In: Rubin RH, Young LS, eds. Clinical Approach to Infection in the Compromised Host. 3rd ed. New York and London: Plenum Medical Book Company, 1994:629.
7. Donnelly JP, DePauw BE. Infections in the immunocompromised host: general principles. In: Mandell GL, Bennett JE, Dolin R, eds. Principles and Practice of Infectious Diseases. 6th ed. New York: Elseiver, Churchill Livingstone, 2005:3421.
8. Holby N, Johansen HK. Ciprofloxacin in sweat and antibiotic resistance. The Copenhagen Study Group on antibiotics in sweat (letter). Lancet 1997; 346:1235.
9. Fischer. Severe combined immunodeficiencies. Immunodef Rev 1992; 3:83.
10. Bachud PY, Calandra T, Francioli P. Bacteremia due to viridans streptococci in neutropenic patients: a review. Am J Med 1994; 97:256.
11. Bow EJ, Loewen R, Chiang MS, et al. Invasive fungal disease in adults undergoing remission-induction therapy for acute myeloid leukemia: the pathogenic role of the antileukemic regimen. Clin Infect Dis 1995; 21:361.

12. Donnelly JP, Maschmeyer G, Daenen S. Selective oral antimicrobial prophylaxis for the prevention of infection in acute leukemia-ciprofloxacin versus co-trimoxazole plus colistin. The EORTC-Gnotobiotic Project Group. Eur J Cancer 1992; 28 A:873.
13. Ellis ME, Al-Abdely H, Sandridge A, et al. Fungal endocarditis: evidence in the world literature, 1965–1995. Clin Infect Dis 2001; 32:50.
14. Canver CC, Patel AK, Kosalcharoen P, et al. Fungal purulent constrictive pericarditis in a heart transplant patient. Ann Thorac Surg 1998; 65:1792.
15. Pierrotti LC, Baddour LM. Fungal and vaginitis, 1995–2000. Chest 2002; 122:302.
16. Miro JM, Engemann JJ, Cabell CH, et al. Intravenous drug use and infective endocarditis: report from the ICE investigators. Sixth National Symposium on Modern Concept in Endocarditis and Cardiovascular Infections. Sitges (Barcelona), Spain, June 2001.
17. Miro JM, del Rio A, Mestres CA. Infective endocarditis intravenous drug abusers and HIV-1 infected patients. Infect Dis Clin NA 2002; 16:273.
18. Losa JE, Miro JM, del Rio A, et al. Infective endocarditis not related to intravenous drug abuse in HIV-1 infected patients: report of eight cases and review of the literature. Clin Microbiol Infect 2003; 9:45.
19. Miro JM, del Rio A, Mestres CA. Infective endocarditis and cardiac surgery and intravenous drug abusers in HIV-1 infected patients. Cardiol Clin 2003; 21:1.
20. Abraham J, Veledar E, Lerakis S. Comparison of frequency of active infective endocarditis by echocardiography in patients with bacteremia with and without human immunodeficiency virus. Am J Cardiol 2003; 91:1.
21. Cicalini S, Forcina G, DeRosa FG. Infective endocarditis in patients with human immunodeficiency virus infection. J Infect 2001; 42:267.
22. Weksler ME. Aging and the immune system. Infect Dis Clin Pract 1995; 3:464.
23. Terpenning MS, Dominguez BL. Endocarditis of oral origin (abstr). In: Proceedings of the International Association for Dental Research 1994 March 9–13. Seattle, Washington.
24. Crossley KB, Peterson PK. Infections in the elderly. Clin Infect Dis 1996; 22:209.
25. Terpenning MS. Infective endocarditis. In: Yoshikawa TT, Norman DC, eds. Infectious Disease in the Aging. Chap. 8. Totowa, New Jersey: Humana Press, 2001:79.
26. Meyers BR, Sherman E, Mendelson MH, et al. Bloodstream infections in the elderly. Am J Med 1989; 86:379.
27. Chassagne P, Perol M-B, Doucette J, et al. Is presentation of bacteremia in the elderly same as in younger patients? Am J Med 1996; 100:65.
28. Terpenning MS, Buggy BP, Kaufmann CA. Infective endocarditis: clinical features in young and elderly patients. Am J Med 1987; 83:626.
29. Selton-Suty C, Hoen B, Gretzinger A, et al. Clinical and bacteriological characteristics of infective endocarditis in the elderly. Heart 1997; 77:260.
30. Gregaratos G. Infective endocarditis in the elderly: diagnosis and management. Am J Geriatr Cardiol 2003; 12:183.
31. Dajani AS, Taubert KA, Wilson W, et al. Prevention of bacterial endocarditis, recommendations by the American Heaart Association. JAMA 1997; 277:1794.
32. Loesche WJ, Schork A, Terpenning MS, et al. Factors which influence levels of selected organisms in saliva of older individuals. J Clin Microbiol 1995; 33:2550.
33. Hockett RN, Loesche WJ, Sodeman TM. Bacteremia in asymptomatic human subjects. Arch Oral Biol 1977; 22:1.
34. Minaganti VR, Cunha BA. Infections associated with uremia and dialysis. Infect Dis Clin NA 2001; 15:385.
35. Descamps-Latscha B, Heberlein A, Nyugen AT, et al. The immune system in end-stage renal disease. Semin Nephrol 1994; 14:253.
36. Lewis SL, Van Epps DE. Neutrophil and monocyte alterations in chronic dialysis patients. Am J Kidney Dis 1987; 9:381.
37. Lewis SL. Fever: thermoregulation and alterations in end-stage renal disease patients. ANNA J 1992; 19:13.
38. Bishara J, Peled N, Samara Z, et al. Infective endocarditis in diabetic and non-diabetic patients. Scand J Infect Dis 2004; 36:795.
39. Moreno R, Zmorano J, Almeira C, et al. Influence of diabetes mellitus and short-and long-term outcome in patients with active infective endocarditis. J Heart Valve Dis 2002; 5:651.

40. Umana E, Ahmed W, Alpert MA. Valvular and perivalvular abnormalities in end-stage renal disease. Am J Med Sci 2003; 325:237.
41. Kessler M, Hoen B, Mayeux D, et al. Bacteremia on patients on chronic hemodialysis. Nephron 1993; 64:95.
42. Bonomo RA, Rice D, Whalen C. Risk factors associated with permanent access-site infections in chronic hemodialysis patients. Infect Control Hosp Epidemiol 1997; 18:757.
43. Beathard GA. Management of bacteremia associated with tunneled-cuffed hemodialysis catheters. 1999; 10:1045.
44. Allon M. Dialysis catheter-related bacteremia: treatment and prophylaxis. Am J of Kidney Dis 2004; 19:1237.
45. Marr KA, Sexton DJ, Conlon PJ, et al. Catheter-related bacteremia and outcome of attempted salvage in patients undergoing hemodialysis. Ann Intern Med 1997; 27:275.
46. Kovalik E, Raymond J, Albers F, et al. The clustering of epidural apices and chronic hemodialysis patients: risks of salvaging access catheters in cases of infection. J Am Soc Nephrol 1996; 7:2264.
47. Kaslow RA, Zellner SR. Infections in patients on maintenance hemodialysis. Lancet 1972; 2:117.
48. Fishbane S, Cunha BA, Shea KW, et al. Vancomycin resistance enterococci in hemodialysis patients. Am J Infect Control 1999; 20:461.
49. Chatzinikolaou I, Finkel K, Hanna H, et al. Antibiotic-coated hemodialysis catheters for the prevention of vascular catheter-related infections: a prospective, randomized study. Am J Med 2003; 115:352.
50. Chow JW, Yu VL. *Staphylococcus aureus* nasal carriage in hemodialysis patients: its role in infections and approaches to prophylaxis. Arch Intern Med 1989; 149:1258.
51. Klutymans J, vanBelkum A, Verbrugh H. Nasal carriage of *Staphylococcus aureus*: epidemiology, underlying mechanisms and associated risks. Clin Microbiol Rev 1997; 10:505.
52. Nissenson AR, Dylan ML, Griffiths RI, et al. Clinical and economic outcome to *Staphylococcus aureus* septicemia in ESRD patients receiving hemodialysis. Am J Kidney Dis 2005; 46:1
53. Cross AS, Steigbigel RT. Infective endocarditis and access site infections in patients on hemodialysis. Medicine 1976; 55:453.
54. Maraj S, Jacobs LE, Kung SC, et al. Epidemiology and outcome of infective endocarditis in hemodialysis patients. Am J Med Sci 2002; 324:254.
55. Doulton T, Sabharwal N, Cairns HS, et al. Infective endocarditis in dialysis patients: new challenges and old. Kidney Int 2003; 64:720.
56. McCarthy JT, Steckleberg JM. Infective endocarditis in patients receiving long-term hemodialysis. Mayo Clin Proc 2000; 10:1008.
57. Leonard A, Raij L, Shapiro FL. Bacterial endocarditis in regularly dialyzed patients. Kidney Int 1973; 4:407.
58. Fernandez-Cean J, Alvarez A, Burguez S, et al. Infective endocarditis in chronic hemodialysis: two treatment strategies. Nephrol Dial Transplant 2002; 17:2226.
59. Shroff GR, Herzog CA, Ma JZ, Collins AJ. Long-term survival of dialysis patients with bacterial endocarditis in the United States. Am J Kidney Dis 2004; 24:1077.
60. Herzog CA, Ma JZ, Collins AJ. Poor long-term survival after acute myocardial infarction among patients on long-term dialysis. N Engl J Med 1998; 339:799.
61. Sandre RM, Shafran SD. Infective endocarditis: review of 135 cases over 9 years. Clin Infect Dis 1996; 22:276.
62. Watanakunakorn C, Tan J, Phair J. Some salients featuring *Staphylococcus aureus* endocarditis. Am J Med 1973; 54:473.
63. Bishara J, Robenshtok E, Weinberger M, et al. Infective endocarditis in renal transplant patients. Transplant Infect Dis 1999; 2:138.
64. Johnson DH, Cunha BA. Infections in cirrhosis. Infect Dis Clin NA 2001; 15:363.
65. Buchbinder NA, Roberts WC. Alcoholism: an important but unemphasized factor predisposing to infective endocarditis. Arch Intern Med 1973; 132:689.
66. Hsu RB, Chen RJ, Chu SH. Infective endocarditis in patients with liver cirrhosis. J Formos Med Assoc 2004; 103:355.
67. Yusuf SW, Syed AS, Swafford J, et al. Culture-positive and culture-negative endocarditis in patients with cancer: a retrospective observational study, 1994–2004. Medicine 2006; 85:86.
68. Edoute Y, Haim N, Rinkevich D, et al. Cardiac valvular vegetations in cancer patients: a prospective echocardiographic study of 200 patients. Am J Med 1997; 102:252.

12 Diagnosis of Infective Endocarditis I

John L. Brusch
Harvard Medical School and Department of Medicine and Infectious Disease Service, Cambridge Health Alliance, Cambridge, Massachusetts, U.S.A.

INTRODUCTION

This chapter reviews the many modalities that are available to diagnose infective endocarditis (IE) with the notable exception of echocardiography. The role of echocardiography will be thoroughly presented in Chapter 14. Separating the discussion of cardiac ultrasound from the other diagnostic methods allows the former to be reviewed by recognized specialists. In the opinion of many, it has become the ascendent method of diagnosing IE. This chapter allows the reader to re-examine the importance of the other available methods, both traditional, such as the blood culture as well as more recent tools, such as various types of molecular methods. There are two major diagnostic goals: (*i*) establishing the existence of IE and (*ii*) defining the causative organism. The latter has major therapeutic implications.

Diagnosis begins with obtaining an accurate history and performing the physical examination. The reader is referred to the chapters for the various types of IE for a more specific discussion of history and physical findings.

HISTORY

Subacute IE is quite indolent in its course. The early clinical symptoms are quite nonspecific (low-grade fever, anorexia, fatigue, and back pain). Usually, they do not suggest any cardiac abnormality (1). Less commonly, subacute disease presents itself with stroke or congestive heart failure. The manifestations of IE usually begin within two weeks of the causative bloodstream infection (BSI) (2). The average interval between the beginning of the bacteremia of IE and establishing the diagnosis of alveolar infection is six weeks. This time span has not improved over the years. The reasons for this delay include: (*i*) the nonspecific presentations of early subacute disease; (*ii*) failure of the patient to seek medical evaluation; (*iii*) failure of the physician to consider the diagnosis of IE until signs and symptoms become more advanced, and (*iv*) the use of antibiotics to treat the symptoms of alveolar infection before the definitive diagnosis is made, which suppresses but does not cure the valvular infection. One needs to inquire about dental work or other invasive procedures. However, most cases of subacute disease are secondary to BSI of daily living.

Acute IE follows a much more aggressive course with high-grade fever and rapidly progressive valvular destruction that leads to congestive heart failure. The physician should inquire about intravenous drug abuse, recent surgical procedures, or placement of intravascular or intracardiac devices.

PHYSICAL EXAM

Fifteen percent of the cases of subacute disease are without fever, especially among the elderly (3). High-grade fever is inevitably a part of acute IE. In the subacute forms, murmurs are always present and do not change character tilts late in the course of disease. In acute IE, they are absent in about one-third of patients with left-sided involvement.

The dermal manifestations of IE (Osler nodes, Janeway lesions, splinter hemorrhages) currently are observed in only approximately 20% of patients. Forty percent of the patients develop arthritis and/or synovitis. The skin and musculo-skeletal findings are usually seen in subacute disease. In both subacute and acute diseases, the patient should be regularly assessed for the early signs of congestive heart failure.

LABORATORY

Blood Cultures

Because of its endovascular location, IE is unique among all infectious processes in that it is capable of producing a continuous bacteremia. This BSI originates in the infected vegetation that enters the bloodstream. The organisms, are cleared to variable degrees by the elements of the reticuloendothelial system that are located in the spleen, liver, and bone marrow (4). The presence of a continuous BSI with a microorganism consistent with valvular infection is sufficient to make the diagnosis of IE. A major challenge to the clinician is properly defining and documenting a continuous BSI. A continuous bacteremia may be defined as two blood cultures positive for the same organism that are obtained at least 12 hours apart or at least three out of four blood cultures positive for the same organism, the first and last of which is separated by at least one hour (5,6). The latter definition recognizes the need to rapidly start empiric antibiotic therapy in acute valvular infection.

In the work-up of valvular infection, there still is a good deal of confusion regarding both the optimal number of blood cultures and the timing of their drawing. One blood culture is often worse than none (7). The lone specimen cannot document a continuous BSI. It is impossible to determine whether an organism, retrieved from a single culture, is a contaminant; up to 50% of positive blood cultures are (8,8a). In 1956, Belli and Waisbren reported that at least five sets of blood cultures should be obtained. This recommendation was based on their observations that when three sets were drawn, only 82% of them were positive (9). A study from the mid-1960s of 789 blood cultures, which were obtained from 206 patients with strep-tococcal IE, showed that the first culture grew the organisms in 96% of the patients. The second raised the retrieval rate to 98% (10). The constancy of the bacteremia of IE facilitates the diagnosis of IE. On the other hand, the low concentration of organ-isms in the bloodstream represents a significant challenge to the detection of the specific pathogen. The concentration of organisms in the BSI of IE is usually <100 CFU/mL of blood. In many cases, the concentration is <10 CFU/mL of blood (10). The most important variable of cultures of blood is not the number of blood cultures performed but the volume of blood that is cultured (11). The greater the volume of blood that is cultured, the greater the microbiological yield. Inoculating 5 mL of blood yields positive cultures in 92% of cases versus a yield of 69% from a sample of 3 mL (12). The optimal total volume of blood to be drawn appears to be 60 mL with 10 mL inoculated into each bottle of a blood culture (20 mL of blood per set) (11). This correlates well with the study that indicated that three sets of blood cultures will detect the organism in greater than 99% of the cases (13). In at least two situations, obtaining more than three sets of blood cultures may be necessary. It is advisable to draw five sets of blood cultures when evaluating the possibility that coagulase-negative staphylococcal (CoNS) BSI represent prosthetic valve endocarditis (PVE). This is because growth of CoNS so frequently represents contamination as well as the fact that the bacteremia of PVE is often intermittent (14). Although still quite unusual, native valve endocarditis because of CoNS needs to be considered when multiple blood cultures are positive for these organisms (15). A more common reason for obtaining extra blood cultures is in the case of patients who are clinically likely to have IE but whose blood cultures are negative and who have recently received antibiotics (see next).

The particular time span over which they are drawn is only significant when antibiotic coverage must be started very rapidly as in the case of acute IE. In the past, detailed instructions were developed to time blood culture draws in relationship to the rise in the patient's temperature. Such approaches were meant to optimize the chance of retrieving the pathogen (3,16). Because the BSI of untreated IE is constant, it makes little sense to try to link the timing of the blood cultures with a rise in fever.

The rate of false-positive blood cultures may approach 50% (8). When caring for an acutely ill patient, it is quite difficult for the physician to avoid treating the positive blood culture. One false-positive blood culture is estimated to result in four days of unnecessary hospitalization (17). Criteria have been established to assist the clinician in determining the significance of a positive blood culture (8,8a). The characteristics of a truly positive blood culture are presented in Table 1. Probably, the most important of these is the particular organism recovered. Is it usually one that is associated with IE? If not, then it should be regarded as a contaminant unless proven otherwise.

As the patient's skin flora is the usual source of a tainted blood culture, a false-positive blood culture usually indicates inadequate preparation of the skin prior to venipuncture (11). Seventy percent isopropyl alcohol is swabbed on the skin (18). After the alcohol dries, a solution of 2% tincture of iodine or an iodophor, which is less irritating, is applied to the same area. The iodine compound is allowed to dry and then the blood for culture should be obtained. Replacing the needle before inoculating the blood into the culture bottle is unnecessary. Each blood culture set should represent a separate venipuncture. There is no evidence that current blood from an artery has a better yield than that collected from the venous circulation. Blood cultures should not be drawn through intravascular lines except for the purpose of documenting infection of the catheter (see Chapter 10). Doing so is associated with a high risk of contamination (19). It is important to emphasize the significance of inoculating 10 mL of blood into each bottle. The 1:10 ratio of blood to broth is beneficial in that it might minimize the suppressive effect of many types of antibiotics (20).

There is no one perfect growth medium available for culturing the pathogens of IE. Traditionally, each set of blood culture bottles consists of an aerobic (trypticase soy) and anaerobic (thioglycolate) broth. The latter's usefulness is not in diagnosing anaerobic IE, which is rare, but in facilitating the recovery of facultative anaerobes,

TABLE 1   Characteristics of True Positive Blood Cultures

Retrieval of organisms highly associated with infective endocarditis
Multiply positive blood cultures for the same organism
Positive blood cultures obtained from a severely ill patient

especially *Abiotrophia* spp. (nutritionally variant streptococci) (12). Certain organisms require specific growth factors. *Abiotrophia* spp. require vitamin B6 or cystine for growth. Commercial media currently contain these factors. *Legionella* spp. are cultured in the buffered charcoal and yeast extract agar with added alpha-ketoglutarate (21). Cultures are incubated at 37°C. Biphasic media had done away with the need for routine subculturing after 18 hours of incubation (19). A further improvement in the techniques of culturing blood is represented by the BACTEC resin containing medium or the BacT/Alert FA medium. These have supplanted the biphasic systems in greater part by their ability to inactivate many types of antibiotics that have been administered prior to obtaining blood cultures. The BACTEC system contains a resin that binds and neutralizes the antibiotic. In addition, the resin particles provide a surface area that appears to promote the growth of staphylococci and some yeasts (22). The BacT/Alert FA medium uses activated charcoal to achieve the same purpose. These systems have supplanted the addition of the anticoagulant sulfopolyanetholsulfonate (SPS) to blood culture bottles (23). SPS blocks the antimicrobial effect of lysozyme and complement as well as interferes with phagocytosis and blocks the action of the aminoglycosides. However, it is inhibitory to bacteria such as *Neisseria* spp.

The technique of lysis centrifugation facilitates the recovery of various types of bacteria and fungi from blood by disrupting the white cells and releasing the pathogens that are contained within (23,24). The lysate is then centrifuged and cultured on the appropriate type of agar. This approach is most useful in detecting intracellular organisms such as *Legionella* spp., fungi, *Staphylococcus aureus*, and *Brucella* spp.

None of these preparations are completely successful in preventing false-negative blood cultures including those produced by the presence of antibiotics in the bloodstream. Automated blood culture systems are able to retrieve the majority of clinically significant organisms within five days as compared with up to three to six weeks that had been recommended previously for manual blood culture systems. This time frame of incubation is true even for most of the very fastidious pathogens such as the HACEK group (*Hemophilus* spp., *Actinobacillus* spp., *Cardiobacterium hominis*, *Eikenella corrodens*, and *Kingella kingii*), *Francisella tularensis*, and *Brucella* (25). Currently, it is not the prolonged incubation times but automated systems and supplemented media that increase the recovery of fastidious organisms from the blood.

Even with these advances in blood culture techniques, culture-negative endocarditis remains a significant challenge to the clinician (5% of all cases of IE) (26–31). This may well be a growing problem due to the indiscriminate use of antibiotics, the increased placement of intracardiac devices, and the growing number in immunosuppressed patients that are susceptible to infections caused by fastidious pathogens. Table 2 presents the most likely causes of culture-negative IE. In the author's experience, previous exposure to antibiotics and sequestered infection are the most commonly encountered categories. As discussed before, newer microbiological techniques markedly lessen the contribution of "hard to grow" organisms to the incidence of culture-negative IE. *Coxiella burnetti* and *Bartonella* spp. (32) are the two most common fastidious organisms currently producing culture-negative IE. For unclear reasons, pathogens of IE, especially *S. aureus*, may penetrate into the interior of the vegetation and leave its surface "sterile." Under these circumstances, the bacteremia ceases, but the organisms continue to replicate and burrow into the base of the valve. Paravalvular abscesses,

TABLE 2 Causes of Culture-Negative Infective Endocarditis

Causes	Comments
Prior antibiotic use	Most frequent cause, at least 35–79% of cases
Sequestration of infection within the thrombus	Surface sterilization phenomena
Fastidious organisms	Fungi, Q-fever, *Tropheryma whipplei*, *Brucella* spp., *Rickettsiae*, *Chlamydiae*, *Legionella*
Right-sided endocarditis	Nonvirulent organisms are filtered out by the lungs
Bacteria-free stage	Untreated infection for more than three months
Mural infective endocarditis in ventricular septal defect	—
Infection related to pacemaker wires	—

Source: From Refs. 26–31.

septal abscesses, or ruptured chordae tendinae may result (33). This phenomenon may be encountered more frequently because of the growing prominence of *S. aureus* IE (34). The delay in making a specific etiologic diagnosis leads to a delay in instituting appropriate antimicrobial therapy, which results negatively on the outcome of valvular infection. The survival rate of patients whose fevers cleared by the seventh day of antimicrobial therapy was 92% as compared with 50% of the individuals who remain febrile (26).

Administration of antibiotics prior to obtaining blood cultures is by far the most common cause of culture-negative IE. Exposure to antibiotics is associated with 35% to 79% of all cases of culture-negative IE. The specific rate is determined by the frequency of fastidious organisms in the local environment. For example where *C. burnetti* is endemic, the importance of prior antibiotic administration diminishes. Pazin et al. (35) demonstrated that the recovery rate of streptococci from the bloodstreams of patients who had received antibiotics in the previous two weeks was 64% compared with 100% of those who were not given antibiotics (35). Antimicrobial agents clear the bacteremia of streptococcal IE within three days of their administration. If these compounds are stopped at that time, blood cultures again become positive within 48 hours. If the course of antibiotics is prolonged, it may take several weeks for the BSI to return (36). In general, the time of the suppression of the bacteremia is directly related to the sensitivity of the particular organism and to the duration of antimicrobial therapy. In the author's experience, the BSI of *S. aureus* IE is suppressed at most for a few days by even two weeks of antibiotic therapy.

Additives to blood of blood culture systems may reverse the inhibitory effect of previously administered antibiotics. The incidence of fungal IE is primarily owing to ever-increasing numbers of immunosuppressed patients and those who are cared for in an intensive care unit (ICU) (37). The diagnosis of fungal endocarditis continues to be difficult despite the significant improvements in culture techniques. This is partly because of the low rate of suspicion for fungal valvular infection. In one large series, only 18% of the cases were suspected at their initial presentation. Routine blood cultures will recover about 50% of *Candida* spp. IE; *Aspergillus* spp. and histoplasma are rarely grown from the blood. Fungal IE must be ruled out in those patients who possess many other signs and symptoms of IE but whose blood cultures remain sterile and who fail to respond to the standard antibiotic regimens for treating bacterial culture-negative endocarditis. When specific fungal culture techniques are used in combination with adjunctive types of tests, the diagnosis of

Candida IE may increase to 95% (11). Culturing the blood of patient in a bottle containing both agar and liquid broth increases the yield of retrieving various types of fungi and *Brucella* (23). Despite the use of the most advanced systems (isolator lysis centrifugation), the recovery rate from the bloodstream of the filamentous fungi, such as *Aspergillus* spp., remains quite low (<30% of cases). Histological culture of large vessel emboli, as well as of suspicious skin lesions, often yields the organism. Serological and DNA techniques that are useful in the diagnosis of fungi is discussed next.

Serological Tests
Serological studies remain useful in the diagnosis of culture-negative IE due to "hard to grow" pathogens. Table 3 presents the pathogens for which serological tests are available. Because of the chronicity of IE, a single significant elevation of IgG antibodies is sufficient for the diagnosis of *C. burnetti*. Antibodies to *C. burnetti* may cross-react with *C. psittaci* and *Bartonella* spp. In short, serological tests are most useful for detecting *C. burnetti* and *Bartonella* spp. As they are the most common fastidious organisms involved in IE, testing for them routinely in cases of culture-negative valvular infection is justified because of their relatively high pretest probability. Antibody tests against the other common listed organisms have the caveats of a low predictive value for IE and frequent cross reactions (38–40). Fifty percent of the cases with staphylococcal IE have increased levels of immunoglobulin (Ig) G antibodies against teichoic acid, which is a major component of the cell wall of *S. aureus*. This test had been proposed as useful for deciding the significance of positive blood cultures that do not meet the definition of the continuous bacteremia. Teichoic acid antibodies may be increased in diseases caused by other gram-positive bacteria. There is often a delay in their appearance. Because of these deficiencies, they are seldom employed currently (41). Serological regulations for fungal IE are thoroughly discussed in a review by MacLeod and Remington (42).

Histological Examination
Histological examination of excised valvular tissue is regarded as the diagnostic "gold standard" of IE. The tissue may be treated by traditional staining methods, or by immunohistological testing (immunoperoxidase, ELISA, immunofluorescent stains) or by 16S rRNA polymerase chain reaction (PCR) amplification sequencing (38,43–45). Similar techniques may be applied to retrieved valvular embolic material. In a study of excised heart valves in patients who were undergoing antibiotic treatment or who had already finished the antibiotic course (45), it was found that

TABLE 3 Serological Testing Clinically Useful and Available for the Diagnosis of Culture-Negative Infective Endocarditis

Organism	Test	Significant titers
Bartonella spp.	Indirect immunofluorescence	1/800
Coxiella burnetti	Indirect immunofluorescence	1/800
Brucella melitensis	Tube agglutination test	>1/160
Legionella pneumophilia	Indirect immunofluorescence	>1/128
Staphylococcus aureus	Counterimmunoelectrophoresis and gel diffusion	Varies

Source: From Refs. 38–41.

the sensitivity of the PCR tests and histological examination were the same (61% and 63%, respectively) with 100% specificity. Cultures were positive in only 13%. The PCR technique identified an organism in 38% of blood culture-negative IE. The low sensitivity of PCR and culture probably is because of the concurrent or previous courses of prolonged antibiotic therapy. These studies do not answer whether a positive PCR indicates an active infection or simply the DNA "tombstones" of killed bacteria. It appears that DNA can be detected after years following a clinical cure. There is previously derived evidence that only positive valvular cultures, not histological findings, should be taken into account in deciding if further antibiotic therapy is required (46).

Abnormalities of Nonspecific Laboratory Tests in Infective Endocarditis

Table 4 lists the abnormalities of nonspecific laboratory tests brought about by IE (47–54). These findings primarily reflect the changes brought about by subacute cases. In acute IE, the rate of leukocytosis would be expected to be much greater than 15%. The erythrocyte sedimentation rate is almost inevitably elevated (mean 57 mm/hr). If it is not, the diagnosis of IE should be in question unless there is congestive heart failure or disseminated intravascular coagulation. A positive rheumatoid factor develops in 50% of the cases that are untreated for six weeks or longer. It can be thought of as the "poor man's circulating immune complex." It disappears with successful therapy. Thirty-five percent of the cases of IE have elevation of circulating immune complexes that are more than that found in any other type of infection (>100 μg/mL). They also resolve with appropriate treatment. Levels of C-reactive protein and procalcitonin also rise and fall during the course of IE. This is modified by the administration of antibiotics. Procalcitonin appears to be more specific by its having higher levels than C-reactive protein and being more elevated during gram-negative valvular infection as well as being more predictive of the need for valvular replacement. The clinical significance of measuring these

TABLE 4 Laboratory Abnormalities of Infective Endocarditis[a]

Abnormality	Percentage of cases
Anemia	70–90
Leukocytosis	20–30
Elevated erythrocyte sedimentation rate	90–100
Histiocytes in the peripheral blood smear	25
Microscopic hematuria	30–50
Proteinuria	50–60
Elevated serum creatinine	10–20
Positive rheumatoid factor	50
Hypergammaglobulinemia	20–30
Circulating immune complexes	65–100
Hypocomplementemia	5–40
Positive lyme serology	?
C-reactive protein	100
Procalcitonin	81–84
Troponin-1	70 (of patients with coronary artery emboli)

[a]Abnormalities found in >15% of the cases.
Source: From Refs. 47–54.

two substances is questionable at the present time. Elevated levels of troponin I reflect myocardial necrosis that is the result of coronary artery emboli that originate in the infected vegetation. It has no prognostic abilities of paravalvular extension or the need for valvular surgery. As would be expected, elevated troponin I levels are seen more frequently in *S. aureus* IE.

Abnormalities of Electrocardiography in Infective Endocarditis

Electrocardiography is useful in identifying the 9% of patients who develop, during the course of their IE, conduction abnormalities and premature ventricular contractions that are secondary to septal abscesses or myocarditis. Seven percent of the patients have these irregularities that are of uncertain age (55). The closeness of both the noncoronary cusp of the aortic valve and the ring of the mitral valve facilitates the spread of infection to the conducting system. Septal abscesses, which arise from the mitral valve, are primarily situated at the lower end of the intraventricular septum and present with a gradual increase in the P-R and Q-T intervals and with left bundle branch block (56). Abscesses that involve the upper septum originate from the aortic valve and often are electrocardiographically silent. They are not present with the evolutionary changes of those of the lower septum. Complete heart block may suddenly appear (57). Repeat electrocardiography is recommended by many to be performed every 48 hours for two weeks in all patients with acute IE, especially that due to *S. aureus*.

Imaging Studies for the Diagnosis of Infective Endocarditis

Radionuclide scans have been developed for both the diagnosis of IE and the detection of its complications. Scanning with Gallium-67 has detected ventricular abscesses and valvular vegetations (58,59). This technique has been found to have a low degree of sensitivity (false-negative 40% of cases). White cells have been tagged with indium-111 as another radionuclide diagnostic modality. Like the gallium scan, it lacks sensitivity and the resolution needed to be clinically useful (60).

Cardiac computed tomography (CT) scans and magnetic resonance imaging (MRI) studies are at the early stages of development for diagnosing IE and its complications such as aortic root abscesses (61,62). With the images of both techniques becoming more rapidly acquired, they will be much more clinically useful in the near future. A CT scan of the spleen should always be obtained in cases of persistent or relapsing IE. Abscesses of this organ often can mimic IE with a continuous bacteremia that is refractory to antibiotics (63).

Cardiac catheterization is seldom necessary for the diagnosis of IE. In the past, it has been used to obtain quantitative cultures as an aid in localizing infection (64,65). The advances in both cultures and echocardiography have markedly lessened the need for catheterization, but it still is friable and plans the surgical approach in the setting of extensive infection. It is generally safe to do. Clearly, the insertion and manipulation of the catheters do not disseminate infection. Advanced heart failure is a relative contraindication.

Diagnostic Criteria of Infective Endocarditis

Discussion of the role of echocardiography in diagnosing and managing IE is thoroughly presented in Chapter 13. This section presents an analysis of the Duke criteria and their usefulness to the clinician in the diagnosis of valvular infections.

TABLE 5 Indications for Echocardiography in Infective Endocarditis

In the work-up of patients who have evidence of continuous bacteremia without a defined source or who have the syndrome of culture-negative endocarditis.
For the detection and characterization of valvular vegetations.
Documentation of valvular dysfunction and the degree of its hemodynamic importance as well as intracardiac complications of shunts or abscesses.
Re-evaluation of patients who are not doing well despite apparently adequate medical management. This would include those with persistent fever or bloodstream infections or worsening valvular dysfunction or overall deterioration.

Source: From Ref. 66.

Because echocardiography is such an essential part of these criteria, Table 5 serves as a reminder to the reader of the indications for performing this diagnostic modality (66).

In this chapter, the various approaches to the diagnosis of IE have been presented. Because of the challenge of determining whether positive blood cultures in the setting of heart disease represents IE or not, guidelines or case definitions have been developed as an aid to the clinician. The first of these was published in 1977 by Pelletier and Petersdorf (48). These investigators proposed three case categories: definite IE, probable IE, and possible IE. These were quite specific but insensitive because the definite category depended on examination of the valvular vegetations. They excluded significant amounts of patients with IE.

Von Reyn et al. (67) adapted the earlier guidelines by adding a rejected category that described cases for which there was a more likely alternative diagnosis. It also required pathological confirmation to include cases into the definite category (67).

The Duke criteria of 1994 adapted the von Reyn guidelines by including echocardiographic findings and adding intravenous drug abuse to the category of predisposing heart conditions (5). In addition, these criteria emphasize the significance of recovery of microorganisms that were typically involved in IE. In 2000, these criteria were modified by adding *C. burnetti* to the major criteria for blood cultures; recommended indications for performing transesophageal echocardiography and redefined category of possible endocarditis to include one major plus one minor criterion or three minor ones (6). Both the original and modified Duke criteria retained pathological criteria: (*i*) demonstration of microorganisms by culture or histology in a vegetation or embolized vegetation or in an intracardiac abscess; (*ii*) the presence of a vegetation or intracardiac abscess with histology consistent with active endocarditis.

Major modified criteria include: (*i*) positive blood cultures—these are defined as recovery of typical organisms (*Streptococcus viridans, Streptococcus bovis*, HACEK group, *S. aureus,* and enterococci) in two out of two sets or persistently positive blood cultures for typical organisms defined as two sets that are obtained >12 hours apart or three blood cultures that were drawn over at least one hour. A single positive culture for *C. burnetti* or phase 1 antibody titer >1/800 is the equivalent of a positive blood culture. (*ii*) Endocardial involvement is defined as new valvular regurgitation or a positive echocardiogram for IE. This is defined as an isolated intracardiac mass in the valve or the supports or in the pathway of regurgitant jets of blood or on implant material, all of which need to be the absence of any alternative anatomical explanation. Endocardial involvement may also be defined as an abscess or new partial dehiscence of prosthetic valves. Transesophageal echocardiograms are recommended for those who have prosthetic valves in place as well as patients who clinically are categorized as having possible IE.

Minor modified criteria include:

1. Predisposing cardiac condition or intravenous drug abuse.
2. Fever >100.4°F (38°C).
3. Arterial emboli, mycotic aneurysms, petechiae, Janeway lesions.
4. Immunological phenomenon such as glomerulonephritis, Osler nodes, blood spots, rheumatoid factor.
5. Microbiology including positive blood cultures but not mean standards of major criteria were serological evidences of active infection with likely microorganisms.

Table 6 presents the diagnostic categories of the modified Duke criteria. The Duke criteria have proven their validity in several clinical studies. In several studies, these standards did not reject one case of pathologically proven IE (68). The following discussion is not aimed to be a comprehensive presentation of the role of echocardiography in IE but as an analysis of the current Duke criteria to explore areas of possible improvement. Although the focus of the Duke criteria is on the echocardiographic findings, it is the microbiological criteria that are most important. The presence of a continuous bacteremia, as defined by the Duke criteria, is, by itself, sufficient to make the diagnosis of IE. There is almost no other process, with the possible exceptions of splenic absceses, mycotic aneurysms, and intravascular lines that have the potential for producing a continuous BSI. An analysis of the individual importance of each of the Duke criteria in diagnosing IE arrived at the conclusion that the major microbiological criteria possessed the highest relative importance (69). On the basis of this reasoning, the possible category makes little sense. This author contends that a patient who exhibits a continuous bacteremia with a typical organism should be placed in the definite category. At the other extreme, three minor criteria constitute too low a threshold because the patient has neither a significant bacteremia nor echocardiographic findings.

By classifying a case as possible, some physicians may feel that initiating antimicrobial therapy at that point is not justified. This author believes that automatic withhold of antibiotic therapy should occur only for rejected cases. The significance of the rejected category is frequently overlooked. As the negative predictive value of the Duke criteria is at least 92%, the clinician can confidently withhold antibiotic

TABLE 6   Diagnostic Categories of Infective Endocarditis of the Modified Duke Criteria

---

Definite—one of the following:
  Positive findings for IE in the pathology or microbiology of the vegetation
  Two major criteria
  One major and three minor criteria
  Five minor criteria
Possible—one of the following:
  One major and one minor criteria
  Three minor criteria
Rejected—one of the following:
  The presence of a definite alternative diagnosis
  Resolution of the signs and symptoms of IE following less than four days of antibiotic therapy
  No pathological evidence had surgery or autopsy following less than four days of antibiotic therapy
  Does not meet the standards for the criteria of possible IE

Abbreviation: IE, infective endocarditis.

therapy for patients who are so categorized and not feel obligated to initiate a therapeutic trial with all its ambiguity and risks (70).

In the presence of a continuous bacteremia, the indications for echocardiography switch from diagnosis to monitoring for or documenting complications (Table 5). A negative echocardiogram does not rule out the possibility of IE. Ten to twenty percent of the cases of IE have a negative transthoracic echocardiogram (TTE) (71). Although transesophageal echocardiograms (TEE) are more sensitive, a negative TEE does not rule out valvular infection (72). This may be because of extremely small vegetations or embolization of the thrombus. If negative, a repeat TEE should be performed within 10 days. The Duke criteria and modified Duke criteria really are most pertinent for the diagnosis of culture-negative IE.

These criteria are more suited for the diagnosis of subacute IE than acute because of the predominance of immunological phenomenon in the subacute form. These criteria do not include CoNS in the definition of microorganisms that are typically involved in IE. They fail to recognize their important role in PVE as well as the possibility of their causing native valve endocarditis. It is a deficiency that will become more significant as time goes on due to the increase in placement of intracardiac devices and intravascular catheters. Algorithms, which have been developed to calculate the significance of CoNS bacteremia, could be incorporated into further modifications of these quite important guidelines (73).

REFERENCES

1. Weinstein L, Rubin RH. Infective endocarditis—1973. Progress Cardiovasc Dis 1974; 16:239.
2. Starkenbaum M, Durack DT, Beeson P. The "incubation period" of subacute bacterial endocarditis. Yale J Biol Med 1977; 50:49.
3. Weinstein L. Infective endocarditis. In: Braunwald E, ed. Heart Disease: A Textbook of Cardiovascular Medicine. 3rd ed. Philadelphia: WB Saunders, 1988:1113.
4. Beeson PB, Brannon ES, Warren JV. Observations on the sites of removal of bacteria from the blood of patients with bacterial endocarditis. J Exp Med 1945; 81:9.
5. Durack DT, Lukes BS, Bright DK. Duke Endocarditis Service. New criteria for diagnosis of infective endocarditis: utilization of specific echocardiographic findings. Am J Med 1994; 96:200.
6. Li JS, Sexton DJ, Mick N, et al. Modified Duke criteria for diagnosis of infective endocarditis. Clin Infect Dis 2000; 30:633.
7. Aronson MD, Bor DH. Blood cultures. Ann Intern Med 1987; 106:246.
8. Bates D, Lee TH. Rapid classification of positive blood cultures: prospective validation of a multivariate algorithm. JAMA 1992; 267:1962.
8a. Weinstein MP. Blood culture contamination: persisting problems and partial progress. J Clin Microbiol 2003; 41:2275.
9. Belli J, Weisbren BA. The number of blood cultures necessary to diagnose most cases of bacterial endocarditis. Am J Med Sci 1956; 232:284.
10. Werner AS, Cobbs CG, Kaye D, Hook EW. Studies on the bacteremia of bacterial endocarditis. JAMA 1967; 202:199.
11. Towns ML, Reller LB. Diagnostic methods: current best practices and guidelines for isolation of bacteria and fungi in infective endocarditis. Infect Dis Clin NA 2002; 16:363.
12. Mermel LA, Maki D. Detection of bacteremia in adults: consequences of culturing an inadequate volume of blood. Ann Intern Med 1993; 119:270.
13. Weinstein MP, Towns ML, Quartey SM, et al. The clinical significance of positive blood cultures in the 1990s: a prospective, comprehensive evaluation of the microbiology, epidemiology and outcome of bacteremia and fungemia in adults. Clin Infect Dis 1997; 24:584.

14. Heimberger T, Duma R. Infections of prosthetic heart valves and cardiac pacemakers. Infect Dis Clin North Am 1989; 3(2):221–245.
15. Baddour LM, Phillips TN, Bisno AL. Coagulase-negative staphylococcal endocarditis: occurrence in patients with mitral valve prolapse. Arch Intern Med 1986; 146:119.
16. Weiss H, Ottenberg R. Relation between bacteria and temperature in subacute bacterial endocarditis. J Infect Dis 1932; 50:61.
17. Bates B, Goldmann L, Lee TH. Contaminant blood cultures and resource utilization. JAMA 1991; 265:365.
18. Weinstein MP. Current blood culture methods and systems: clinical concepts, technology and interpretation of results. Clin Infect Dis 1996; 23:40.
19. Miller M, Casey J. Infective endocarditis: new diagnostic techniques. Am Heart J 1978; 96:123.
20. Murray PR, Traynor P, Hopson D. Critical assessment of blood culture techniques: analysis of recovery of complicated facultative anaerobes, strict anaerobic bacteria and fungi in aerobic and anaerobic blood culture bottles. J Clin Microbiol 1992; 30:1462.
21. Weinstein L, Brusch JL. Diagnosis. In: Weinstein L, Brusch JL, eds. Infective Endocarditis. New York: Oxford University Press, 1996:236.
22. Spaargaren J, van Boven CPA, Voorn GP. Effectiveness of resins in neutralizing antibiotic activities in Bactec Plus Aerobic/F culture medium. J Clin Microbiol 1998; 36:3731.
23. Washington JA. The microbiological diagnosis of infective endocarditis. J Antimicrobiol Chemother 1987; 20(suppl A):29.
24. Archibald LK, McDonald LC, Addison RM, et al. Comparison of BACTEC MYCO/F LYTIC and WAPOLE ISOLATOR 10 (lysis-centrifugation) systems for detection of bacteremia, mycobacteremia and fungemia in a developing country. J Clin Microbiol 2000; 38:2994.
25. Baron EJ, Scott JD, Tompkins LS. Prolonged incubation and extensive subculturing do not increase recovery of clinically significant microorganisms from standard automated blood cultures. Clin Infect Dis 2005; 41:1677.
26. Van Scoy RE. Culture-negative endocarditis. Mayo Clin Proc 1982; 57:149.
27. Pesanti EL, Smith IM. Infective endocarditis with negative blood cultures: an analysis of 52 cases. Am J Med 1979; 66:43.
28. Barbari EF, Cockerill FR, Steckleburg JM. Infective endocarditis due to unusual or fastidious microorganisms. Mayo Clin Proc 1997; 72:532.
29. Hoen B, Selton-Suty C, Lacassin F, et al. Infective endocarditis in patients with negative blood cultures: analysis of 88 cases from a one-year nationwide survey in France. Clin Infect Dis 1995; 20:501.
30. Keefer CS. Subacute bacterial endocarditis: active cases without bacteremia. Ann Intern Med 1937; 11:714.
31. Libman E. The clinical features of cases of subacute bacterial endocarditis that spontaneously become bacteria-free. Am J Med Sci 1913; 146:625.
32. Broqui P, Raoult D. Endocarditis due to rare and fastidious bacteria. Clin Microbiol Rev 2001; 14:177.
33. McFarland MM. Pathology of infective endocarditis. In: Kaye D, ed. Infective Endocarditis. 2nd ed. New York: Raven Press, 1992:57.
34. Roberts WC. Characteristics of consequences of infective endocarditis (active or healed or both) learned from morphologic studies. In: Rahimtoola SH, ed. Infective Endocarditis. New York: Grune and Stratton, 1978:55.
35. Pazin GJ, Saul S, Thompson ME. Blood culture positivity: suppression by outpatient antibiotic therapy in patients with bacterial endocarditis. Arch Intern Med 1982; 57:149.
36. Weinstein L. Infective endocarditis. In: Braunwald E, ed. Heart Disease: A Textbook of Cardiovascular Medicine. 3rd ed. Philadelphia: WB Saunders, 1988:1113.
37. Ellis ME, Al-Abdely H, Standridge A, et al. Fungal endocarditis: evidence the world literature, 1965–1995. Clin Infect Dis 2001; 32:50.
38. Houpikian P, Raoult D. Diagnostic methods: current best practices and guidelines for identification difficult-to-culture pathogens in infective endocarditis. Infect Dis Clin NA 2002; 16:377.
39. Raoult D, Casalta JP, Richet H, et al. Contribution of systematic serologic testing in diagnosis of infective endocarditis. J Clin Microbiol 2005; 43:5238.

40. Fournier PE, Raoult D. Nonculture laboratory methods for the diagnosis of infectious endocarditis. Curr Infect Dis Rep 1999; 1:136.
41. Christensson B, Hedstrom S, Kronvall G. Clinical significance of serologic methods in the diagnosis of staphylococcal septicemia and endocarditis. Scand J Infect Dis 1983; 41(suppl 140):140.
42. Mc Leod R, Remington J. Fungal endocarditis. In: Rahmitoola SH, ed. Infective Endocarditis. New York: Grune and Stratton, 1978:119.
43. Broqui P, Dumler JS, Raoult D. Immunohistologic demonstration of *Coxiella burnetti* in the valves of patients with Q fever endocarditis. Am J Med 1994; 97:451.
44. Rovery C, Greub G, Lepidi H, et al. The search detection of bacteria on cardiac valves of patients with bacterial endocarditis. J Clin Microbiol 2005; 43:163.
45. Greub G, Lepidi H, Rovery C, et al. Diagnosis of infectious endocarditis in patients undergoing valve surgery. Am J Med 2005; 118:230.
46. Morris AJ, Drinkovic D, Pottumarthy S, et al. Gram stain, culture and histopathological examination for heart valves removed because of infective endocarditis. Clin Infect Dis 2003; 36:697.
47. Kaye K, Kaye D. Laboratory findings including blood cultures. In: Kaye D, ed. Infective Endocarditis. 2nd ed. New York: Raven Press, 1992:20.
48. Pelletier LL, Petersdorf RG. Infective endocarditis: a review of 125 cases from the University Of Washington Hospitals, 1963–1972. Medicine (Baltimore) 1977; 56:287.
49. Weinstein L, Schlesinger J. Pathoanatomic, pathophysiologic and clinical correlates in endocarditis. N Engl J Med 1979; 291:832.
50. Kaufman RH, Thompson J, Valentjin RM, et al. The clinical implications and pathogenic significance of circulating immune complexes in infective endocarditis. Am J Med 1981; 71:17.
51. Kael AT, Volkman DJ, Gorevic PD, et al. Positive lyme serology in subacute bacterial endocarditis. JAMA 1990; 162:967.
52. Watkin RW, Lang S, Smith JM, et al. Role of troponin I in active infective endocarditis. Am J Cardiol 2004; 94:1.
53. Mueller C, Huber P, Laifer G, et al. Procalcitonin and the early diagnosis of infective endocarditis. Circulation 2004; 109:1707.
54. Kocazeybek B, Kucukoglu S, Oner YA. Procalcitonin and C-reactive proteins in infective endocarditis: correlation with etiology and prognosis. Chemotherapy 2003; 49:76.
55. Dinubile M, Calderwood S, Steinhaus DA, et al. Cardiac conduction abnormalities complicating native valve active infective endocarditis. Am J Cardiolol 1986; 58:1213.
56. Sanson J, Slodki S, Gruhn JG. Myocardial abscesses. Am Heart J 1963; 66:301.
57. Weinstein L. Life-threatening infective endocarditis. Archiv Intern Med 1986; 46:953.
58. Wiseman J, Rouleau J, Rigo R, et al. Gallium-67 myocardial imaging for the detection of bacterial endocarditis. Radiology 1976; 120:135.
59. Sachdev M, Peterson GE, Jollis JG. Imaging techniques for the diagnosis of infective endocarditis. Infect Dis Clin NA 2002; 16:319.
60. McDermott BP, Mohan S, Thermidor M. The lack of diagnostic value of the indium scan in acute bacterial endocarditis. Letter to the editor. Am J Med 2004; 8:621.
61. Cowan J, David P, Reid D, et al. Aortic root abscess complicating bacterial endocarditis demonstration by computed tomography. Br Heart J 1994; 52:591.
62. Winkler M, Higgins C. MRI of perivalvular infectious pseudoaneurysms. Am J Radiol 1986; 47:253.
63. Magilligan DJ Jr. Splenic abscess. In: Magilligan DJ Jr, Quinn E, eds. Endocarditis—Medical and Surgical Management. New York: Marcel Decker, 1986:197.
64. Welton D, Young J, Raizner A. Value and safety of cardiac catheterization during active infective endocarditis. Am J Cardiol 1979; 44:1306.
65. Mills J, Abbot J, Utley JR, et al. Role of cardiac catheterization in infective endocarditis. Chest 1977; 72:576.
66. Cheitlin MD, Armstrong WF, Aurigemma GP, et al. ACC/AHA/ASE 2003 guideline update the clinical application of echocardiography: summary article: A report of the American College of Cardiology/American Heart Association Task Force on Practice Guidelines (ACC/AHA/ASE Committee to Update the 1997 Guidelines for the Clinical Application of Echocardiography). Circulation 2003; 108:1146.

67. Von Reyn CF, Levy BS, Arbeit RD, et al. Infective endocarditis: an analysis based on strict case definitions. Ann Intern Med 1981; 94:505.
68. Sandre RM, Shafron SD. Infective endocarditis: review of 135 cases over 9 years. Clin Infect Dis 1996; 22:276.
69. Rognon R, Kehtari R, Francioli P. Individual value of each of the Duke criteria for the diagnosis of infective endocarditis. Clin Microbiol Infect 1999; 5:396.
70. Dodds GA 3rd, Sexton DJ, Durack DT, et al. Negative predictive value of the Duke criteria for infective endocarditis. Am J Cardiol 1996; 77:403.
71. Stratton JR, Werner JA, Pearlman AS, et al. Bacteremia and the heart: serial echocardiographic findings in 80 patients with documented or suspected bacteremia Am J Med 1982; 73:851.
72. Sochowski RA, Chan K-L. Implication of negative results on monoplane transesophageal echocardiographic study in patients with suspected infective endocarditis. J Am Coll Cardiol 1993; 21:216.
73. Tokars JL. Predictive value of blood cultures positive for coagulase-negative staphylococci: implications for patient care and health-care quality. Clin Infect Dis 2004; 39:333.

13

Echocardiography

Davinder S. Jassal
Cardiac Ultrasound Laboratory, Division of Cardiology, Massachusetts General Hospital and Harvard Medical School, Boston, Massachusetts, U.S.A., and Bergen Cardiac Care Center, Division of Cardiology, St. Boniface General Hospital, Winnipeg, Manitoba, Canada

Michael H. Picard
Cardiac Ultrasound Laboratory, Division of Cardiology, Massachusetts General Hospital and Harvard Medical School, Boston, Massachusetts, U.S.A.

INTRODUCTION

Infective endocarditis is a diagnostic and therapeutic challenge that is associated with high patient morbidity and mortality (1). The diagnosis and management of infective endocarditis has changed dramatically over the past 40 years, in particular the use of echocardiography (2,3). Since the initial description of valvular vegetations by M Mode echocardiography in 1973 (4), this noninvasive imaging technique has assumed an increasingly important role in the evaluation of a patient with infective endocarditis.

Echocardiography serves two important roles. The first involves assisting in the diagnosis of the condition by the identification of valvular masses. The echocardiographic appearance of vegetations has been added as one of the major Duke diagnostic criteria (3). Additionally, echocardiography is useful for the detection and characterization of the hemodynamic consequences of infection.

Although the role of echocardiography is well-established in the diagnosis and management of native valve and prosthetic valve endocarditis, the recent introduction of nonvalvular cardiovascular devices has expanded its utility (5). Echocardiography will play a defining role in the management of these infections involving a variety of cardiovascular prostheses and devices that are used to replace or assist damage of the cardiovascular system (5).

DIAGNOSIS OF INFECTIVE ENDOCARDITIS

Despite advances in imaging technology in the current millennium, the initial diagnosis of infective endocarditis (IE) remains a clinical one. Criteria for the diagnosis of endocarditis were initially proposed by Pelletier et al. in 1977 followed by von Reyn et al. in 1981 (6,7). Although both diagnostic criteria are reasonably specific, they lack sensitivity. Subsquently in 1994, the Duke criteria for the diagnosis of IE was established using major and minor criteria in a manner analogous to the Jones criteria for rheumatic heart disease (3,8). Aside from positive blood cultures and a new regurgitant murmur, echocardiographic findings became one of the major Duke criteria providing objective evidence of endocardial involvement (3). Specifically, these include:

1. Oscillating intracardiac mass, on valve or supporting structures, or in the path of regurgitant jets, or on implanted material, in the absence of an alternative anatomic explanation, or

2. Abscess, or
3. New partial dehiscence of a prosthetic valve.

Abnormal echocardiographic findings not fulfilling these definitions such as nonspecific valvular thickening are considered as minor criteria. If the patient has two major, one major and three or five minor, there is a high probability of having infective endocorditis (3).

ECHOCARDIOGRAPHIC APPROACH: TRANSTHORACIC VS. TRANSESOPHAGEAL ECHOCARDIOGRAPHY

Due to the noninvasive nature and low cost associated with transthoracic echocardiography (TTE), it remains the initial procedure of choice in patients suspected of having IE (9). The diagnostic yield of TTE in the detection of vegetations is influenced by a myriad of factors, including image quality, size of the vegetation, location of vegetation, reflectivity of vegetation, presence of inherent valvular disease or valvular prosthesis, experience of the examiner, and pretest probability of endocarditis (9).

On two-dimensional echocardiography, a vegetation is defined as an abnormal reflective, irregular mass attached to the valve leaflet, with independent motion (10). Vegetations tend to develop on the upstream side (low pressure) of the affected valve; such as the atrial side of the mitral valve and the ventricular side of the aortic valve. The size of the vegetation can vary from a millimeter to several centimeters in dimension. In most cases however, vegetation must be at least 3 mm to 6 mm in size to be reliably detected by TTE (10). With respect to size, fungal vegetations are larger than bacterial vegetations, tending to embolize more readily (11). Additionally, tricuspid valve vegetations are larger than those located on the left-sided cardiac valves (12).

Although TTE is the initial imaging modality of choice in the clinical suspicion of endocarditis, transesophageal echocardiography (TEE) is more sensitive and specific for both the detection of valvular vegetations and their complications. The sensitivity for the detection of vegetations increases to 95% using TEE imaging (13–16). Due to the higher frequency transducer, structures of interest being closer to the transducer and reduction of impediments to the ultrasound signal, TEE imaging often provides dramatic improvement in visualization of the valve (13–16). As image quality tends to be superior from the transesophageal approach, small normal variants of valve anatomy may be appreciated and should not be interpreted as abnormalities (15). Anatomic abnormalities that may mimic infective endocarditis on echocardiography include (15):

1. Thrombus
2. Papillary fibroma
3. Aortic valve Lambl's excrescence
4. Beam-width artifact from calcified valve
5. Marantic endocarditis
6. Myxomatous mitral valve.

According to the ACC/AHA guidelines for the clinical application of enhocardiography, a TTE is typically used initially in individuals with native valves, whereas TEE should be used as the primary diagnostic imaging modality in patients with prosthetic valves (17).

While the identification of a vegetation is helpful in establishing the diagnosis of acute IE, specific characteristics of the mass by echocardiography are also useful when stratifying patients at risk. The prognostic characteristics of vegetation mobility, extension to adjacent nonvalvular structures, and degree of calcification have been extensively studied (18–21). Sanfillipo et al. (18) evaluated 219 patients with vegetations and identified that both mobility and involvement of extravalvular structures were significant predictors of complications, including heart failure, cerebrovascular accident, and need for valve replacement. Thus, the identification and characterization of vegetation by echocardiography is fundamental in the diagnosis and prognosis of patients with IE.

NATIVE VALVE ENDOCARDITIS
Aortic Valve
The aortic valve is a common site of involvement in IE. Predisposing factors include a bicuspid aortic valve, rheumatic deformation of the leaflets, and calcification observed in the elderly (2). An echogenic mass attached to the ventricular side of the aortic leaflet with independent motion and prolapse into the left ventricular outflow tract is diagnostic for a valvular vegetation (Figs. 1,2). Aside from an infective aortic valve mass, one must entertain a Lambl's excrescence in the differential diagnosis (2). In contrast to the bulky mobile mass of vegetation, a Lambl's excrescence is typically a short, thin, filamentous projection off a valve leaflet (Fig. 3). Larger Lambl's lesions, however, are more difficult to differentiate from vegetations. As there are presently no echocardiographic features of noninfective lesions that can reliably differentiate them from infective lesions, the correct diagnosis lies in correlating echocardiographic findings with the clinical scenario and microbiological findings.

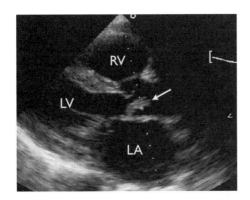

FIGURE 1 A transthoracic parasternal long axis view illustrating vegetation (*arrow*) involving the aortic valve during systole. *Abbreviations*: LA, left atrium; LV, left ventricle; RV, right venticle.

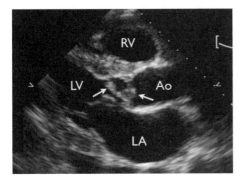

FIGURE 2 A transthoracic parasternal long axis view illustrating vegetation (*arrows*) involving the aortic valve during diastole. *Abbreviations*: LA, left atrium; LV, left ventricle; RV, right ventricle; Ao, aorta.

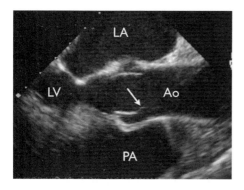

FIGURE 3   A transesophageal long axis view of the aorta with demonstration of a Lambl's excrescence on the right coronary cusp of the aortic valve (*arrow*). *Abbreviations:* LV, left ventricle; LA, left atrium; PA, pulmonary artery; Ao, aorta.

Mitral Valve

As compared with any other valve, the mitral valve is more frequently involved in IE (2). Predisposing factors include rheumatic deformation of the mitral leaflets and myxomatous degeneration (2). Diagnostic features of mitral valve vegetations include rapid independent motion, prolapsing into the left atrium in systole with evidence of valve dysfunction (Figs. 4, 5). On occasion, mitral valve vegetations can become large enough to obstruct the mitral inflow orifice, mimicking the characteristic echocardiographic features of mitral stenosis. Other things to

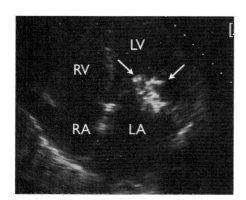

FIGURE 4   A large vegetation (*arrows*) involving the posterior mitral leaflet on transthoracic echocardiography (apical four-chamber view). *Abbreviations*: LA, left atrium; LV, left ventricle; RA, right atrium; RV, right ventricle.

(A)   **(B)**

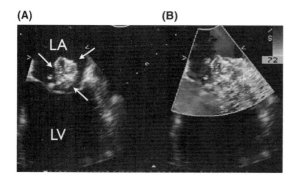

FIGURE 5   (*See color insert*) (**A**) Mitral valve vegetation. The large vegetation (*arrow*) involving the mitral valve is seen on a systolic frame of transesophageal echocardiography. (**B**) Color Doppler imaging reveals moderate mitral regurgitation. *Abbreviations*: LA, left atrium; LV, left ventricle.

entertain in the differential diagnosis of a mitral valve mass include a severely myxomatous leaflet, a partial flail leaflet, thickened rheumatic valve, or a ruptured papillary muscle (2).

Tricuspid Valve

Tricuspid valve endocarditis commonly occurs in intravenous drug abusers (12), but can occur in other conditions associated with bacteremia. Such predisposing factors include alcohol abuse, virulent skin infections, and infected venous catheters (12). The right ventricular inflow view is often diagnostic, demonstrating large, mobile echoes attached to the atrial side of a tricuspid leaflet with prolapse into the right atrium during systole (Figs. 6–8). The vegetations on the tricuspid valve are usually larger then on other values especially when due to *Staphylococcus aureus* infection. Due to the mobility of these vegetations, septic pulmonary emboli are a frequent complication of tricuspid valve endocarditis (22).

Pulmonic Valve

Isolated pulmonic valve endocarditis is an extremely rare diagnostic entity (23). The clinical suspicion of pulmonic valve endocarditis should be entertained in any febrile patient with multiple pulmonary emboli. In echocardiographic studies, intravenous drug use (IVDU), pulmonary artery catheterization, and congenital

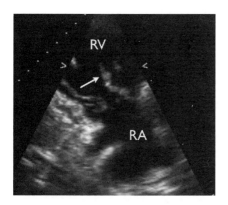

FIGURE 6 A transthoracic echocardiographic right ventricular inflow view demonstrating a large vegetation (*arrow*) on the tricuspid valve. *Abbreviations*: RA, right atrium; RV, right ventricle.

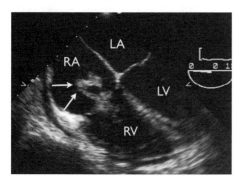

FIGURE 7 A systolic frame of transesophageal four-chamber view illustrating a large serpeginous vegetation (*arrow*) attached to the tricuspid valve. *Abbreviations*: LA, left atrium, LV, left ventricle; RA, right atrium, RV, right ventricle.

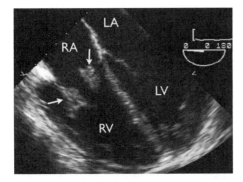

FIGURE 8 A diastolic frame of transesopha-geal four-chamber view illustrating vegetations (*arrows*) attached to the two leaflets of tricuspid valve. *Abbreviations*: LA, left atrium; LV, left ventricle; RA, right atrium, RV, right ventricle.

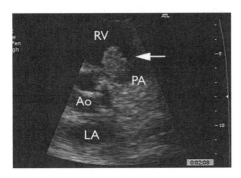

FIGURE 9 A transthoracic short axis view of the aorta illustrating vegetation on the pulmonic valve (*arrow*). *Abbreviations:* Ao, aorta; LA, left atrium; PA, pulmonary artery; RV, right ventricle. *Source*: From Ref. 23.

malformations (i.e., pulmonic stenosis, patent ductus arteriosus, and Tetralogy of Fallot) can predispose an individual to the development of isolated pulmonic valve endocarditis (24). IVDU patients develop pulmonic valve endocarditis about 10 times less frequently than the tricuspid valve (12). Although visualization of the pulmonic valve is at times suboptimal due to intervening lung tissue and the inability to obtain a cross-sectional view of the valve, TTE can often provide the diagnostic information (Fig. 9) (25). In addition to the typical parasternal views of the right ventricular outflow tract, the pulmonic valve can be visualized from the subcostal view.

PROSTHETIC VALVE ENDOCARDITIS

IE of prosthetic valves, both bioprosthetic and mechanical, is often a diagnostic dilemma. The identification of vegetations on prosthetic valves is difficult to detect using echocardiography compared with native valve endocarditis (26). The active infectious process involving mechanical prosthetic valves usually begins in the peri-valvular area at the annular insertion site (Figs. 10–13) (26,27). Necrosis of the supporting annular tissue with loosening of the sutures may lead to dehiscence of the sewing ring (26,27).

A number of imaging artifacts associated with the prosthetic valve can mimic echocardiographic findings of vegetations. Distinguishing small vegetations from the prosthetic material (i.e., sutures) can be extremely difficult (Fig. 14). Both throm-bus and pannus may have a similar appearance and cannot be readily discernable from infectious vegetative material (Fig. 15) (26,27). Also, strands can be observed

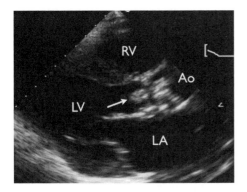

FIGURE 10 A diastolic frame of transthoracic parasternal long axis image illustrating vegetation (*arrow*) attached to the bioprosthetic Carpentier-Edwards aortic valve. *Abbreviations*: Ao, aorta; LA, left atrium; LV, left ventricle; RV, right ventricle.

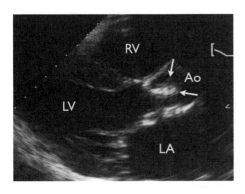

FIGURE 11 A systolic frame of transthoracic parasternal long axis view illustrating vegetation (*arrows*) attached to the bioprosthetic Carpentier-Edwards aortic valve. *Abbreviations*: Ao, aorta; LA, left atrium; LV, left ventricle; RV, right ventricle.

by TEE imaging of prosthetic valves, particularly in the early postoperative months, and must be distinguished from vegetations (26,27). Typically, the lesion size, patient's clinical presentation, and microbiological information can help distinguish between vegetation and fibrous strands.

The sewing ring and support structures of bioprosthetic and mechanical valves are strongly reflective and create "acoustic" shadows where no diagnostic image is noted. This will prevent vegetation detection within the valve apparatus or its distal shadow. The reverberations and shadowing in particular affect transthoracic imaging of the mitral prosthesis from apical views, where the left atrial side of

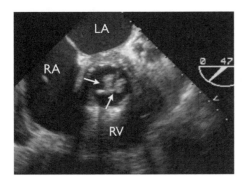

FIGURE 12 An aortic valve vegetation is demonstrated on the short axis view of a bioprosthetic Carpentier-Edwards valve on transesophageal echocardiography. *Abbreviations*: LA, left atrium; PA, pulmonary artery; RA, right atrium.

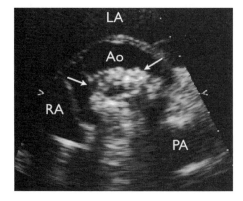

FIGURE 13 A tranesophageal short axis view of a St. Jude mechanical valve in the aortic position with multiple vegetations (*arrows*). *Abbreviations*: Ao, aorta; LA, left atrium; PA, pulmonary artery; RA, right atrium.

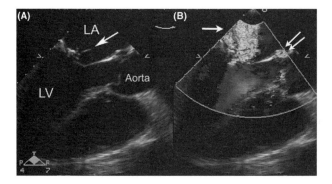

FIGURE 14 (*See color insert*) A transesophageal long axis view of a patient with dehiscence of a mitral annular ring (**A**, B mode image; **B**, Color Doppler). A linear echodensity arises from the posterior portion of the ring consistent with a torn suture (**A**: *arrow*). The posterior portion of the mitral valve ring is dehisced with severe mitral regurgitation (**B**: *single arrow*). A fistulous channel is identified in the intervalvular fibrosa between the aorta and the left atrium (**B**: *double arrow*) with a moderate amount of shunt by color Doppler. *Abbreviations*: LA, left atrium; LV, left ventricle.

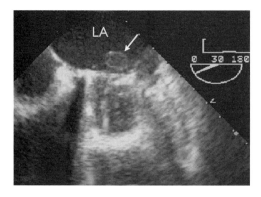

FIGURE 15 A systolic frame of transesophageal long axis view of a patient with a mechanical mitral valve with a thrombus (*arrow*). *Abbreviation:* LA, left atrium.

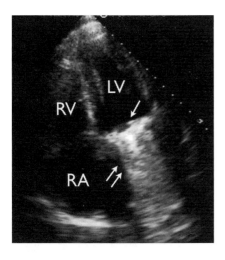

FIGURE 16 A transthoracic apical four-chamber view illustrating a St. Jude mechanical valve (*single arrow*) in the mitral position with shadowing of the left atrium (*double arrow*) owing to reverberations from the valve.

the valve is masked by the prosthesis (Fig. 16). As a result, the paravalvular infection or abscess in the mitral annulus and/or the resulting valvular regurgitation may be missed (26) by TTE imaging.

Acoustic shadowing of the aortic valve prosthesis is less of a problem by TTE as the degree of significant aortic regurgitation may be evaluated clearly from the apical and parasternal views. Transthoracic echocardiography is rarely sufficient to exclude the diagnosis of endocarditis in patients with prosthetic valves in whom there is a high index of suspicion of an active infectious process. As such, whenever prosthetic valve endocarditis is suspected, and TTE, if performed, is negative, TEE imaging should be strongly considered (17). In a large series of prosthetic valve endocarditis, while TTE demonstrated a sensitivity of 57% and specificity of 63%, TEE imaging demonstrated a sensitivity of 86% and a specificity of 88% (26).

COMPLICATIONS OF ENDOCARDITIS
Valvular Regurgitation
In infective endocarditis, the acute development of valvular regurgitation can precipitate heart failure. On two-dimensional echocardiography, the destruction of the valve leaflet by the infectious process in addition to the distortion of the line of closure by the vegetative mass can be visualized (2,9). Assessment of the degree of valvular regurgitation in endocarditis is further delineated by using pulse, color flow, and continuous wave Doppler (10,28).

In the setting of aortic valve endocarditis, perforation of the aortic leaflet, flail cusp, or both may occur in up to 50% of all cases (29). Severe aortic insufficiency as estimated by continuous wave Doppler has been associated with a poor prognosis (Fig. 17) (30). Perforation of the mitral valve leaflet is less common, occurring in only 15% of all patients with mitral valve endocarditis (Fig. 18) (10).

Abscess
Extension of the acute infectious process from the valve leaflets to the surrounding tissue is a natural step in IE. Typically, abscess development occurs around the valve

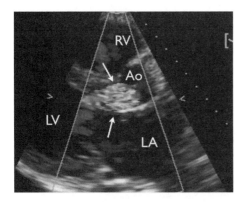

FIGURE 17 (*See color insert*) A transthoracic parasternal long axis view demonstrating severe aortic insufficiency (*arrows*) owing to acute infective endocarditis of the native aortic valve. *Abbreviations*: Ao, aorta; LA, left atrium; LV, left ventricle; RV, right ventricle.

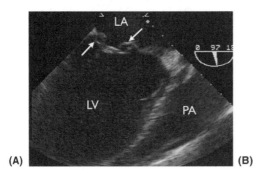
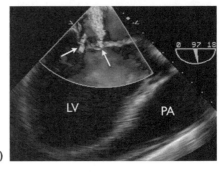

(A)   (B)

FIGURE 18 A transesophageal echocardiographic long axis view illustrating aneurysms of the mitral valve leaflets due to acute infective endocarditis; (**A**) with perforation resulting in (**B**) (*See color insert*) two separate jets of mitral regurgitation as seen on color. *Abbreviations*: LA, left atrium; LV, left ventricle; PA, pulmonary artery.

annulus adjacent to the infected leaflet tissue, being more common with the aortic than the mitral valve (29–31). In native aortic valve endocarditis, abscess development usually occurs through the weakest portion of the annulus, near the membranous portion of the interventricular septum (Figs. 19, 20) (31). The sensitivity and specificity of TTE for abscess detection is 67% and 100%, respectively, compared

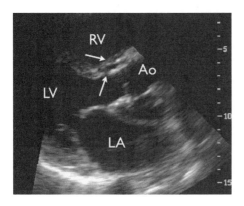

FIGURE 19 A transthoracic parasternal long axis view from a patient with a bioprosthetic aortic valve illustrating an aortic root abscess involving the right coronary cusp (*arrows*). *Abbreviations*: Ao, aorta; LA, left atrium; LV, left ventricle; RV, right ventricle.

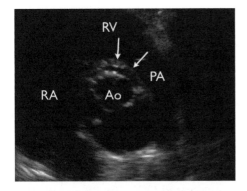

FIGURE 20 A transthoracic parasternal short axis view of the aorta illustrating an aortic abscess involving the tissue adjacent to the left and right coronary cusps of the aortic valve. *Abbreviations*: Ao, aorta; PA, pulmonary artery; RA, right atrium; RV, right ventricle.

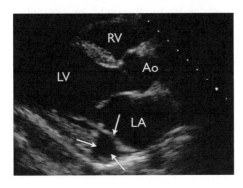

FIGURE 21 A transthoracic parasternal long axis view demonstrating a pseudoaneurysm (*arrows*) of the posterior mitral valve annulus owing to acute infective endocarditis. *Abbreviations*: Ao, aorta; LA, left atrium; LV, left ventricle; RV, right ventricle.

with 93% and 98% for TEE imaging (31). Involvement of the aortic annulus may extend into the contiguous anterior mitral valve leaflet as represented by the increased thickness of the leaflet tissue, vegetation, leaflet perforation, or fistula in the intervalvular fibrosa.

The development of a mitral ring abscess is less common. A mitral annular abscess appears as an increased thickening and central lucency in the posterior aspect of the mitral annulus in the left ventricular wall (31). This may lead to the development of a pseudoaneurysm of the left ventricle, which may persist after the infection is treated (Figs. 21, 22).

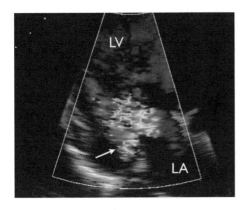

FIGURE 22 (*See color insert*) A transthoracic apical three-chamber view with color illustrating color flow into the pseudoaneurysm (*arrow*). *Abbreviations*: LA, left atrium; LV, left ventricle.

Intracardiac Fistula

Both cardiac abscesses and mycotic aneurysms may rupture into adjacent structures, thus creating intracardiac fistulous tracts (1,9). The fistulous communications may be single or multiple, extending from the aorta to either the right ventricle, the right atrium or left atrium (1,9). Using color Doppler, the site of the communication is usually well-defined and continuous-wave Doppler can demonstrate the high systolic flow velocity within the fistulous communication (Fig. 14).

NONVALVULAR CARDIOVASCULAR DEVICE-RELATED INFECTIONS

In recent years, intracardiac devices in addition to prosthetic valves have become more prevalent in the treatment of heart disease. Thus, their role as a risk factor for the development of infective endocarditis has increased (5,32). As the use of such devices increases, especially in the elderly population, the incidence of associated intracardiac infection is expected to rise (5,32).

Pacemaker/Implantable Cardiac Defibrillators

Infections of pacemakers and implantable cardiac defibrillators (ICD) have reported to range from 0.2% to 12% and are considered a serious complication of pacing therapy due to the inherent difficulties in the management of cardiac device endocarditis and the adverse outcome (33–43).

Initial cases of pacemaker endocarditis were described in the early 1970s (34,35). In pacemaker-/ICD-infective endocarditis, vegetation formation can occur either on the tricuspid valve (Fig. 23), or along the course of the electrode (Figs. 24, 25), including the endocardium of the right atrium or right ventricle (36,37).

Several studies have examined the role of echocardiography in the diagnosis of implantable cardiac devices including pacemakers and defibrillators (38–40). In patients with suspected IE of implanted antiarrhythmic devices, TEE is superior to transthoracic imaging (38,39). Vilacosta et al. (39) performed a prospective study comparing the utility of either TTE or TEE to visualize vegetation attached to pacemakers in their cohort of 10 patients. Lead vegetations were identified in only two patients by TTE and seven patients by TEE. Of the seven patients identified with IE by TEE, five underwent surgery confirming the findings (39). The superiority of TEE imaging is due to the complete interrogation of the superior vena cava and the upper part of the right atrium as many of these pacemaker infections occur in this region (38,39). The detection of lead vegetations by TTE has a sensitivity of 22–30% whereas by TEE the sensitivity is 95% (36,39–44).

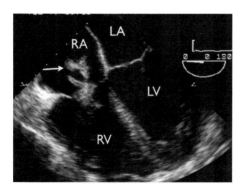

FIGURE 23   A transesophageal four-chamber view illustrating vegetations on the tricuspid valve after removal of the temporary pacemaker wire. *Abbreviations*: LA, left atrium; LV, left ventricle; RA, right atrium; RV, right ventricle.

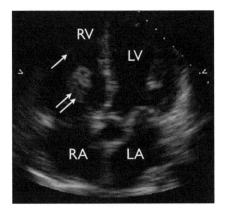

FIGURE 24 A transthoracic apical four-chamber view illustrating a pacemaker wire (*single arrow*) with vegetation adherent to the wire (*double arrows*). *Abbreviations*: LA, left atrium; LV, left ventricle; RA, right atrium; RV, right ventricle.

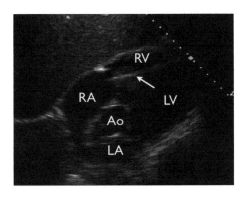

FIGURE 25 A transthoracic subcostal view demonstrating a mass of vegetations on the implantable cardiac defibrillators lead. *Abbreviations*: Ao, aorta; LA, left atrium; LV, left ventricle; RA, right atrium; RV, right ventricle.

Vascular Conduits

The use of combined prosthetic aortic conduits and valve implantation for the repair of ascending aortic root aneurysms has increased over the past decade. First described by Bentall and de Bono (45), the procedure can be modified to include a second tubular graft with anastomoses to the coronary arteries as suggested by Cabrol et al. (46).

Due to the characteristic increase in the reflections from the prosthetic patch materials, detection of vegetations on vascular conduits is difficult. Using the combined approach of TTE and TEE, abnormal mobility can be detected using two-dimensional imaging and dehiscence or obstruction can by confirmed by Doppler techniques. Imaging goals in the diagnosis of conduit endocarditis include direct visualization of the entire conduit, the anastomoses between conduit and aorta, and finally the prosthetic valve (47).

Atrial Septal Defect Closure Devices

Of the various complications described following implantation of an atrial septal defect (ASD) closure device, the two least common include thrombus formation (Fig. 26) and infection. Only five cases of IE involving ASD closure devices have been described in the literature to date (48–51). The ACC/AHA guidelines for IE prophylaxis do not recommend antibiotics for patients with ASD (52). Following the implantation of ASD closure devices, the prescription and duration of prophylactic antimicrobial therapy is physician-dependent.

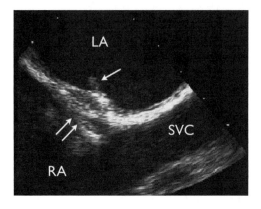

FIGURE 26 A transesophageal echocardiographic bicaval view demonstrating a thrombus (*single arrow*) on an Amplatzer closure device of the interatvie septum (*double arrows*). *Abbreviations*: LA, left atrium; RA, right atrium; SVC, superior vena cava.

Ventricular-Assist Devices

Mechanical circulatory support with left ventricular-assist devices (LVAD) has been used successfully as both a bridge to heart transplantation and as destination therapy in end-stage heart failure (53). In a study of 68 individuals studied for up to 2.5 years of follow-up, one-third of LVAD became infected within three months of implantation (32). LVAD endocarditis, defined as infection of the LVAD surface in contact with blood, is associated with a high mortality rate, particularly as these patients with severe heart failure have limited reserve (54,55). The pathogen can colonize the inner surfaces of the device and grafts as a bloodstream infection, or the outer surfaces of the device and drivelines as a localized infection. The role of echocardiography (both TTE and TEE) is to carefully inspect these potential sites of infection and ensure unobstructed flow from the inflow LVAD cannula in the left ventricular apex to the outflow cannula in the aorta (Fig. 27A,B). In most cases of LVAD endocarditis, prompt device debridement, removal, and replacement is necessary (56).

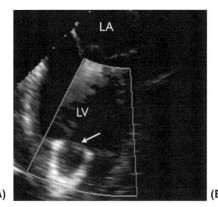
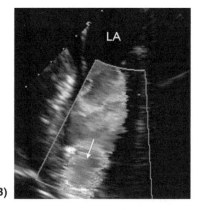

(A)   (B)

FIGURE 27   (*See color insert*) (**A**) transeophageal long axis view of the left ventricle demonstrating an inflow left ventricular-assist devices cannula at the left ventricular apex (*arrow*). (**B**) transesophageal long axis view of the left ventricle demonstrating unobstructed flow into the left ventricular-assist devices cannula on color Doppler (*arrow*). *Abbreviations:* LA, left atrium; LV, left ventricle.

CLINICAL UTILITY

Although echocardiography has been incorporated into the diagnostic algorithm of patients with suspected acute IE, systematic usage in clinical practice remains ill-defined. The low cost and wide availability of TTE can lead to the potential for overuse in patients with bacteremia.

Based on major and minor clinical and laboratory criteria, Jassal et al. have classified patients with suspected native valve IE as high likelihood (two major or one major and three minor), moderate likelihood (one major or three minor) or low likelihood of having the disease (Table 1) (57). In patients with a high clinical likelihood of infective endocarditis, the practical role of TTE for diagnostic purposes is low. In the same context, echocardiography is often requested for patients with transient fever, a nonregurgitant murmur, or both who have a very low likelihood for the disease, with low diagnostic yield (5,57,58).

Strict adherence to indications for TTE and TEE may help to facilitate more accurate diagnosis in those patients with moderate likelihood of the disease (57). Any patient suspected of having IE by clinical criteria should be screened by TTE. When the images are of good quality and the study is negative, an alternative

TABLE 1 Integrating Clinical and Laboratory Data for Rational Use of Echocardiography in Patients with Suspected Native Valve Infective Endocarditis

---

Clinical criteria for diagnosis of infective endocarditis (adapting Duke Criteria)
Major criteria
Positive blood cultures for infective endocaritis:
  Typical microorganisms for infective endocarditis, including viridans strep, *Streptococcus bovis*, HACEK (*Hemophilus* spp., *Actinobacillus* spp., *Cardiobacterium hominis*, *Eikenella corrodens*, and *Kingella kingii*), or community-acquired *Staphylococcus aureus* or enterococcus OR
  Microorganisms from persistent positive blood cultures, at least two positive cultures drawn >12 hours apart
Evidence of endocardial involvement:
  New valvular regurgitation on clinical exam (worsening or changing of pre-existing murmur not sufficient)
Minor criteria
Predisposition: predisposing heart condition or intravenous drug use
Fever: temperature >38°C on two separate occasions
Vascular phenomena: major arterial emboli, septic pulmonary infarcts, mycotic aneurysms, intracranial hemorrhage, conjunctival hemorrhages, Janeway lesions
Immunological phenomenon: glomerulonephritis, Osler's nodes, Roth's spots, and rheumatoid arthritis
Microbiological evidence: positive blood cultures but do not a meet a major criteria as defined before
Serological evidence of active infection with organism consistent with endocarditis
  High likelihood: two major or one major and three minor clinical criteria
  — Transthoracic (TTE) and transesophageal echocardiography (TEE) to assess prognosis or complications
  Moderate likelihood: one major or three minor clinical criteria
  — TTE as initial test. If the echo is positive, then treat appropriately
  — TEE if the patient has high-risk echocardiographic features on TTE or if clinical suspicion remains after negative or nondiagnostic TTE
  Low likelihood: firm alternative diagnosis
  — No echocardiography for diagnosis. Look for and treat alternative diagnosis

---

Source: From Ref. 57.

diagnosis should be sought if the clinical suspicion is low. If on the other hand, the clinical suspicion is high, TEE should be performed. TEE should also be performed in those in whom the results of the TTE are equivocal owing to structural abnormalities or poor acoustic window and yet clinical suspicion is moderate to high. In this situation, if TEE is initially negative, a re-evaluation of the clinical data is warranted and a repeat TEE in 7 to 10 days might be necessary if the clinical suspicion remains moderate to high (57). In Table 1, an algorithm for the appropriate use of echocardiography in patients with varying clinical likelihoods of endocarditis is presented.

SUMMARY

IE continues to be a diagnostic and therapeutic challenge. Echocardiography plays a key role in the diagnosis, management, and prognosis of these patients.

REFERENCES

1. Bayer AS, Bolger AF, Taubert KA, et al. Diagnosis and management of infective endocarditis and its complications. Circulation 1998; 98:2936–2948.
2. Evangelista A, Gonzalez-Alujas. Echocardiography in infective endocardits. Heart 2004; 90:614–617.
3. Durack DT, Lukes AS, Bright DK, et al. New criteria for diagnosis of infective endocarditis: utilization of specific echocardiographic findings. Duke Endocarditis Service. Am J Med 1994; 96:200–209.
4. Dillon JC, Feigenbaum H, Konecke LL, et al. Echocardiographic manifestations of valvular vegetations. Am Heart J 1973; 86(5):698–704.
5. Baddour LM, Bettmann MA, Bolger AF, et al. Nonvalvular cardiovascular device-related infections. Circulation 2003; 108:2015–2031.
6. Pelletier LL Jr, Petersdorf RG. Infective endocarditis: a review of 125 cases from the University of Washington hospitals, 1963–1972. Medicine (Baltimore) 1977; 56:287–313.
7. Von Reyn CF, Levy BS, Arbeit RD, et al. Infective endocaridits: an analysis based on strict case definitions. Ann Intern Med 1981; 94:505–518.
8. Lukes AS, Bright DK, Durack DT, et al. Diagnosis of infective endocarditis. Infect Dis Clin North Am 1993; 7:1–8.
9. Murphy JG, Foster-Smith KF. Management of complications of infective endocarditis with emphasis on echocardiographic findings. Infect Dis Clin North Am 1993; 7:153–156.
10. Yvorchuk KJ, Chan KL. Application of transthoracic and transesophageal echocardiography in the diagnosis and management of infective endocarditis. J Am Soc Echocardiogr 1994; 14:294–308.
11. Pierrotii LC, Baddour LM. Fungal endocarditis, 1995–2000. Chest 2002; 122(1):302–310.
12. Hecht SR, Berger M. Right-sided endocarditis in intravenous drug users: prognostic features in 102 episodes. Ann Intern Med 1992; 117:560–566.
13. Shively BK, Gurule FT, Roldan CA, et al. Diagnostic value of transesophageal compared with transthoracic echocardiography in infective endocarditis. J Am Coll Cardiol 1991; 18:391–397.
14. Pedersen WR, Walker M, Olson JD, et al. Value of transesophageal echocardiography as an adjunct to transthoracic echocardiography in evaluation of native and prosthetic valve endocarditis. Chest 1991; 100:351–366.
15. Shapiro SM, Young E, DeGuzman, et al. Transesophageal echocardiography in diagnosis of infective endocarditis. Chest 1994; 105:377–382.
16. Birmingham GD, Rahko PS, Ballantyne F. Improved detection of infective endocarditis with transesophageal echocardiography. Am Heart J 1992; 123:774–781.
17. Cheitlin MD, Alpert JS, Armstrong WF, et al. ACC/AHA guidelines for the clinical application of echocardiography: a report of the American College of Cardiology/American Heart Association task force on practice guidelines (committee on clinical application

of echocardiography) developed in collaboration with the American Society of Echocardiography. Circulation 1997; 95:1686–74.

18. Sanfillipo A, Picard M, Newell J, et al. Echocardiographic assessment of patients with infectious endocarditis: predictions of risk for complications. J Am Coll Cardiol 1991; 18:1191–1199.

19. Heinle S, Wilderman N, Harrison K, et al. Value of transthoracic echocardiography in predicting embolic events in active infective endocarditis. Am J Cardiol 1994; 74:799–801.

20. Tischler M, Vaitkus P. The ability of vegetation size on echocardiography to predict complications: a meta-analysis. J Am Soc Echo 1997; 10:562–568.

21. Sachdev M, Peterson GE, Jollis JG. Imaging techniques for diagnosis of infective endocarditis. Cardiol Clin 2003; 21:185–195.

22. San Roman JA, Vilacosta I, Zamorano JL, et al. Transesophageal echocardiography in right-sided endocarditis. J Am Coll Cardiol 1993; 21:1226–1230.

23. Jassal DS, Chiasson M, Rajda M, et al. Isolated pulmonic valve endocarditis. Can J Cardiol 2005; 21(4):365–366.

24. Rowley KM, Clubb KS, Walker Smith GJ, et al. Right-sided infective endocarditis as a consequence of flow-directed pulmonary-artery catheterization. N Engl J Med 1984; 311:1152–1156.

25. Shapiro SM, Young E, Ginzton LE, et al. Pulmonic valve endocarditis as an underdiagnosed disease: role of transesophageal echocardiography. J Am Soc Echocardiogr 1992; 5:48–51.

26. Daniel WG, Mugge A, Grote J, et al. Comparison of transthoracic and transesophageal echocardiography for the detection of abnormalities of prosthetic and bioprosthetic valves in the mitral and aortic positions. Am J Cardiol 1993; 71:210–215.

27. Alam M, Rossman HS, Sun I. Transesophageal echocardiographic evaluation of St. Jude Medical and bioprosthetic valve endocarditis. Am Heart J 1992; 123:236–239.

28. Zogbhi WA, Enriquez-Sorano M, Foster E, et al. Recommendations for evaluation for the severity of native valvular regurgitation with two-dimensional and Doppler echocardiography. J Am Soc Echocardiogr 2003; 16:777–802.

29. Leung DY, Cranney GB, Hopkins AP, et al. Role of transesophageal echocardiography in the diagnosis and management of aortic root abscess. Br Heart J 1994; 72:175–181.

30. Vuille C, Nidorf M, Weyman, et al. Natural history of vegetations during successful medical treatment of endocarditis. Am Heart J 1994; 128:(6 Pt 1):1200–1209.

31. Chan KL. Early clinical course and long-term outcome of patients with infective endocarditis complicated by perivalvular abscess. Can Med Assoc J 2002; 167:19–24.

32. Rose EA, Geligns AC, Moskowitz AJ, et al. Long-term use of a left-ventricular assist device for end-stage heart failure. New Engl J Med 2001; 345:1435–1443.

33. Arber N, Pras E, Copperman Y, et al. Pacemaker endocarditis: report of 44 cases and review of the literature. Medicine 1994; 73:288–305.

34. Schwartz IS, Pervez N. Bacterial endocarditis associated with a permanent transvenous cardiac pacemaker. JAMA 1971; 218:736–737.

35. Corman LC, Levison ME. Sustained bacteremia and transvenous cardiac pacemakers. JAMA 1975; 233:264–266.

36. Klug D, Lacroix D, Savoye C, et al. Systemic infection related to endocarditis on pacemaker leads: clinical presentation and management. Circulation 1997; 95:2098–2107.

37. Duval X, Selton-Suty C, Alla F, et al. Endocarditis in patients with a permanent pacemaker: a 1-year epidemiological survey on infective endocarditis due to valvular and/or pacemaker infection. CID 2004; 39:69–74.

38. Tighe DA, Tejada LA, Kirchhoffer JB, et al. Pacemaker lead infection: detection by multiplane transesophageal echocardiography. Am Heart J 1996; 131:616–618.

39. Vilacosta I, Sarria C, Roman JA, et al. Usefulness of transesophageal echocardiography for diagnosis of infected transvenous permanent pacemakers. Circulation 1994; 89: 2684–2687.

40. Chua JD, Wilkhoff BL, Lee I, et al. Diagnosis and management of infections involving implantable electrophysiologic cardiac devices. Ann Intern Med 2000; 133:604–608.

41. Chamis AL, Peterson GE, Cabell CH, et al. *Staphylococcus aureus* bacteremia in patients with permanent pacemakers or implantable cardioverter-defibrillators. Circulation 2001; 104:1029–1033.

42. Caoub P, Leprince P, Nataf P, et al. Pacemaker infective endocarditis. Am J Cardiol 1998; 82:480–484.
43. Victor F, De Place C, Camus C, et al. Pacemaker lead infection: echocardiographic features, management and outcome. Heart 1999; 81:82–87.
44. Del Rio A, Anguera I, Miro JM, et al. Surgical treatment of pacemaker and defibrillator lead endocarditis. The impact of electrode lead extraction on outcome. Chest 2003; 124:1451–1459.
45. Bentall H, De Bono A. A technique for complete replacement of ascending aorta. Thorax 1968; 23:338–339.
46. Cabrol C, Pavie A, Gandjibakhch I, et al. Complete replacement of the ascending aorta with reimplantation of the coronary arteries. J Thorac Cariovasc Surg 1981; 8:309–315.
47. Dent J, Kaul S. Utility of tranesophageal echocardiography in the diagnosis of aortic conduit endocarditis in patients who have undergone the Cabrol procedure. J Am Soc Echocardiogr 1992; 5:434–436.
48. Sievert H, Babic UU, Hausdorf G, et al. Transcatheter closure of atrial septal defect and patent formane ovale with the ASDOS device (a multi-institutional European trial). Am J Cardiol 1998; 82:1405–1413.
49. Bullock AM, Menahem S, Wilkinson JL. Infective endocarditis on an occluder closing an atrial septal defect. Cardiol Young 1999; 9:65–67.
50. Goldstein JA, Beardslee MA, Xu H, et al. Infective endocarditis resulting from cardioSEAL closure of a patent foramen ovale. Catheter Cardiovasc Interv 2002; 55:217–220.
51. Balasundaram RP, Anadaraja S, Juneja R, et al. Infective endocarditis following implantation of Amplatzer atrial septal occluder. Indian Heart J 2005; 57:167–169.
52. Dajani As, Taubert KA, Wilson W, et al. Prevention of bacterial endocarditis. Recommendations by the American Heart Association. JAMA 1997; 277:1794–1801.
53. Radovancevic B, Vrtovec B, Frazier OH. Left ventricular assist devices: an alternative to medical therapy for end-stage heart failure. Curr Opin Cardiol 2003; 18(3):210–214.
54. Holman WL, Pambouskian SV, Blood M, et al. Managing device infections: are we progressing or is infection an insurmountable obstacle? ASAIO J 2005; 51(4):452–455.
55. Holman WL, Park SJ, Long JW, et al. Infection in permanent circulatory support: experience from the REMATCH trial. J Heart Lung Transplant 2004; 23(12):1359–1365.
56. Karchmer AW, Longworth DL. Infections of intracardiac devices. Cardiol Clin 2003; 21:253–271.
57. Jassal DS, Lee C, Silversides C, et al. Can structured clinical assessment using a modified Duke's criteria improve appropriate use of echocardiography in patients with suspected infective endocarditis? Can J Cardiol 2003; 19(8):1017–1022.
58. Jassal DS, Hassan A, Buth KJ, et al. Surgical management of infective endocarditis. J Heart Val Dis 2006; 15:115–121.

14

Medical Management

John L. Brusch

Harvard Medical School and Department of Medicine and Infectious Disease Service, Cambridge Health Alliance, Cambridge, Massachusetts, U.S.A.

INTRODUCTION

There has been no other bacterial infection, with the exception of bacterial meningitis, whose clinical course has been so favorably altered by the availability of antimicrobial agents than that of infective endocarditis (IE). This disease was always fatal, although the patient could live well beyond a year with untreated subacute IE, (1). Antistreptococcal vaccines and various types of dyes (gentian violet) were unsuccessfully employed. The availability of the first sulfonamide, sulfanilamide, in 1936 marked the beginning of the modern antimicrobial era. Although it had impressive results against many types of infections, it had little effect on IE. By administering penicillin, the physician, who used to be a mere observer of the inevitable, was able to cure 90% of cases of streptococcal IE. This chapter focuses both on the principles and specifics of the antibiotic management of the various types of IE. The therapeutic precepts of antibiotic management of IE have been slowly, and sometimes painfully, accrued over the decades. The rules are constantly evolving with the availability of newer types of intravascular and intracardiac devices, more potent immunosuppressive agents, and newer classes of antibiotics.

Before the hostile nature of the infected vegetation to antibiotics was fully understood, it was observed that 20% of patients with *Streptococcus viridans* relapsed when penicillin was given for 14 days. This occurred despite the exquisite sensitivity of the streptococcus to penicillin in vitro. There was no relapse of patients who had received 30 days of the antibiotic (2,3).

When the tetracyclines and chloramphenicol became available in the early 1950s, they were used singly or together with penicillin to treat subacute IE. When used alone, there was marked symptomatic improvement of the patient, but a very high rate of relapse when the agent was stopped. It became clear that they interfered with the cure rate of penicillin. The time-kill curves in rabbits demonstrated that chloramphenicol interferes with the rate of killing (bactericidal effect) of *S. viridans* by penicillin (4,5).

The explanation for these observations was provided in 1972 by Durack and Beeson in their landmark studies of the pathogenesis of bacterial endocarditis (6,7). These investigators established the incredible intravegetation density of bacteria that ranges from 10^9 to 10^{10} colony forming units (CFU)/g. Not only did the pathogens exist in great numbers, but they were also in a markedly reduced metabolic and reproductive state, as determined by the decreased uptake of l-alanine into the bacterial walls. Their indolent condition makes them less susceptible to the bactericidal agents that have their peak effect on actively replicating bacteria. Morphological changes may also occur in the bacteria deep within the vegetation. Under these conditions, they may produce exopolysaccharides that may act as an additional barrier to the movement of penicillin into the cell wall (8,9).

The vegetation of subacute IE contains a cellular reaction of primarily mononuclear cells, lymphocytes, and histiocytes. The fibrin meshwork of the thrombus interferes with their migration and phagocytic functions of the few polymorphonuclear leukocytes that are present in the vegetation (10). Under such conditions, it is understandable why bactericidal drugs are required to sterilize the vegetation. The failure of bacteriostatic antibiotics is apparent by a very high rate of relapse or by initial unresponsiveness of the valvular infection. Relapse is often associated with the development of resistance to clindamycin or to the macrolides (11,12). In the present time, linezolid and quinpristin/dalfopristin appear to be the first exceptions to the necessity of using only bactericidal drugs to treat IE.

For almost 70 years, it has been appreciated that the ability of antimicrobial agents to cure IE is greatly dependent on their ability to achieve therapeutic levels within the thrombus. The ineffectiveness of sulfonamides is not only attributed to their bacteriostatic nature but also to their poor penetration of the vegetation (13,14). The measurement of the minimal inhibitory concentration (MIC) and minimal bactericidal concentration (MBC) may not be indicative of the concentration of the antibiotic that is needed to inhibit or kill the pathogens within the vegetation. In one experimental model, the concentration of ceftriaxone needed to sterilize the vegetation of the infecting *Escherichia coli* was 220 times greater than the MBC of that drug in broth (15).

There is very limited data available of antibiotic concentrations within human valvular vegetations obtained at surgery (16). The results indicate that there is close approximation of antibiotic levels in serum, in valvular tissue, and in the vegetation. To overcome the inherent difficulties and limitations of human tissue levels, several experimental systems have been developed. Weinstein et al. developed a rabbit model to study the penetration of various antibiotics into a fibrin thrombus that had been implanted subcutaneously (17,18). There was a delay documented in the movement of the drug between the bloodstream and the clot. The penetration of the compound was inversely proportional to its degree of protein binding, and directly proportional to its peak level in serum. A significant criticism of this model was that it was not designed to detect any uneven distribution of the antibiotic within the fibrin clot.

Other models were developed that were based on studying the pharmacokinetics of various types of antibiotics in valvular vegetations induced in rabbits (19,20). As opposed to the aforementioned model, the penetration of various antimicrobial agents into the thrombi was not delayed. Infection actually promoted their entry into the clot. The conclusion was that antibiotic penetration was not a major impediment to sterilizing the vegetations of IE.

Cremieux and Carbon studied the distribution of antibiotics within cardiac vegetations by means of autoradiographic techniques (21). This model identified three patterns of penetration: (*i*) that which was limited to the periphery of the fibrin clot; (*ii*) that which progressively penetrated from the periphery to the core of the thrombus; and (*iii*) that which resulted in a homogeneous distribution. The specific determinants of these patterns were unable to be identified. The highly protein-bound antibiotics, ceftriaxone and teicoplanin, possessed limited penetration. Another highly protein-bound compound, daptomycin, moved into the surface of the clot quite readily but not into its center. This was felt due to its preferential binding to a protein within the external layering of the fibrin matrix (22,22a). This concentration gradient correlated with increased bacterial survival at the core. The concentration of organisms in the interior differed from those in the periphery by as much as log 10 CFU/g. Additionally, there were significant ultrastructural morphological differences between the bacteria found in these two areas.

Another significant variable in the performance of an antibiotic within the vegetation is its degree of postantibiotic effect (PAE). It is the term that describes the continued suppression of bacterial multiplication after the level of the antibiotic falls below the MIC of the agent (23,24). The PAE is both bacteria- and antibiotic-specific. The aminoglycosides, fluoroquinolones, and tetracyclines exhibit this effect against many gram negatives. The duration of the PAE for gram negatives ranges from two to six hours. The beta-lactam drugs, with the exception of imipenem, do not exhibit this effect against the gram negatives. They do have an abbreviated PAE (less than two hours) against many gram positives. This effect is not just an in vitro phenomenon. The PAE does appear to have biological validity, as demonstrated in various animal models of IE. The most important determinants of the PAE are the concentration of the antimicrobial agent and the length of time that the organism is exposed to it. Other contributing factors are the pH of the environment and combinations of antibiotics. The mechanism has not been well-established. It does not appear to be the result of residual antibiotic, but may be attributed to sublethal damage produced by the agent. When the PAE is absent, as in the case of a beta-lactam drug treating a gram-negative urinary tract infection, the concentration of the antibiotic must remain always above its MIC in order to suppress the growth of the pathogen. One cannot simply apply the in vitro measurements of PAE to a specific patient. For example, the duration of the PAE of imipenem, observed during the treatment of *Pseudomonas aeruginosa* IE in rats, is significantly decreased by the same mechanisms that influence the MIC of the same antibiotic. The aminoglycosides may be less affected in this situation than the beta-lactams (25,26).

In IE, the goal of therapy is to achieve a level of antibiotic that remains within the vegetation long enough to eradicate the infection within the thrombus. The dosing schedules of treating the various types of organisms associated with IE are based on a combination of clinical observation, experimental models, and pharmacokinetic values derived from humans and animals. Barza et al. observed that a given amount of an antimicrobial agent, administered by bolus, produces higher levels in the vegetation than does the same amount given continuously by drip (17). The optimum dosing interval of antibiotics, used in the treatment of IE has not been well-established for many of those most commonly used. One model of *Staphylococcus aureus* IE demonstrated that methicillin, given every four to eight hours, resulted in the best outcomes. The same daily dosage of methicillin was completely ineffective if administered every 12 hours (27). This same system affirmed the data of Barza that a bolus infusion was therapeutically superior to a continuous one. The optimum dosage interval is primarily dependent on three variables: (*i*) the duration of time during which serum levels of the antibiotic are higher than the MBC; (*ii*) the duration of the PAE; and (*iii*) the value of 1 "log growth time." The dosage interval of beta-lactam drugs must be increased in the elderly because of age-related dysfunction of the renal tubules.

Quite early in the antibiotic era, it was established that four weeks of penicillin treatment of *S. viridans* IE achieved 100% cure without relapses. The results of two weeks of penicillin therapy fell far short of this (see earlier for details) (2,3). Only when a two-week regimen of penicillin is combined with streptomycin does the cure and relapse rate approximate that of four weeks of penicillin alone (28). For most organisms and most types of antibiotics, four weeks of therapy is more than adequate. The major exceptions are prosthetic valve endocarditis (PVE) (Chapter 9 and Chapter 15); fungal IE; multiply resistant and other types of micro-organisms, especially when they are associated with metastatic infection. There is a growing tendency to prolong the course of uncomplicated IE on the basis of "more may be better," with little risk to the patient. The author's experience indicates otherwise. A good example of this is the case of the patient who was a good response treated for streptococcal endocarditis one month with. However, penicillin was continued for six weeks. During this therapeutic extension, the patients became superinfected with a mixture of *P. aeruginosa* and other gram-negative bacteria (29).

Orally administered penicillin, in combination with streptomycin has been documented to cure streptococcal IE (21,30). It is the author's belief that the intravenous route of administration for most types of antibiotics, used for the treatment of IE, is mandatory. The oral route often results in serum concentrations of antimicrobials that are subtherapeutic and may vary day-to-day. This is true both in normal healthy volunteers and in those who are ill. Additionally, the gastrointestinal symptoms of oral antibiotics may well contribute to a high degree of noncompliance. Giving antibiotics by mouth does not appear to lessen many of their complications, especially that of suprainfection, which occurs at a rate quite similar to that of intravenously administered compounds (31).

In the treatment of bacterial valvular infection, the MIC and MBC must be determined for the usual panel of antimicrobial agents used against the isolated pathogen. The Kirby Bauer agar diffusion disc tests offer only quantitative and not qualitative sensitivity information. The Schlicter test or serum bactericidal test (SBT) was the first in-vitro approach to determine the effectiveness of an antibiotic regimen in the management of IE (32). The SBT measures the greatest dilution of the peak and trough levels in the serum of an antibiotic against a standard concentration of the infecting organism. It is not clear whether the determination of the peak or trough SBT is more valid. This uncertainty is attributed to the lack of standardization of the inoculum and the diminution of the protein-binding effect, when the antibiotic is diluted in either serum or broth (33). Both a peak SBT 1/64 and a trough value of 1/32 are predictive of clinical success. Failure to achieve these levels does not make either clinical or microbiological failure inevitable. Aiming to achieve levels of 1/64–1/32 may pose a significant risk of ototoxicity and nephrotoxicity. There is little correlation between the SBT and the bactericidal concentration of the antibiotic in the vegetation of animals (34). The SBT is not useful in measuring the therapeutic efficacy of various combinations of antibiotics. For example, pairing gentamicin with ceftriaxone may decrease the concentration of the aminoglycosides to a level below that which is required to produce synergy. The presence of synergistic combinations is best documented by the determination of "killing curves."

The SBT test should be primarily used in patients with: (*i*) a poor clinical response to apparently appropriate therapy; (*ii*) IE caused by unusual pathogens; and (*iii*) a change in the route of administration of the antibiotic (35). In all patients, blood cultures should be drawn several days in the therapy to insure clearance of the bloodstream infections (BSI). Table 1 presents the essential principles of antibiotic therapy of IE.

EXTRA-HOSPITAL TREATMENT OF INFECTIVE ENDOCARDITIS

Three to fourteen percent of cases of IE are managed outside the hospital for at least some part of their entire antibiotic course (36,37). In 1993, Durack predicted that up to 50% of patients with IE would be treated with outpatient parenteral antimicrobial therapy (OPAT) (38). It can be delivered at home or at an infusion center. With the rise of *S. aureus* endocarditis and its associated complications, it is unlikely that

TABLE 1 Basic Principles of Antibiotic Therapy of Infective Endocarditis

The necessity of using bactericidal antibiotics because of the "hostile" environment of the infected vegetation[a].

The MIC and MBC of the administered antibiotic against the isolated pathogen needs to be determined in order to insure adequate dosing of the agent.

Generally, intermittent dosing of an antibiotic provides superior penetration of the thrombus as compared with a continuous infusion. Its penetration into the tissue is directly related to its peak level in serum.

All patients with infective endocarditis should be treated in a healthcare facility for the first 1–2 weeks to monitor their hemodynamic stability.

In cases of potential acute infective endocarditis, antibiotic therapy should be started immediately after 3–5 sets of blood cultures have been drawn. Preferably all of them should be obtained within 1–2 hours, so as to allow the expeditious commencement of antibiotic therapy.

The selection of antibiotic/antibiotics needs to be made empirically on the basis of physical examination and clinical history.

In cases of potential subacute infective endocarditis, antibiotic treatment should not be started until the final culture and sensitivity data are available. A delay of 1–2 weeks in doing so does not adversely affect the final outcome.

The usual duration of therapy ranges from 4 to 6 weeks. A 4-week course is appropriate for an uncomplicated case of native valve endocarditis. A shorter course of 2 weeks may be appropriate in certain cases (see text). Six weeks are required for the treatment of prosthetic valve endocarditis, and in those infections with large vegetations, such as those associated with infection by members of the HACEK family.

[a]Linezolid and quintristin/dalfopristin appear to be exceptions to this principle.
Abbreviations: HACEK, *Hemophilus* spp., *Actinobacillus* spp., *Cardiobacterium hominis*, *Eikenella corrodens*, and *Kingella kingii*; MBC, minimal bactericidal concentration; MIC, minimal inhibitory concentration.

there would be such an increase in extra-hospital care. As discussed in Chapter 11, many of the same complications of antibiotic administration, which occur in the hospital, take place in other venues too. However, for the well-selected patient, management of IE outside the hospital offers tremendous economic, psychological, and social advantages. The development of various types of ambulatory infusion devices, and the availability of antibiotics, which require once-a-day dosing, have helped make home infusions practical (39). The penicillins and most of the cephalosporins require multiple daily dosing to achieve maximum therapeutic levels. Once-a-day antimicrobial agents that are suitable for the treatment of IE include the aminoglycosides, ceftriaxone, ertapenem, many of the quinolones, daptomycin, vancomycin, amphotericin, and caspofungin. Before the availability of antibiotics with long half-lives, outpatient therapy of IE was limited to those drugs that could be administered orally. This restricted outpatient therapy appropriate for penicillin sensitive strains of *S. viridans*. The case reports that orally administered linezolid has cured IE in certain cases has made outpatient therapy potentially even more accessible (40). Another desirable quality in an agent being considered for OPAT is the lack of the need for its serum levels to be measured for monitoring whether they are therapeutically adequate and/or potentially toxic. In most situations, the aminoglycosides are not good candidates for home administration for both these reasons (41). The clinician needs regularly obtained and promptly reported results of the aminoglycoside and the serum levels in order to prevent nephrotoxicity. This is just not feasible to be achieved always. A possible exception might be the case when gentamicin is given in synergistic and not therapeutic doses. Because the amount of antibiotic administered is significantly less, there is probably lesser toxicity threat.

Candidates for home therapy must be carefully evaluated. They must be in stable physical and mental health, and have the capacity to learn self-administration of the drug. There must be another responsible person in the home setting to monitor the patient for a consequence of IE, such as a stroke. For obvious reasons, the patient must have no history of intravenous drug abuse (IVDA). In addition, candidates for OPAT must be stable cardiovascularwise without any degree of cardiac failure. They should not be considered potential candidates for possible imminent valvular surgery or drainage of a paravalvular abscess (38,42–45). Outpatient parenteral antimicrobial therapy should be considered for uncomplicated cases of left-sided IE that are attributed to susceptible micro-organisms. Even these patients should be hospitalized during the first weeks of therapy when the greatest amount of life-threatening complications are expected to occur. Outpatient parenteral antimicrobial therapy then serves as the continuation phase of their treatment. When these standards are met, extra-hospital therapy of IE, as compared with hospital therapy, is less costly, is well-tolerated by the patient, and has good clinical outcomes (46). Patients with right-sided IE can probably be discharged from the hospital in less than two weeks. Given the fact that most of these are IVDA, compliance with OPAT is a major issue, in addition to the risk of their using the intravascular access as a route of administration of recreational drugs. Oral antibiotic therapy of right-sided IVDA IE had some success with combinations of the quinolones and rifampin (47). The increase in methicillin-resistant *Staphylococcus aureus* (MRSA) made this option a less appealing one. Linezolid or a derivative antibiotic may be useful in this situation.

RESPONSE TO ANTIMICROBIAL CHEMOTHERAPY

The most important parameter to monitor during the initial treatment phase of IE is the response of the patient's temperature to the antibiotic regimen. Significant fever that persists for more than seven to ten days into the therapy should be of concern (48–53). Fifty to seventy-five percent of all patients become afebrile by the one-week mark of the initiation of antibiotic therapy. The response rate increases by another approximately 20% by the end of two weeks. A slower defervescence may indicate a less responsive organism, such as *S. aureus* or *P. aeruginosa*. Fifty percent of the patients with *S. viridans* IE became afebrile within seven days of treatment with penicillin gentamicin. The remainder did so by three weeks. This distribution would indicate a biphasic susceptibility of these isolates to antimicrobial agents. Persistent fever past three weeks is not an absolute indication for a change in the antimicrobial regimen. It does call for a complete reassessment of the patient's diagnosis and treatment. Thirty-three to forty-five percent of the cases with prolonged fever are attributed to intracardiac complications (paravalvular abscesses and myocardial abscesses). In some series, up to 28% are due to drug reactions (drug fever or drug toxicity to end organs) (50). The remainder consists of extracardiac complications (splenic absceses); mycotic aneurysms of the disease; nosocomial infections (complications of intravascular catheters) disease; complications of IVDA IE (pulmonary emboli, continued use of intravenous recreational drugs during hospitalization); *Clostridium difficile* colitis; suprainfections fungal and recurrent emboli from large valvular vegetations.

Blumberg reported on 36 patients with fever unresponsive to the administered antibiotic regimen despite favorable sensitivity tests (52). There was no relationship between the fever pattern and its cause. A thorough evaluation revealed several processes, including myocardial abscesses and large (>1 cm in diameter) friable vegetations. In three individuals, there was no other possible cause of continued fever than the valvular infection itself. These patients finally became afebrile after the involved valve was removed. In this series, cerebral mycotic aneurysms presented the most difficult diagnostic challenge. They are usually unrecognized prior to their rupture.

When fever persists despite what is apparently appropriate antibiotic therapy, blood cultures should be repeated to document that the BSI has cleared. Echocardiography should be obtained, initially a transthoracic echocardiogram (TTE). If this is not diagnostic, then a transesophageal echocardiogram (TTE) should be performed in order to visualize the most common cause of persistent fever, a suppurative intracardiac complication. Subsequently, extracardiac (mycotic aneurysms), nosocomial (line-related and *C. difficile* colitis), splenic abscesses, and unrelated causes should be searched for. Drug fever, in reality, is a diagnosis of exclusion. Very rarely does it present itself with eosinophilia. Leukocytosis or a shift to the left is inconsistent with a benign drug fever.

MORTALITY OF INFECTIVE ENDOCARDITIS

In 1992, Mansur reviewed 300 episodes of IE in 227 patients, which occurred between 1978 and 1986 (54). Two-thirds of these cases had significant complications when on antibiotic therapy. This was true for individuals with native or prosthetic valve infections. These investigators postulated that undesirable outcomes in IE were related to increase in complications. They defined these as embolic, cardiac, and immunological. Their appearance was not necessarily associated with the microbiological course of the valvular infection. Cardiac failure developed in one-third of the patients. This is consistent with other studies that estimate that congestive failure is present in 15–65% of the patients (55). This report documents that congestive heart failure is less often a cause of death than it was in the past. Formerly, cardiac decompensation was the leading cause of death (56). This diminution is most likely the result of the current aggressiveness in diagnosis and surgical correction of valvular decompensation at a relatively early stage. The central nervous system was the second most frequent site of infection with mycotic aneurysms and cerebral absceses. The valve IE and prosthetic valve IE had identical rates of cerebral embolism and intracerebral mycotic aneurysms. Twenty-one percent of patients had the sepsis syndrome, with *S. aureus* being the most commonly associated organism. Drug reactions occurred in 14% of patients. Although cardiac complications were reported more frequently, death most often occured in those with cerebral involvement or sepsis. This is understandable in light of the difficulty in diagnosing cerebral infections in IE, especially mycotic aneurysms, and the high mortality rate of sepsis owing to any cause. The mortality rate in IE of intracranial mycotic aneurysms approaches 60%. If detected prior to rupture, this figure is 30%. After their rupture, mortality is at least 80%. Mycotic aneurysms of the cerebral vessels develop in 2–10% of patients with IE (57,58). Cerebral angiography is the diagnostic modality of choice. However, it is hard to justify its use as a screening test in every patient with IE. Magnetic resonance imaging (MRI) appears promising in this role. Table 2 presents the mortality rates among patients with native IE due to various organisms (59). Mortality of individuals, who require cardiac surgery is presented in Chapter 15.

In a recent retrospective study of patients with left-sided native valve endocarditis, the overall rate of death was 25% (49). The investigators identified five

TABLE 2   Mortality Rates of Left-Sided Native Valve Infective Endocarditis
Due to Various Organisms

Organism	Mortality rates (%)
Streptococcus viridans and Streptococcus bovis	4–16
Enterococci	15–25
Staphylococcus aureus	25–47
Groups B, C, G streptococci	13–50
Coxiella burnetti	5–37
Pseudomonas aeruginosa, Enterobacteriaceae, fungi	>50

Source: From Ref. 59.

independent mortality risk factors to which they gave a weighted score (Table 3). Prediction of the six-month mortality can be calculated from the total score of the risk factors (Table 4). The validity of this model has been verified.

The mortality rate of PVE, prior to 1980, was 70% and 45% for early and late types, respectively. With the recognition that aggressive surgery is necessary in most cases of PVE, mortality has decreased to between 15% and 25%, with no relationship to whether the infection is of early or late onset (60). The role of surgery is more thoroughly discussed in Chapter 15.

RELAPSE AND RECURRENCE OF INFECTIVE ENDOCARDITIS

Relapse of IE usually occurs approximately two months after the completion of the antibiotic course (61). The risk for relapse is highly associated with the specific pathogen. There appears to be no rate of relapse in patients with *S. viridans* IE, who have been treated with penicillin for four weeks (62). *Staphylococcus aureus* (4%); enterococci (8–20%), especially involving the mitral valve, gram negatives, especially *P. aeruginosa* and fungal infections have a higher rate of relapse and a much higher rate of initial therapeutic failures (4,59). Surgery for PVE does not seem to lessen the relapse rate. Overall, the relapse rate for PVE is 10%, and is 6% to 15% in surgical cases (63).

TABLE 3   Risk Factors for Death in Complicated Native Valve Endocarditis

Mortality risk factors	Weighted score
Abnormal mental status	4
Charlson comorbidity score of 2	3
Moderate to severe congestive heart failure	3
Non-*Streptococcus viridans* pathogens	6 for *Staphylococcus aureus*; 8 for other organisms
Medical therapy alone	5

TABLE 4   Calculation of Six-Month Mortality Due to Complicated
Left-Sided Native Valve Endocarditis

Total weighted score	Six-month mortality rate (%)
Equal to or less than 6 points	6
7–11 points	17
12–15 points	31
Greater than 15 points	63

processes, including myocardial abscesses and large (>1 cm in diameter) friable vegetations. In three individuals, there was no other possible cause of continued fever than the valvular infection itself. These patients finally became afebrile after the involved valve was removed. In this series, cerebral mycotic aneurysms presented the most difficult diagnostic challenge. They are usually unrecognized prior to their rupture.

When fever persists despite what is apparently appropriate antibiotic therapy, blood cultures should be repeated to document that the BSI has cleared. Echocardiography should be obtained, initially a transthoracic echocardiogram (TTE). If this is not diagnostic, then a transesophageal echocardiogram (TTE) should be performed in order to visualize the most common cause of persistent fever, a suppurative intracardiac complication. Subsequently, extracardiac (mycotic aneurysms), nosocomial (line-related and *C. difficile* colitis), splenic abscesses, and unrelated causes should be searched for. Drug fever, in reality, is a diagnosis of exclusion. Very rarely does it present itself with eosinophilia. Leukocytosis or a shift to the left is inconsistent with a benign drug fever.

MORTALITY OF INFECTIVE ENDOCARDITIS

In 1992, Mansur reviewed 300 episodes of IE in 227 patients, which occurred between 1978 and 1986 (54). Two-thirds of these cases had significant complications when on antibiotic therapy. This was true for individuals with native or prosthetic valve infections. These investigators postulated that undesirable outcomes in IE were related to increase in complications. They defined these as embolic, cardiac, and immunological. Their appearance was not necessarily associated with the microbiological course of the valvular infection. Cardiac failure developed in one-third of the patients. This is consistent with other studies that estimate that congestive failure is present in 15–65% of the patients (55). This report documents that congestive heart failure is less often a cause of death than it was in the past. Formerly, cardiac decompensation was the leading cause of death (56). This diminution is most likely the result of the current aggressiveness in diagnosis and surgical correction of valvular decompensation at a relatively early stage. The central nervous system was the second most frequent site of infection with mycotic aneurysms and cerebral absceses. The valve IE and prosthetic valve IE had identical rates of cerebral embolism and intracerebral mycotic aneurysms. Twenty-one percent of patients had the sepsis syndrome, with *S. aureus* being the most commonly associated organism. Drug reactions occurred in 14% of patients. Although cardiac complications were reported more frequently, death most often occured in those with cerebral involvement or sepsis. This is understandable in light of the difficulty in diagnosing cerebral infections in IE, especially mycotic aneurysms, and the high mortality rate of sepsis owing to any cause. The mortality rate in IE of intracranial mycotic aneurysms approaches 60%. If detected prior to rupture, this figure is 30%. After their rupture, mortality is at least 80%. Mycotic aneurysms of the cerebral vessels develop in 2–10% of patients with IE (57,58). Cerebral angiography is the diagnostic modality of choice. However, it is hard to justify its use as a screening test in every patient with IE. Magnetic resonance imaging (MRI) appears promising in this role. Table 2 presents the mortality rates among patients with native IE due to various organisms (59). Mortality of individuals, who require cardiac surgery is presented in Chapter 15.

In a recent retrospective study of patients with left-sided native valve endocarditis, the overall rate of death was 25% (49). The investigators identified five

TABLE 2   Mortality Rates of Left-Sided Native Valve Infective Endocarditis
Due to Various Organisms

Organism	Mortality rates (%)
Streptococcus viridans and Streptococcus bovis	4–16
Enterococci	15–25
Staphylococcus aureus	25–47
Groups B, C, G streptococci	13–50
Coxiella burnetti	5–37
Pseudomonas aeruginosa, Enterobacteriaceae, fungi	>50

Source: From Ref. 59.

independent mortality risk factors to which they gave a weighted score (Table 3). Prediction of the six-month mortality can be calculated from the total score of the risk factors (Table 4). The validity of this model has been verified.

The mortality rate of PVE, prior to 1980, was 70% and 45% for early and late types, respectively. With the recognition that aggressive surgery is necessary in most cases of PVE, mortality has decreased to between 15% and 25%, with no relationship to whether the infection is of early or late onset (60). The role of surgery is more thoroughly discussed in Chapter 15.

RELAPSE AND RECURRENCE OF INFECTIVE ENDOCARDITIS

Relapse of IE usually occurs approximately two months after the completion of the antibiotic course (61). The risk for relapse is highly associated with the specific pathogen. There appears to be no rate of relapse in patients with *S. viridans* IE, who have been treated with penicillin for four weeks (62). *Staphylococcus aureus* (4%); enterococci (8–20%), especially involving the mitral valve, gram negatives, especially *P. aeruginosa* and fungal infections have a higher rate of relapse and a much higher rate of initial therapeutic failures (4,59). Surgery for PVE does not seem to lessen the relapse rate. Overall, the relapse rate for PVE is 10%, and is 6% to 15% in surgical cases (63).

TABLE 3   Risk Factors for Death in Complicated Native Valve Endocarditis

Mortality risk factors	Weighted score
Abnormal mental status	4
Charlson comorbidity score of 2	3
Moderate to severe congestive heart failure	3
Non-*Streptococcus viridans* pathogens	6 for *Staphylococcus aureus*; 8 for other organisms
Medical therapy alone	5

TABLE 4   Calculation of Six-Month Mortality Due to Complicated
Left-Sided Native Valve Endocarditis

Total weighted score	Six-month mortality rate (%)
Equal to or less than 6 points	6
7–11 points	17
12–15 points	31
Greater than 15 points	63

Recurrence of non-IVDA IE is less than 10% (64,65). Less than 10% of previously infected prosthetic valves become reinfected (60). Congenital heart disease is the most frequent underlying disorder, followed by rheumatic heart disease and mitral valve prolapse, for the development of recurrent non-IVDA IE (66,67).

The use of illicit drugs is the greatest risk factor for recurrent IE; 40% of the cases of IVDA IE recur. A review of the overall cases of recurrent IE documented that reinfection was three times higher in men than in women. Forty-three percent of the total cases were attributed to the continued use of intravenous drugs. The interval between the episodes of endocarditis was less than the IVDA-initiated disease. In all types of the cases of recurrence, there was little association between the first and second pathogens, except among IVDA, where *S. aureus* predominates (68).

CARE AFTER COMPLETION OF ANTIBIOTIC THERAPY

For any patient with a past history of IE, three sets of blood cultures should be obtained before starting antibiotic therapy. The patient should be followed closely for evidence of congestive heart failure. Good oral hygiene practices should be followed, and antimicrobial prophylaxis should be given before invasive procedures (58).

TREATMENT OF SPECIFIC ORGANISMS
Non-Enterococcal Streptococcal Infective Endocarditis

The *S. viridans* group and *Streptococcus bovis* are responsible for up to 40% of all cases of native valve endocarditis (NVE). Most of these are quite sensitive to penicillin (MIC <0.12 µg/mL) (58). These organisms are characterized as intermediately sensitive to penicillin if their MIC is between 0.12 and 0.5 µg/mL (69,70). Highly penicillin-resistant organisms are those that have their MIC >0.5 µg /ml or >1 µg/ mL depending on the source. Moellering advocates for the latter value. High-grade resistance to penicillin appears to be to be the result of an alteration in the penicillin-binding protein (71). These categories of penicillin sensitivity do have clinical significance. Some 13.4% of blood culture isolates of *S. viridans* possess high-level resistance to penicillin, 17% of which are highly resistant to ceftriaxone (MIC >2 µg/ mL) (72). Prophylactic administration of penicillin appears to be a major cause of the development of high-grade resistance. Approximately 20% of the isolates of *S. viridans* are tolerant to penicillin. (73). Tolerance is a laboratory phenomenon in which the MBC of antibiotic exceeds its MIC by at least a factor of 10. Combining penicillin with an aminoglycoside leads to more effective killing in vitro of these tolerant strains.

Abiotrophia spp. (nutritionally variant streptococci) produce 5% to 10% of cases of IE that are caused by penicillin-sensitive streptococci (74). All isolates are tolerant to penicillin. The MIC for this organism is >1 µg/mL in 33% of patients (75). There is a higher mortality and relapse rate caused by these penicillin-resistant isolates (76). Third-generation cephalosporins and carbapenems are more active than penicillin. Infective carditis, due to these organisms, is treated in the same fashion as enterococcal valvular infections.

Streptococcus viridans are also sensitive to the cephalosporins, especially the third-generation cephalosporins and vancomycin (77). Ceftriaxone has become the most frequently used therapy against *S. viridans* IE because of the flexibility in its once-a-day administration. It may be given intravenously or a intramuscularly. Strains of *S. viridans* that are tolerant to penicillin and all *Abiotrophia* isolates should be treated with the combination of a beta-lactam antibiotic and synergistic doses of gentamicin. *Abiotrophia* spp. are equally tolerant to the cephalosporins (ceftriaxone), vancomycin, and amoxicillin (78). Strains of *S. viridans* that are highly resistant to penicillin are also resistant to ceftriaxone.

Aminoglycosides by themselves have no effect on *S. viridans*. The addition of either gentamicin, netilmicin, or streptomycin to a beta-lactam, most commonly ceftriaxone, results in synergy. Synergy is demonstrated, both in vitro and clinically, for sensitive, resistant, and tolerant strains of *S. viridans* and for the tolerant isolates of *Abiotrophia* spp. (79). *Streptococcus viridans*, which are highly resistant to penicillin, are often resistant to streptomycin and a kanamycin. Gentamicin appears to be of value in treating IE caused by *S. viridans* that is resistant to streptomycin and kanamycin, but sensitive to penicillin.

Currently, the most popular regimen against penicillin-sensitive streptococcal IE is ceftriaxone and gentamicin (69). This combination regimen makes it suitable for home infusion and enables a two-week course of therapy of uncomplicated IE owing to the sensitive *S. viridans* (80). Because of the ready availability of serum levels, gentamicin has become the preferred aminoglycoside. When it is combined with a beta-lactam for the purpose of a shorter course of therapy or for the treatment of tolerant or resistant *S. viridans*, it may be administered in once-a-day dosing (3 mg/kg) or in divided doses every eight or 12 hours. Once-a-day dosing of aminoglycosides has now become a recognized therapeutic option (58). Single daily dosing is more appropriate for home administration. Increased concentrations in serum of the aminoglycoside improves the killing rate of *S. viridans*. A high peak level in serum also leads to increased levels within the vegetation. Given once a day, gentamicin undergoes a washout period from the renal cortex. This regimen may also decrease the risk of nephrotoxicity (80,81,82). Generally, a four-week course of therapy is required in treating *S. viridans/S. bovis* IE. A two-week course is allowable under certain circumstances (Table 5).

In the past, Weinstein had treated all cases of *S. viridans* IE in nonallergic patients with penicillin alone. There were no treatment failures and no relapses within six months (83). With the development of more resistant or less sensitive *S. viridans* and *S. bovis*, the ability to use penicillin alone is quickly diminishing. In a sense, these gram-positive organisms are beginning to resemble enterococci in their sensitivity patterns. In an experimental model, the addition of gentamicin or streptomycin to the beta-lactam results in more rapid clearance from the infected vegetation (84). The treatment of *S. viridans*, highly resistant to penicillin (MIC >1 µg/mL, is problematic. The use of extraordinary doses of penicillin (36 million units per day for four weeks) combined with an aminoglycoside has had some success against some isolates. The addition of the aminoglycoside to penicillin has failed in others.

TABLE 5 Conditions Necessary for a Two-Week Teatment Course
of *Streptococcus viridans* or *Streptococcus bovis* IE with a Beta-Lactam
Antibiotic and an Aminoglycoside

Penicillin-sensitive isolates
Native valve endocarditis
Symptoms of infective endocarditis lasting less than 3 months
No intracardiac complications
No extracardiac involvement
Low risk of developing aminoglycoside associated ototoxicity or nephrotoxicity

Source: From Refs. 72, 82.

The use of glycopeptides against these strains has had the the must success (72). Linezolid is promising for the treatment of these isolates. The antibiotic sensitivity pattern of *S. bovis* closely resembles that of *S. viridans*. The MBC of penicillin against *S. bovis* is usually <0.2 µg/mL. The treatment regimens for *S. bovis* IE are the same as those for *S. viridans* (85).

In patients with minor allergic reactions, cephalosporins are a good alternative. Individuals with a history of serious allergic reactions (urticaria anaphylaxis) would benefit most from the administration of linezolid or vancomycin. Linezolid has not been recognized officially for this role. Unless one has experience, the author does not recommend sensitizing the patient because of the risks involved. Except for linezolid and quinpristin/dalfopristin, bacteriostatic antibiotics such as erythromycin or clindamycin should generally be avoided (see earlier discussion). On the basis of anecdotal evidence, erythromycin appears to be a more effective agent in the treatment of IE. Clindamycin should be considered a third-line antibiotic in treating valvular infections. It often fails to sterilize the vegetation and puts the patient at risk for the development of *C. difficile* colitis (86).

Group A streptococci remain quite sensitive to penicillin G. Infective endocarditis, caused by *Streptococcus pyogenes,* responds to intravenous penicillin alone (3 million units every four hours for four weeks) (87). Groups B, C, and G are less sensitive to penicllin than group A. It is advisable to treat these organisms with 20 million units of penicillin or 2 g of ceftriaxone daily for four to six weeks with the addition of gentamicin for the first two weeks (88).

Increasing isolates of *S. pneumoniae* (MIC of penicillin-sensitive pneumococci = 0.6 µg/mL) have become relatively (MIC 0.1–1.0 µg/mL) or highly resistant (MIC >2 µg/mL) to penicillin. Antibiotic regimens must be dependent on sensitivity testing. Treatment choices are also influenced by the fact whether meningitis is associated with the valvular infection or not (89,90). Penicillin-sensitive pneumococcal IE is treated with penicillin G with a dosage regime of four million units IV every four hours or ceftriaxone 2 g IV every 12 hours or cefotaxime for g IV every six hours, whether meningitis is present or not. These regimens remain the same for relatively penicillin-resistant isolates if meningitis is not present. For the treatment of relatively resistant pneumococcal IE, which is complicated by meningitis, and for all cases produced by highly resistant isolates, vancomycin is added to the cephalosporins. It has not been established whether the addition of an aminoglycoside to beta-lactam antibiotic or vancomycin has any beneficial effects in the treatment of pneumococcal IE with or without concurrent meningitis (72).

Table 6 presents the antibiotic regimens for the treatment of selected non-enterococcal streptococci. They are based on the the American Heart Association guidelines. These are quite similar to those of the British Society for Antimicrobial Chemotherapy and the European Society of Cardiology (91,92).

Enterococcal Infective Endocarditis

Enterococcus faecalis and *Enterococcus faecium* are the most clinically important of the 12 species of the genus, *Enterococcus,* accounting for 90% of enterococcal infections. They produce 87.5% and 12.5%, respectively, of cases of enterococcal endocarditis (93,94). Enterococci have presented significant problems in resistance since the beginning of the antibiotic era. They are intrinsically resistant to penicillins owing to their low-affinity binding proteins (95). Changes in these sites have been identified among people who had never been exposed to any antibiotics (96).

TABLE 6   Guidelines for Antimicrobial Therapy of Nonenterococcal Streptococcal Native Valve Infective Endocarditis[a]

Antibiotic	Dosage regimen
A. Penicillin-sensitive *Streptococcus viridans* and *Streptococcus bovis*[b]	
Penicillin G[1]	Penicillin G 20,000,000 U IV in 4 divided doses for 4 weeks
Penicillin G[1] and Gentamicin[c]	Penicillin 20,000,000 U IV in 4 divided doses for 2 weeks Gentamicin 3 mg/kg given q24 h as a single dose or in divided doses q8 h for 2 weeks (Ceftriaxone 2 g IV/IM for 4 weeks may be used in patients with mild reactions to penicillin).
or Ceftriaxone	Ceftriaxone 2 g IV/IM for 4 weeks (may be used in patients with mild reactions to penicillin)
B. Penicillin-resistant or tolerant S. viridans and S. bovis[b,d]	
Penicillin G[1] or Ceftriaxone	Penicillin G 24,000,000 U IV in 4 divided doses for 4 weeks and ceftriaxone 2 g IV/IM for 4 weeks
Gentamicin	Gentamicin 3 mg/kg given q24 h as a single dose or in divided doses q8 h for 2 weeks
C. Abiotrophia spp. and group B streptococci[b]	
Penicillin G[1] and Gentamicin	Penicillin G 20,000,000 U IV in 4 divided doses for 6 weeks Gentamicin 3 mg/kg given q24h as a single dose or in divided doses q8 h for 2 weeks

[1]Vancomycin 30 mg/kg IV q12 h in patients highly allergic to penicillin.
[a]For patients with normal renal function.
[b]See text for definition.
[c]Short-course therapy (see text).
[d]Regimen is appropriate for treatment of prosthetic valve endocarditis with penicillin-sensitive or resistant *S. viridans* or *S. bovis*.
Abbreviations: PO, postoral; IV, intravenous; IM, intramuscular.

Enterococcus faecium possesses both a more frequent and greater magnitude of resistance to the penicillins than does *E. faecalis*. It had been labeled the "nosocomial pathogen of the 1990s" (97). Although it did not live up to this prediction, falling behind the rapid rise of *S. aureus*, it remains a major challenge to the clinician. The MIC of penicillin/ampicillin for *E. faecalis* ranges from 1 to 4 µg/mL, whereas that for *E. faecium* lies between 16 and 64 µg/mL (95,98). One-third of *E. faecium* possesses an MIC for penicillin of >200. Enterococci are completely resistant to the cephalosporins.

The success rate of treating enterococcal IE with penicillin alone was <40%. Hunter, in 1947, documented that the combination of penicillin and streptomycin was curative in approximately 85% of cases (99). In 1971, Moellering published studies that elucidated the mechanism of synergy. The resistance of the enterococci to aminoglycosides is secondary to the inability of these antimicrobials to penetrate into the interior of the bacterial cell, and attach to the ribosomal target (99). Penicillin and other cell-wall active antibiotics facilitate the entry of the aminoglycoside by damaging the integrity bacteria's cell wall (100). It is the aminoglycosides that actually kill the enterococcus (101). Synergistic combinations have become the mainstay of the treatment of enterococcal IE. Ampicillin along with an aminoglycoside has become the most frequently used synergistic combination in the United States. This is attributed probably to both the relative unavailability of parenteral penicillin and the perception that ampicillin is significantly more effective against enterococcal strains, which is not the case. In reality, ampicillin in twofold dilution is more effective than penicillin G. This difference is not significant. Because of increased allergic reactions to ampicillin, the guidelines of the European Society of Cardiology recommend the use of penicillin G (8). Over time, these pathogens have developed resistance to one or more of the components of the synergistic pair.

Most of the enterococci are sensitive to vancomycin. The MBC of vancomycin is at least 10 times higher than the MIC. This gap in sensitivity makes vancomycin a bacteriostatic compound when used alone against enterococci. However, it is synergistic with the aminoglycosides (102).

Not all cell-wall active antibiotics are synergistically active with the aminoglycosides. The cephalosporins and the antistaphylococcal penicillins fail to do so when they are combined with an aminoglycoside (103). The contributing factors to this are: (*i*) their low intrinsic activity against the enterococci; (*ii*) their increased protein binding; and (*iii*) the presence of inactive metabolites (4). Those antibiotics, which interfere with bacterial protein synthesis (macrolides, chloramphenicol, and tetracyclines) are not synergistically active with the aminoglycosides.

In vitro, rifampin is quite active against enterococcal spp. When this agent is used alone, micro-organisms rapidly develop resistance. Another marked disadvantage of rifampin is that it antagonizes the action of ampicillin (4). Although enterococci appear sensitive to trimethoprim/sulfamethoxazole in vitro, this antimicrobial agent appears to have little effect in vivo. This is attributed to the fact that enterococci can make use of preformed folic acid from their host, unlike other bacteria (104).

Synergistic combinations have become the keystone of treatment of enterococcal IE. Development of resistance to any of the agents of the synergistic combination negates this theraputic approach. Over the last 20 years, several new patterns of enterococcal resistance have appeared. These include (*i*) high-level resistance to the aminoglycosides; (*ii*) non–penicillinase-mediated resistance to penicillins (MIC >128 µg/mL), (*iii*) penicillinase-mediated resistance; and (*iv*) vancomycin resistance (105).

In 1979, isolates of *E. faecalis*, highly resistant to the aminoglycoside, including kanamycin, amikacin, netilmicin, and most importantly gentamicin, were first identified (106). Up to 50% to 60% of nosocomial isolates of enterococci currently have high-grade resistance to gentamicin (107), which is attributed to plasmid-induced production of an enzyme with two functional regions that produce acetyltransferase and phosphotransferase. Twenty-five percent of the strains remain susceptible to streptomycin (105). In 1983, enterococcal strains, which show high-grade resistance to both gentamicin (MIC >500 µg/mL) and streptomycin (MIC >2000 µg/mL), were identified (108). Synergistic combinations simply do not exist for the treatment of these strains. Discussion of enterococcal resistance to other aminoglycosides is presented in an excellent review by Chow (109).

Enterococci have developed resistance to ampicillin and penicillin above their baseline level (MIC of ampicillin = 1–4 µg/mL; MIC of penicillin = 2–8 µg/mL). The mechanism involved in the case of *E. faecalis* is the production of penicillinase, similar to that of *S. aureus*, but in such smaller amounts that it is hard to detect by standard Kirby–Bauer techniques (110). These isolates are susceptible to the beta-lactamase inhibitor agents, such as ampicillin-sulbactam. Many of these are also resistant to gentamicin.

Enterococcus faecium has developed a marked increase in the MIC of ampicillin due to a nonpenicillinase mechanism, probably on the basis of an altered penicillin-binding protein (111). The MIC usually ranges from 8 to 32 µg/mL. Under these circumstances, the MIC may well exceed 256 µg/mL.

High-level enterococcal vancomycin resistance (MIC >64 µg/mL) first appeared in 1988. It is the most challenging of all the enterococcal resistance patterns, because it typically presents in the isolates of *E. faecium* that often are resistant to ampicillin as well (112). Enterococci are the third most common cause of nosocomial BSI and 27.5% of enterococci, isolated in the intensive care unit setting, are resistant to vancomycin (113). Resistance to both vancomycin and teicoplanin is a growing problem. These strains are often sensitive to daptomycin (114). The topic of screening for enterococcal resistance to the penicillins, vancomycin, and aminoglycosides has been well-presented by Barbara Murray (115).

Enterococci also have the ability to develop resistantce to the newer agents that have been developed to meet the increasing problem of resistance of gram-positive organisms. Linezolid, the first clinically available member of the oxazolidinone class, has good in-vitro activity against both *E. faecium* and *E. faecalis*. Resistance to this agent, on the basis of mutations of the enterococcal 23S ribosome, has been reported, usually developing after 21 days of therapy (116,117,117a). It is superbly absorbed by the oral route even in patients receiving tube feedings. Although cases of IE have been treated successfully when the antibiotic is administered orally, this should not become a routine practice (117b). In stable patients, the author has converted to the oral route after two weeks of intravenous therapy. Resistance has been documented in patients without any previous exposure to this drug (118). Quinupristin-dalfopristin (QD), a streptogramin antibiotic, is bacteriostatic against vancomycin-resistant *E. faecium*, but has no effect on the more common *E. faecalis* (119). Daptomycin belongs to the lipopeptide class of antibiotics. Unlike linezolid and QD, it is rapidly bactericidal against *S. aureus*, streptococci, and enterococci, even to those isolates that are resistant to vancomycin, QD, and linezolid. It is synergistic with gentamicin against *S. aureus* and enterococci (Table 7) (120,121,121a). Tygecycline, a glycylcycline, is promising for the treatment of resistant enterococci and staphylococci (122). In the future, these four agents would be called upon more frequently to deal with the ongoing problem of resistant enterococci. Before the development of these newer agents, chloramphenicol had a degree of success in treating vancomycin-resistant enterococcal BSI (123). Because of its toxicity, it should only be employed under extraordinary circumstances.

The standard therapy of enterococcal IE is synergistic regimen composed of a cell-wall active antibiotic and gentamicin. Streptomycin may be substituted for in 25% of isolates that are resistant to gentamicin. There is no justification in using an aminoglycoside with a cell-wall active antibiotic, if the isolates are resistant to that aminoglycoside. The specific dose of gentamicin necessary to achieve synergy

TABLE 7 Antibiotic Treatment Options for the Treatment of Endocarditis Due to Highly Resistant Gram-Positive Organisms[a]

Antibiotic dosage
Linezolid 600 mg q12 h (either PO or IV)[b]
Quinpristin/dalfopristin 7.5 mg/kg q8 h
Daptomycin 6 mg/kg q24 h[c]

[a]See text for indications.
[b]Effectiveness of the PO route may be approximated to that of the IV route (see text).
[c]This higher dose (usual dose = 4 mg/kg q 24 h) is probably required to treat IE due to *Staphylococcus aureus* and enterococci.
Abbreviations: PO, postoral; IV, intravenous.
Source: From Ref. 242.

is not clear. Some advocate a total daily dose of 4.5 mg/kg in eight-hour divided doses. Others advocate the use of 3 mg/kg per day, divided into three doses. The smaller amount may produce less nephrotoxicity, at the same time as it achieves the minimally necessary level in the serum to achieve synergy (3 µg/mL) (124). Anecdotal experience supports the use of once-a-day dosing of aminoglycosides to achieve synergy. Such an approach does facilitate the extrahospital administration of antibiotics. In a recent series of patients with both native and prosthetic valve IE, a successful outcome was reached with a median duration of cell-wall active antibiotic and aminoglycoside therapy of 42 and 15 days, respectively. If these results are substantiated, two weeks of synergistic therapy followed by two to four weeks of monotherapy with a cell-wall active antibiotic would be adequate (124a). Successful therapy of resistant enterococcal IE is dependent on the recognition, in the infecting enterococcus, of the presence of resistance to one or more components of a potentially synergistic combination. For the treatment of enterococcal IE that is resistant to all the aminoglycosides, ampicillin, given by continuous infusion, to achieve a serum level of 16 µg/mL, was considered to be the best therapeutic option (115). Ampicillin was felt to be superior to vancomycin. Imipenem, ciprofloxacin, or ampicillin-sulbactam were alternative approaches (125).

Presently, linezolid, QD, or daptomycin should be the initial approach to treating aminoglycoside-resistant enterococci (Table 7). There are small clinical series and experimental models that indicate that linezolid, QD, and daptomycin may be synergistic with the aminoglycosides and cell-wall active antibiotics (126). To achieve cure of a case of enterococcal IE, for which there is no synergistic combination of antibiotics available, it is often necessary to perform valvular surgery sooner than later. Table 8 summarizes the treatment regimens for enterococcal IE.

Staphylococcus aureus Infective Endocarditis

There are many questions that have to be answered in choosing the most appropriate treatment of *S. aureus* IE. Is the isolate MRSA? Is the valvular infection solely right-sided? Is prosthetic material involved?

Although most strains of *S. aureus* were quite sensitive to penicillin at the beginning of the antibiotic era, only 10% remain sensitive today. One cannot rely on the Kirby–Bauer sensitivity tests to identify penicillin-resistant *S. aureus*. Susceptibility must be confirmed by measuring the MIC and MBC of penicillin against the isolate. Those that are sensitive are inhibited by <0.1 µg/mL (127).

Penicillin resistance is on the basis of three mechanisms: (*i*) penicillinase production; (*ii*) altered penicillin-binding proteins (MRSA); and (*iii*) tolerance. The semisynthetic penicillins, oxacillin, or nafcillin, are the antibiotics of choice to treat methicillin-sensitive *S. aureus* (MSSA). These are therapeutically equivalent on the basis of both animal and clinical studies (128). Oxacillin may cause elevated liver function tests. This usually is of little significance. Prolonged administration of nafcillin may lead to leukopenia. Nafcillin does have a major advantage in that it is excreted almost entirely by the biliary tract, and hence does not need to be adjusted in renal failure (129). Oxacillin can clear 99% of BSI, caused by MSSA, in two to six days (130). The relapse rate is approximately 5%. First-generation cephalosporins, such as cefazolin, may be substituted in those with a history of a minor reaction to the penicillins. There have been isolated case reports of failure of cefazolin. Theoretically, cephalosporins may be inferior to the semisynthetics because they are more susceptible to the beta-lactamases of *S. aureus* (inoculum effect) (131).

TABLE 8 Treatment of Enterococcal Native Valve Infective Endocarditis

Type of resistance	Regimen[a]
(1) None	Penicillin G (18–30 million units/24 h IV)[b] given in 4-hr equally divided doses or Ampicillin (12 g/24 h IV) given in 4-hr equally divided doses or Vancomycin (30 mg/kg/24 h IV) given in 2 equally divided doses plus Gentamicin (3 mg/kg/24 h IV/IM)
(2) Resistant to penicillins owing to beta-lactamase production	Ampicillin-sulbactam (12 g/24 h IV)[b] given in 4 equally divided doses or Vancomycin (30 mg/kg/24 h) given in 2 equally divided doses
(3) Intrinsic penicillin resistance[c,d]	Vancomycin (30 mg/kg/24 h) given in 2 equally divided doses plus Gentamicin (3 mg/kg/24 h)
(4) Resistance to vancomycin and to aminoglycosides[c,d]	
(A) *Enterococcus faecium*	Linezolid (1200 mg/24 h IV/PO)[c,e] given in 2 equally divided doses or Quinupristin-dalfopristin (22.5 mg/kg/24 h IV)[c,e] given in 3 equally divided doses
(B) *Enterococcus faecalis*	Linezolid (1200 mg/24 hrs IV/PO)[c,e] given in 2 equally divided doses or Imipenem (2 g/24 h) plus Ampicillin (12 g/24 h IV)

[a]For adults with normal renal function.
[b]Four weeks duration in symptoms less than three months; six weeks if symptoms more than three months.
[c]For both native and prosthetic valve endocarditis.
[d]May require emergent valve surgery for cure.
[e]Treatment should extend for at least eight weeks.
Abbreviations: PO, postoral; IV, intravenous; IM, intramuscular.
Source: From Refs. 58, 59.

The particular pharmacokinetics of the beta-lactamases and that of the antibiotic make it unlikely that a significant quantity of cefazolin is inactivated. This agent does offer the option of intramuscular management of uncomplicated *S. aureus* IE in those patients with inadequate intravenous access.

There are two major indications for the use of vancomycin in the treatment of *S. aureus* IE: (*i*) significant allergy to the beta-lactam agents and (*ii*) MRSA as the causative agent. The risk of ototoxicity and nephrotoxicity, which is caused by vancomycin, markedly increases when an aminoglycoside is added (132). There is agreement in the usefulness of measuring levels of vancomycin in serum either to insure adequate therapeutic levels or safe ones (133). Because of increasing MIC of vancomycin for *S. aureus*, the traditional target of trough concentrations of 5% to 10 µg/mL are felt to be inadequate by many and should be adjusted upward (10–15 µg/mL). The author, in general, believes that trough levels of vancomycin should be obtained in patients who have end-stage renal disease, who are receiving other nephrotoxic drugs, who are morbidly obese, or who have a fluctuating renal function. In addition, in treating IE with vancomycin, trough levels should be higher than generally recommended (15–20 µg/mL). Of course, renal function should be the major consideration in aiming for a high trough level. Vancomycin must be administered over at least one hour intravenously to avoid the generalized flushing reaction due to pharmacological release of histamine from mast cells.

It has been long acknowledged that vancomycin is not the therapeutic equivalent of the semisynthetic penicillins (135–138). It is not as rapidly bactericidal as nafcillin against the high concentrations of bacteria that are found within the infected vegetation. Small and Chambers reviewed 13 cases of MSSA IE that were treated with vancomycin. The failure rate was 35%. In another study, 7/10 episodes of MSSA bacteremia that occurred after treatment with vancomycin for *S. aureus* BSI relapses.

Animal models have suggested that the addition of an aminoglycoside to a penicillin or vancomycin may produce the synergistic effect by clearing *S. aureus* from the bloodstream and vegetation much more rapidly than when a single antibiotic is used (139). A retrospective review of the effect of a beta-lactam drug with or without an aminoglycoside in individuals with *S. aureus* IVDA IE indicated no difference in the death rate for each group (140). A similar study in non-IVDA IE came to the same conclusions (141). The most thorough one, a multicenter study involving IVDA and non-IVDA patients, looked at the effect of the combination of nafcillin, given for six weeks, along with gentamicin for the first two weeks (142). There was no difference in the fatality rate between the two groups. In IVDA IE and non-IVDA IE, the combination lessened the duration of BSI. In all those who received both antibiotics, the median duration of fever was less than those that received nafcillin alone (five days vs. three days). Azotemia was significantly greater in those treated with the penicillin and gentamicin.

In 1988, Chambers et al. cured 94% of cases of staphylococcal right-sided IVDA with two weeks of nafcillin plus tobramycin (143). These patients had a very low incidence of metastatic infection or valvular damage. The original design for the study included therapy with vancomycin plus tobramycin. Because of its high failure rate, this arm of the study was stopped. Vancomycin does not appear to be suitable, even when combined with gentamicin. It is for short-term cure of right-sided IE. Later, Chambers' findings were confirmed in IVDA with cloxacillin and either gentamicin or amikacin. Many of these had AIDS (moderately decreased CD4 count) and large tricuspid vegetations (143a). In the 1980s, there was great interest in treating uncomplicated right-sided IVDA IE with an oral regimen, such as ciprofloxacin and rifampin; this combination had a good deal of success with cure rates of approximately 90% (143b). Short-course therapy of MRSA in a right-sided endocarditis is not appropriate. The rise in the resistance of both MSSA and MRSA to be quinolones has made oral therapy less likely to be successful with this class of drugs.

Because these studies have been hampered by relatively small numbers and significant difficulties in achieving true randomization of patients with multiple underlying conditions, it is reasonable to add gentamicin to a semisynthetic penicillin so as to sterilize the vegetation as quickly as possible, and hence limit valvular damage. Conversely, it would be appropriate to add aminoglycoside to monotherapy when the patient is not responding clinically or failing to clear the BSI.

Combination therapy may also be indicated for treating tolerant *S. aureus*. These are strains of *S. aureus* for which the MBC of a cell-wall active antibiotic is much greater than the corresponding MIC (144). Some reports have it that 40% of the isolates of *S. aureus* from BSI are tolerant. They are difficult to detect as only about 7% of a newly isolated bacterial colony may exhibit the property. The strains seem to be deficient in autolytic enzymes, and hence are at least semiresistant to the cell-wall active antibiotics. The addition of synergistic doses of gentamicin appears to compensate for this deficiency. Some series indicate that tolerant *S. aureus* IE has a more complicated clinical course (145). Other studies have failed to identify any difference in their rate of killing by beta-lactam drugs (146). Similar to combination therapy of MSSA, the addition of gentamicin increases the rate of sterilization of the vegetations, but does not lead to a clear-cut improvement in clinical outcome. Again, the clinician is faced with a decision to add gentamicin to a cell-wall active antibiotic (excepting vancomycin) on the basis of inconclusive supportive evidence. It must always be kept in mind that in staphylococcal IE, an incomplete response to appropriate antibiotic therapy is the consequence of an unidentified focus of infection either intracardiac or extracardiac (147).

Rifampin has a property that, all things being equal, would make it a leading candidate for treating *S. aureus* IE. It is able to penetrate into white blood cells and other phagocytes, and is an intracellular pathogen. Its ability to sterilize to staphylococcal abscesses more rapidly than any other antibiotic reflects this characteristic (148). When employed as monotherapy, these organisms quickly become resistant. This is prevented by adding a semisynthetic penicillin. Unfortunately, there is evidence, albeit conflicting, that rifampin decreases the bactericidal activity of the penicillinase-resistant penicillins and quinolones (149,150). The current recommendation is to avoid routine use of rifampin in treating *S. aureus* NVE.

Trimethoprim-sulfamethoxazole has had quite a mixed record in the treatment of MSSA IE. Markowitz (151) demonstrated that it was effective against MRSA IE, but failed to eradicate valvular infections caused by MSSA.

Teicoplanin is a glycopeptide antibiotic that is often discussed in the treatment of gram-positive endocarditis. It is not available in the United States. It probably will never be approved for use in this country for the treatment of *S. aureus* IE because it was inferior to vancomycin in several clinical trials (151a).

Although experience with them is limited, linezolid, QD, and daptomycin are becoming more viable alternatives to vancomycin for the treatment of MSSA IE. In the author's opinion, these appear to have more effectiveness in treating staphylococcal IE than the glycopeptide. In general, the older bacteriostatic antibiotics such as clindamycin and erythromycin should be avoided in the treatment of MSSA IE.

The treatment of MRSA IE poses several challenges. It is difficult to recognize the presence of methicillin resistance because only one organism out of 10^5 may be resistant (heteroresistance). Care must be taken in culturing for this staphylococcal variant (152). Vancomycin remains the mainstay of therapy. However, patients with MRSA IE have persistent BSI for nine days (six days for MSSA), and remain febrile for seven days after initiation of vancomycin. The addition of rifampin makes no difference, or may be antagonistic (136). Gentamicin is synergistic with vancomycin both in vitro and in vivo (105). The clinical significance of this is still not clear. A recent study of isolates of MRSA that were in vitro sensitive but failed to respond to vancomycin, indicated that vancomycin's rate of killing these organisms was markedly diminished (153). Community-acquired MRSA IE may respond to trimethoprim-sulfamethoxazole as does right-sided non–community acquired MRSA (151). Clindamycin should be avoided even for the treatment of community-acquired MRSA IE because of its inconsistent success in treating valvular infections (154).

Linezolid, QD, dactinomycin, effective against MRSA and *S. aureus* isolates that are completely resistant vancomycin-resistant staphylococcus aureus (VRSA) or intermediately resistant to vancomycin intermediate staphylococcus aureus (VISA) (Table 7) (155,156). Of these three, the author has the most personal experience in using linezolid in the treatment of MRSA IE. Linezolid and QD appear to be exceptions to the longstanding rules that bacteriostatic drugs are inferior agents in the treatment of IE. There is evidence that administration of linezolid by continuous infusion results in the antibiotic having an in vivo bactericidal effect on experimental vegetations (157,158). Certainly, linezolid has had failures (159). A certain amount of these may be attributed to low serum levels (160). In experimental models, combining linezolid with subinhibitory concentrations of imipenem has produced synergy against MRSA (161). The most concerning side effects of linezolid are anemia, leucopenia, and thrombocytopenia. The anemia and leukopenia appear to be the result of marrow suppression, somewhat like that of chloramphenicol. It usually is reversible. The thrombocytopenia appears to be the result of an immune-mediated process that may be reversed with intravenous immunoglobulin (162). It usually develops after 10 days of treatment. These blood dyscrasias are the most common cause for discontinuing the antibiotic. The serotonin syndrome is quite an unusual event during linezolid administration. Quinupristin-dalfopristin has been combined with vancomycin to achieve success in treating a variety of severe *S. aureus* infections, and had failed monotherapy with vancomycin (163). There appears to be somewhat less experience with daptomycin. It has demonstrated excellent bactericidal activity against multidrug-resistant *S. aureus*, and was recently approved by the Food and Drug Administration (FDA) for the treatment of MSSA and MRSA BSI and right-sided IE (121,123). The basis of the approval was a prospective, randomized and controlled registration trial of *S. aureus* bacteremia and endocarditis. The data, submitted to the FDA, do not support the treatment of left-sided *S. aureus* IE. Table 9 summarizes the treatment of MSSA and MRSA IE.

The antibiotic regimen for the treatment of staphylococcal PVE is determined by the in vitro sensitivity tests and not whether the isolate is *S. aureus* or coagulase-negative staphylococci (CoNS) (Table 9) (164). At least 11 species of CoNS had been implicated in various human infections. The most clinically important are the isolates of *Staphylococcus epidermidis* (165) that account for 50% of PVE (166). Coagulase-negative staphylococci has several unique properties that give it unique advantages in infecting medical devices, including the production of slime (glycocalyx) and resistance to many classes of antibiotics (Chapters 9 and 10). Many isolates of community-acquired *S. epidermidis* are quite sensitive to the beta-lactam drugs. Fifty-eight percent of healthcare-acquired infections are resistant to them (167).

Approximately 7% of NVE is caused by CoNS (168). They usually are indolent organisms similar to viridans streptococci. The mortality rates vary from 13% to 20%, despite appropriate treatment. This may reflect the fact that most patients had significant underlying valvular disease. *Staphylococcus lugdunensis* is a species of CoNS that is quite aggressive in attacking native valves . It can result in rapid valvular destruction and a mortality rate of up to 70% (169). The treatment of CoNS NVE is the same as that for *S. aureus* (58).

Coagulase-negative staphylococci infect prosthetic valves or other prosthetic material, most commonly during the time of their implantation. These organisms are generally resistant to cephalosporins and penicillins. Most are sensitive to rifampin (170). Isolates of CoNS can become resistant to this agent in a one-step process when they are present in high density, such as that occuring in PVE (171). Resistance of *S. epidermidis* to the penicillinase-resistant penicillins is on the same basis as that of MRSA. Like MRSA, these isolates are heterogeneous and should be screened for by the same methods used to identify MRSA (172). In the past, almost

TABLE 9 Antibiotic Therapy of *Staphylococcus aureus* Infective Endocarditis (IE)[a]

Valve type (IE type)	Antibiotic	Dosage
Native (MSSA)	Oxacillin[b] +/– Gentamicin Or	Oxacillin 2 g IV q4 h for 4–6 weeks +/– gentamicin 3 mg/kg q 24 h as a single dose or in divided doses q8 h for 5 days
	Vancomycin[c,d] +/– Gentamicin Or	Vancomycin 15 mg/kg IV q12 h for 4–6 weeks +/– gentamicin 3 mg/kg q24 h as a single dose or in divided doses q8 h for 5 days
	Cefazolin +/– Gentamicin	Cefazolin 1.5 g IV q8 h for 4–6 weeks (in patients with mild allergies to penicillin) +/– gentamicin 3 mg/kg q24 h as a single dose or in divided doses q8 h for 5 days
Prosthetic (MSSA)	Oxacillin[b] or Vancomycin or Cefazolin and	Oxacillin 2g IV q4h for 4-6 weeks or Vancomycin 15 mg/kg IV q12h for 4-6 weeks or cefazolin 1.5 g IV q8 h for 4–6 weeks in patients with mild allergies to penicillin
	Rifampin And	Rifampin 300 mg PO q8 h for 6 weeks
	Gentamicin	Gentamicin 3 mg/kg q24 h as a single dose or in divided doses q8 h for 2 weeks
Native (MRSA)	Vancomycin[d]	Vancomycin 15 mg/kg IV q12 h for 4–6 weeks
Prosthetic (MRSA)[e]	Vancomycin[d] and	Vancomycin 15 mg/kg IV q12 h for 4–6 weeks
	Rifampin and	Rifampin 300 mg PO q8 h for 6 weeks
	Gentamicin	Gentamicin 3 mg/kg q24 h as a single dose or in divided doses q8 h for 2 weeks

[a]For patients with normal renal function.
[b]May substitute nafcillin at equal doses for patients in significant renal failure.
[c]For patients with severe penicillin allergy.
[d]Substitute linezolid in critically ill patients or those with significant renal failure (refer to discussion in text and Table 7).
[e]If the isolate is resistant to the aminoglycosides, a quinolone to which it is proven sensitive may be substituted.
Abbreviations: MSSA, methicillin-sensitive *Staphylococcus aureus*; MRSA, methicillin-resistant *Staphylococcus aureus*; PO, postoral; IV, intravenous; IM, intramuscular.
Source: From Refs. 58, 164.

all of the aminoglycosides have been bactericidal for CoNS. Currently, a significant minority of *S. epidermidis* (at least 30%) has become resistant to one or more members of this class of antibiotics (170). From experimental models and human case series, it is clearly apparent that rifampin is the critical component of the antibiotic regimen. This is probably because it is the only antibiotic that can continue to be bactericidal against CoNS that are embedded in a glycocalyx (173). The importance of protecting rifampin with another antibiotic was first demonstrated in animals by Kolbasa in 1983 (174). Karchmer and Archer reached the same conclusion in patients with methicillin-resistant *S. epidermidis* (MRSE) (175). Two groups of patients were studied. One was given vancomycin plus rifampin for six weeks; the other was treated with the same antibiotics plus gentamicin for the first two weeks. The outcomes were similar in both. However, 37% of patients, who did not receive gentamicin, developed resistance to rifampin. Peak levels of vancomycin should range

TABLE 10 Therapy for Coagulase-Negative Staphylococcal Infection of Prosthetic Valves or Other Prosthetic Material[a,b]

Antibiotic	Dosage regimen
Vancomycin and	15 mg/kg q12 h for 6 weeks
Rifampin and	300 mg PO q8 h for 6 weeks
Gentamicin	3 mg/kg q24 h IV as a single dose or in divided doses q12 h for 2 weeks

[a]80% of isolates recovered within the first year after valve replacement are resistant to the beta-lactam antibiotics. After this period, 30% are resistant. Sensitivity to the penicillins must be confirmed, because standard sensitivity testing may not detect resistance. If the isolate is sensitive, oxacillin or cefazolin may be substituted.
[b]If the organism is resistant to the aminoglycosides, a quinolone to which it is proven sensitive, should be substituted.
Abbreviations: PO, postoral; IV, intravenous; IM, intramuscular.
Source: From Refs 58, 164.

between 30 and 35 µg/mL because of the high MIC encountered in MRSE (176). If the isolate is sensitive to an aminoglycoside, it should be administered for the first two weeks to augment the bactericidal activity of the other agents, and to decrease the risk of developing resistance to rifampin. When methicillin-sensitive CoNS is present, a semisynthetic penicillin should be substituted for vancomycin (170) Table 10. In the face of aminoglycoside resistance, a fluoroquinolone should be used instead in the combination regimen. Karchmer prefers to hold off beginning rifampin until the patient has been treated for two days with two effective "anti-CoNS" antibiotics. If there is only one effective antibiotic available, then it should be given for three days prior to starting rifampin.

Gram-Negative Organisms
There has been a marked increase in the incidence of gram-negative IE since the 1960s. Approximately 5% of NVE and 50% of PVE are attributed to these organisms (177). Most common gram negatives are the HACEK group (*Hemophilus* spp., *Actinobacillus* spp., *Cardiobacterium hominis*, *Eikenella corrodens*, and *Kingella kingii*), the *Enterobacteriaceae*, *P. aeruginosa*, and *Salmonella* spp. Valvular infection with any one of these can be associated with a mortality rate of up to 80%. This is attributed to several factors: (*i*) the high incidence of impaired host defenses (cirrhosis, IVDA); (*ii*) the presence of intracardiac prosthetic material; (*iii*) the low incidence of gram-negative IE makes it difficult to carry out controlled trials to discover optimum treatment for many of these pathogens; and (*iv*) the necessity of using antibiotics with a low therapeutic/toxicity ratio (the aminoglycosides) (178).

The development of the third-generation cephalosporins, broad-spectrum penicillins and the carbapenems have provided more options for the treatment of gram-negative IE. They have has also created new clinical challenges. The increase in the use of the third part to the right generation cephalosporins has led to a marked increase in infections due to *Enterobacter* sp. They are now the third most common organisms involved in nosocomial gram-negative infections, surpassed only by *E. coli* and *P. aeruginosa* (178,179). *Enterobacter* spp. have also become more resistant to the newer cephalosporins. Because these cephalosporinases are not expressed constitutively, but must be induced by exposure to cephalosporins, they often evade detection in the clinical microbiology laboratory. Enterobacter spp. are the primary source of the cephalosporinases, as they are the most common colonizers of the bowel. The gastrointestinal tract appears to be the source of infection of both patients and healthcare workers (180). *Pseudomonas* spp., *E. coli*, and *Klebsiella pneumoniae* possess similar beta-lactamases that can inactivate the third-generation cephalosporins and broad-spectrum penicillins. These developments have had a significant impact on the antibiograms for many types of healthcare facilities (181). Other types of inducible beta-lactamases are able to inactivate beta-lactamase inhibitors, such as clavulanic acid and sulbactam (182). These are a serious threat to the antibacterial drugs, such as ticarcillin/clavulanic acid and ampicillin/sulbactam. Limiting the use of the third-generation cephalosporins is the most direct way of controlling the problem of extended spectrum beta-lactamases. In treating IE that is caused by an organism with the potential of producing an inducible cephalosporinase, strong consideration should be given to using a broad-spectrum penicillin combined with an aminoglycoside or with aztreonam. The addition of the penicillin augments the therapeutic activity of the aminoglycoside (183). The beta-lactam component contributes to the ability to continue the bactericidal effect when the level of the aminoglycoside goes below its MBC for the infecting organism. The use of "double beta" (2 beta-lactam drugs) regimens may serve as a potent stimulus for the induction of cephalosporinases (178). Aztreonam and the quinolones provide additional options for the treatment of IE due to *Enterobacteriaceae* (*E. coli*, *Klebsiella*, *Enterobacter*, *Serratia*, *Citrobacter*, *Providencia Salmonella*, and *Proteus*) (184). Development of resistance among various gram-negative organisms to the quinolones has been well-documented (185). The carbapenems (imipenem, meropenem, and ertapenem) along with fourth-generation cephalosporins provide the best coverage against organisms that produce the extended spectrum beta-lactamases (186).

In summary, the antibiotics of choice in treating IE due to the *Enterobacteriaceae* are the carbapenems, aztreonam, certain broad-spectrum penicillin/beta-lactamase inhibitor (piperacillin/tazobactam) and the third-generation cephalosporins (caveat of inducing cephalosporinases). In most instances, one of these should be combined with an aminoglycoside. Doing so increases their effectiveness in sterilizing the vegetation of IE (Table 11) (183). By themselves, ampicillin cefazolin are quite effective in the treatment of IE caused by *E. coli* and *Proteus mirabilis* (187). These organisms may be an appropriate exception to the need to employ a combination regimen in the treatment of gram-negative IE. Third-generation cephalosporins are probably the drugs of choice for treating salmonella IE followed by the quinolones (188).

Serratia valvular infections, especially left-sided IVDA IE, often require surgery for cure despite appropriate antibiotic treatment (189). These organisms possess a high degree of resistance factors that by one mechanism or other produce resistance to penicillins, carbapenems, aminoglycosides, a fluoroquinolone, and trimethoprim/sulfamethoxazole (190,191). Close attention must be paid to the in vitro sensitivity data when choosing an antibiotic regimen to treat IE caused by *Serratia marcescens*. The treatment of *S. marcescens* NVE is one of the most challenging therapeutic areas of IE.

The greatest degree of experience in treating *P. aeruginosa* IE is among IVDA. The prognosis of parenteral preparation drug uses with this type of IE is markedly better than that of non-IVDA. The importance of a synergistic effect and the need for above-average doses of tobramycin on the outcome of *Pseudomonas* valvular infection was recognized in the 1970s (192). These investigators discovered that the addition of carbenicillin to a very large dose of gentamicin (8 mg/kg/day) significantly decreased the fatality rate in these patients. Lack of a synergistic effect

TABLE 11 Suggested Representative Antibiotic Therapy of Infective Endocarditis Caused by Enterobacteriaceae and the HACEK Organisms

Organism	Antibiotic	Dosage regimen[a,b,c]
Escherichia coli and Proteus mirabilis	Ampicillin +/– Gentamicin Or Ceftriaxone Or Ciprofloxacin	12 g/day 5 mg/kg/day 1–2 g/day 400 mg IV q12 h
Enterobacter spp. and Klebsiella spp.	Ticarcillin/Clavulanic acid	6 g (ticarcillin) IV of q6 h
Citrobacter spp.[d], Providencia spp.	Meropenem Or Ceftriaxone Or Cefipime Plus Gentamicin	2 g IV q8 h 2 g IVq 12 h 2 g mq12 h 5 mg/kg/day
Serratia marcescens[e]	Cefipime Or Imipenem Or Ciprofloxacin Plus Amikacin Ceftriaxone	2 g IV q8 h 1 g IV q6 h 400 mg IV q12 h 7.5 mg/kgIV q12 h 2 g IVq12 h
Salmonella spp.	Or Ciprofloxacin	400 mg IV q12

[a]For patients with normal renal function.
[b]Duration of therapy, at least six weeks.
[c]Final selection must be based on sensitivity testing.
[d]Citrobacter freundi most resistant species of Citrobacter.
[e]High frequency of multidrug resistance. Amikacin sensitivity usually preserved. Plasmid-mediated resistance to third- and fourth-generation cephalosporins and carbapenems. Extended spectrum beta-lactamases encountered. Quinolone resistance occurs.

between the two agents was highly predictive of failure. Tobramycin should be the aminoglycoside of choice against serious *P. aeruginosa* infections, as the MBC of this agent is two to four times lower than that of gentamicin. Twelve micrograms per millilitre is the aimed peak level (193). Although such large doses of aminoglycoside are used, these patients do not appear to be at any higher risk of nephrotoxicity than those given more average doses. Therapy should be continued for at least six weeks. Animal models of this disease provide some possible reasons why such intensive antibiotic dosing must be included. These include: (*i*) constitutive production of beta-lactamases by the organism; (*ii*) relative aminoglycoside resistance emerging during therapy; (*iii*) lack of postantibiotic effect by beta-lactam drugs; and (*iv*) protection of *Pseudomonas* by its glycocalyx environment (194).

The HACEK group includes *Hemophilus* spp., *A. actinomycetemcomitans*, *C. hominis*, *E. corrodens*, and *K. kingii*. Of these, *Hemophilus parainfluenza* and *Hemophilus aphrophilus* are the ones most often involved in valvular infections

(195). Many of these are sensitive to ampicillin. Isolates are capable of producing a variety of beta-lactamases. Because of their nutritional requirements, members of the HACEK are difficult to cultivate, especially in automatic susceptibility testing systems (196). Because of this, it must be assumed that the isolates are resistant to monotherapy with ampicillin. Aminoglycosides have been combined with ampicillin, with success in the past, to treat HACEK IE. The antibiotics of current choice are the third-generation cephalosporins. Ampicillin/sulbactam is an appropriate alternative to cephalosporins. Quinolones are only recommended for those patients who are intolerant to these beta-lactam antibiotics (58,197). Hopefully, by avoiding the use of aminoglycosides, the patient will be at lower risk of nephrotoxicity.

Brucella Infective Endocarditis
Infective endocarditis is the most frequent cause of death in individuals with brucellosis (198,199). There has been no definite agreement on the correct antibiotic or dosage regimen for its treatment. The combination of doxycycline with rifampin and sulfamethoxazole-trimethoprim for a prolonged period of time is a reasonable approach. The older approach of streptomycin and rifampin is still employed by many (198). Because its diagnosis is often delayed, the complication rate is high and surgery is often required.

Neisseria Gonorrhea Infective Endocarditis
Neisseria gonorrhea is by far the most common *Neisseria* spp. involved in IE. The organism remains generally quite sensitive to penicillin (20 million units/day intravenously for four weeks), but resistant strains have been recognized more frequently (200,201). It would be prudent to initially administer a third-generation cephalosporin until reliable sensitivity data is available.

Gram-Positive Bacilli
Corynebacteria Infective Endocarditis
There has been a significant increase in IE owing to corynebacteria, especially *Corynebacteria jeikeium*. These organisms primarily infect prosthetic valves with rare involvement of native valves (202). Isolates are often resistant to many classes of antibiotics, including penicillins, cephalosporins, and the aminoglycosides. Vancomycin alone or combined with gentamicin, if the isolate is sensitive, appears to be the treatment of choice (203). The combination of vancomycin and gentamicin is most justified for the treatment of early-onset PVE. The mortality rate of this disease is 73% as compared with 11% of late-onset PVE.

Listeria Monocytogenes
Infective endocarditis is an unusual complication of *L. monocytogenes* (<10% of cases) (204–206). The organism is sensitive in vitro to a number of antibiotics, including, penicillin, ampicillin, gentamicin, erythromycin, tetracyclines, chloramphenicol, and trimethoprim sulfamethoxazole. Ampicillin by itself is effective in treating many types of *Listeria* infection. However, it appears to have delayed bactericidal activity. For this reason, it is recommended that gentamicin be added to enhance its bactericidal activity. Native valve endocarditis requires six to eight weeks of treatment, and PVE, even longer. *Listeria* may require valvular surgery for cure. The mortality rate of both types is similar (approximately 40%).

Q-Fever Infective Endocarditis

As in the case of many of the causes of culture-negative endocarditis, the delay in diagnosis and treatment of Q-fever IE (approximately one year) is the basis of failure of medical therapy alone and the need of eventual valvular surgery (207–209). Prolonged therapy must be used because many agents, such as the tetracyclines, are bacteriostatic. In addition, *Coxiella burnetti* lives in a protected, intracellular environment. Treatment regimens should include doxycycline and chloroquine. By alkalinizing the intracellular environment, chloroquine potentiates the action of doxycycline. This approach may be more effective than the synergistic combination of a quinolone and doxycycline (210). Treatment should be extended for at least 12–18 months. Some advocate treating for the life of the patient if the infected valve has not been removed. This is based on the fact that, the organism has been identified in surgical specimens after five years of therapy with tetracyclines. Others advocate continuing antibiotics until the phase-1 immunoglobulin (Ig) G antibody is <1/200.

Bartonella Infective Endocarditis

Since its initial description in 1993, there are somewhat more than 100 cases reported in the literature (211–213). It makes up about 3% of the cases of culture-negative endocarditis. *Bartonella quintana* and *Bartonella henselae* are responsible for a vast majority of cases. Because of its "newness" and relatively small amount of cases, there is no sufficient data to make definitive treatment recommendations. There is evidence that administration of aminoglycosides results in a higher recovery rate and a lower relapse rate than other antibiotics. Other regimens include combining beta-lactam antibiotics with either aminoglycosides or doxycycline (211). Overall, 87% of patients recover with treatment; 2% suffer a relapse; and the death rate is 12%.

T. whippelii Infective Endocarditis

The diagnosis of Whipple's IE is often made serendipitously on the histological examination of resected valvular tissue (214). A currently recommended regimen for the treatment of the valvular infection of Whipple's disease consists of penicillin or ceftriaxone for four weeks. This would be followed by oral trimethoprim sulfamethoxazole for one year (215).

Culture-Negative Infective Endocarditis

Cases of culture-negative IE that are not associated with the previous use of anti-biotics, should receive coverage for enterococci, MSSA, gram-negative anaerobes and for fastidious organisms. Consideration should be given for coverage of MRSA, especially in IVDA or those with intravascular devices in place. The recommended treatment of culture-negative NVE consists of ampicillin-sulbactam plus gentamicin or vancomycin plus gentamicin plus ciprofloxacin. Culture-negative early PVE is treated with vancomycin plus gentamicin plus cefepime plus rifampin. The regimen for treating late PVE is the same as that for treating culture-negative NVE (58). These recommendations differ significantly from previous ones. The author's opinion is that if there is reasonable suspicion of MRSA as the pathogen in culture-negative NVE, vancomycin or linezolid should be substituted for ampicillin-sulbactam. The length of time to defervescence on the aforementioned regimens is negatively correlated with survival. Ninety-two percent of those who became afebrile within seven days of the start of antibiotics, survived aginst only 50% of those whose fever lasted longer than seven days. Major emboli and congestive heart

TABLE 12   Therapy of Various Types of Infective Endocarditis[a]

Organism	Antibiotic regimen	Alternative regimen
Culture negative	Ampicillin 2 g IV q4 h for 4 weeks[b] And Gentamicin 5 mg/kg q24 h IV given in a single dose or in divided doses q8 h for the first 2 weeks And Oxacillin 2 g IV q4 h for 4 weeks Or If MRSA is suspected or prosthetic material is present, vancomycin 30 mg/kg q 12 h for 4 weeks	
Pseudomonas	Ticarcillin 3 g IV q4 h for 6 weeks2 And Tobramycin 5 mg/kg q24 h IV given in a single dose or in divided doses q8 h	Ceftazidime[c] 2 g IV q8 h for 6 weeks Or Aztreonam[d] 2 g IV q6 h for 6 weeks And Tobramycin 5 mg/kg IV q24 h given in a single dose or in divided doses q8 h
HACEK group	Ampicillin 2 g IV q4 h for 4–6 weeks[b] And Gentamicin 5 mg/kg q24 h as a single dose or in divided doses q8 h	Cefotaxime[c] 2 g IV q8 h for 4–6 weeks And Gentamicin 5 mg/kg q24 h given in a single dose or in divided doses

[a]For patients with normal renal function.
[b]Preferred regimen (see text).
[c]In patients with mild penicillin allergy.
[d]In patients with severe penicillin allergy.
Abbreviations: HACEK, *Hemophilus* spp., *Actinobacillus* spp., *Cardiobacterium hominis*, *Eikenella corrodens*, and *Kingella kingii*; IV, intravenous.

failure were the major causes of death in unresponsive culture-negative IE (216,217). Tables 11–13 present suggested treatment regimens for various types of gram-negative abdominal infections.

Fungal Infective Endocarditis
The incidence of fungal IE is clearly on the rise owing to increasing numbers of the immunocompromised and of IVDA; growing volumes of cardiac surgery and increased use of broad-spectrum antibiotics (218). *Candida* spp. are the most commonly isolated fungi from valvular infections (50%). Presently, they are equally divided between *Candida albicans* and non–*albicans*. In the past, only 17.6% of patients survived (219), and today 40% survive when treated medically and surgically (220). This modest improvement may be attributed to more rapid diagnoses brought about by improved diagnostic techniques (221). Mortality in *Aspergillus* IE is close to 100% despite appropriate antifungal therapy and prompt surgical intervention (222). When treated with amphotericin alone, the cure rate in the cases of IE owing to Histoplasma, a much less virulent fungus, is 47% (223) . With modern methods of blood culturing, false-negative blood cultures in cases of *Candida* IE occur less than 30% of the time. This rate is certainly higher than that for bacterial IE, but better than what has been reported in the past. The continued poor survival rate is attributed to: (*i*) the difficulty in diagnosing fungal IE in a timely fashion; (*ii*) the dysfunctional host defenses of many patients; (*iii*) until recently, limited variety of

TABLE 13 Representative Antibiotic Therapy of Various Forms of Infective Endocarditis[a,b]

Organism	Dosage regimen
Corynebacterium jeikium	Vancomycin 1 g q 12 h IV Plus Gentamicin 1 mg/kg q 8 h
Listeria monocytogenes	Ampicillin 12 g/day Plus Gentamicin 1.7 mg/kg q8 h
Coxiella. burnetii	Doxycycline 100mg IV/PO bid Plus Chloroquine 200 mg tid[c]
Brucella spp.	Doxycycline 100 mg bid PO Plus Rifampin 900 mg/day PO Plus Trimethoprim-sulfamethoxazole 160/800 mg PO tid
Bartonella spp.	Ceftriaxone 2 g/day for 6 weeks, gentamicin 1 mg/kg q8 h ×14 days Plus Doxycycline 100 mg IV ×6 weeks

[a]For patients with normal renal function.
[b]Given for at least six weeks.
[c]See text for duration of therapy.
Abbreviations: PO, postoral; IV, intravenous.

effective antifungal agents; (*iv*) presence of large and friable vegetations that often embolize and invade the myocardium; and (*v*) relapse of infection years after apparently successful therapy (224).

Amphotericin was the first effective agent for the treatment, and remains the most frequently recommended in this treatment of fungal IE. It faces real challenges in the eradication of *Candida* from the meshwork of fibrin that compose the valvular vegetation. The fibrin appears to protect the fungus from the concentrations of the antifungal that are fungicidal to the *Candida* spp. in vitro. In the end, amphotericin decreases the numbers of fungi, but does not completely eradicate them (225–227). Some non-*albicans* species of *Candida* are more resistant to amphotericin. Although there have been scattered reports of cure with antimicrobial alone, this approach cannot be generally recommended. The IE of Histoplasma may be an exception. The recognition of the inadequacy of medical therapy alone is the basis for the recommendation that surgery for both fungal and PVE should be performed after one to two weeks of amphotericin therapy (228) (Chapter 15). The addition of 5-flucytosine to amphotericin may improve the results of medical therapy. This pairing has not consistently produced synergism. In an animal model, the combination does not sterilize the vegetation (226). Amphotericin B lipid complex or amphotericin B lysosomal complex has been used to avoid the various toxicities of amphotericin deoxycholate. These modifications of amphotericin do not have any clear-cut therapeutic advantage. After surgery, amphotericin or fluconazole (see next) should be continued for six weeks or even longer (Chapter 15) because of the difficulty in eradicating the valvular bed of the remaining fungi.

The development of fluconazole has made some significant contributions in the treatment of *Candida* IE. It has been associated with cures by itself; it is, far better tolerated than amphotericin, and its oral absorption make it practical for long-term suppression (229–232). In an experimental model, the presence of thrombin-induced

TABLE 14   Resistance Patterns of *Candida* Species

Candida Species	Sensitivity to antifungals[a]
Candida albicans	Sensitive to all classes of antifungals
Candida glabrata	Potentially resistant to all azole antifungals, and relatively resistant to amphotericin
Candida parapsilosis	Sensitive to all classes of antifungals, but may be relatively resistant to caspofungin
Candida krusei	Resistant to fluconazole. May be relatively resistant to amphotericin
Candida lusitaniae	Resistant to amphotericin

[a]Standardization of testing has not been established for echinocandins.

platelet microbicidal proteins potentiates the effect of fluconazole against *C. albicans* (233). Overall, fluconazole appears to be inferior to amphotericin in the treatment of Candida IE, both on a clinical and experimental basis (234). Itraconazole may have some value in the treatment of Aspergillus IE (235,236). The role of other azoles, including voriconazole and caspofungin, in the treatment of fungal IE, is unclear and not been defined. Caspofungin does appear promising for the treatment of *Candida* spp. There is growing evidence of successful treatment of *Candida* endocarditis by caspofungin with and without the use of amphotericin B (237,238). However, there are failures reported as well. These must be kept in prospective as amphotericin B certainly has been an imperfect antifungal agent. A recent study demonstrated that caspofungin was at least the equal of amphotericin B in treating invasive candidiasis (239). With the increased availability of antifungal agents, susceptibility testing has become essential in choosing medical therapy. Unfortunately, there are no generally accepted standards established for the echinocandins (240,241) (Table 14). Table 15 presents an approach to the management of patients at risk for candidal IE.

TABLE 15   Approach to the Patient at Risk for Candidal Endocarditis

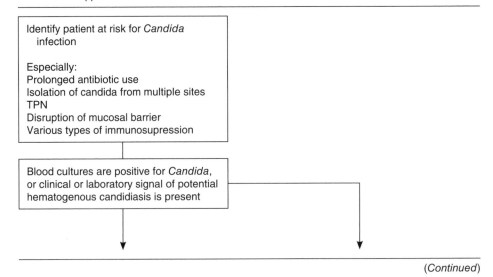

TABLE 15   Approach to the Patient at Risk for Candidal Endocarditis (*Continued*)

Patient is hemodynamically stable, does not have high-grade candidemia, and does not appear to have organ infection		Patient is hemodynamically unstable, has high-grade candidemia, or shows evidence of organ infection	
Remove all venous catheters, or leave venous catheter in place initially, and consider removal if clinical condition deteriorates or does not improve after two days of therapy, and obtain echocardiogram to look for valvular vegitations.		Remove all venous catheters, and obtain echocardiogram to look for valvular vegetations. Treat any associated syndromes of hematogenous candidiasis (e.g., endophthalmitis, pericarditis, suppurative thrombophlebitis, endocarditis).	
Patient is infected or colonized by *Candida albicans*, *Candida tropicalis*, *Candida parapsiolsis*.	Patient is infected or colonized by *Candida krusei*, *Candida glabrata*, or *Candida lusitaniae*	Patient is infected or colonized by *C. albicans*, *C. tropicalis*, *C. parapsiolsis*.	Patient is infected or colonized by *C. krusei*, *C. glabrata*, or *C. lusitaniae*
Give fluconazole, 600–800 mg/day IV for 2–3 days, then, if possible, lower dosage to 400 mg/day PO. Treat for 7–10 days (patient should be free of signs and symptoms of infection for 5 days before treatment is ended).	Capsofungin or voriconazole preferred to the older regimin of amphoterecin +/− flucytosine. Treat for 5–7 days (patient should be free of signs and symptoms of infection for 5 days before treatment is ended).	Give amphotericin B at full dosage. Consider adding flucytosine, 25 mg/day PO in two divided doses. Also consider adding G-CSF, 300 µg/day). Capsofungin or Voriconazole may be preferable. Treat for 10–14 days and then evaluate for need of valvular replacement.	Capsofungin or voriconazole may be preferable to the older regimen of amphoterecin B +/− flucytosine. Consider adding G-CSF, 300 µg/day. Treat for 10–14 days and then evaluate for need of valvular replacement.

Abbreviations: IV, intravenous; IM, intramuscular.
Source: Adapted from Refs. 243 and 244.

REFERENCES

1. Weinstein L, Brusch JL. The historical development of antimicrobial and surgical therapy of infective endocarditis. In: Weinstein L, Brusch JL. Infective Endocarditis, chapter 2. New York: Oxford University Press, 1996:17.
2. Christie RV. Penicillin in subacute bacterial endocarditis: report of the medical research council on 269 patients treated in 14 centers appointed by the penicillin clinical trust committee. Br Med J 1948; 1:1.
3. Hamburger M, Stein L. *Streptococcus viridans* subacute bacterial endocarditis: two week treatment schedule with penicillin. JAMA 1952;149:542.
4. Weinstein L, Brusch JL. Medical management. In: Weinstein L, Brusch JL . Infective Endocarditis, chapter 13. New York: Oxford University Press, 1996:25.
5. Carizosa J, Kobsa WD, Kaye D. Antagonism between chloramphenicol and penicillin in streptococcal endocarditis in rabbits. J Lab Clin Med 1975; 85:307.

6. Durack DT, Beeson PB. Experimental bacterial endocarditis I. Colonization of a sterile vegetation. Br J Exp Pathol 1972; 53:44.

7. Durack DT, Beeson PB. Experimental bacterial endocarditis. II. Survival of bacteria in endocardial vegetations. Br J Exp Pathol 1972; 53:50.

8. Frehel C, Hellio R, Cremieux AC, et al. Nutritionally variant streptococci develop ultrastructural abnormalities during experimental endocarditis. J Microb Pathog 1988; 4:247.

9. Dall L, Bernes WG, Lane JW, et al. Enzymatic modifications of glycocalyx in the treatment of experimental endocarditis due to viridans streptococci. J Infect Dis 1987; 156:736.

10. Libman E, Friedberg CK. Subacute Bacterial Endocarditis. Oxford: Oxford University Press, 1941.

11. Watanakunakorn C. Clindamycin therapy for *Staph aureus* endocarditis: clinical relapse and development of resistance to clindamycin, lincomycin and erythromycin. Am J Med 1976; 60:419.

12. Levinson M. Treatment of endocarditis due to viridans streptococci in experimental models. In: Bisno A, ed. Treatment of Infective Endocarditis, chapter 2. New York: Grune and Stratton, 1981.

13. Friedman M. A study of the fibrin factor in relation to subacute endocarditis. J Pharmacol Exp Ther 1938; 63:173.

14. Nathanson MH, Liebhold RA. Diffusion of sulfonamides and penicillin into fibrin. Proc Soc Exper Biol Med 1946; 52:83.

15. Joly V, Pangon B, Vallois JM, et al. Value of antibiotic levels in serum and cardiac vegetations are predicting antibacterial effect of ceftriaxone in experimental *Escherichia coli* endocarditis. Antimicrob Agents Chemother 1987; 31:1632.

16. Daschner FD, Frank V. Antimicrobial drugs in human cardiac valves and endocarditis lesions. J Antimicrob Chemother 1988; 12:776.

17. Barza M, Brusch J, Bergeron MG, et al. Penetration of antibiotics into fibrin loci in vivo. III. Intermittent versus continuous infusion and the effect of probenecid. J Infect Dis 1974; 129:73.

18. Barza M, Weinstein L. Penetration of antibiotics into fibrin loci in vivo. I comparison of penetration of ampicillin into fibrin clots, absceses and "interstitial fluid". J Infect Dis 1974; 129:59.

19. Contrepois AJ, Callois JM, Garaud JJ, et al. Kinetics and bactericidal effect of gentamicin and latamoxef (moxalactam) in experimental *Escherichia coli* endocarditis. J Antimicrob Chemother 1986; 17:227.

20. McColm AA, Ryan DM. Penetration of beta-lactam antibiotics into cardiac vegetations, aorta and heart muscle in experimental *Staphylococcus aureus* endocarditis: comparison of sets as a team, cefuroxime and methicillin. J Antimicrob Chemother 1985; 16:349.

21. Cremieux AC, Carbon C. Pharmacokinetics and pharmacodynamic requirements for antibiotic therapy of experimental endocarditis. Antimicrob Agents Chemother 1992; 36:2069.

22. Cremieux AC, Maziere B, Valois JM, et al. Evaluation of antibiotic diffusion into cardiac vegetations by quantitative autoradiography. Infect Dis 1989; 159:938.

22a. Michiels MJ, Bergeron MG. Differential increased survival of staphylococci and limited ultrastructural changes in the core of infective fibrin clots after daptomycin administration. Antimicrob Agents Chemother 1996; 40:203.

23. Vogelman B, Gudmundson S, Leggett J, et al. Correlation of antimicrobial pharmacokinetic parameters with therapeutic efficacy in an animal model. J Infect Dis 1988; 158:831.

24. Drusano GL. Role of pharmacokinetics in the outcome of infection. Antimicrob Agents Chemother 1988; 32:289.

25. Ingerman MJ, Pitsakis PG, Rosenberg AF, et al. The importance of pharmacodynamics in determining the dosing interval in therapy for experimental *Pseudomonas* endocarditis in the rat. J Infect Dis 1986; 153:707.

26. Franciolli M, Bille J, Glauser MP, et al. Beta-lactam resistance mechanisms of methicillin-resistant *Staphylococcus aureus*. J Infect Dis 1991; 163:514.

27. Gengo F, Schentag J. Rate of methicillin penetration into normal heart valves and experimental endocarditis lesions. Antimicrob Agents Chemother 1982; 21:456.

28. Malacoff RF, Frank E, Andriole VT. Streptococcal endocarditis (nonenterococcal, non-Group A): single vs combination therapy. JAMA 1979; 241:1807.

29. Weinstein L, Goldfield M, Chang TW. Infection occurring during chemotherapy: a study of the frequency, type and predisposing factors. N Engl J Med 1954; 261:247.
30. Tan JS. Successful two-week treatment schedule for penicillin-susceptible *Streptococcus viridans* endocarditis. Lancet 1971; 2:1340.
31. Weinstein L, Schlesinger J. Treatment of infective endocarditis. Prog Cardiovasc Dis 1973; 6:275.
32. Schlicter J, MacLean H, Milzo A. Effective penicillin therapy in subacute bacterial endocarditis and other classic infections. Am J Med Sci 1949; 217:600.
33. Weinstein MP, Stratton CW, Ackley A, et al. Multicentre collaborative evaluation of a standardized serum bactericidal test as a prognostic indicator in infective endocarditis. Am J Med 1985; 78:262.
34. Mellors JW, Coleman DL, Andriole VT. Value of the serum bactericidal test in management of patients with bacterial endocarditis. Eur J Clin Microbiol 1986; 5:67.
35. Vosti K. Serum bactericidal test: past, present and future use in the management of patients with infections. In: Remington JS, Swartz MN, eds. Current Clinical Topics in Infectious Diseases. Boston: Blackwell Scientific, 1990:43, 10.
36. Rubinstein E. Cost implications of home care in serious infections. Hosp Formul 1993; 28:46.
37. Tice AD. Outpatient parenteral antimicrobial therapy. In: Mandell GL, Bennett JE, Dolin R, eds. Principles and Practice of Infectious Diseases. 6th ed, chapter 45. Philadelphia: Elseiver, 2005:629.
38. Durack D. Endocarditis. In: Tice AD, ed. Outpatient Parenteral Antibiotic Therapy: Management of Serious Infections. New York: HP Publishing Company, 1993:6.
39. Tice AD. Infusion devices. In: Tice AD. Handbook of Outpatient Parenteral Therapy for Infectious Diseases. New York: Scientific American Medicine, 1997.
40. Babcock HM, Ritchie DJ, Christiansen E, et al. Successful treatment of vancomycin-resistant *Enterococcus* endocarditis with oral Linezolid. Clin Infect Dis 2001; 32:1373.
41. Moore RD, Liebman PS, Smith CR. Clinical response to aminoglycoside therapy: importance of the ratio of peak concentrations to minimal inhibitory concentrations. J Infect Dis 1987; 155:93.
42. Brown RB. Selection and training of patients for outpatient intravenous antibiotic therapy. Rev Infect Dis 1991; 13(suppl 2):S147.
43. Monteiro CA, Cobbs CG. Outpatient management of infective endocarditis. Curr Infect Dis Rep 2001; 3:319.
44. Andrews MM, von Reyn CF. Patient selection criteria in management guidelines for outpatient parenteral antibiotic therapy for native valve endocarditis. Clin Infect Dis 2001; 15:203.
45. Tice AD, Rehm SJ, Dalovisio JR, et al. Practice guidelines for outpatient parenteral antimicrobial therapy. Clin Infect Dis 1651; 4:38.
46. Heldman AW, Hartert TV, Ray SC, et al. Oral antibiotic treatment of right-sided staphylococcal endocarditis in injection drug users: prospective randomized comparison with parenteral therapy. Am J Med 1996; 101:68.
47. Wolter JM, Cagney RA, McCormack JG. A randomized trial of home vs hospital intravenous antibiotic therapy in adults with infectious diseases.
48. Davenport J, Hart G. Prosthetic valve endocarditis 1976–1987: antibiotic, anticoagulation and stroke. Stroke 1990; 21:993.
49. Hasburn R, Vikram HR, Barakart LA, et al. Complicated left sided native valve endocarditis in adults: risk classification for mortality. JAMA 2003; 289:1933.
50. Ledermann MM, Sprague L, Wallis RS, Ellner JJ. Duration of fever during treatment of infective endocarditis. Medicine (Baltimore) 1992; 71:52.
51. Douglas A, Moore-Gillon J, Eykyn S. Fever during treatment of infective endocarditis. Lancet 1986; 1:1341.
52. Blumberg E, Robbins N, Adimora A, et al. Persistent fever in association with infective endocarditis. Clin Infect Dis 1992; 15:93.
53. Lichtlen P. General principles of conservative treatment of infective endocarditis. In: Horstkotte D, Bodnar E, eds. Infective Endocarditis. Aylesberg, Becks, England: ICR Publishers, 1991:85.

54. Mansur A, Grinberg M, Lemoda-Luz P, et al. Complications of infective endocarditis: a reappraisal in the 1980s. Arch Intern Med 1992; 152:2428.
55. Tornos MKP, Permanyer-Miralda G, Montserrat O. Long term complications of native and of infective endocarditis in non-addicts. Ann Intern Med 1992; 117:567.
56. Garvey GJ, Neu HC. Infective endocarditis-an evolving disease: a review of endocarditis at the Columbia-Presbyterian Medical Center 1968–1973. Medicine 1978; 57:105.
57. Molinari GF, Smith L, Goldstein MN, et al. Pathogenesis of cerebral mycotic aneurysms. Neurology 1974; 23:325.
58. Baddour LM, Wilson WR, Bayer AS, et al. Infective endocarditis: diagnosis, antimicrobial therapy in management of complications. A statement for health-care professionals from the Committee on Rheumatic Fever, Endocarditis and Kawasaki disease, Council on Cardiovascular Disease in the Young and the Councils On Clinical Cardiology, Stroke and Cardiovascular Surgery and Anesthesia, American Heart Association-executive summary. Circulation 2005; 111:3167.
59. Karchmer AW. Infective endocarditis. In: Zips DP, Libby P, Bonow RO, Braunwald E, eds. Braunwald's Heart Disease: A Textbook of Cardiovascular Medicine. 7th ed. Chpt 58, 1645.
60. Lytle BW, Priest BP, Taylor PC, et al. Surgery for acquired heart disease: surgical treatment for prosthetic valve endocarditis. J Thorac Cardiovasc Surg 1996; 111:198.
61. Wilson W, Guiliani E, Danielson G, et al. Management of complications of infective endocarditis. Mayo Clin Proc 1982; 57:162.
62. Lerner PI, Weinstein L. Infective endocarditis in the antibiotic era. Engl J Med 1966; 247:199.
63. Karchmer AW, Longworth DW. Infections of intracardiac devices. Infect Dis Clin NA 2002; 16:477.
64. Morris AJ, Drinkovic D, Pottumarthy S, et al. Gram stain, culture and histopathological examination findings for heart valves removed because of infective endocarditis. Clin Infect Dis 2003; 36:697.
65. Dajani A, Bisno A, Chung T, et al . Prevention of bacterial endocarditis: recommendations of the American Heart Association. JAMA 1990; 264:2919.
66. Levinson M, Kaye D, Mandell G, et al. Characteristics of patients with multiple episodes of bacterial endocarditis. JAMA 1980; 211:1355.
67. Welton DE, Young JB, Gentry WO, et al. Recurrent infective endocarditis: analysis of predisposing factors and clinical features. Am J Med 1979; 66:932.
68. Baddour LM. Twelve year review of recurrent native valve endocarditis. a disease of the modern antibiotic era. Rev Infect Dis 1980; 10:1163.
69. Roberts R. Streptococcal endocarditis: the viridans and beta-hemolytic streptococci. In: Kaye D, ed. Infective Endocarditis. 2nd ed. New York: Raven Press, 1992:191.
70. Moellering RC Jr. Treatment of endocarditis caused by resistant streptococci. In: Horstkotte D, Bodnar E, eds. Infective Endocarditis. London: ICR Publishers, 1991:102.
71. Karchmer AW, Moellering RC Jr, Maki DC, et al. Single antibiotic therapy for streptococcal endocarditis. JAMA 1979; 241:1801.
72. Hoen B. Special issues of the management of infective endocarditis caused by Gram-positive cocci. Infect Dis Clin NA 2002; 16:437.
73. Pulliam L, Inokuchi S, Hadley WK, et al. Penicillin tolerance in experimental streptococcal endocarditis. Lancet 1979; 2:957.
74. Roberts RB, Kreiger AG, Schiller NL, et al. Viridans streptococcal endocarditis: the role of various species including pyridoxal-dependent streptococci. Rev Infect Dis 1979; 1:955.
75. Tuohy MJ, Procop GW, Washington J. Antimicrobial susceptibility of *Abiotrophia adiacens* and *Abiotrophia defectiva*. Diagn Microbiol Infect Dis 2000; 38:189 .
76. Bouvet A. Human endocarditis due to nutritionally variant streptococci: *Streptococcus adjacena* and *Streptococcus defectivus*. Eur Heart J 1995; 16(suppl B):24.
77. Rahal JJ, Myers BR, Weinstein L. Treatment of bacterial endocarditis with cephalothin. N Engl J Med 1968; 279:1305.
78. Holloway Y, Dankert J. Penicillin tolerance in nutritionally variant streptococci. Antimicrob Agents Chemother 1982; 22:1073.

79. Stamboulian D, Bojhevi P, Arevalo C. Antibiotic management of patients with endo-carditis due to penicillin-susceptible streptococci. Rev Infect Dis 1991; 13(suppl 2):S160.
80. Roberts SA, Lang SDR, Ellis- Pegler RB. Short-course treatment of penicillin-susceptible viridans streptococcal infective endocarditis with penicillin and gentamicin. Infect Dis Clin Prac 1993; 2:191.
81. Prins J, Buller H, Kuijper E, et al. Once vs. thrice daily gentamicin in patients with serious infections. Lancet 1993; 341:355.
82. Phair J, Tan J, Venezio F .Therapy of infective endocarditis due to penicillin susceptible streptococci: duration disease is a major determinant of outcome in treatment of infective endocarditis. In: Bisno A, ed. Treatment of Infective Endocarditis. New York: Grune and Stratton, 1981.
83. Weinstein L. Infective Endocarditis. In: Braunwald E, ed. Heart Disease : A Textbook of Cardiovascular Medicine. 3rd ed, chapter 34. Philadelphia: WB Saunders 1988.
84. Sande MA, Irvin RG. Penicillin-aminoglycoside synergy in experimental streptococcal viridans endocarditis. J Infect Dis 1974; 129:572.
85. Moellering RC Jr, Krogstad D. Antibiotic resistance in enterococci. In: Schlessinger D, ed. Microbiology. Washington: American Society for Microbiology, 1979:293.
86. Weinstein L, Brusch JL. Medical management. In: Weinstein L, Brusch, JL. Infective Endocarditis, chapter 13. New York: Oxford University Press, 264.
87. Baddour LM. Infective endocarditis caused by beta-hemolytic streptococci. Clin Infect Dis 1998; 26:66.
88. Wilson W, Geraci J. Antimicrobial therapy for penicillin-sensitive streptococcal infective endocarditis: two regimens treatment of infective endocarditis. In: Bisno A, ed. Treatment of Infective Endocarditis. New York: Grune and Stratton, 1981:61.
89. Martinez E, Miro JM, Almirante B, et al. The effect of penicillin resistance of *Streptococcus pneumoniae* on the presentation, prognosis in treatment of pneumococcal endocarditis in adults. Clin Infect Dis 2002; 35:130.
90. Aronin SI, Mukherjee SK, West JC, Cooney EL. Review of pneumococcal endocarditis in the penicillin era. Clin Infect Dis 1998; 26:165.
91. Horstkotte D, Follath F, Gutschik E, et al. Guidelines on prevention, diagnosis and treatment of infective endocarditis: executive summary; Task Force on Infective Endocarditis of the European Society of Cardiology. Eur Heart J 2004; 25:267.
92. Elliott TS, Foweraker J, Gould FK, et al. Guidelines for the antibiotic treatment of endocarditis in adults: report of the Working Party of the British Society for Antimicrobial Chemotherapy. J Antimicrob Chemother 2004; 54:971.
93. Ruoff KL, Maza L, Murtagh MJ, et al. Species identities of enterococci related from clinical specimens. J Clin Microbiol 1990; 28:435.
94. Anderson DJ, Murdoch DR, Sexton DJ, et al. Risk factors for infective endocarditis in patients with enterococcal bacteremia: a case-control study. Infection 2004; 32:72.
95. Williamson R, LeBourgenec C, Gutmann L, et al. One or two low affinity penicillin binding proteins may be responsible for the range of susceptibility of Enterococcus faecium to benzylpenicillin. J Gen Microbiol 1985; 131:1933.
96. Zighlboim-Daum S, Moellering RC Jr. Mechanisms and significance of antimicrobial resistance in enterococci. In: Actor Daneo-Moore L, Higgins ML, et al, eds. Antibiotic Inhibition of Bacterial Cell Surface Assembly and Function. Washington DC: American Society of Microbiology, 1988:505.
97. Spera R, Farber B. Multiply-resistant Enterococcus faecium : The nosocomial pathogen, of the 1990's. JAMA 1992, 268, 2563.
98. Moellering RC Jr, Korzeniowski OM, Sande MA, et al. Species-specific resistance to antimicrobial synergism in *Streptococcus faecium* and *Streptococcus faecalis*. J Infect Dis 1979; 140:203.
99. Hunter TH. Use of streptomycin in the treatment of bacterial endocarditis. Am J Med 1947; 2:436.
100. Moellering RC Jr, Weinberg AN. Studies on antibiotic synergism against enterococci. II Effect of various antibiotics on the uptake of C14-labeled streptomycin by enterococci. J Clin Invest 1971; 50:2580.
101. Murray B. The life and times of the enterococcus. Clin Microbiol Rev 1992; 3:46.

102. Watanakunakorn C, Bakie C. Synergism of vancomycin-gentamicin and vancomycin-streptomycin against enterococci. Antimicrob Agents Chemother 1973; 4:120.
103. Marier RL, Joyce N, Andriole VY. Synergism of oxacillin and gentamicin against enterococci. Antimicrob Agents Chemother 1975; 8:571.
104. Grayson ML, Thauvin C, Eliopoulos GM, et al. Failure of trimethoprim-sulfamethoxazole therapy in experimental enterococcal endocarditis. Antimicrob Agents Chemother 1990; 34:1792.
105. Kaye KS, Engemann JJ, Fraimow HS, Abrutyn E. Pathogens resistant to antimicrobial agents: epidemiology, molecular mechanisms and clinical management. Infect Dis Clin NA 2004; 18:467.
106. Horodniceanu T, Bouquelert L, EL- Solh N, et al. High level, plasmid-borne resistance to gentamicin in *Streptococcus faecalis* subsp. zymogens. Antimicrob Agents Chemother 1979; 16:686.
107. Paterson JE, Zervos MJ. High-labeled gentamicin resistance in enterococcus: microbiology, genetic basis and epidemiology. Rev Infect Dis 1990; 12:644.
108. Mederski-Samoraj BD, Murray BE. High level resistance to gentamicin in clinical isolates of enterococci. J Infect Dis 1983; 147:751.
109. Chow JW. Aminoglycoside resistance in enterococci. Clin Infect Dis 2000; 31:586.
110. Murray BE. Beta-lactamase-producing enterococci areas. Antimicrob Agents Chemother 1992; 36:2355.
111. Fontana R, Ligozzi M, Pittaluga F, Satta G. Intrinsic penicillin resistance in enterococci. Microb Drug Resist 1996; 2:209.
112. Coque TM, Tomayko JF, Ricke SC, et al. Vancomycin-resistant enterococci from nosocomial, community and animal sources in the United States. Antimicrob Agents Chemother 1996; 40:2605.
113. National Nosocomial Infections Surveillance (NNIS) System Report, data summary from January 1992 through June 2003, issued August 2003. Am J Infect Control 2003; 31:481.
114. Lutticken R, Kunstmann G. Vancomycin-resistant *Streptococcaceae* from clinical material. Zbi Bakt Hyg 1988; A:267, 379.
115. Murray BE. Antibiotic resistance among enterococci: current problems and management strategies. In: Remington J, Swartz M, eds. Current Clinical Topics in Infectious Diseases. Cambridge MA: Blackwell Scientific, 1991:94.
116. Meka VG, Gold HS. Antimicrobial resistance to linezolid. Clin Infect Dis 2004; 39:1010.
117. Prytowsky J, Siddiqui F, Chosay J, et al. Resistance to linezolid: characterization of mutations in rRNA and comparison to their occurrences in vancomycin-resistant enterococci. Antimicrob Agents Chemother 2001; 45:2154.
117a. Beringer P, Nguyen M, Hoem N, et al. Absolute bioavailability and pharmacokinetics of linezolid in hospitalized patients given enteral feedings. Antimicrob Agents Chemother 2005; 49:3676.
117b. RavindranV, Kaye J, Kaye GC, Meigh RE. Successful use of oral linezolid is a single active agent in endocarditis unresponsive to conventional antibiotic therapy. J Infect 2003; 47:164.
118. Lundstrom TS, Sobel JD. Antibiotics for Gram-positive bacterial infections: vancomycin, quinupristin-dalfopristin, linezolid and daptomycin. Infect Dis Clin NA 2004; 18:651.
119. Jones RN, Ballow CH, Biedenbach DJ, et al. Antimicrobial activity of quinupristin-dalfopristin (RP 59500 . Synercid) tested against 28,000 recent clinical isolates from 200 medical centers in the United States and Canada. Diagn Microbiol Infect Dis 1998; 31:437.
120. Tally FP, DEBruin MF. Development of daptomycin for Gram-positive infections. J Antimicrob Chemother 2000; 46:523.
121. Critchley IA, Draghi DC, Sahm DF, et al. Activity of daptomycin against susceptible in multidrug resistance Gram-positive pathogens collected in the Secure study (Europe) during 2000–2001. J Antimicrob Chemother 2003; 51:639.
121a. Cha R, Rybak MJ. After mice and against multiple drug-resistant staphylococcus and enterococcus isolates in an in vitro pharmacodynamic model with simulated endocardial vegetations. Diagn Microbiol Infect Dis 2003; 47:539.

122. Cercenado E, Cercenado S, Gomez JA, Bouza E. In vitro activity of tigecycline (GAR 936) a novel glycylcycline, against vancomycin-resistant enterococci and staphylococci with diminished susceptibility to glycopeptides. J Antimicrob Chemother 2003; 52:138.

123. Lutenbach E, Schuster MG, Bilker WB, Brennan PJ. The role of chloramphenicol in the treatment of bloodstream infections due to vancomycin-resistant Enterococcus. Clin Infect Dis 1998; 27:1259.

124. Wilson WR. Antimicrobial therapy of streptococcal endocarditis. J Antimicrob Chemother 1987; 20(suppl A):147.

124a. Olaison L, Schadewitz K. The Swedish Society for Infectious Diseases Quality Assurance Study Group for Endocarditis: enterococcal endocarditis in Sweden, 1995–1999: can shorted therapy with aminoglycosides be used? Clin Infect Dis 2002; 34:159.

125. Weinstein L, Brusch JL. Medical management. In: Weinstein L, Brusch JL, chapter 13. Infective Endocarditis. New York: Oxford University Press, 1996:256.

126. Thompson RL, Lavin B, Talbot GH. Endocarditis due to vancomycin resistant *Enterococcus faecium* in an immunocompromised patient: cure by administering combination therapy with Quinpristin/dalfopristin and high dose ampicillin. South Med J 2003; 96:818.

127. Sande M, Korzeniowski O. The antimicrobial therapy of staphylococcal endocarditis and treatment of infective endocarditis. In: Bisno A, ed. Treatment of Infective Endocarditis. New York: Grune and Stratton, 1981:113.

128. Egert J, Carrizosa J, Kaye D. Comparison of methicillin, nafcillin or oxacillin and therapy of *Staphylococcus aureus* endocarditis in rabbits. J Lab Clin Med 1977; 89:126.

129. Brusch JL, Barza M, Brown RB, et al. comparative, genetics of 13 antibiotics in dogs. Infection 1976, 4(suppl 2):S82.

130. Korzeniowski O, Sande M. The National Collaborative Endocarditis Study Group: combination antimicrobial therapy for *Staphylococcus aureus* endocarditis in patients addicted to parenteral drugs and in nonaddicts. A prospective study. Ann Intern Med 1982; 97:496.

131. Chambers H. Antibiotic treatment of staphylococcal endocarditis. In: Horstkotte D, Bodnar E, eds. Infective Endocarditis. London: ICR Publishers, 1991:110.

132. Moellering RC Jr, Krogstad DJ, Greenblatt DJ. Vancomycin therapy in patients with impaired renal function: a nomogram for dosing. Ann Intern Med 1981; 94:343.

133. Freeman CD, Quintilliani R, Nightingale CH. Vancomycin therapeutic drug monitoring: is it necessary. Ann Pharmacother 1993; 27:594.

134. American Thoracic Society; Infectious Disease Society of America. Guidelines for the management of adults with hospital-acquired, ventilator-associated and healthcare-associated pneumonia. Am J Respir Crit Care Med 2005; 171:388.

135. Gopal V, Bisno AL, Silverblatt FJ. Failure of vancomycin treatment in *Staphylococcus aureus* endocarditis: in vivo and in vitro observations. JAMA 1976; 236:1604.

136. Levine DP, Fromm BS, Reddy BR. Slow response to vancomycin for vancomycin plus rifampin in methicillin-resistant *Staphylococcus aureus* endocarditis. Ann Intern Med 1991; 1/15:674.

137. Small PM, Chambers HF. Vancomycin for *Staphylococcus aureus* endocarditis in intravenous drug abusers. Antimicrob Agents Chemother 1998; 34:1227.

138. Harstein AL, Mulligan ME, Morthland VH, et al. Recurrent *Staphylococcus aureus* bacteremia . J Clin Microbiol 1991; 30:670.

139. Sande MA, Courtney KB. Nafcillin-gentamicin synergism in experimental staphylococcal endocarditis. J Lab Clin Med 1976; 88:118.

140. Abrams B, Sklaver A, Hoffman T, et al. Single combination therapy of staphylococcal endocarditis in intravenous drug abusers. Ann Intern Med 1979; 90:789.

141. Watanakunakorn C, Baird IM. Prognostic factors in *Staphylococcus aureus* endocarditis and results of therapy with penicillin and gentamicin. Am J Med Sci 1977; 273:133.

142. Korzeniowski O, Sande MA. The National Collaborative Endocarditis Study Group. Combination antimicrobial therapy for *Staphylococcus aureus* endocarditis in patients addicted to parenteral drugs and non addicts: a prospective study. Ann Intern Med 1982; 97:496.

143. Chambers HF, Miller T, Newman MD. Right-sided *Staphylococcus aureus* endocarditis in intravenous drug abusers—two week combination therapy. Ann Intern Med 1988; 109:619.

143a. Ribera E, Gomez Jimenez J, Cortes E, et al. Effectiveness of oxacillin with and without gentamicin in short-term therapy for right-sided *Staphylococcus aureus* endocarditis: a randomized, controlled trial. Ann Intern Med 1996; 125:969.

143b. Dworkin RJ, Lee BL, Sande MA, Chambers HS. The treatment of right-sided *Staphylococcus aureus* endocarditis in intravenous drug abusers with ciprofloxacin and rifampicin. Lancet 1989; 2:1071.

144. Mayhall CG, Medoff G, Marr TT. Variation in the susceptibility of strains of *Staphylococcus aureus* to oxacillin, cephalothin and gentamicin. Antimicrobial Agents Chemother 1976; 10:707.

145. Rajashekaraiah K, Rice T, Rao V, et al. Clinical significance of tolerant strains of *Staphylococcus aureus* in patients with endocarditis. Ann Intern Med 1988; 93:796.

146. Watanakunakorn C. Antibiotic-tolerant *Staphylococcus aureus*. Antimicrob Ag Chemother 1978; 4:561.

147. Sheagren J. *Staphylococcus aureus*, the persistent pathogen (second of two parts). N Engl J Med 1984; 310:1437.

148. Mandell GL, Vest TK. Killing of intraerythrocytic *Staphylococcus aureus* by rifampin: in vitro and in vivo studies. J Infect Dis 1972; 125:486.

149. Zinner SH, Lagast H, Klatersky J. Anti-staphylococcal activity rifampin with other antibiotics. J Infect Dis 1981; 144:365.

150. Weinstein L, Brusch JL. Medical management. In: Weinstein L, Brusch JL. Infective Endocarditis, chapter 13. New York: Oxford University Press, 1996:276.

151. Markowitz N, Quinn E, Saravolatz L. Trimethoprim-sulfamethoxazole compared with vancomycin for the treatment of *Staphylococcus aureus* infection. Ann Intern Med 1992; 117:390.

151a. Kaatz G, Sen S, Dorman N, et al. Merging teicoplanin resistance during therapy of *Staphylococcus aureus* endocarditis. J Infect Dis 1990; 162:103.

152. Karchmer AW. Staphylococcal endocarditis: laboratory and clinical basis for antibiotic therapy. Am J Med 1985; 78(suppl 6b):116.

153. Sakoulas G. Relationship of MIC and bactericidal and 70 to efficacy of vancomycin for treatment of methicillin resistant *Staphylococcus aureus* bacteremia. J Clin Microbiol 2004; 42:2398.

154. Watanakunakorn C. Clindamycin therapy of *Staphylococcus aureus* endocarditis: clinical relapse development of resistance to clindamycin, lincomycin and erythromycin. Am J Med 1976; 60:419.

155. Tenover FC, Biddle JW, Lancaster MV. Increasing resistance to vancomycin and other glycopeptides in *Staphylococcus aureus*. Emerg Infect Dis 2001; 7:327.

156. LaPlante KL, Rybak MJ. Impact of high-inoculum *Staphylococcus aureus* on the activities of nafcillin, vancomycin, linezolid and dactinomycin alone and in combination with gentamicin, in an vitro pharmacodynamic model. Antimicrob Agents Chemother 2004; 48:4665.

157. Batard JC, Perez L, Boutoille D, et al. In vivo efficacy of continuous infusion versus intermittent dosing of linezolid compared to vancomycin in a methicillin-resistant *Staphylococcus aureus* rabbit endocarditis model. Antimicrob Agents Chemother 2002, 46, 3706.

158. Bassetti M, DiBiagio A, DelBono V, et al. Successful treatment of methicillin-resistant *Staphylococcus aureus* endocarditis with linezolid. Int J Antimicrob Agents 2004; 24:83.

159. Ruiz ME, Guerrero IC, Tuazon. Endocarditis caused by methicillin-resistant *Staphylococcus aureus*: treatment failure with linezolid. Clin Infect Dis 2002; 35:1018.

160. Sperber SJ, Levine JF, Gross PA. Persistent MRSA bacteremia in a patient with low linezolid levels. Clin Infect Dis 2003; 36:675.

161. Jacqueline C, Navas D, Batard E, et al. In vitro and in vivo synergistic activities of linezolid combined with subinhibitory concentrations of imipenem against methicillin-resistant *Staphylococcus aureus*.

162. Bernstein WB, Trotta RF, Rector JT, et al. Mechanisms for linezolid-induced anemia and thrombocytopenia. Ann Pharmacother 2003; 37:517.

163. Scotton PG, Rigoli R, Vaglia A. Combination of quinipristin/dalfopristin and glycopeptides in severe methicillin-resistant staphylococcal infections failing previous glycopeptides regimens. Infection 2002; 30:161.

164. Karchmer AW. Infections of prosthetic heart valves. In: Waldvogel F, Bisno AL, eds. Infections Associated with Indwelling Medical Devices. 3rd ed. Washington D.C.: American Society for Microbiology, 2000:145.
165. Kloss W. Coagulase-negative staphylococci. Clin Microbiol Newslett 1982; 4:75.
166. Kloss W. Natural populations of the genus *Staphylococcus*. Ann Rev Microbiol 1982; 34:559.
167. Patrick C. Coagulase-negative staphylococci: pathogens with increasing clinical significance. J Pediatr 1990; 116:497.
168. Chu VH, Cabell CH, Abrutyn E, et al. Native valve endocarditis due to coagulase-negative staphylococci: report of 99 episodes from the International Collaboration on Endocarditis database. Clin Infect Dis 2004; 39:1527.
169. Vandenesch F, Ettiene J, Reverdy ME, et al. Endocarditis due to *Staphylococcus lugdunensis*: report of 11 cases and review. Clin Infect Dis 1993; 17:871.
170. Karchmer AW, Archer GL, Dimukes WE. In *Staphylococcus epidermidis* causing prosthetic valve endocarditis: microbiologic and clinical observations as guides to therapy. Ann Intern Med 1983; 98:447.
171. Archer GL. Antimicrobial susceptibility and detection of resistance among *Staphylococcus epidermidis* isolates recover from patients with infections of indwelling foreign devices. Antimicrob Agents Chemother 1978; 14:353.
172. Chambers HF. Coagulase-negative staphylococcal resistant to beta-lactam antibiotic in vivo produces penicillin-binding protein 2a. Antimicrob Ag Chemother 1987; 31:1919.
173. Richards GK, Gagnon RF, Obst G, Kostiner GB. The affected peritoneal dialysis solutions on rifampin action against *Staphylococcus epidermidis* in the fluid and biofilm phases of growth. Perit Dial Intern 1993; 13(suppl 2):S341.
174. Kobasa WD, Kaye KL, Schapiro T, et al. Therapy for experimental endocarditis due to *Staphylococcus epidermidis*. Rev Infect Dis 1983; 5:5533.
175. Karchmer AW, Archer GL. The Endocarditis Study Group: methicillin-resistant *Staphylococcus epidermidis* prosthetic valve endocarditis: a therapeutic trial in Programs and Abstracts of the Twenty- Fourth Interscience Conference of Antimicrobial Agents and Chemotherapy, Washington D.C., 1984.
176. Whitener C, Caputo G, Weitkamp M, et al. Endocarditis due to coagulase-negative staphylococci: microbiologic, epidemiologic and clinical considerations. In: Wilson W, Stecklebert JJ, eds. Infective Endocarditis in Infective Dis Clin NA. 1993:7.
177. Cohen PS, Maguire JH, Weinstein L. Infective endocarditis caused by gram negative bacteria: a review of the literature, 1945–1977. Prog Cardiovasc Dis 1980; 22:205.
178. Sanders C. New beta-lactams: new problems for the internist. Editorial. Ann Intern Med 1991; 115:650.
179. Sanders WE Jr, Sanders CC. Inducible beta-lactamases: clinical and epidemiologic implications for use of newer cephalosporins. Rev Infect Dis 1988; 10:830.
180. Tancrede CH, Andremont AO, Leonard FC. Epidemiology of Enterobacteria resistant to cefotaxime in hospital. J Antimicrob Chemother 1984; 14(suppl B):53.
181. Rice LB, Willey SH, Papanicolau GA, et al. The break its intensity resistance caused by extended-spectrum beta-lactamases at a Massachusetts chronic care facility. Antimicrob Agents Chemother 1990; 34:2193.
182. Sanders CC, Iaconis JP, Bodey GP, et al. Resistance to ticarcillin-potassium clavulanate among clinical isolates of the family Enterobacteriaceae: Role of PSE – 1beta-lactamase and high levels of TEM-1 and SHV-1 and problems with false susceptibility in disk diffusion tests. Antimicrob Agents Chemother 1988; 32:1365.
183. Levison ME, Kobasa WD. Mezlocillin and ticarcillin alone and combined with gentamicin in the treatment of experimental *Enterobacter aerogenes* endocarditis. Antimicrob Agents Chemother 1984; 25:683.
184. Kobasa WD, Kaye D. Aztreonam, cefoperazone and gentamicin in the treatment of experimental Enterobacter carotid knees endocarditis in rabbits. Antimicrob Agents Chemother 1988; 24:321.
185. Bayer AS, Hirano L, Yih J. Development of beta-lactam resistance and increased quinolone MIC's during therapy of experimental *Pseudomonas* endocarditis. Antimicrob Agents Chemother 1988; 32:231.

186. Chambers HF. Other beta-lactam antibiotics. In: Mandell GL, Bennett JE, Dolin R, eds. Principal and Practice of Infectious Diseases, chapter 21. Philadelphia: Elseiver, 2005:311.
187. Weinstein L, Schlessinger J. Treatment of infective endocarditis-1973. Prog Cardiovasc Dis 1973; 16:275.
188. Rodriguez C, Olcoz MT, Izquierdo G, et al. Endocarditis due to ampicillin-resistant non typhoid Salmonella. Cure with a third generation cephalosporin. Rev Infect Dis 1990; 12:817.
189. Mills J, Drew D. *Serratia marcescens* endocarditis. Ann Intern Med 1976; 85:397.
190. Cooper R, Mills J. *Serratia* endocarditis. Arch Intern Med 1980; 140:199.
191. Hejazi A, Falkiner FR. *Serratia marcescens.* J Med Microbiol 1997; 46:903.
192. Reyes MP, Brown WJ, Lerner AM. Treatment of patients with *Pseudomonas* endocarditis with high dose aminoglycoside and carbenicillin therapy. Medicine 1978;57:57.
193. Reyes MP, Lerner AM. Current problems in the treatment of infective endocarditis due to *Pseudomonas aeruginosa.* Rev Infect Dis 1983; 5:314.
194. Fowler VG, Scheld WM, Bayer AS. Endocarditis and intravascular infections. In: Mandell GL, Bennett JE, Dolin R, eds. Principal and Practice of Infectious Diseases, chapter 74. Philadelphia: Elseiver, 2005:1000.
195. Lynn DJ, Kane JG, Parker RH. Haemophilus parainfluenza and influenza endocarditis: a review of forty cases. Medicine 1977; 56:115.
196. Bryan JP, Pankey GA. Haemophilus paraphrophilus endocarditis. South Med J 1986; 79:480.
197. Wilson WR, Karchmer AW, Dajani AS, et al. Antibiotic treatment of adults with infective endocarditis due to streptococci, enterococci, staphylococci and HACEK microorganisms. JAMA 1995; 74:1706.
198. Flugelman M, Galvan E, Genchetrit E, et al. Crucial doses in patients with heart disease: when should endocarditis be diagnosed? Cardiology 1990; 77:313.
199. Young EJ. Brucellosis: current epidemiology, diagnosis and management. Curr Top Infect Dis 1995; 15:115.
200. Weisner P, Handsfield H, Holmes K. Though antibiotic resistance gonococci causing disseminated infection. N Engl J Med 1973; 288:1221.
201. Bush L, Boscia J. Disseminated multiple antibiotic resistant gonococcal infection: needed changes in antimicrobial therapy. Ann Intern Med 1987; 197:692.
202. Murray BE, Karchmer AW, Moellering RC Jr. Diphtheroid prosthetic valve endocarditis. Am J Med 1980; 69:838.
203. Cauda R, Tamburrini E, Ventura G, et al. Infective vancomycin therapy for corynebacteria pseudodiphtheriticum endocarditis. South Med J 1987; 80:1598.
204. Nieman RE, Lorber B. Listeriosis and adults: a changing pattern. Report of 8 cases and review of the literature, 1968–1978. Rev Infect Dis 1980; 2:207.
205. Gallagher PG, Watanakunakorn D. *Listeria monocytogenes* endocarditis: A review of the literature 1950–1986. Scand J Infect Dis 1988; 20:359.
206. Marco F, Almela M, Nolla-Salas J, et al. In vitro activities and 3 to antimicrobial agents against *Listeria monocytogenes* strains isolated from Barcelona , Spain. Diagn Microbiol Infect Dis 2000; 38:259.
207. Varma MPS, Adgey AAJ, Connolly JH. Chronic Q fever endocarditis. Br Heart J 1980; 43:695.
208. Fenallar F, Fournier P-E, Garrier M, et al. Risk factors and prevention of Q fever endocarditis. CID 2001; 33:312.
209. Raoult D, Etienne J, Massip P, et al. Q fever endocarditis in the South France. J Infect Dis 1987; 155:570.
210. Raoult D, Houpikian P, Tissot-Dupont H, et al. Treatment of Q fever endocarditis: comparison of two regimens containing doxycycline and ofloxacin or hydroxychloroquine. Arch Intern Med 1999; 59:167.
211. Raoult D, Fournier PE, Vendenesch F, et al. Outcome and treatment of *Bartonella endocarditis.* Arch Intern Med 2003; 163:226.
212. Raoult D, Fournier PE, Drancourt M, et al. Diagnosis of 22 new cases of *Bartonella endocarditis.* Ann Intern Med 1996; 125:646.

213. Fournier PE, Lelievre H, Eykyn SJ, et al. Epidemiologic and clinical characteristics of *Bartonella quintana* and *Bartonella henselae* endocarditis: a study of 48 patients. Medicine (Baltimore) 2001; 80:245.
214. Fenollar F, Lepidi H, Raoult D. Whipple's endocarditis: review of the literature and comparisons with Q fever, *Bartonella* infection and blood culture positive endocarditis. Clin Infect Dis 2001; 33:1309.
215. Brouqui P, Raoult D. Endocarditis due to rare and fastidious bacteria. Clin Microbiol Rev 2001; 14:177.
216. Tunbel A, Kaye D. Endocarditis with negative blood cultures. N Engl J Med 1992; 325:1215.
217. Persand V. Two unusual cases of mural endocarditis with a review of the literature. Am J Clin Pathol 1970; 53:832.
218. Leaf H, Simberkoff M. Fungal endocarditis . In: Hortkotte D, Bodnar E, eds. Infective Endocarditis. London: ICR Publishers, 1991:180.
219. McLeod R, Remington JS. Fungal endocarditis. In: Rahimtoola SH, ed. Infective Endocarditis. New York: Grune and Stratton, 1978:211.
220. Ellis ME, Al Abdely H, Sandridge A, et al. Fungal endocarditis: evidence in the world literature, 1965–1995. Clin Infect Dis 2001; 32:50.
221. Selig MS, Speth CP, Kozinn PJ, et al. Patterns of *Candida* endocarditis following cardiac surgery: importance of early diagnosis and therapy (an analysis of 91 cases). Prog Cardiovasc Dis 1974; 27:125.
222. El-Hamasmy I, Durrleman N, Stevens LM, et al. *Aspergillus* endocarditis after cardiac surgery. Ann Thorac Surg 2005; 80:359.
223. Kouhaty DS, Stalker JB, Munt PW. Nonsurgical treatment of histoplasma endocarditis involving a bioprosthetic valve. Chest 1991; 1:253.
224. Smith BM, Hoeprich PD, Huston AC, et al. Activity of two polyene and two imidazole antimicrobics on *Candida albicans* and fibrin clots. J Lab Clin Med 1983; 102:126.
225. Rubinstein E, Noreiga E, Simberkoff MS, et al. Tissue penetration of amphotericin B in *Candida* endocarditis. Chest 1974; 66:376.
226. Sande MA, Bowman CR, Calderone RA. Experimental *Candida albicans* endocarditis: characterization of the disease and response to therapy. Infect Immun 1977; 17:140.
227. Melgar GR, Nasser RM, Gordon SM, et al. Fungal prosthetic valve endocarditis in 16 patients: an 11 year experience in a tertiary care hospital. Medicine (Baltimore) 1997; 76:94.
228. Nasser RM, Melgar GR, Longworth DL, Gordon SM. Incidence and risk of developing fungal prosthetic valve endocarditis after nosocomial candidemia. Am J Med 1997; 103:25.
229. Pappas PG, Rex JH, Sobel JD, et al. Guidelines for treatment of candidiasis. Clin Infect Dis 2004; 38:161.
230. Czwerwiec FS, Bilsker MS, Kamerman ML, Bisno AL. Long-term survival after fluconazole therapy of *Candida* prosthetic valve endocarditis. Am J Med 1993; 94:545.
231. Yeaman MR, Cheng D, Desai B, et al. This susceptibility to thrombin-induced platelet microbicidal proteinase associated with increased fluconazole efficacy against experimental endocarditis due to *Candida albicans*. Antimicrob Agents Chemother 2004; 48:3051.
232. Castiglia M, Smego RA Jr, Sames EL. Candida endocarditis and amphotericin B. intolerance: potential role for fluconazole. Infect Dis Clin Pract 1994; 3:248.
233. Baddour LM. Long-term suppressive therapy for fungal endocarditis (letter, comment). Clin Infect Dis 1996; 23:1338.
234. Witt M, Bayer A. Comparison of fluconazole and amphotericin B for prevention and treatment of experimental *Candida* endocarditis. Antimicrob Agents Chemother 1991; 35:2481.
235. Gumbo T, Taege AJ, Mawhorter S, et al. Aspergillus valve endocarditis in patients without prior cardiac surgery. Medicine 2000; 79:261.
236. Longman LP, Martin MV. A comparison of the efficacy of itraconazole, amphotericin B and 5-fluorocytosine in the treatment of *Aspergillus fumigatis* endocarditis in the rabbit. J Antimicrob Chemother 1987; 20:719.

237. Jiminez-Expopsito MJ, Torres G, Baraldes A, et al. Native valve endocarditis due to *Candida glabrata* treated without valvular replacement: a potential role for caspofungin in the induction maintenance treatment. Clin Infect Dis 2004; 39:e70.

238. Rajendram R, AlP NJ, Mitchell AR, et al. Candida prosthetic valve endocarditis cured by capsofungin therapy without valve replacement. Clin Infect Dis 2005; 40:e72.

239. Moudgal V, Little T, Boikov D, Vasquez JA. Mulechinocsandin –multiazole-resistant *Candida parasilosis* isolates serially obtained during therapy for prosthetic valve endocarditis. Antimicrob Agents Chemother 2005; 49:767.

240. Mora-Duarte J, Betts R, Rotstein C, et al. Comparison of Capsofungin and amphotericin B for invasive candidiasis. N Engl J Med 2002; 347:2020.

241. Hospenthal DR, Murray CK, Rinaldi MG. The role of antifungal susceptibility testing in therapy of candidiasis. Diag Microbiol Infect Dis 2004; 48:153.

242. Sakoulas G, Eliopoulos GM, Alder J, et al. Efficacy of Daptomycin in experimental endocarditis due to methicillin-resistant *Staphylococcus aureus*. Antimicrob Agents Chemother 2003; 47:714.

243. Anaisse EJ, Bishara AB, Solomkin JS. Fungal Infection. ACS Surgery, 2005.

244. Souba WW, Fink MP, Jurkovich GJ, et al. New York: Web Professional Publishing, 2005:1486–1487.

15

Surgical Treatment of Native Valve and Prosthetic Valve Infective Endocarditis

John L. Brusch

Harvard Medical School and Department of Medicine and Infectious Disease Service, Cambridge Health Alliance, Cambridge, Massachusetts, U.S.A.

INTRODUCTION

The first reported surgical cure of infective endocarditis (IE) was the repair of a ventricular septal defect and removal of a tricuspid vegetation, which was infected with *Candida albicans*, by Kay et al. in 1960 (1). In 1965, Wallace et al. (2) removed an aortic valve that was persistently infected with *Serratia marcescens*. Despite treatment with colistin and kanamycin, the patient remained febrile, his bacteremia continued, and his aortic regurgitation became more severe. After three weeks of medical treatment, the infected valve was removed and replaced with Starr-Edwards prosthesis. The surgical specimen was notable for massive, soft vegetations that involved the perforated left and right coronary cusps. Operative cultures were positive for *S. marcescens*. The patient recovered without complication and remained free of disease. These surgeons observed sagely: "The results of a combined program of intense antimicrobial therapy and resection of the infected valve produced encouraging results in the correction of the hemodynamic abnormality." They did add a qualifying statement: "In selected cases, active endocarditis need not be considered a reason for valvular replacement." This last statement was the first to recognize the major challenge of cardiac surgery performed in the treatment of IE, knowing when an operative procedure should be undertaken. The discussion of the indications for surgery in IE is the major focus of this chapter.

Approximately 15–25% of patients with IE undergo surgical treatment. This figure is the same for cases from tertiary-care institutions and community hospitals (3,4). Twenty-five to thirty percent of surgeries are performed during the acute phase of valvular infection, 20% to 40% later in the course of the disease (5–7). Since the availability of cardiac surgery, the mortality rate of IE has decreased from 30% to 20% of the cases. This reduction has been most dramatic in cases due to *Staphylococcus aureus* for which the death rate has declined from 60% to 30% (5). Because there has been an increase in cases due to extremely resistant organisms, such as *S. aureus*, enterococci, gram-negatives, and fungi, the absolute number of deaths because of IE has not declined. Fifty percent of certain types of infection do not respond to intensive medical and surgical treatment. This situation plays a great part in the increase in both intra- and extracardiac complications of IE that are caused by the increasing involvement of aggressive pathogens combined with a concurrent rise in the number of impaired hosts (8–10). In the last 20 years, there has been a progressively better definition of the indications for cardiac surgery in IE. Transthoracic echocardiography (TTE) contributed significantly to the development of surgical indications. Transesophageal echocardiography (TEE) has allowed these to be even more "fine-tuned" (11–13). It is important to emphasize that the decision

TABLE 1 Indications for Surgery in Native Valve and Prosthetic Valve Infective Endocarditis

Congestive heart failure
Persistent infection
Intracardiac fistulas penetrating into the pericardium
Rupture of the sinus of Valsalva aneurysm
Septal perforation
Paravalvular abscess
Aortic or sinus of Valsalva aneurysms
Staphylococcal prosthetic valve endocarditis
Early prosthetic valve endocarditis
Progressive paravalvular leak
Fungal endocarditis
Infection with difficulty to treat organisms
Enlarging vegetation despite one to two weeks of antimicrobial therapy

to perform surgery should not be based on echocardiographic findings alone. Echocardiographic results should be interpreted in light of careful follow-up examination, response of fever to antimicrobial therapy, and clearance of the bloodstream infection (BSI). The preoperative duration of antibiotic therapy has little, if any, effect on operative mortality (14,15). Besides the treatment of the primary valvular infection, the reasons to administer antibiotics before surgery are to suppress/eradicate bacteria from the sewing base of the implanted valve and to prevent BSI secondary to the surgical debridement.

The major indications for surgery, both in the past and present, are persistent infection and congestive heart failure (CHF) (13,16,17). In left-sided IE, CHF is the most common reason for surgical intervention; in right-sided, it is persistent infection. This is understandable given the fact that significant damage to the tricuspid valve has little of the hemodynamic effect than damage to the aortic or mitral valves has. The major indications for cardiac surgery are presented in Table 1. Several systems have been developed that utilize a scoring system to calculate the necessity for surgical intervention (18,19). The author believes that the decision for surgical intervention should be based primarily on the clinical features of the case and not a set of scoring guidelines. This is especially true for the echocardiographic characteristics of the patient. Although there is correlation between the ultrasound findings and the clinical course of the patient, the echocardiographic findings are usually not good enough to justify surgery by themselves. There are no completely accepted parameters that accurately determine the risk of an embolizing vegetation. Significant, but often overlooked factors are the experience of the cardiac surgeons and the level of postoperative management provided by the hospital (20).

Michael et al. defined the need for and timing of surgery into three stages: *stage 1*—surgery that is required for severe aortic regurgitation begins after bacteriological cure of IE is achieved; *stage 2*—elective surgery, during antimicrobial therapy, of patients who have developed cardiac failure that responds rapidly to medical management, and *stage 3*—emergent surgery of patients who develop severe complications such as intractable CHF or persistent bacteremia (21). Hasbun et al. (22) developed a similar system but with four stages. Simply stated, some complications require surgery emergently, urgently, or electively (22). Olaison and Pettersson (5) have recently prioritized the indications for surgery into three categories: (*i*) emergency surgery performed on the same day; (*ii*) urgent surgery performed within one to two days; and (*iii*) elective surgery simply described as "earlier is usually better." In the discussion of the individual surgical indications, reference will be made to Olaison and Pettersson's three categories. In order to give some perspective to the significance of the surgical indicators, it is important to be aware of the most frequent causes of death in IE. In decreasing importance, they are: neurologic events, CHF, emboli, rupture of a mycotic aneurysm, complications of cardiac surgery, failure of antimicrobial therapy, and prosthetic valve endocarditis (PVE) (23).

CONGESTIVE HEART FAILURE

Congestive heart failure is the most frequent cause for surgery in IE. Prior to the availability of cardiac surgical techniques, 91% of IE-associated fatalities were due to CHF (24). Medical therapy, alone, results in a death rate of 75% in patients with moderate to advanced CHF. Appropriate surgical intervention can reduce this to 25% (7,18,). Heart failure accounts for up to 75% of surgical procedures in IE (25). Mills et al. (26) were among the first to recognize the significant role surgery could play in treating the CHF of IE. In their uncontrolled series, only one out of 15 patients who were treated medically were alive in six months. Nine of the 14 who received both medical and surgical therapies were still alive. These findings were confirmed by Croft (27). Survival of the patients who received medical and surgical therapies was clearly superior: 56% versus 11% of those who were treated medically. Published in 1997, a meta-analysis of nine retrospective studies, involving 300 patients in significant heart failure, demonstrated a 60% versus 29% advantage in the survival rate of dual therapy (28). A major criticism of all these studies of native valve endocarditis (NVE) is that they did not take into account comorbidities such as kidney failure and cerebrovascular disease that prevented a surgical approach. Although this potential bias favors the surgically treated groups, the striking difference between the two approaches most likely still remains significant. The difference in survival from PVE-associated CHF, in those treated medically and in those treated medically and surgically, parallels that of NVE. At six months, mortality in the former group approaches 100%. In the surgical cohort, 45–85% are alive at this point (29). For *S. aureus* PVE, a multivariate analysis of the effectiveness of a combined surgical and medical approach compared with a medical approach has been conducted (29a). Even with the adjustment of the patients' comorbidities, surgery resulted in a 20-fold decrease in patient deaths.

The individuals who benefited most from surgery are those present with the new onset of significant congestive failure and are operated upon within four days of the beginning of treatment (15,30). The decision to operate is based on the hemodynamic factors and not the course of the valvular infection. In patients not in failure, the length of preoperative antibiotic therapy has no bearing on intraoperative death (15). The operative mortality of urgent surgery in patients without clinical CHF ranges from 6% to 11%. This rate increases to 17% to 33% for those in failure (30a). Over time, valvular insufficiency rises to ventricular dilatation and further insufficiency. This spiral of deterioration converts mild CHF to severe failure usually within the first month of antibiotic therapy.

There are a few valid reasons for delay in operating. The most important of these is patients with IE who have already suffered a recent stroke. Forty-four percent of patients, who have had a nonhemorrhagic embolic stroke within seven days, will have further cerebral deterioration following cardiac surgery. Seventeen percent of the individuals will have cortical deterioration when surgery is performed between eight and 14 days after the initial insult. After two weeks, the chance of worsening brain function is <10%. If stroke had been hemorrhagic, neurological worsening would continue at 20% for at least one month (30b). Other reasons include extracardiac infections such as splenic abscesses. Age itself is not a contraindication to surgery. Age-associated coronary artery disease often must be defined before valvular surgery can be performed. Clinically apparent myocardial infarction occurs in 3% of the cases during treatment and is responsible for 1% of the deaths. The infarcts are because of emboli that obstruct the coronary circulation. Loss of myocardium is a major contributor to postoperative CHF (30c,30d).

Severe aortic regurgitation results in more severe and more rapidly progressive CHF than does mitral valve incompetence. Clinical signs of significant heart failure, in the presence of aortic regurgitation, demand an immediate cardiac surgery consultation (31). Acute aortic regurgitation with evidence of early closure of the anterior leaflet of the mitral valve represents an uncomplicated overload of the left ventricle that calls for urgent (same day) surgery (32). Progressive heart failure, in conjunction with acute aortic or mitral valve incompetence, likewise demands early surgery. During the first week, the findings of significant valvular incompetence by Doppler echocardiography is not reliably predictive of the need of urgent surgery. Conversely, the absence of echocardiographic findings of valvular incompetence during the first week does not guarantee that the patient will not develop significant incompetence in the future. Often in early acute aortic regurgitation, the auscultatory findings are quite unimpressive. Somewhat paradoxically, pre-existing aortic insufficiency may respond to medical management during active phase of IE. Severe mitral regurgitation less often needs urgent surgical correction, but will ultimately require it. The CHF, which is associated with IE, is usually caused by perforation of the valvular cusps of a native valve or a bioprosthetic one (33). Unusually, it may be because of obstruction of valvular orifice by a large vegetation, rupture mitral chordae tendineae, the formation of fistulous intracardiac shunts, or prosthetic valve dehiscence. Pulmonary valve or tricuspid valve insufficiency, because of IE, seldom require surgery unless pulmonary hypertension is present (32).

In the presence of IE-associated CHF, the clinician must be aware of two caveats. Paradoxically, pre-existing aortic insufficiency may respond to medical management during the active phase of IE unless the valvular infection worsens the pre-existing regurgitation. When judging the severity of congestive failure, the presence of other contributing factors, such as anemia, and renal failure, must be taken into account when assessing the patient for surgery.

PERSISTENT INFECTION/PERSISTENT BACTEREMIA

Failure to clear the BSI of IE after seven days of appropriate antimicrobial therapy is generally associated with a poorer than average clinical outcome (34). When metastatic infection has been ruled out, persistent fever usually represents an intracardiac complication (56%) (5). By itself, fever is not synonymous with persistent infection. The physician must view this one vital sign in the context of the patient's entire clinical picture. Recurrent fever, which usually presents itself three to four weeks into apparently successful therapy, is usually because of hypersensitivity reactions to antibiotics, especially the beta-lactams (35). When fever is persistent and/or associated with continued BSI, surgery can significantly decrease the fatality rate from 34–90% to 9–13% (36). If the underlying valvular structure is competent, stand to removal of large vegetations does away with the sources of possible emboli and allows repair of the damaged leaflets (37). This approach is most frequently used in intravenous drug abusers (IVDA) IE. Bacterial infection of the tricuspid valve can be treated either by excision of the entire valve or of one or two of its leaflets (34).

Persistent infection is almost inevitable in individuals with fungal IE. Valve replacement should be undertaken as soon as possible in these cases. However, the fatality rate remains high for candidal IE (42%) despite dual therapy. Eighty-seven percent of *Aspergillus* IE succumb (38); these dismal outcomes are most likely because of high rates of embolization, metastatic infections (70% of cases overall), perivalvular, and myocardial abscesses (39). Early surgical intervention may improve long-term outcomes. Tricuspid valvulectomy is often adequate to eradicate right-sided fungal endocarditis. End-organ damage, from fungal emboli, may improve with local removal.

Despite the dramatic success of the very first placement of a prosthetic valve for definitive treatment of IE, there has been great concern that the implanted valve itself may become infected (2). In great part, this original surgery was successful because the patient had received several weeks of preoperative antibiotics. Surgical outcomes are much better when the patient has been partially or fully treated (40). In patients with evidence of active IE, early postoperative deaths were 11.5%. Two percent suffered recurrences within a few months of the surgery. Long-term reinfection of the prosthetic valve occurs in 20% to 40% of IVDA and in 5% of nondrug abusers (36). Congestive heart failure, age, renal failure, and staphylococcal IE were positively correlated with a poor result. There was no increased risk associated with the number of valves infected, whether they were prosthetic or not, and the particular valves involved. These figures have been confirmed in other studies (41,42).

These outcomes can be correlated with the histological findings and cultures of the excised tissue (43). Cultures were positive in 41% of the individuals who had received only a few days of preoperative antibiotics. This is compared with 10% and 12% of patients who had completed, respectively, 50% or 100% of their intended course. Gram stains may remain positive for months after microbiological cure and so do not serve as good indicators of active infection.

Cases of culture-negative endocarditis, which continue to be febrile after seven to 10 days of antibiotic therapy, should undergo a TEE and possibly a magnetic resonance angiogram to look for the very likely possibility of a paravalvular infection. A less likely cause of persistent fever in these patients is that the empiric antibiotic regimen is ineffective against the infecting organisms (44). If extracardiac sources of fever were ruled out, many would advocate surgery in this situation even in the absence of a definable intracardiac source.

Surgery is mandated in all cases of PVE when there is indication that the infection has spread to the adjacent myocardium. Evidence of spread includes heart failure, development of regurgitant murmurs, fever that continues despite appropriate antimicrobial therapy, and conduction abnormalities on electrocardiography. Peivalvular infections are especially common in early PVE and infections of an aortic prosthesis. Coagulase-negative staphylococci and *S. aureus* together account for approximately 50% of early PVE. Essentially all of these types of infection spread to the perivalvular areas with a valvular ring abscess (essentially a paravalvular abscess) and/or valvular dehiscence in 60% of the cases (45–48). The surgical approach leads to greater than six-month survival of patients, especially those with CHF (64% vs. 0%) and less relapses than a medical treatment alone does. The recurrence of PVE ranges from 6% to 15%. Repeat surgery must be performed to treat recurrent PVE or dysfunction of the prosthesis in up to 25% of the patients (6,29,45). Early surgery and antibiotic therapy constitute the best approach to *S. aureus* PVE (11).

Mitral valve repair is an option for partially treated or completely healed disease, seldom for active IE. It should be considered in IVDA to be unreliable in taking any correlation and who are at risk of recurrent IE because of their high rate of recidivism in using illicit drugs (49,50).

Certain types of PVE have a reasonable chance of being treated with antibiotics alone. Factors that are predictive of a nonsurgical cure include: (*i*) late-onset PVE (>12 months after implantation); (*ii*) infection with nonaggressive organisms (*Streptococcus viridans* and members of the HACEK group); (*iii*) absence of perivalvular invasion; (*iv*) infection of a mitral prosthetic valve; (*v*) early detected bioprosthetic valve IE; and (*vi*) prompt institution of antibiotic therapy (45,51). Mitral PVE results in less perivalvular infection than aortic PVE. Because IE of bioprosthetic valves involves the valvular leaflets but not the sewing ring, it is somewhat easier to treat. These cells are also less likely to become infected within the first 24 months after their implantation. There does not seem to be any difference in the risk of infection when either type of prosthetic valve is implanted in the setting of IE (51a). Individuals who are treated for PVE medically without surgery need to be closely monitored with repeated TEEs for at least two months postoperatively (30a).

An unresolved issue is the duration of antimicrobial therapy after valve implantation. This is dependent on several factors including: the length of time preoperative antibiotics were administered; the susceptibility to antibiotics of the pathogens; the culture status of the excised tissue; and the condition of the valve sewing bed (52,53). The European Society of Cardiology recommends that the patient receive a full course of antibiotics if the operative cultures are positive. If there is no growth, a full course of treatment (including the preoperative duration) should be administered. Karchmer's approach is similar with modifications. All patients with PVE should receive a full course of antibiotic therapy postoperatively when the Gram stain of the excised material is positive despite the culture being negative. Also, if the valve is sewn into a debrided abscess cavity, then a full postoperative course of appropriate antibiotics be given.

VALVULAR VEGETATIONS

The significance of valvular vegetations, besides the fact that they are the focus of infection, is a major area of controversy in the management of IE (Table 3). The concern focuses on the risk of embolization that they pose. As valvular vegetations are detectable in up to 78% of cases of IE, this probably presents the most common challenge to the clinician in managing the patient with IE (54). The incidence of clinically apparent arterial emboli in IE is approximately 43%. About 27% to 65% of emboli involve the cerebral circulation (55–58). Twenty-five percent of deaths from IE are because of emboli. Seventy-five percent of clinically apparent emboli occur before the onset of antibiotic therapy (59). It is very likely that the incidence of emboli of all types is significantly greater than reported. This is based on the estimation by Olaison and Pettersson that as the brain receives approximately 14% of total cardiac output and suffers 50% of all emboli, it stands to reason that emboli to other sites are grossly underdetected (5).

It has been hoped that echocardiography would identify specific characteristics of vegetations that would be predictive of embolization and to identify those patients who would benefit from preventive surgery. Early studies, which employed TTE, did not prove a clear association between the presence of valvular vegetations and the risk of embolization (60). The study of Mugge et al. utilized both TTE and TTE. It found that 47% of IE patients with vegetations that were >10 mm in diameter and were located on native mitral valves suffered emboli. Only 19% of the individuals with smaller vegetations evidenced embolization. Vegetations found at other sites did not appear to have potential for embolization. There appeared to be no significant correlation between valvular thrombi and the development of CHF and death. Bayer (62) did report an association between heart failure and vegetations >10 mm. Studies have indicated that vegetations located on the anterior leaflet of the mitral valve have the highest rate of emboli (37%) (63). This is probably because of extraordinary mechanical stress placed on this leaflet that may lead to the breaking up and eventual embolization of the vegetation. Another study demonstrated the correlation between embolization and extremely mobile and large vegetations (>15 mm). *Staphylococcus aureus* IE was another risk factor (58). However, in this study, there appeared to be no connection between mitral location and embolization. Another series demonstrated that large vegetations were predictive of embolic events only in patients with *S. viridans* IE (54). Other findings conclude that IE produced by *S. aureus* has the highest incidence of embolization (64). Other patient characteristics that have been implicated in an increased risk for embolization include atrial fibrillation, PVE, and a history of previous embolus (54).

A recent meta-analysis indicates that systemic embolization was increased in the presence of vegetations >10 mm compared with those with valvular thrombi of 10 mm (37% vs. 19%) (65). More definitive studies support the association correlation between embolization and : (*i*) vegetations >10 mm, (*ii*) those located on the anterior leaflet of the mitral valve, and (*iii*) those with increased mobility (58,65,66). It is important to emphasize that there is no proof that operating on patients with these characteristics actually pre-empts embolization (27).

Potentially, a more valid prognostic characteristic would be the response of the vegetation to antimicrobial therapy. For both NVE and PVE, the risk of embolization markedly decreases during the first two weeks of antimicrobial therapy from 13 to 18 events/1000 treatment days to three to seven events/1000 treatment days (30,54). Rohmann documented that an increase or even stability in the size of the vegetation >8 mm in diameter was predictive of an extended period of healing. This prolonged time of valvular repair was associated with a higher incidence of embolization, CHF, and death. The dictum that surgery should be performed in patients who have had two or more major embolic episodes during antimicrobial therapy needs to be questioned. Surgery should be strongly considered when there have been recurrent emboli past the two-week mark of beginning antimicrobial agents and a large vegetation is still present, especially if it is on the anterior leaflet of the mitral valve, is quite mobile, and is enlarged. In this situation, the development of other complications, such as a paravalvular abscess, were ruled out by a TEE.

Is there a role for valvular surgery as a measure to prevent embolization? "Vegetation size alone is really an indication for surgery" (44). Of course if there is concurrently a significant degree of heart failure, surgery should be performed for this reason. The decision to operate should be one based on a comprehensive review of all the clinical factors interpreted in the light of the aforementioned information accrued over 30 years. Table 2 presents possible indications for valvular surgery for prevention of primary or secondary embolic events.

TABLE 2   Indications for Valvular Surgery for the Primary and Secondary
Prevention of Embolic Events in Infective Endocarditis

Vegetation located on the anterior leaflet of mitral valve
Vegetation >10 mm in diameter
Mobile vegetation
Atrial fibrillation
Enlarging vegetation despite antimicrobial therapy
Staphylococcus aureus infective endocarditis
Previous embolization
Recurrent embolization during the first two weeks of antimicrobial therapy

PARAVALVULAR/EXTRAVALVULAR EXTENSIONS
OF INFECTIVE ENDOCARDITIS

Spread of valvular infection into the base of the valve and further into the myocardium occurs in 10% to 14% of the individuals with NVE and 45% to 60% of the cases of PVE (52). In NVE, it is more frequent in aortic valve involvement. Aortic IE and IVDA are the two major risk factors for the development of paravalvular abscesses (67). Pettersson and Carbon summarize the pathogenesis of paravalvular abscesses and their complications (68). Cellulitis, which spreads from the base of the valve, evolves to form abscess. Hemodynamic forces working on the weakened, infected paravalvular tissue produce pseudoaneurysms. Pseudoaneurysms also may be the result of trained abscesses. The same process may travel around the circumference of the valve in a "horseshoe" manner. This may lead to separation of the aortic and mitral valve annulus from the ventricle or period. Fistulas are the result of abscesses burrowing into a ventricle or atria. When they burrow into the pericardial space, death almost inevitably ensues. Heart block is the result of interventricular septal involvement.

The major clinical clues to the existence of a paravalvular abscess are the presence of an unexplained persistent fever despite appropriate antibiotics and the development of pericarditis. For diagnosis, a TEE should done. It is much more sensitive in diagnosing invasive infection, in either NVE or PVE, than a TTE (sensitivity of 87% vs. 30%) (see Chapter 13). Fistulas are best detected by Doppler echocardiography. If echocardiography fails to detect the suspected abscess, the use of magnetic resonance imaging may be fruitful. Although it is relatively insensitive in detecting paravalvular abscess (28% to 53%), electrocardiography is quite specific (69–72). Dinubile (16) developed criteria for determining the needs for urgent surgery in IE. These are based on the characteristics of heart block: (*i*) the new onset or progression of established heart block; (*ii*) aortic valve IE; (*iii*) persistence of block for at least one week after beginning treatment with antimicrobial agents; and (*iv*) identifying and eliminating other causes of abnormal conduction (e.g., digoxin or verapamil). There is a fairly high rate of false-positive TEEs in PVE.

As discussed, emergent surgery is quite beneficial with a low reinfection rate. Often, radical surgery must be performed to extirpate large absences at the root of the aorta. This brings about the real risk of damage to the conduction system, which can result in postoperative atrioventricular block (A-V) block. The goal of surgery is threefold: debridement, drainage, and reconstruction. Reconstruction of the involved area is often the most challenging. The success of the implanted valve, both in a hemodynamic and an infectious disease sense, depends to a great degree on the viability of the tissue into which the valve ring is sewn. There are several newer techniques that have had been useful in reconstructing a viable bed. A few patients may not require surgery because of the uncomplicated nature of the abscesses.

METASTATIC COMPLICATIONS OF INFECTIVE ENDOCARDITIS

Mycotic aneurysms affect 2% to 15% of the patients with IE (Table 4) (73). They most commonly involve the sinus of Valsalva or the supravalvular proximal thoracic aorta (74). One to five percent of the cases of IE are complicated by cerebral mycotic aneurysms. Additional sites are the abdominal arteries, the coronary arteries, and the pulmonary arteries. Mycotic aneurysms may also develop in the legs, small bowel, valvular leaflets, and the annulus of the mitral valve.

This discussion will focus on cerebral mycotic aneurysms (75). Their incidence has not decreased with the availability of antibiotics. They usually appear clinically late in the course of IE. Mycotic aneurysms of IE are most commonly the result of deposition of infected emboli in the vaso vasorum, usually associated with *S. viridans* IE. Less often, they may be because of septic emboli, most often involving *S. aureus*, to the lumen of the artery (76). Usually, they are deposited at the branch points of the cerebral arteries. *Streptococcus viridans* is responsible for more mycotic aneurysms than *S. aureus*. However, those that are associated with the latter pathogen have a higher rate of rupture.

The diagnosis of mycotic aneurysms is very challenging, and the consequences of rupture are so devastating. The median interval between the diagnosis of valvular infection and the clinical appearance of rupture/hemorrhage is 18 days (range 0 to 35 days) (77). At times, there may be herald signs such as seizures, transient focal deficits, focal headache, and aseptic meningitis (due to small leaks). Sudden development of homonomous hemianopsia is a particularly useful sentinel event in an individual who is IE. Unfortunately, many of these signs and symptoms are relatively nonspecific for patients with IE (Chapter 6). Guidelines for cerebral arteriography have been developed to assist the physician in deciding when imaging is necessary (78). Eighty percent of the patients with a ruptured mycotic aneurysm died compared with 30% of those whose lesions do not (79). Wilson et al. (80) identified mycotic aneurysms/cerebral hemorrhage in seven patients (80). All had developed severe headaches and visual field defects. The mycotic aneurysms

TABLE 3 Cardiac Complications of Acute Infective Endocarditis After Mitral, Aortic, and Mitral-Aortic Valve Replacement

	MVR (%)	AVR (%)	DVR (%)	Average (%)
Periprosthetic dehiscence	60	80	91	76.7
Interference of vegetation and valve occluder	9	7	25	9.7
Cardiac failure	37	48	67	46.6
Myocarditis/pericarditis	11	14	16	13.6
Intracardiac fistulas/abscesses	11	11	25	12.6
Conduction disturbances	23	20	50	24.3
Ventricular arrhythmias	3	5	8	4.9
Septic thromboembolism	25	21	58	27.2

Abbreviations: AVR, aortic value replacement; DVR, mitral–aortic valve replacement; MVR, mitral valve replacement.
Source: From Ref. 19.

had been detected on computed tomography (CT) scan by the telltale signs of perivascular information consistent with a small degree of leakage. Based on this experience, these authors recommended that CT scanning be performed on all IE patients who have developed headaches and other premonitory neurological symptoms (especially homonomous hemianopsia). When the scan is equivocal or negative but clinical suspicion is strong, arteriography should be performed.

Certainly, CT scanning should be an essential part of the screening process of patients with neurological symptoms of any type prior to planned cardiac surgery. Ten to 50 percent of intracranial hemorrhages on the CT scan are the result of to ruptured mycotic aneurysms (81). When a cerebral bleed is visualized, the next step is to perform cerebral angiography in order to identify the ruptured mycotic aneurysm that should be treated with resection, clipping our embolization before cardiac surgery is undertaken. Operative mortality is increased significantly in the presence of a hemorrhagic infarct but not in an ischemic one. In a nonhemorrhagic stroke, valve replacement can be undertaken 72 hours after the event. Because of the significantly increased risk of hemorrhage during surgery of a hemorrhagic infarction, there should be a three-week interval between the bleed and surgery (82). Both focal neurologic deficits and diffuse processes, such as encybalitis are associated with poor surgical outcomes but also more diffuse neurological processes such as encephalitis (83). This increase probably reflects that seen in any type of surgery in the patient and is unable to follow simple commands postoperatively.

It has been recommended that all cerebral aneurysms, due to valvular infection, should be excised because of the risk of fatal rupture. At least 30% of them heal with medical treatment (30a,84) alone. The period of greatest risk for aneurysmal leakage or rupture is during the first two weeks of antimicrobial therapy. It is unusual but still possible that an aneurysm that has not changed its appearance could rupture after successful antimicrobial treatment. Intact aneurysms should be followed angiographically every two weeks during the time of antibiotic therapy. Of course, anticoagulation should be avoided during this time of observation. If they enlarge, surgery is mandatory (85–87). To complicate matters, an unknown percentage of asymptomatic aneurysms may, early on, enlarge but then become thrombosed (85). Although they have enlarged, they no longer present a real risk of rupture. Surgery of the intact mycotic aneurysm is called for only when it continues to grow despite several weeks of antimicrobial therapy or only when there is no evidenced-based medicine to aid the clinician in deciding whether to operate on a single, stable-appearing aneurysm that persists after therapy. Most experts would propose removal of the aneurysm if it could be performed with minimal chance of damage to the patient's brain. A major factor that favors surgical removal is a peripheral location. Removal of those that are located close to the midline of the brain pose much more of a risk of permanent, surgically induced neurological damage (88).

Mycotic aneurysms of the peripheral circulation are approached in a very similar fashion to those of the cerebral circulation (30b). If the collateral circulation is adequate, there is no need for a bypass graft. If at all possible, prosthetic devices should be avoided in order to minimize the risk of infection. This is especially true for mycotic aneurysms of the abdominal aorta and its branches. When resection is impossible to achieve, embolization of these arteries should be considered (89,90).

Multiple cerebral abscesses <1 cm in diameter usually respond to antimicrobial therapy. Larger ones require drainage. This should be done prior to undertaking any type of cardiac surgery as the abscess may give rise to a BSI with the potential to infect the implanted valve (91).

Splenic abscesses complicate from 3% to 5% of cases of IE (92). Their presence must always be ruled out before valve replacement is undertaken because of purported persistent IE. Ultrasonography and CT scanning does not always differentiate between sterile infarcts and abscesses. Continued fever and enlargement of the defect is consistent with a purulent collection. In aspiration of the spleen, yields of polymorphonuclear cells and/or microorganisms is confirmatory. In the past, a splenectomy would be done at this point as continuation of antibiotics is usually unsuccessful. Currently, drainage by a percutaneously placed catheter often is effective. If this approach fails or there are multiple apices, a splenectomy is required (93). Table 5 summarizes the ranking of indications for surgery in active IE.

ANTICOAGULATION IN INFECTIVE ENDOCARDITIS

In 1947, Thill and Meyer treated patients with subacute bacterial endocarditis with a combination of penicillin and dicumarol (94). This idea was based on animal studies that showed that anticoagulation could potentiate the antibacterial activity of penicillin by decreasing the size of the vegetation (95). There was an unacceptably high incidence of cerebral hemorrhage in the patients receiving anticoagulation. The advent of prosthetic valves highlighted the safety issue of using anticoagulation in active IE. Wilson et al. studied the role of coumadin in PVE. Thirty percent of the patients, who were not hard anticoagulation, separate significant neurological complications (96). Another study confirmed these findings (97). Another series indicated that cerebral events more commonly occurred in those receiving coumadin (98). A more recent study focused on the difference in outcome between *S. aureus* NVE and *S. aureus* PVE. The vast majority of those with PVE were on anticoagulation and were maintained on heparin during hospitalization (99). The findings indicated that the risk of hemorrhagic transformation of embolic strokes (50%) was so high that anticoagulation of any type should be discontinued until several weeks into the course of antimicrobial treatment.

The author agrees with the approach that in patients with PVE (mechanical valves) maintenance anticoagulation should be continued (52). It has no ability to prevent valvular emboli in PVE or NVE. If an infarct, either hemorrhagic or nonhemorrhagic, occurs, then the anticoagulation needs to be stopped. It would be reasonable to substitute heparin for coumadin during the first two weeks of

TABLE 4 Noncardiac Complications of Acute Infective Endocarditis After Mitral, Aortic, and Mitral-Aortic Valve Replacements

	MVR (%)	AVR (%)	DVR (%)	Average (%)
Persistent sepsis (>72 hr)	27	20	25	20.4
Hematuria/protienuria	51	54	58	53.4
Acute renal failure	14	16	25	16.5
Mycotic aneurysms	6	4	0	3.9
Diffuse vasculitis	9	7	25	9.7
Nonembolic involvement of the central nervous system	23	2	30	22.3

Abbreviations: AVR, aortic value replacement; DVR, mitral–aortic valve replacement; MVR, mitral valve replacement.
Source: From Ref. 19.

TABLE 5 Ratings of Indications for Surgery in Acute Infective Endocarditis[a]

+++++	++++	+++	++	+
Severe CHF	"Kissing" infection of anterior leaflet of mitral and aortic valves	Compensated CHF on medical therapy	Subclinical CHF	Nonstreptococcal IE
Fungal endocarditis (except due to *Histoplasma* spp.)		Recurrent emboli	Single embolic episode	Vegetation in echocardiography
Persistent sepsis (>72 hrs) despite antimicrobial therapy			Isolated IE of aortic valve or of more than one valve	Isolated IE of mitral valve
Rupture of aneurysm of sinsus of Valsalva			Small perivalvular dehiscence	
New onset of atrioventricular block conduction disturbances, myocardial abscess, significant perivalvular dehiscence, or observed tilting movements of the valve[b]				

+ + + + +, highest ranking; +, lowest ranking.
[a]Surgery rarely indicated for right-sided ranking.
[b]Pertains to prosthetic valve endocarditis.
Abbreviations: CHF, congestive heart failure; IE, infective endocarditis.
Source: From Refs. 10,16,17, and 93.

treatment, the time of the highest risk of embolization. The advantage of intravenous heparin is its quick reversibility when the infusion is stopped. When thrombosis develops in extracardiac areas, appropriate anticoagulation should be instituted. Especially in deep vein thrombosis of the legs, the use of an umbrella in the inferior vena cava would be a good alternative to coumadin.

There have been some experimental studies that indicate that aspirin might lessen the virulence of *S. aureus* IE and decrease the frequency of emboli in *S. aureus* IE (100). A randomized study showed that aspirin had no positive effect on the course of *S. aureus* IE (101).

REFERENCES

1. Kay JH, Bernstein S, Feinstein D, et al. Surgical cure of *Candida albicans* endocarditis with open-heart surgery. N Engl J Med 1961; 264:907.
2. Wallace AG, Young WG, Osterhout S. Treatment of acute bacterial endocarditis by valve excision and replacement. Circulation 1965; 31:450.
3. McAnulty J, Rahimtoola S. Surgery for infective endocarditis. JAMA 1979; 242:77.
4. Watanakunakorn C, Burbert T. Infective endocarditis in a large community teaching hospital 1980–1990: a review of 210 episodes. Medicine 1993; 72:90.
5. Olaison L, Pettersson G. Current best practices and guidelines: indications for surgical intervention in infective endocarditis. Infect Dis Clin NA 2002; 16:453.
6. Jault F, Gandjbakch I, Rama A, et al. Active native valve endocarditis: determinants of operative death in late mortality. Ann Thorac Surg 1997; 63:1737.
7. Larbalestier R, Kinchla N, Aranki S, et al. Acute bacterial endocarditis: optimizing surgical results. Circulation 1992; 86(SII):68.
8. Bayliss R, Clarke C, Oakley CM. The microbiology and pathogenesis of infective endocarditis. Br Heart J 1983; 50:513.
9. Walsh TJ, Hutchins GM, Bulkley BH, et al. Fungal infections of the heart: analysis of 51 autopsy cases. Am J Cardiol 1980; 45:357.
10. Carvagal A, Frederisken W. Fatal endocarditis due to *Listeria monocytes*. Rev Infect Dis 1988; 10:616.
11. Wolff M, Witchitz S, Chastang C, et al. Prosthetic valve endocarditis in the ICU. Prognostic factors of overall survival in a series of 122 cases and consequences for treatment decision. Chest 1995; 108;688.
12. Verheul H, Renee B, Vanden Brink A, et al. Effective changes in management of active infective endocarditis on outcome in a 25 year period Am J Cardiol 1993; 72:682.
13. D'Agostino R, Miller D, Stinson E. Valve replacement in patients with native valve endocarditis: what really determines operative outcome. Ann Thorac Surg 1985; 40:429.
14. Agnitjori AK, McGiffin DC, Galbraith AJ, et al. Aortic valve infection. Risk factors for death and recurrent endocarditis after aortic valve replacement. J Thorac Cardiovasc Surg 1995; 110:1708.
15. Olaison L, Hogevick H, Myken P, et al. Early surgery in infective endocarditis. Q J Med 1996; 89:267.
16. DiNubile MJ. Surgery in active endocarditis. Ann Intern Med 1980; 96:650.
17. Karp RB. Role of surgery in infective endocarditis. Cardiovasc Clin 1987; 17:141.
18. Alsip SG, Blackstone EH, Kirklin JW. Indications for cardiac surgery in patients with active infective endocarditis. Am J Med 1985; 78(suppl 6B):138.
19. Horstkotte D, Schulte H, Bircks W. Factors influencing prognosis and indication for surgical intervention in acute native valve endocarditis. In: Horstkotte D, Bodnar E, eds. Infective Endocarditis. London: ICR Publishers, 1991:187a.
20. Horstkotte D, Bircks W, Loogen F. The infective endocarditis of native prosthetic valves-the case for prompt surgical intervention? A retrospective analysis of factors affecting survival. Z Kardiol 1986; 75(suppl 2):168.
21. Michael P, VitouxB, Hage A. Early and delayed surgery in acute native valve endocarditis. In: Horstkotte D, Bodner E, eds. Infective Endocarditis. London: ICR Publishers, 1991:22.

22. Hasbun R, Vikram HR, Barakat LA, et al. Complicated subsided native valve endocarditis in adults: risk classification for mortality. JAMA 2003; 29:1933.

23. Fowler VG, Scheld WM, Bayer AS. Endocarditis and intravascular infections. In: Mandell GL, Bennett JE, Dolin R, eds. Principles and Practice of Infectious Diseases. 6th ed. Philadelphia: Elsevier, 2005:1001.

24. Pellitier LI, Petersdorf RG. Infective endocarditis: a review of 125 cases of the University of Washington Hospitals, 1963–1972. Medicine (Baltimore) 1977; 56:287.

25. Blaustein AS, Lee JR. Indications for and timing of surgical intervention in infective endocarditis. Cardiol Clin 1996; 14:393.

26. Mills J, Utley J, Abbott J. Heart failure in infective endocarditis: predisposing factors, course and treatment. Chest 1974; 66:151.

27. Croft CH, Woodward W, Elliott A, et al. Analysis of surgical versus medical therapy in active complicated native valve endocarditis. Am J Cardiol 1983; 51:1651.

28. Moon M R, Stinson EB, Miller DC. Surgical treatment of endocarditis. Prog Cardiovasc Dis 1997; 40:239.

29. Lytle BW, Priest BP, Taylor PC, et al. Surgery for acquired heart disease: surgical treatment of prosthetic valve endocarditis. J Thorac Cardiovasc Surg 1996; 111:198.

29a. John MVD, Hibberd PL, Karchmer AW, et al. *Staphylococcus aureus* prosthetic valve endocarditis: optimal management and risk factors for death. Clin Infect Dis 1998; 26:1302.

30. Alestig K, Hogevik H, Olaison L. Infective endocarditis: a diagnostic and therapeutic challenge for the new millennium. Scand J Infect Dis 2000; 32:343.

30a. Bayer AS, Bolger AF, Taubert KA, et al. Diagnosis and management of infective endocarditis and its complications (AHA scientific statement) Circulation 1998; 98:2936.

30b. Eishi K, Kawazoe K, Kuriyama T, et al. Surgical management of infective endocarditis associated with renal complications: multicenter retrospective study in Japan. J Thorac Cardiovasc Surg 1995; 110:1745.

30c. Buchbinder NA, Roberts WC. Left-sided valvular active infective endocarditis: a study of forty-five necropsy patients. Am J Med 1972; 53:20.

30d. Menzies C. Coronary embolism with infarction in bacterial endocarditis. Br Heart J 1961; 23:464.

31. Karalis D, Blumberg E, Vilaro J. Prognostic significance of valvular regurgitation in patients with infective endocarditis. Am J Med 1991; 90:193.

32. Olaison L, Pettersson G. Current best practices and guidelines indications for surgical intervention in infective endocarditis. Cardiol Clin 2003; 21:235.

33. Buchbinder NA, Roberts WC. Left sided valvular active endocarditis—a study of 45 necropsy patients. Am J Med 1972; 53:20.

34. Yee ES, Khonsari S. Right sided infective endocarditis: valvuloplasty, valvulotomy or replacement. J Cardiovasc Surg 1989; 30:744.

35. Olaison L, Belin L, Hogevick H, et al. To incidence of beta-lactam-induced delayed hypersensitivity and neutropenia during treatment of infective endocarditis. Arch Intern Med 1999; 159:607.

36. Weinstein L, Brusch JL. Surgical management. In: Weinstein L, Brusch JL, eds. Infective Endocarditis. New York: Oxford University Press, 1996:308.

37. Stimmel B, Donoso E, Dack S. Comparison of infective endocarditis in drug addicts and nondrug uses. Am J Cardiol 1973; 32:924.

38. Ellis ME, Al-Abdely H, Sandridge A, et al. Fungal endocarditis: evidence in the world literature, 1965–1995. Clin Infect Dis 2001; 32:50.

39. McLeod R, Remington JS. Fungal endocarditis. In: Rahimtoola SH, ed. Infective Endocarditis. New York: Grune and Stratton, 1978:211.

40. Bauernschmitt R, Jakob HG, Vahl C-F, et al. Operation for infective endocarditis: results after implantation of mechanical valves. Ann Thorac Surg 1998; 65:359.

41. David TE, Bos J, Christakin CT. Heart valve operations in patients with active infective endocarditis. Ann Thorac Surg 1990; 49:701.

42. Lee EM, Schapiro LM, Wells FC. Conservative operation for infective endocarditis of the mitral valve. Ann Thorac Surg 1998; 65:1087.

43. Morris AJ, Drinkovic D, Pottumarthy S, et al. Gram stain, culture and histopathological examination findings for heart valves removed because of infective endocarditis. Clin Infect Dis 2003; 36:697.
44. Karchmer AW. Infective endocarditis. In: Zipes DP, LibbyP, Bonow RC, Braunwald E, eds. Braunwald's Heart Disease: A Textbook of Cardiovascular Medicine. 7th ed. Philadelphia: Elsevier, 2005:1650.
45. Calderwood SB, Swinski LA, Karchmer AW, et al. Prosthetic valve endocarditis. Analysis of factors affecting outcome of therapy. J Thorac Cardiovasc Surg 1986; 92:776.
46. Gordon SM, Serkey JM, Longworth DL, et al. Early-onset prosthetic valve endocarditis: the Cleveland Clinic experience 1992–1997. Ann Thorac Surg 2000; 69:1388.
47. Vongppatanasin W, Hills LD, Lange RA. Prosthetic heart valves. N Engl J Med 1996; 335:407.
48. Yu VL, Fang GD, Keys TF, et al. Prosthetic valve endocarditis: superiority of surgical valve replacement versus medical therapy only. Ann Thorac Surg 1994; 58:1073.
49. Zegdi R, Debieche M, Latremouille C, et al. Long-term results of mitral valve repair in active endocarditis. Circulation 2005; 111:2532.
50. Dreyfus G, Serraf A, Jabara VA, et al. Valve repair in acute endocarditis. Ann Thorac Surg 1990; 49:706.
51. Truninger K, Attenhofer Jost CH, Seifert B, et al. Long-term follow-up of prosthetic valve endocarditis: what characteristics identify patients who were treated successfully with antibiotics alone. Heart 1999; 82:714.
51a. Ivert TSA, Dismukes WE, Cobbs GG, et al. Prosthetic valve endocarditis. Circulation 1984; 69:223.
52. Karchmer AW. Infections of prosthetic heart valves. In: Waldvogel F, Bisno AL, eds. Infections Associated with Indwelling Medical Devices. Washington D.C.: American Society for Microbiology, 2000:145.
53. Horstkotte D, Follath F, Gutschik E, et al. Guidelines and prevention, diagnosis and treatment of infective endocarditis executive summary; The Task Force of Infective Endocarditis of the European Society of Cardiology. Eur Heart J 2004; 25:267.
54. Steckleberg JM, Murphy JG, Ballard D, et al. Emboli in infective endocarditis: the prognostic value of echocardiography. Ann Intern Med 1991; 114:635.
55. Argulu A, Asfav I. Management of infective endocarditis: 17 years experience. Ann Thorac Surg 1987; 43:144.
56. Weinstein L, Schlessinger JJ. Pathoanatomic, pathophysiologic and clinical correlation in endocarditis. N Engl J Med 1974; 291:839.
57. Weinstein L, Schlessinger JJ. Pathoanatomic, pathophysiologic and clinical correlation in endocarditis. N Engl J Med 1974; 291:1122.
58. DiSalvo G, Habib G, Pergola V, et al. Echocardiography predicts embolic events in infective endocarditis. J Am Coll Cardiol 2001; 37:1069.
59. Heiro M, Nikoskelainen J, Engblom E, et al. Neurologic manifestations of infective endocarditis. A 17-year experience in a teaching hospital in Finland. Arch Intern Med 2000; 160:2781.
60. Thompson KR, Nanda NC, Gramiak R. Reliability of echocardiography in the diagnosis of infectious endocarditis. Radiology 1977; 125:473.
61. Mugge A, Daniel WG, Frank G, et al. Echocardiography in infective endocarditis: the assessment of the prognostic implications of vegetation size determined by the transthoracic and transesophageal approach. J Am Coll Cardiol 1989; 14:631.
62. Bayer AN, Blomquist IK, Bello E. Tricuspid valve endocarditis due to *Staphylococcus aureus*. Correlation of two-dimensional echocardiography with clinical outcomes. Chest 1988; 93:247.
63. Rohman S, Erbel R, Gorge G, et al. Clinical relevance of vegetation localization by transesophageal echocardiography in infective endocarditis. Eur Heart J 1992; 13:446.
64. Stafford WJ, Petch J, Radford DJ. Vegetations in infective endocarditis: clinical relevance and diagnosis by cross sectional echocardiography. Br Heart J 1985; 53:310.
65. Tischler MD, Vaitkus PT. The ability of vegetation size and echocardiography to predict clinical complications: a meta-analysis. J Am Soc Echocardiogr 1997; 10:562.

66. Mangoni ED, Adinolfi LE, Tripodi MF, et al. Risk factors for "major" embolic events in hospitalized patients with infective endocarditis. Am Heart J 2003; 146:311.

67. Omari B, Shapiro S , Gintzon L, et al. Predictive risk factors for periannular extension of native valve endocarditis: clinical and echocardiographic analyses. Chest 1989; 96:1273.

68. Pettersson G, Carbon. The Endocarditis Working Group of the International Society of Chemotherapy: recommendations for the surgical treatment of endocarditis. Clin Microbiol Infect 1998; 4:3S.

69. Blumberg EA, Karalis DA, Chandrasekaran K, et al. Endocarditis-associated paravalvular abscess. Do clinical parameters predict the presence of abscess? Chest 1995; 107:898.

70. Meine TJ, Nettles RE, Anderson DJ, et al. Cardiac conduction abnormalities in endocarditis defined by the Duke criteria. Am Heart J 2001; 142:280.

71. Dinubile M. Heart block during bacterial endocarditis: a review of the literature and guidelines for surgical intervention. Am J Med Sci 1989; 287:30.

71. Douglas A, Moore-Gillen J, Ekyns S. Fever during treatment of infective endocarditis. Lancet 1989; 1:1341.

72. Daniel WG, Mugge A, Martin RP, et al. Improvement in the diagnosis of abscesses associated with endocarditis by transesophageal echocardiography. N Engl J Med 1991; 324:795.

73. Roach MR, Drake CG. Ruptured cerebral aneurysms caused by microorganisms. N Engl J Med 1963; 273:246.

74. Feigl D, Feigl A, Edwards JE. Mycotic aneurysms of the aortic root: a pathologic study of 20 cases. Chest 1986; 90:553.

75. Weinstein L, Brusch JL. Surgical management. In: Weinstein L, Brusch JL, eds. Infective Endocarditis. New York: Oxford University press, 1996:310.

76. Masuda J., Yutani C, Waki R, et al. Histopathological analysis of the mechanisms of intracranial hemorrhage complicating infective endocarditis. Stroke 1992; 22:843.

77. Frazee JG, Cahan LD, Winter J. Bacterial intracranial aneurysms. J Neurosurg 1980; 53:633.

78. Salgado AV, Furlan AJ, Keys TF. Mycotic aneurysm, subarachnoid hemorrhage and indications for cerebral angiography in infective endocarditis. Stroke 1987; 18:1057.

79. Bohmfalk GL, Story JL, Wissinger JP, et al. Bacterial intracranial aneurysm. J Neurol Surg 1978; 48:369.

80. Wilson WR, Lie JT, Houser OW, et al. The management of patients with mycotic aneurysms. Curr Clin Top Infect Dis 1981; 2:151.

81. Gillinov AM, Shah RV, Curtis WE, et al. Valve replacement in patients with endocarditis acute neurologic deficit. Ann Thorac Surg 1996; 61:1125.

82. Ting W, Silverman N, Levitsky S. Valve replacement in patients with endocarditis and cerebral septic emboli. Ann Thorac Surg 1991; 51:18.

83. Parrino PE, Kron IL, Ross SD, et al. Does a focal neurologic deficit contraindicate operation in a patient with endocarditis? Ann Thorac Surg 1999; 67:59.

84. Pruitt A, Rubin R, Karchmer AW, et al. Neurologic complications of bacterial endocarditis. Medicine 1978; 57:329.

85. Cobbs G, Livingston E. Special problems in the management of infective endocarditis. In: Bisno A, ed. Treatment of Infective Endocarditis. New York: Grune and Stratton, 1981:141.

86. Cantu RC, LeMay M, Wilkinson HA. The importance of repeated angiography in the treatment of mycotic-embolic intracranial aneurysms. J Neurosurg 1966; 25:189.

87. Wilson WR, Giuliani ER, Danielson GK, et al. The management of complications of infective endocarditis. Proc Mayo Clinic 1982; 57:152.

88. Phuong LK, Link M,Widjicks E. The management of intracranial infectious aneurysms: a series of 16 cases. Neurosurgery 2002; 51:1145.

89. Mundth ED, Darling RC, Alvarado RH, et al. Surgical management of mycotic aneurysms and the complications of infection in vascular reconstructive surgery. Am J Surg 1969; 117:460.

90. Porter L, Houston M., Kadir S. Mycotic aneurysms of the hepatic artery: treatment with arterial embolization. Am J Med 1979; 67:697.

91. Ziment I. Nervous system complications in bacterial endocarditis. Am J Med 1969; 47:593.

92. Mansur AJ, Greinberg M, Lamos de Luz P, Bellotti G. The complications of infective endocarditis: A reappraisal in the 1980s. Arch Intern Med 1992; 152:2428.
93. Magilligan D. Cardiac surgery in infective endocarditis. In: Horstkotte D, Bodnar E, eds. Infective Endocarditis. London: ICR Publishers, 1991:210.
94. Thill C, Meyer O. Experience with penicillin and dicumarol in the treatment of subacute bacterial endocarditis. Ann J Med Sci 1947; 13:500.
95. Freedman L, Valoni J. Experimental infective endocarditis. Progr Cardiovasc Dis 1979; 22:169.
96. Wilson W, Geraci J, Danielson G. Anticoagulant therapy and central nervous system complications in patients with prosthetic valve endocarditis. Circulation 1978; 57:1004.
97. Karchmer AW, Dismukes WE, Buckley MJ, et al. Late prosthetic valve endocarditis: clinical features influencing therapy. Am J Med 1978; 64:199.
98. Carpenter J, McAllister C, U.S. Army Collaborative Group. Anticoagulation in prosthetic valve endocarditis. South Med J 1983; 76:1372.
99. Tornos P, Almirante B, Mirabet S, et al. Infective endocarditis due to *Staphylococcus aureus*: deleterious effect of anticoagulant therapy. Arch Intern Med 1999; 159:473.
100. Kupperwasser LI, Yeaman MR, Nast CC, et al. Salicylic acid attenuates serial incident in vascular infections by targeting global regulatory pathways in *Staphylococcus aureus*. J Clin Invest 2003; 112:222
101. Chan KL, Dumesnil JG, Cujec B, et al. A randomized trial of aspirin on the risk of embolic event in patients with infective endocarditis. J Am Coll Cardiol 2003; 42:775.

16 Prophylaxis of Infective Endocarditis

John L. Brusch

*Harvard Medical School and Department of Medicine and Infectious Disease
Service, Cambridge Health Alliance, Cambridge, Massachusetts, U.S.A.*

INTRODUCTION

Despite the availability of antibiotics, the incidence of infective endocarditis (IE)
has not decreased. It has actually increased in certain populations (nosocomial/
healthcare-associated IE) (1). Realization of this relative failure of traditional antibiotic prophylaxis is a compelling argument to re-examine our approach in preventing valvular infections. A pragmatic starting point would be to understand the types
of IE that we are currently able to prevent and the potential benefits and risks
for doing so. The goal of this chapter is to critically appraise the current recommendations for prevention of IE and to suggest how the practitioner may be able to
appropriately modify them for a specific patient. The numerous guidelines, which
have been developed by the American Heart Association (AHA) (2) and others over
the years (3,3a), had never been intended to be strict rules or clinical pathways.
Their intent has been to direct the reader to those cardiac conditions that require
antimicrobial prophylaxis, to identify those invasive procedures that present a real
risk to these patients, and to make suggestions concerning the appropriate dosage
regimens of various antibiotics that are used to prevent valvular infection. They are
"… not intended as a standard of care or as a substitute for clinical judgment" (2).
Because of their infrequent issue, they cannot remain current with the changing
epidemiology of the disease.

  Prophylaxis for the prevention of IE needs to become more than just the use of
antibiotics to prevent valvular infection due to invasive procedures. About 15% to
25% of the cases of IE are because of a variety of invasive procedures. Coupled with
this is the fact that of those individuals who develop IE due to an invasive procedure;
only 50% had been identified as appropriate for antibiotic prophylaxis (4–7).
Under these circumstances, only about 10% of the cases of IE can be prevented by
the current prophylactic approaches, assuming that antimicrobial prophylaxis is
100% effective. The 1997 prophylaxis guidelines of the AHA emphasize their limited
potential for preventing valvular infection. They state: "A reasonable approach
should consider the following: the degree to which the patient's underlying condition creates the risk of endocarditis; the apparent risk of bacteremia with the procedure (as defined in these recommendations); the potential adverse reactions of the
prophylactic antimicrobial agent to be used; and the cost benefit aspects of the
recommended prophylactic regimen." In the absence of randomized controlled
human trials, the guidelines' recommendations are based on in vitro susceptibility
of common pathogens in IE, animal models of prophylaxis, and retrospective study
of endocarditis cases with special attention to failures of antibiotic prophylaxis.

  It is the author's opinion that most clinicians who prescribe antimicrobial
prophylaxis have never read the guidelines in their entirety and so have missed
these important points about their intent. This may contribute to the relatively
low adherence to these guidelines by the practitioners. Shortly after the introduction

of the 1997 guidelines, a study was undertaken to identify the compliance of physicians to their recommendations. The patients were identified as high risk, intermediate risk, and low risk for the development of IE following an invasive procedure (8). Sixty-six percent of the patients in the high- and intermediate-risk categories received prophylaxis. Antibiotic prophylaxis was also prescribed for those who were in the negligible risk category. This degree of adherence is consistent with other studies (9–11). Another factor contributing to the application of the guidelines for antibiotic prophylaxis is the reliance of the physicians on echocardiographic findings to determine underlying cardiac risk. A recent survey was made of physicians' reliance on echocardiographic findings in use of antibiotic prophylaxis (12). Eighty-one percent of the respondents considered echocardiography to be the most important factor in their choice of prophylaxis. Twenty-seven percent paid more attention to the clinical findings. Family physicians were found to be more tied to the echocardiographic studies than the internists. In short, the reliance of echocardiographic findings must be taken into account when formulating updates of guidelines for the use of antibiotic prophylaxis. Over the years, the guidelines have shifted away from parenteral therapy to orally administered antibiotics. This has been done to increase compliance in the dentist's office. As more resistant pathogens develop in the community, such oral regimens may produce marginal or ineffective levels of antibiotics in the blood.

MECHANISMS OF ANTIBIOTIC PROPHYLAXIS

Bayer identified three steps in the pathogenesis of IE that are potentially susceptible to the administration of prophylactic antibiotics (13): (i) eradication of microorganisms from the bloodstream before they can adhere to the thrombus; (ii) prevention of adherence to the sterile platelet-fibrin thrombus; and (iii) inhibiting the growth of the adherent bacteria and facilitating their killing by the host's defenses before they multiply and penetrate within the vegetation. This last step may be the most significant (5,7). Prevention of IE by antibiotics is not always due to their bactericidal action. Sub-bactericidal levels may also protect against infection of the thrombus (14). This is most likely because of interference of adherence. Animal models have demonstrated that streptococcal IE can be prevented if penicillin is administered just prior to or up to 30 minutes after the introduction of bacteria into the bloodstream (5,15). This effect disappears if the antibiotic is given six hours after the appearance of bacteria in the blood. Penicillinase can also negate the protective effect of penicillin. This model supports that the site of prophylactic action of antibiotics is either eradicating bacteria before they can "set up housekeeping" on the platelet fibrin-thrombus or after they have adhered to the vegetation. At least, two animal studies have demonstrated the efficacy of prophylaxis (16).

No study has ever demonstrated unequivocally that prophylactic antibiotics prevent the development of IE after invasive procedures in humans. There are relatively strong indications that they do. In one pediatric study, the overall incidence of positive blood cultures for *Streptococcus viridans* was lower in patients receiving amoxicillin versus those who were not (33% vs. 84%) (17). Another study involving prosthetic heart valves showed that IE occurred in 2.7% of untreated individuals versus none who received antibiotics just prior to undergoing an invasive procedure (18). It is truly difficult to prove the efficacy of antibiotic prophylaxis in human studies because the risk is very small. In a recent French study, it was estimated that the risk of developing IE in patients with prosthetic valves in place and those with significant predisposing native valve conditions who were unprotected during dental procedures was 1 in 10,700 and 1 in 46,000, respectively (19). The authors concluded that a large amount of prophylaxis would have to be given to protect a few. Definitive controlled studies in humans will never be conducted because of ethical and legal considerations.

Failures of appropriately administered antibiotics are well-documented. The largest series was from 1983 (20). Most of the failures occurred during dental procedures. Seventy-five percent were caused by *S. viridans*. Only 12% of cases of IE did receive appropriate prophylaxis. All isolates of *S. viridans* were sensitive to the administered antibiotic. Erythromycin was given to 15% of the patients. However, it was implicated in two failures of prophylaxis. This may have been because of marginal absorption of the drug (21). Gastrointestinal intolerance may have contributed to poor compliance. Mitral valve prolapse (MVP) was the most common underlying cardiac pathology in this group. Penicillin-resistant flora may develop in individuals taking a variety of antibiotics frequently. This possibility should be taken into account when selecting a specific prophylactic regimen.

Inadequate knowledge of susceptible individuals concerning the risk presented by various procedures very likely contributes to failure to prevent IE. One series reported that 78% of patients remembered having received instructions about prophylaxis, but only 20% retained any specific knowledge (22). This can be especially tragic in children with congenital heart disease. In this particular population, insufficient knowledge concerning prophylaxis has been well-documented (23).

A disproportionate focus has been put on preventing iatrogenic disease with antimicrobial prophylaxis. Preventing the most common sources of transient bloodstream infection (BSI) has been neglected. Poor oral hygiene appears to be the most frequent cause of spontaneous bacteremia (10). Significant dental pathology, especially gingivitis, has been identified in about 50% of the patients at risk of developing IE (24). Although the need to maintain excellent oral hygiene in at risk patients has been emphasized by the AHA, the nonpharmacologic approaches to the prevention of IE have not been widely practiced (2,7,25). Table 1 presents these recommendations. The risk of bacteremia, which is associated with mastication or brushing of the teeth, is directly related to the overall health of the periodontal tissue (26).

Nonpharmacological approaches to reducing transient BSI from sites other than the oral cavity include: (*i*) avoiding enemas; (*ii*) minimizing invasive procedures especially including placement of intravascular devices (central lines); (*iii*) avoid manipulating skin lesions; (*iv*) fully investigate any unexplained febrile illness in patients who are at risk; (*v*) avoid administering antibiotic in febrile patients who are at risk of developing IE without first conducting a thorough evaluation; (*vi*) maintenance of bowel regularity; and (*vii*) proper insertion and maintenance of intravascular access devices (Table 2).

TABLE 1 Nonpharmacological Approaches to Decreasing
Bacteremias from the Oral Cavity

Meticulous dental care
Regular brushing of the teeth
Flossing with waxed floss
Avoidance of irrigation devices (e.g., Waterpik)
Avoidance of dental trauma
Rinsing of the mouth regularly with an antiseptic
No dental work within two to three weeks after a cardiac procedure

TABLE 2 Recommendations for the Prevention of Intravascular Catheter-Related Infections

General
  Not recommended
    Preventive strategies incorporating therapeutic antimicrobial agents
During catheter insertion
  Strongly recommended
    Full-barrier precautions during central venous catheter insertion
    Subcutaneous tunneling of short-term catheters inserted in the internal jugular or
      femoral veins when catheters are not used for blood drawing
    Contamination shield for pulmonary artery catheters
    Insertion site preparation with chlorhexidine-containing antiseptics
    Prophylaxis with vancomycin and other therapeutic agents
  Recommended
    Subclavian vein, rather than jugular or femoral vein, catheter insertion
  Consider
    Insertion site preparation with tincture of iodine
    Full-barrier precautions during insertion of midline, peripheral artery, and pulmonary
      artery catheters
  Not recommended
    Femoral vein catheter insertion
Catheter maintenance
  Strongly recommended
    Provide-iodine ointment applied to hemodialysis catheter-insertion sites
    Specialized nursing teams caring for short-term peripheral venous catheters at institutions
      with a high incidence of infection
    Chlorhexidine-silver sulfadiazine-impregnated short-term central venous catheters
    Minocycline-rifampin-impregnated short-term central venous catheters
    Antiseptic chamber-filled hub or hub-protective antiseptic sponge for central venous catheters
      with an expected duration of approximately two weeks
    Povidone-iodine-saturated sponge enclosed in plastic casing fitted around the central venous
      catheter hubs
    Assess need for intravascular catheters on a daily basis; remove catheters as soon as
      possible after intended use
    Adequate nurse-to-patient ratio in ICUs
    Change needleless system, the device and end cap if present on a regular basis in
      accordance with the manufacturers' guidelines and reduce contact with nonsterile water
  Continuing quality improvement programs to improve compliance with catheter care guidelines
    Disinfect catheter hubs and sampling ports before accessing
    Low-dose heparin for patients with short-term central venous catheters
    Low-dose warfarin for patients with long-term central venous catheters
    Pulmonary artery catheters heparin-bonded with benzalkonium chloride. Povidone-iodine
      ointment applied to nontunneled, long-term central venous or midline catheter-insertion
      sites of immunocompromised patients with heavy *Staphylococcus aureus* carriage
      (i.e., patients with AIDS and cirrhosis)
    Specialized nursing teams caring for catheters used for TPN
  Recommended
    Gauze dressings preferred if excessive oozing of blood from the insertion site
  Consider
    Antiseptic chamber-filled hub or hub-protective antiseptic sponge for central venous catheters
      in ICUs
  Not recommended
    Routine replacement of central venous catheters
    Mupirocin ointment applied to the insertion site
    Triple antibiotic ointments applied to the insertion sites
    Silver-impregnated, subcutaneous collagen-cuffed central venous catheters
    In-line filters for prevention of catheter infection

Abbreviations: ICU, intensive care unit; TPN, total parenteral nutrition.
Source: From Ref. 61.

TABLE 3 Estimated Risk of Catheter-Associated Bloodstream Infection for Different Types of Vascular Access

Catheter type	Bloodstream infections (1000 device days)
Short plastic peripheral	<2
Arterial	10
Central venous	
Multilumen	30
Swan-Ganz	10
Hemodialysis	50
Long-term	
PICCs (peripherally inserted central catheters)	2
Cuffed central catheters (Hickman®, Broviac®)	2
Subcutaneous central venous ports (Infusaport, Port-A-Cath®)	<1

Source: From Ref. 27.

Intravascular devices have become so significant in the pathogenesis of IE (Chapters 6 and 10). Intravascular catheters are associated with rates of BSI of 4% to 14% accounting for at least 120,000 cases of nosocomial bacteremia per year. Central catheters produce 30% to 90% of BSI found in critical care units (27). Rates of BSI markedly increase past four days after their insertion. Sixteen percent of the patients with prosthetic valves in place will develop prosthetic valve endocarditis (PVE) secondary to a BSI acquired in the hospital (28). These devices are the primary sources of *Staphylococcus aureus* BSI (Table 3). Because *S. aureus* can infect normal valves, any patient who experiences a BSI with this pathogen is at risk of developing IE no matter whether there are predisposing cardiac conditions or not.

CARDIAC RISK FACTORS FOR THE DEVELOPMENT OF INFECTIVE ENDOCARDITIS

Table 4 identifies patients who are at intermediate and high risk based on potential outcome if valvular infection does occur. All other cardiac conditions fall into the

TABLE 4 High-Risk and Moderate Cardiac Conditions Associated with Endocarditis

Cardiac condition	Patient's level of risk
Acquired valvular dysfunction (rheumatic heart disease, degenerative valvular disease)	Moderate
Complex cyanotic congenital heart disease[b]	High
Hypertrophic cardiomyopathy	Moderate
Mitral valve prolapse with valvular regurgitation and/or thickened leaflets	Moderate
Previous bacterial endocarditis[a]	High
Prosthetic heart valves	High
Surgically corrected pulmonary shunts or conduits	High
Other congenital cardiac conditions	High

[a]Probably the highest risk category.
[b]Excludes secundum atrial septal defects and surgical repair of atrial septal defects and patent ductus arteriosus beyond six months. These do not require prophylaxis.
Source: From Ref. 2.

negligible category for which prophylaxis is not warranted. The most frequent predisposing condition and greatest risk to the patient is recurrent native valve endocarditis (NVE), intravenous drug abuser (IVDA), or non-IVDA-associated (29). The most definable cause of recurrent IE is IVDA. However, more than 50% of the cases have no obvious predisposition to repeated valvular infections except previous cases of IE.

Generally, individuals with congenital heart disease require antibiotic prophylaxis. The major exceptions are those with isolated ostium secundum defects always closer to major septal defects in the distant past or six weeks after ligature of a patent ductus arteriosus. Small ostium secundum defects do not require prophylaxis because of the lack of a significant pressure gradient between the two atria.

The incidence of IE within 60 days of valve implantation ranges from 0.3% to 0.5%. For the rest of the patient's life, the annual rate is between 0.5% and 1% (30). After 60 days, the most likely organisms to infect the valve are oral streptococci. Because of this, a thorough dental survey should be performed and necessary procedures carried out prior to elective valve surgery. The most important contributing factor is the degree of gingivitis just as it is in people with oral-associated NVE. The risk of rheumatic fever-damaged valves developing IE approximates that of prosthetic valves (0.4% yearly) (31).

The lifetime risk for developing IE of patients with idiopathic hypertrophic subaortic stenosis (hypertrophic cardiomyopathy) is 5% (32). This abnormality has been deemed to pose a moderate risk for the patient. The American College of Cardiology (ACC)/AHA 1998 guidelines recommend prophylaxis for this condition only when there is a latent or resting obstruction (33).

The role of antibiotic prophylaxis in MVP remains controversial despite the efforts of the 1997 AHA guidelines to clarify this situation. In some series, MVP underlies 29% of the subacute cases (34). When cases associated with IVDA are excluded, these patients have an incidence of IE from zero to five to eight times higher than that of the general population (35). Because MVP is present in approximately 5% of the population, it is clear that not all examples of this valvular variant are at an increased risk of infection. In fact, that MVP "represents a spectrum of valvular changes and clinical behavior" (2) adds to the difficulty in deciding on the factors that determine the need for antibiotic prophylaxis (36). Dehydration, tachycardia, and an increased adrenergic state can produce transient MVP not associated with any structural abnormalities. The presence of a regurgitant murmur, and not a click, is strongly associated with the risk of developing IE (20,34). This is because it is the jet of mitral regurgitation that leads to the turbulence of blood flow that produces sterile fibrin-platelet and thrombi. Abnormal valve motion causes the click but not the required disordered blood flow. Myxomatous degeneration causes a type of MVP (37). In this condition, the valve leaflets thicken with deposition of the proteoglycan substances. These deposits increase with age. Thickening of the anterior mitral valve is associated with significant regurgitation, which is sometimes intermittent (38). Three percent of these patients will eventually develop valvular infection. Another risk factor for the development of IE in MVP is being a male older than 45 years (39). According to some, these two characteristics could be considered adequate reasons to give antimicrobial prophylaxis. This is because the systolic murmur may be intermittent but significant (40). The 1998 ACC/AHA guidelines could not state that antibiotic prophylaxis was inappropriate for patients in MVP without findings of valvular regurgitation. This is because of the concern that such patients may be at an increased risk of developing IE. On the other hand, the ACC/AHA guidelines clearly state that antibiotic prophylaxis is not warranted in patients with only physiological mitral regurgitation that is evident on echocardiography but not on auscultation (33).

Similar in many aspects to MVP is papillary dysfunction that produces atrioventricular regurgitation (41). For the purposes of prophylaxis, the author considers it a type of MVP.

The 1997 guidelines do not directly address a major cardiac risk factor for the development of IE, the degenerative cardiac lesions. These include calcified mitral annulus, calcific nodular lesions, and thrombi secondary to myocardial infarction. These occur primarily in the elderly and affect both mitral and aortic valves. The degenerative lesions underlie approximately 50% of NVE of the elderly (42,43). Except for IVDA IE, endocarditis has become a disease of the older people. The importance of the murmurs, which these degenerative processes produce, is minimized because they have been previously recognized. When studied echocardiographically, these murmurs usually are not hemodynamically significant. Thus, they are considered as a benign part of aging and not an underlying condition that gives rise to valvular vegetations. Awareness of this situation helps explain that a significant amount of cases of IE have no known underlying cardiac disease process (44). With the tendency of physicians to base the need for antibiotic prophylaxis on the results of an echocardiogram (see before), these patients infrequently receive preprocedure prophylaxis. Cases of IE in the elderly have greater rates of morbidity and mortality than those in the younger individuals (45). The degenerative lesions should be classified at least as an intermediate risk factor.

BACTEREMIC-PRODUCING PROCEDURES THAT REQUIRE ANTIMICROBIAL PROPHYLAXIS

Although transient BSIs are essential for the pathogenesis of IE, not all invasive procedures that generate them require antimicrobial prophylaxis for patients who were susceptible to the development of IE. *Escherichia coli* BSIs pose no risk for the patient with rheumatic valvular disease as gram-negative NVE is quite unusual. For the patient at risk, those measures that result in bacteremias with *S. viridans*, an organism closely associated with IE, do require antibiotic coverage. There are other variables that are correlated with an increased risk of BSIs. Those procedures that cause a great deal of bleeding are more likely to mobilize bacteria into the bloodstream. This is especially true for dental/oral surgical procedures. Procedures, especially biopsies of mucosal surfaces, which are performed with rigid instruments, are associated with a higher incidence of bacteremia than those employing flexible ones (Table 5). The duration of BSI is a significant factor in determining the risk for developing IE. The bacteremia must last for at least 15–30 minutes to initiate infection of a susceptible cardiac structure (46). The more trauma to the soft tissue and bleeding, the longer does the bacteremia last.

Antibiotic prophylaxis is called for in those dental procedures that generate a good deal of bleeding (Table 6). Edentulous individuals have developed *S. viridans* IE. This is probably related to leave fitting dentures that have created an ulceration act that acts as a portal of entry for the streptococcus into the bloodstream (47).

Endoscopy procedures rarely lead to endocarditis (48). Their rate of generating BSIs is low (2–5%) and is composed of organisms that have little potential for causing IE. Significantly higher rates of BSI are seen in esophageal dilatation of strictures and sclerotherapy of esophageal varices (12–31%) (49). Other gastrointestinal and

TABLE 5 Risk of Bacteremia Associated with Various Procedures

Low (0–20%)	Moderate (20–40%)	High (40–100%)	Organism
	Tonsillectomy		
Bronchoscopy (rigid)			
Bronchoscopy (flexible)			Streptococcus spp. or Staphylococcus epidermidis
Endoscopy			S. epidermidis, Streptococci, and diphtheroids
Colonoscopy			Escherichia coli, Bacteroides sp., and S. epidermidis
Barium enema			Enterococci and aerobic gram-negative rods
	Transurethral resection of the prostate		Coliforms, Enterococci, and Staphylococcus aureus
Cystoscopy			Coliforms and gram-negative rods
		Traumatic dental procedures	Streptococcus viridans
Liver biopsy (in setting of cholangitis)			Coliforms and Enterococci
	Sclerotherapy of esophageal varices		S. viridans, gram-negative rods, and S. aureus
Esophageal dilatation		Esophageal dilatation	S. aureus and S. viridans
	Suction abortion		S. viridans and anaerobes
Transesophageal echocardiography			Streptococcus spp.

Source: From Refs. 2, 48.

genitourinary procedures, which warranty prophylaxis, are presented in Table 6. The reader is advised to refer to the 1997 guidelines for an excellent discussion of bacteremic-producing procedures.

REGIMENS FOR ANTIBIOTIC PROPHYLAXIS

The targets of the 1997 guidelines are *S. viridans* and the enterococci. *Streptococcus viridans* is the predominant pathogen in dental-associated IE and the *Enterococcus* the premier organism of genitourinary/gastrointestinal tract valvular infections.

Amoxicillin is the mainstay of prophylaxis in dental, oral, respiratory tract, and esophageal procedures in intermediate- and high-risk patients and of intermediate-risk patients undergoing gastrointestinal and genitourinary procedures as it is well-absorbed and still retains significant activity against the targeted pathogens. How long it will remain effective against the enterococci is problematic as these pathogens become more resistant to antimicrobial therapy (Chapter 14). The 1997 guidelines do not mandate but make optional antibiotic coverage for gastrointestinal and genitourinary tract procedures. In patients with a history of minor penicillin allergies, cephalexin or cefadroxil may be used. Otherwise, azithromycin or clarithromycin are

TABLE 6 Medical Procedures for which Endocarditis Prophylaxis Is Recommended

Dental compresses[a]
  Dental extractions
  Dental implants
  Root canals
  Initial placement of orthodontic bands
  Intraligamentary local anesthetic injections
  Periodontal procedures
  Prophylactic cleaning of teeth or implants if bleeding anticipated
  Subgingival placement of antibiotic fibers or strips
Gastrointestinal tract[b]
  Biliary tract surgery
  Endoscopic retrograde cholangiography with biliary obstruction
  Esophageal stricture dilatation
  Sclerotherapy for esophageal varices
  Surgical operations that involve intestinal mucosa
Genitourinary tract
  Cystoscopy
  Prostatic surgery
  Urethral dilatation
Respiratory tract
  Bronchoscopy with a rigid bronchoscope
  Surgical operations that involve respiratory mucosa
  Tonsillectomy and/or adenoidectomy

[a]Prophylaxis recommended for patients with high- and intermediate-risk cardiac conditions.
[b]Prophylaxis recommended for high-risk patients; optional for intermediate-risk patients.
Source: From Ref. 2.

reasonable alternatives. Clindamycin is also proposed as an alternative agent to amoxicillin. The author believes that the use of clindamycin be sharply curtailed because of the epidemic of *Clostridium difficile* colitis (50). Erythromycin has been dropped from the most recent guidelines because of its erratic gastrointestinal absorption (21) and documented failures of prophylaxis (see previous discussion).

Exactly 2.0 g of amoxicillin is currently recommended to be given one hour before the procedure with no postprocedure dose. Avoiding the need for a second dose is aimed at improving compliance. It is justified by somewhat limited human and animal studies that indicate that the preprocedure dosage produces prolonged serum levels, which exceed the minial inhibitory concentration (MIC) of most streptococci. In addition, there appears to be a prolonged inhibitory phase that lasts from six to 14 hours (51,52). Clearly, a more sustained inhibitory effect is produced by a postprocedure dose of antibiotics (2,53). It is the author's practice to do this in patients in high-risk groups such as patients with prosthetic valves in place. Tables 7 and 8 present the specifics of the prophylactic regimens discussed before.

Because PVE is such a catastrophic event, the author believes that whenever possible intravenous prophylactic antibiotics (vancomycin and gentamicin) should be employed. At the least, one postprocedure dose should be given. Linezolid may be an oral alternative to parenteral dosing in high-risk patients, especially the ones with prosthetic valves in place (54).

When unanticipated bleeding occurs, there is some evidence derived from animal studies that providing an appropriate antibiotic within two hours following the procedure will be effective (55). It is important that antibiotic prophylaxis be

TABLE 7 Prophylactic Antibiotic Regimens for Dental/Oral, Respiratory Tract, and Esophageal Procedures

Drug	Dosing regimen
Amoxicillin	2.0 g PO 1 hr before procedure
Ampicillin[a]	2.0 g IM or IV within 30 min before procedure
Azithromycin[b] or Clarithromycin[b]	500 mg PO 1 hr before procedure
Clindamycin[b,c]	600 mg PO 1 hr before procedure
Cephalexin[d] or Cefadroxil[d]	2.0 g PO 1 hr before procedure
Cefazolin[d,e]	1 g IV within 30 min before procedure
Clindamycin[c,e]	600 mg IV within 30 min before procedure
Azithromycin[e,f]	500 mg IV within 30 min before procedure

[a]For patients unable to take oral medications.
[b]For patients allergic to penicillin.
[c]Generally should avoid its use because of risk of *Clostridium difficile* colitis.
[d]For use in patients with minor penicillin allergies.
[e]For use in patients allergic to penicillin and unable to take oral medications.
[f]As a substitute for clindamycin; not in the official 1997 American Heart Association (AHA) guidelines reference.
Abbreviations: IM, intramuscular; IV, intravenous.
Source: From Ref. 2.

given within two hours following the procedure. If four hours elapse, the window of opportunity for prophylaxis has closed.

Amoxicillin and other beta-lactam antibiotics should not be used as prophylaxis in patients who are receiving penicillin for the prevention of rheumatic fever or who have recently been given penicillins and cephalosporins within a few weeks

TABLE 8 Prophylactic Antibiotic Regimens for Genitourinary and Gastrointestinal Procedures

Patients	Antibiotic regimen
High-risk patients	Ampicillin 2.0 g IM or IV within 30 min of starting the procedure; 6 hr later 1.0 g IM or IV or amoxicillin 1.0 g orally + Gentamicin 1.5 mg/kg within 30 min of starting the procedure
High-risk patients allergic to ampicillin/amoxicillin	Vancomycin 1.0 g IV over 1–2 hr; complete infusion within 30 min of starting the procedure + Gentamicin 1.5 mg/kg within 30 min of starting the procedure
Moderate-risk patients	Amoxicillin 2 .0 g PO 1 hr before procedure; ampicillin 2.0 g IM or IV within 30 min of starting the procedure
Moderate-risk patients allergic to ampicillin/ amoxicillin	Vancomycin 1.0 g IV over 1–2 hr; complete infusion within 30 min of starting the procedure

Abbreviations: IM, intramuscular; IV, intravenous; PO, postoral.

of the procedure. Isolates of *S. viridans*, resistant to penicillin, have been recovered from these patients. These resistant *S. viridans* have been documented to cause IE (56). The use of benzathine penicillin, administered monthly, appears to induce penicillin resistance less frequently (57). Withholding penicillins for approximately two weeks will cause the oral flora to revert back to normal (58).

There is a real need to refine the criteria for which preprocedure antimicrobial prophylaxis is absolutely necessary. Patients die from anaphylaxis to the penicillins. Mitral valve prolapse stands as a good example of the potential of overadministration of antibiotic prophylaxis. Clemens and Ransoho estimated that for every two to three cases of IE, associated with MVP, which was prevented, there was one fatal anaphylactic reaction (59). An analysis by Bor and Himmelstein arrived at similar conclusions and advocated for the use of less allergic drugs, such as erythromycin, to provide prophylaxis for this condition (60).

REFERENCES

1. Bouza E, Menasalvas A, Munoz P, et al. Infective endocarditis—a prospective study at the end of the 20th century: new predisposing conditions, new etiologic agents and still a high mortality. Medicine 2001; 80:298.
2. Dajani AS, Taubert KA, Wilson W, et al. Prevention of bacterial endocarditis: recommendations by the American Heart Association. Circulation 1997; 96:358.
3. Gould FK, Elliott TS, Foweraker J, et al. Guidelines for the prevention of endocarditis: Report of the working party of the British society of antimicrobial chemotherapy. J Antimicrob Chemother 2006 (E-pub ahead of print).
3a. Antibacterial prophylaxis for dental, GI and GU procedures. Med Lett Drugs Ther 2005; 47:59.
4. Shulman ST. Prevention of infective endocarditis: the view from the United States. J Antimicrob Chemother 1987; 20(suppl A):111.
5. Durack V. Prevention of infective endocarditis. N Engl J Med 1995; 332:38.
6. Weinstein L, Rubin R. Infective endocarditis—1973. Prog Cardiovasc Dis 1973; 16:239.
7. van der Meer JTM, Thompson J, Valkenburg HA, Michel MF. Epidemiology of bacterial endocarditis in the Netherlands II. Antecedent procedures and use of prophylaxis. Arch Intern Med 1992; 152:1869.
8. Seto TB, Kwiat D, Taira DA, et al. Physicians' recommendations to patients for use of antibiotic prophylaxis to prevent endocarditis. JAMA 2000; 284:68.
9. Boyle N, Gallagher C, Sleeman D. Antibiotic prophylaxis for bacterial endocarditis: a study of knowledge and application of guidelines among dentists and cardiologists. J Ir Dent Assoc 2006; 51:232.
10. Weinstein L, Brusch JL. Prophylaxis. In: The Weinstein L, Brusch JL eds. Infective Endocarditis. New York: Oxford University Press, 1996:322.
11. Brusch JL. Appraisal of the current recommendations for antibiotic prophylaxis of infective endocarditis.APUA Newslett 1999; 17:2.
12. Singh SM, Joyner CD, Alter DA. The importance of echocardiography in physicians' support of endocarditis prophylaxis. Arch Intern Med 2006; 166:549.
13. Bayer AS. New concepts in the pathogenesis and modalities of chemoprophylaxis of native valve endocarditis. Chest 1989; 96:893.
14. Glauser MP, Bernard JP, Moreillon P. Successful single-dose amoxicillin prophylaxis against experimental streptococcal endocarditis: evidence for two mechanisms of protection. J Infect Dis 1983; 147:568.
15. Glauser MP, Francioli P. Relevance of animal models to the prophylaxis of infective endocarditis. J Antimicrob Chemother 1987; 20(suppl A):87.
16. Malverni R, Francioli PB, Glauser MP. Comparison of single and multiple doses of prophylactic antibiotics in experimental streptococcal endocarditis. Circulation 1987; 76:376.
17. Lockhart PB, Brennan MT, Kent ML, et al. Impact of amoxicillin prophylaxis on the incidence, nature and duration of bacteremia in children after intubation and dental procedures. Circulation 2004; 109:2878.

18. Horstkotte D, Rosin H, Friedreichs W, Loogen F. Contribution for choosing the optimal prophylaxis of bacterial endocarditis. Eur Heart J 1987; 8(suppl J):379.

19. Duval X, Alla F, Hoen B, et al. Estimated risk of endocarditis in adults with predisposing cardiac conditions undergoing dental procedures with or without antibiotic prophylaxis. Clin Infect Dis 2006; 42:e102.

20. Durack D, Bisno A, Kaplan A. An apparent failure of endocarditis prophylaxis: analysis of 52 cases submitted to a national registry. JAMA 1983; 250:2318.

21. Meier B, Luthy R, Siegenthaler W. Endokarditis–Pophylaxe mit Amoxicillin, Clindamycin oder Erythromycin. Schweiz Med Wochenschr 1984; 114:1252.

22. Pitcher DW, Papouchado M, Channer KS, et al. Endocarditis prophylaxis: do patients remember advice and know what to do? Br Med J 1986; 293:1539.

23. Caldwell RI, Hurwitz CA, Girod DA. Subacute bacterial endocarditis in children. Am J Dis Child 1971; 122:312.

24. Holbrook WP, Willey RF, Shaw TRD. Dental health in patients susceptible to infective endocarditis. Br Med J 1981; 283:371.

25. Tzukert AA, Leviner E, Sela M. Prevention of infective endocarditis: not by antibiotics alone. Oral Surg, Oral Med, Oral Pathol 1986; 62:385.

26. Everett E, Hirschmann J. Transient bacteremia and endocarditis prophylaxis: a review. Medicine 1977; 56:61.

27. Brusch JL. Infective endocarditis in critical care. In: Cunha B, ed. Infectious Diseases in Critical Care Medicine. New York: Marcel Dekker, 1998:387.

28. Fang G, Keys T, Gentry L. Prosthetic valve endocarditis resulting from nosocomial bacteremia. Ann Intern Med 1993; 119:560.

29. Baddour LM. Twelve year review of recurrent native-valve infective endocarditis: a disease of the modern antibiotic era. Rev Infect Dis 1988; 10:1163.

30. Eliopoulos GM. Enterococcal endocarditis. In: Kaye D, ed. Infective Endocarditis. New York: Raven Press, 1992:209.

31. Doyle EF, Spagnuolo M, Taranta A, et al. The risk of bacterial endocarditis during antirheumatic prophylaxis. JAMA 1967; 2001:129.

32. Chagnac A, Rudnike C, Loebel H. Infectious endocarditis in idiopathic hypertrophic subaortic stenosis: report of three cases and review of the literature. Chest 1982; 81:346.

33. Bonow RO, Carbello B, deLeon AC Jr, et al. ACC/AHA guidelines for the management of patients with valvular heart disease: executive summary: A Report of the American College of Cardiology/American Heart Association Task Force on Practice Guidelines (Committee on Management of Patients with Valvular Heart Disease). Circulation 1998; 98:1949.

34. MacMahon S, Hickey A, Wilcken D. Risk of infective endocarditis in mitral valve prolapse with and without precordial systolic murmurs. Am J Cardiol 1989; 58:105.

35. Clemens JD, Horwitz RI, Jaffe CC, et al. A controlled evaluation of the risk of bacterial endocarditis in persons with mitral-valve prolapse. N Engl J Med 1982; 307:776.

36. Carabello BA. Mitral valve disease. Curr Prob Cardiol 1993; 7:423.

37. Zuppiroli A, Rinaldi M, Kramer-Fox R, et al. Natural history of mitral valve prolapse. Am J Cardiol 1995; 75:1028.

38. Weissman NJ, Pini R, Roman MJ, et al. In vivo mitral valve morphology and motion in mitral valve prolapse. Am J Cardiol 1994; 73:1080.

39. Devereaux RB, Hawkins I, Kramer-Fox R, et al. Complications of mitral valve prolapse: disproportionate occurrence in men and older patients. Am J Med 1986; 81:751.

40. Devereaux RB, Frary CJ, Kramer-Fox R, et al. Cost-effectiveness of infective endocarditis prophylaxis for mitral valve prolapse with or without a mitral regurgitant murmur. Am J Cardiol 1994; 74:1024.

41. Bayer R. Antibiotic prophylaxis and regurgitant murmurs. Letter. Ann Intern Med 1990; 112:148.

42. Sipes JN, Thompson RL, Hook EW. Prophylaxis of infective endocarditis: a re-evaluation. Ann Rev Med 1977; 28:371.

43. McKinsey DS, Ratts TE, Bisno AL. Underlying cardiac lesions in adults with infective endocarditis. The changing spectrum. Am J Med 1987; 82:681.

44. Venezio FR, Westenfelder GO, Cook FV, et al. Infective endocarditis in a community hospital. Arch Intern Med 1982; 142:789.

45. Terpenning MS, Buggy BP, Kauffman CA. Infective endocarditis: clinical features in young and elderly patients. Am J Med 1987; 83:626.
46. Baltch A, Schaffer C, Hammer M. Bacteremia following dental cleaning in patients with and without penicillin prophylaxis. Am Heart J 1982; 104:1135.
47. Goodman J, Kolhouse J, Koenig M. Recurrent endocarditis in an edentulous man. South Med J 1973; 66:352.
48. Hirota WK, Petersen K, Baron TH, et al. Guidelines for antibiotic prophylaxis for GI endoscopy. Gastrointest Endosc 2003; 58:475.
49. Nelson DB, Sanderson SJ, Azar MM. Bacteremia with esophageal dilatation. Gastrointest Endosc 1998; 48:563.
50. Francloli P, Glavser MP. Successful prophylaxis of experimental streptococcal endocarditis with single doses of sublethal concentrations of penicillins. J Antimicrob Chemother 1985; 15:297.
51. Fluckiger U, Francioli P, Blaser J, et al. Role of amoxicillin serum levels for successful prophylaxis of experimental endocarditis due to tolerant streptococci. J Infect Dis 1994; 169:397.
52. Dajani AS, Bawdon RE, Berry MC. Oral amoxicillin as prophylaxis for endocarditis: what is the optimal dose? Clin Infect Dis 1994; 18:157.
53. Fluckiger U, Moreillon P, Blaser J, et al. Stimulation of amoxicillin pharmacokinetics in humans for the prevention of streptococcal endocarditis in rats. Antimicrob Agent Chemother 1994; 38:2846.
54. Athanassopoulos G, Pefanis A, Sakka V, et al. Linezolid prophylaxis against experimental aortic valve endocarditis due to *Streptococcus oralis* or *Enterococcus faecalis*. Antimicrob Agent Chemother 2006; 50:654.
55. Berney P, Francioli P. Successful prophylaxis of experimental streptococcal endocarditis with single-dose amoxicillin administered after bacterial challenge. J Infect Dis 1990; 161:281.
56. Parillo J, Borst G, Mazur M. The endocarditis due to resistant viridans streptococci during oral penicillin chemoprophylaxis. N Engl J Med 1979; 300:294.
57. Sprunt K. Role of antibiotic resistance in bacterial endocarditis. In: Kaplan EL, Taranta AV, eds. Infective Endocarditis. AHA Monograph No. 52 Dallas: American Heart Association, 1997:17.
58. Leviner E, Tzukert AA, Benoliel R, et al. Development of resistance oral viridans streptococci after administration of prophylactic antibiotics: time management in the dental treatment of patients susceptible to infective endocarditis. Oral Surg, Oral Med, Oral Pathol 1987; 64:417.
59. Clemens JD, Ransohoff DR. A quantitative assessment of pre-dental antibiotic prophylaxis for patients with mitral valve prolapse. J Chronic Dis 1984; 37:531.
60. Bor DH, Himmelstein DU. Endocarditis prophylaxis for patients with mitral valve prolapse: a quantitative analysis. Am J Med 1984; 76:711.
61. For Disease Control and Prevention. Guidelines for the prevention of intravascular catheter-related infections. MMWR 2002; 51:1.

17 The Mimics of Endocarditis

Burke A. Cunha
Winthrop University Hospital, Mineola, New York, U.S.A.

OVERVIEW

Endocarditis may be classified clinically by acuteness of onset, whether it involves a native or prosthetic valve, by the host it occurs in, or by the infecting organism. Subacute bacterial endocarditis (SBE) is usually caused by organisms of relatively low virulence and occurs in patients with cardiac valvular damage. As the name suggests, SBE is subacute in onset and is rarely, if ever, a medical emergency. Patients with SBE may be complicated by aseptic embolic phenomenon to the central nervous system coronary arteries, spleen, or kidneys. The most common pathogen in SBE is the viridans streptococci. Any one of the viridans streptococci may cause SBE, and pathogenic potential is proportional to thickness of the mucopolysaccharide capsule. The diagnosis of SBE rests on positive blood cultures due to organisms that are known causes of SBE. The bacteremia in SBE is continuous and blood cultures are persistently positive. Patients with SBE also invariably have a heart murmur if the valves of the heart are involved in the infectious process. Temperatures in SBE are ≤102°F. Peripheral manifestations, Roth spots, splenomegaly, or splinter hemorrhages may also be present, particularly in those individuals who have a long interval between the onset of their symptoms and the diagnosis of endocarditis (1–3).

Acute bacterial endocarditis (ABE) refers to acute endocarditis most often caused by *Staphylococcus aureus*. The onset of ABE, as its name suggests, is acute with temperatures ≥102°F (excluding intravenous drug abusers). ABE is often a medical emergency because it is frequently complicated by heart block, septic embolic phenomenon, that is, brain abscess, septic pulmonary emboli, splenic abscesses, or myocardial abscesses. Because ABE pathogens are virulent, they are capable of attacking normal heart valves, often resulting in valvular dysfunction and acute heart failure. As with SBE, ABE is also characterized by a continuous bacteremia because of *S. aureus*. In contrast to SBE, the murmur of ABE is either new in onset or changes its intensity over time (1,4,5).

There are other variants of infectious endocarditis (IE) including prosthetic valves, that is, prosthetic valve endocarditis (PVE) and "culture-negative endocarditis" (CNE). PVE presents subacutely with low virulent pathogens, for example, SBE or acutely ABE if because of virulent pathogens. The same complications occur in PVE as with native valve SBE or ABE. "Culture-negative endocarditis" is a separate clinical entity. The term "culture-negative endocarditis" should only be applied when the signs/symptoms of endocarditis are in patients with a heart murmur, valvular vegetation, and peripheral manifestations of SBE/ABE. The presence of a murmur, fever, and vegetation by cardiac echocardiography are insufficient to diagnose CNE. It should only be considered if a patient has fever, cardiac vegetation, and heart murmur with peripheral manifestations (1,2,6,7).

MIMICS OF ENDOCARDITIS

The clinical diagnosis of endocarditis is based on fever, heart murmur, high-grade/ continuous bacteremia, vegetation on either transthoracic echocardiography (TTE) or transesophageal echocardiography (TEE) with or without peripheral manifestations. Any disorder that presents itself with one or more of these findings may readily be confused with SBE or ABE. There are many disorders which with a cardiac murmur and fever, without a high grade/continuous bacteremia may mimic SBE or ABE. The disorders most likely to mimic endocarditis include myocarditis, marantic endocarditis, Libman-Sacks endocarditis [because of systemic lupus erythematosus (SLE)], and atrial myxomas. Disorders with Roth spots or splinter hemorrhages include collagen vascular diseases, that is, SLE, severe anemia, Dressler's syndrome, and nail trauma. Splenomegaly with fever may occur with a variety of infectious disorders, but relatively few would be confused diagnostically with SBE or ABE. Acute malaria, although presenting itself with fever, possibly a heart murmur because of severe anemia, or splenomegaly, would rarely, if ever, be confused with endocarditis. By far, the three most common clinical disorders mimicking endocarditis are marantic endocarditis, SLE, and atrial myxomas (1,2,6,8).

Marantic Endocarditis

Marantic endocarditis refers to patients' murmur, cardiac vegetation, and negative blood cultures. Marantic endocarditis may be considered a variant of CNE. Marantic endocarditis, that is, the finding of a murmur and cardiac vegetation in the absence of bacteremia, may occur following treated/untreated SBE/ABE. Vegetations also occur on cardiac valves due to a variety of noninfectious conditions, for example, Libman-Sacks endocarditis of SLE. Clinicians overly depending on echocardiography for the diagnosis of endocarditis may be misled by marantic endocarditis. Vegetations are only of diagnostic significance for valvular infection of they are present in the setting of a high-grade/continuous bacterenia, the hallmark of infective endocarditis. Cardiac vegetations without positive blood cultures are not diagnostic of CNE. Patients with marantic endocarditis are afebrile in contrast to most patients with SBE or ABE who are febrile, even if elderly. The diagnostic approach to the patient with presumed endocarditis should begin with positive blood cultures, that is, high-grade/continuous bacteremia. Blood cultures should be positive in a high percentage (75–100%) of the specimens taken, particularly if the organism cultured is staphylococci. Excluding PVE, *Staphylococcus epidermidis*, and other coagulase-negative staphylococci (CoNS) rarely cause endocarditis on native valves. If CoNS are excluded, then the degree of culture positivity with *S. aureus* and the rapidity of blood culture positivity determine the clinical significance of *S. aureus* bacteremia in relationship to endocarditis. Febrile patients with a cardiac murmur have no other obvious source for staphylococci bacteremia. Patients with *S. aureus* 1/4 or 1/8 blood cultures are not diagnostic of endocarditis. Positive blood cultures with a negative TTE or TEE indicate bacteremia, not endocarditis. Similarly, vegetation on TTE/TEE with negative blood cultures in the absence of peripheral endocarditis manifestations is diagnostic of marantic endocarditis until proven otherwise (3,6,9–12).

Viral Myocarditis

Viral myocarditis may mimic endocarditis. Myocarditis often presents with fever, murmur, and peripheral embolic phenomenon. A heart murmur in viral myocarditis may be related to fever/cardiac dilation. Patients often have cardiomegaly in contrast to patients with endocarditis who usually do not unless they have pre-existing congestive heart failure (CHF). Viral myocarditis occurs most commonly in young adults in contrast to elderly patients with CHF/cardiomegaly that are often present in older patients. The peripheral white blood cell (WBC) count is not highly elevated in SBE. Leukopenia/thrombocytopenia may be present in patients with viral myocarditis in contrast to SBE/ABE. The degree of fever is unhelpful in differentiating viral myocarditis from SBE/ABE. In both viral myocarditis and SBE, the erythrocyte sedimentation rate (ESR) is elevated. The ESR is moderately elevated in viral myocarditis, but may exceed 100 mm/hr in SBE. The elevation of the ESR is a function of time in endocarditis. For this reason, patients with ABE usually have ESRs in the range of 40–60 mm/hr, whereas those with SBE have higher ESR elevations often in the range of 80–120 mm/hr. Echocardiography in patients with viral myocarditis shows no vegetations and blood cultures are negative (excluding skin contaminants). The absence of a high-grade/continuous bacteremia, and lack of vegetation on echocardiography effectively rules out viral myocarditis as a mimic of endocarditis (6,13).

Systemic Lupus Erythematosus

Systemic lupus erythematosus is a multisystem collagen vascular disease easily confused with SBE. Unlike, SBE, the course of SLE is characterized by flares and remissions. SLE patients with flare are more likely to be confused with IE then during remissions. Like endocarditis, flares of SLE are usually accompanied by fever. In an acute SLE flare, temperatures may be ≥102°F mimicking ABE and during remission temperatures with SLE if present are ≤102°F mimicking SBE. In common with SBE, SLE may be accompanied by splenomegaly. Because SLE is a chronic relapsing disorder, SLE is often complicated by the anemia of chronic disease. Patients with SBE frequently have anemia of chronic disease as well. Uncommonly, patients with SLE have "verrucous vegetations" on one or more cardiac valves. These vegetations are termed Libman-Sacks endocarditis in patients with SLE. In Libman-Sacks endocarditis, vegetations are responsible for the murmurs and the vegetations on cardiac echocardiography (6,8,14).

Patients with SLE may be complicated by lupus cerebritis mimicking aseptic emboli in SBE or septic emboli in ABE. They frequently have renal involvement manifested by glomerular nephritis or immune complex-mediated renal insufficiency. Patients with SBE often have renal involvement secondary to infarction, immune complex-mediated renal failure, or focal glomerular nephritis (microscopic hematuria). Systemic lupus erythematosus patients with vasculitis may have tender finger tips mimicking the Osler nodes. However, patients with SLE do not have Janeway lesions typical of ABE. Fundoscopic findings in SLE typically are that of cytoid bodies or cotton wool spots, whereas Roth spots are the usual finding in SBE. Splinter hemorrhages are rare with SLE. Even with Libman-Sacks verricous vegetations, the incidence of endocarditis in SLE is extremely low. Fortunately, the single most important diagnostic criterion in SBE is continuous bacteremia, which is clearly absent in SLE. The absence of high-grade/continuous bacteremia in SLE patients even with fever, heart murmur, vegetation on echocardiography, splenomegaly, and embolic phenomenon clearly distinguishes SBE from SLE (6,8,14).

Atrial Myxomas

Left atrial myxomas are rare but, when present, mimic SBE. Atrial myxomas, particularly, left atrial myxomas, if sessile, can variably obstruct the left ventricular outflow tract, resulting in a murmur. The murmur from a left atrial myxoma may be constant in nonsessile myxomas and may vary in intensity with sessile atrial myxomas. As neoplasms, atrial myxomas are frequently accompanied by fever, a cardinal manifestation of SBE. Atrial myxomas present themselves subacutely, as do patients with SBE, and are often complicated by embolic phenomenon in the same distribution as those with SBE. Emboli to the CNS, spleen, kidneys, or extremities may occur with atrial myxomas, as with SBE. Patients with atrial myxomas have echocardiographic findings that are often confused with the vegetation of endocarditis. In atrial myxoma, some laboratory abnormalities may suggest endocarditis, that is, highly elevated ESR. Among the disorders associated with an ESR ≥100 mm/hr are malignancies, SLE, and SBE. The increased rheumatoid factors (RF) or biologically false-positive VDRLs are not common in SBE laboratory present with atrial myxomas. Noninvasively, atrial myxoma is suggested by the presence of polyclonal gammopathy on serum protein electrophoresis (SPEP). There are relatively few conditions that are associated with a polyclonal gammopathy on SPEP, and only a left atrial myxoma and SLE would be considered in the differential diagnosis of SBE mimics. With atrial myxomas, polyclonal gammopathy of SPEP is present; polyclonal gammopathy is helpful in distinguishing it from SBE. SBE is not associated with a polyclonal gammopathy on SPEP. Patients with atrial myxomas do not have splenomegaly or Roth spots, but often have peripheral splinter hemorrhages. The definitive way to differentiate atrial myxomas from endocarditis is by blood cultures. The incidence of endocarditis with atrial myxomas is exceedingly rare. The absence of a continuous bacteremia in patients with atrial myxoma clearly distinguishes this endocarditis mimic from true infective endocarditis (3,6,15–19).

CONCLUSION

Endocarditis may be mimicked by a variety of noninfectious and infectious disorders. Endocarditis is defined by the presence of an otherwise unexplained high-grade/continuous bacteremia, a cardiac murmur, and a cardiac vegetation on cardiac echocardiography. Because endocarditis is complicated by embolic phenomenon (either aseptic in SBE or septic in ABE), disorders, which are accompanied by embolic phenomenon, may mimic SBE. The disorders most likely to be confused with SBE are marantic endocarditis, SLE, viral myocarditis, and atrial myxomas. These disorders may present with a combination of findings that may initially suggest endocarditis until blood culture results are known (1,3,6,8).

Other disorders that may mimic endocarditis are so rare that they are not common causes of diagnostic confusion, that is, thrombotic thrombocytopenic purpura (TTP). Clinically, TTP presents itself with fever, mental confusion, and anemia, all common manifestations of SBE. However, the anemia of TTP is microangiopathic in contrast to the anemia of SBE, which is the anemia in chronic disease. If the patient is severely anemic in TTP, then splinter hemorrhages and a cardiac murmur may be present, suggesting the possibility of SBE. TTP is easily ruled out as a mimic of endocarditis by the absence of high-grade/continuous bacteremia and the absence of vegetation by TTE or TEE (6).

An important clinical feature that helps to differentiate endocarditis from its mimics is fever. The absence of fever is helpful in distinguishing marantic from infective endocarditis. Marantic endocarditis is a difficult differential diagnostic problem because it has many features in common with IE and may be complicated by embolic phenomena. Because patients with marantic endocarditis have a murmur and vegetation on cardiac echocardiography, the unwary are easily mislead early in the diagnostic process before blood culture results become available. IE is a rare complication with marantic endocarditis. Vegetations on heart valves not because of SBE may represent the residual of antecedent SBE or may be the result of some other process. Systemic lupus erythematosus frequently mimics endocarditis. Patients with SLE often have some of the cardinal findings found of SBE, that is, fever, heart murmur (secondary to fever/anemia), vegetations (Libman-Sacks verrucous vegetations) splenomegaly, renal insufficiency, painful finger tips (mimicing Osler's nodes), and/or emboli to the CNS (SLE cerebritis). These patients may also have an elevated ESR. Systemic vasculitis may be positive for antinuclear cytoplasma antibodies (ANCA) as in SBE (20,21). Fortunately, SBE is rare with Libman-Sacks endocarditis (3,14).

Cardiac tumors, particularly left atrial mxyomas, frequently mimic endocarditis. Atrial myxomas may be present with cardiac echocardiographic findings, which may resemble vegetations. Patients with atrial myxomas have fever and a heart murmur depending upon the location of the myxoma in the left atrium. Patients with atrial myxoma have fever and embolic phenomenon including splinter hemorrhages. In atrial myxomas, the ESR is also highly elevated, frequently ≥100 mm/hr, which is seen in very few conditions, one of which is SBE. Two laboratory tests clearly distinguish atrial myxoma from endocarditis, that is, absence of a continuous bacteremia in atrial myxoma clearly differentiates it from SBE, and polyclonal gammopathy on SPEP. In SBE, the SPEP is normal and high-grade/continuous bacteremia is present. The polyclonal gammopathy on the SPEP and atrial mxyoma represent a polyclonal immune response to the intracardiac tumor and is useful diagnostically in differentiating mxyomas from SBE (6,22,23) (Table 1).

Because the diagnosis of IE rests upon demonstrating an otherwise unexplained high-grade/continuous bacteremia with a cardiac murmur and vegetation, the two tests that discriminate between the mimics of endocarditis and SBE are high-grade/continuous bacteremia and vegetation on cardiac echocardiography. There are pitfalls to be avoided in misinterpreting the significance of blood cultures and valvular vegetations. The most common causes of echocardiographic confusion are valvular calcifications of the aortic/mitral valve and intracardiac tumors.

TABLE 1 Mimics of Infective Endocarditis: Clinical and Laboratory Features

Mimics of endocarditis	Bacteremia	Cardiac vegetation	Fever	Splenomegaly	Emboli	↑ ESR	Abnormal SPEP[a]
Marantic endocarditis	−	+	−	−	±	−	−
Viral myocarditis	−	−	+	−	±	+	−
SLE (Libman-Sacks endocarditis)	−	+	+	±	−	+	+
Atrial myxoma	−	±	+	−	+	+	+
Infectious endocarditis	+	+	+	±	±	+	−

[a]Polyclonal gammopathy on SPEP.
Abbreviations: ESR, erythrocyte sedimentation rate; SLE, systemic lupus erythematosus; SPEP, serum protein electrophoresis.

Blood culture positivity must be interpreted carefully. Up to 25% of peripherally drawn blood cultures may be contaminated with skin flora, for example, streptococci (CoNS, *S. aureus*) during the venipuncture. In a patient without a prosthetic valve, fever, or heart murmur, the presence of 1/4–1/8 positive blood cultures with an organism that is part of the normal skin flora has no diagnostic significance. Even 2/4 blood cultures with *S. aureus* may represent contamination if the venipuncture was performed with poor aseptic technique, but repeat blood cultures will be negative.

Certain organisms have diagnostic significance even if they are present in only a single blood culture associated with endocarditis, that is, *Listeria, Brucella, Hemophilus* spp., and the like. The significance of other organisms in blood cultures is difficult to interpret, that is, enterococci. Enterococci may contaminate blood cultures during the venipuncture process because of the proximity in bed-ridden patients of rectum/fecal flora and the geographical proximity of the anticubital fossa. Differentiating enterococcal bacteremia from a gastrointestinal or genitourinary source in a patient with a pre-existing heart murmur may be a difficult diagnostic problem. Excluding these situations, the presence of continuous bacteremia in the absence of any other intravascular focus of infection is the fundamental first step in the diagnosis of endocarditis (1–3,24).

The secondary confirmatory step is to demonstrate cardiac vegetation by cardiac echocardiography. In spite of the increased sensitivity and specificity of TEE over TTE, it is preferable to screen patients with positive blood cultures suggesting SBE by TTE instead of a TEE. Transesophageal echocardiography is invasive and potentially dangerous and more expensive than TTEs. Used for the diagnosis of endocarditis, TEE is excellent in ruling in or ruling out endocarditis and normal valves. It has an advantage when a perivalvular abscess is suspected or if the patient has PVE. If the patient with suspected SBE, has a completely negative TTE in terms of there being no vegetations present, then the TEE adds no additional information. Conversely, if the TTE has questionable vegetation, then it is not unreasonable to get a TEE to clarify the situation and determine if vegetation is actually present. It should not be used as a screening tool for the reasons mentioned, and a totally negative TTE for vegetations has sufficient sensitivity and specificity to be rest assured that the patient does not have a cardiac vegetation, and indeed does not have endocarditis (25–27).

Indium scanning has been used in the diagnosis of SBE. Enhanced indium uptake in the cardiac area depends somewhat on vegetation size. In ABE, indium scans are unhelpful diagnostically and are negative even in the presence of large vegetations. Gallium or indium scanning may be helpful in the diagnosis of viral myocarditis (6,13,28,29).

The most common mimic of endocarditis because of SLE, myocarditis, myxomas, or marantic endocarditis, must be differentiated from SBE/ABE as well as CNE. Because CNE is infectious as a result of fastidious organisms, clinicians should be particularly careful to avoid confusing marantic endocarditis and CNE. In contrast to SBE/ABE, bacteremia is not present in marantic endocarditis or CNE, but both may present with a murmur, vegetation on cardiac echocardiography, and embolic phenomenon (30–33). Fever favors the diagnosis of CNE, but a definitive diagnosis depends on identifying the infectious agent of CNE by special culture techniques for fastidious organisms, for example, *Legionella, Brucella*, fungi, or by serologic tests, for example, *Chlamydia psittaci* and Q-fever (1–3,6,30–33).

ILLUSTRATIVE CASES OF MIMICS OF ENDOCARDITIS

The diagnosis of endocarditis depends on the presence of three findings: continuous/high-grade bacteremia (due to a known endocarditis pathogen), heart murmur, and vegetation as demonstrated by cardiac echocardiography. If any of these conditions are absent, the patient does not have endocarditis. A low-grade or noncontinuous bacteremia may represent skin contamination during venipuncture when the blood cultures are collected or a transient bacteremia. The presence of a murmur is necessary for the diagnosis of endocarditis. Finally, vegetation must be demonstrated by cardiac echocardiography. Mimics of endocarditis occur when one or more of these necessary pre-requisites are missing. For example, vegetation without a heart murmur or high-grade/continuous bacteremia is not indicative of endocarditis. Even the presence of a heart murmur plus vegetation in the absence of a continuous/high-grade bacteremia is not diagnostic of endocarditis. *Staphylococcus aureus*, *S. epidermidis*, or *Streptococcus viridans* bacteremias which are not high-grade (3/4 or 4/4)/continuous are diagnostic of endocarditis when a murmur and cardiac vegetation are present. The following illustrative cases do not fulfill the three necessary clinical requisites for the diagnosis of endocarditis and for this reason may be considered mimics of endocarditis.

Illustrative Case # 1 ■ Patient # 1 is a 58-year-old male who is admitted to the hospital for rate control of his atrial flutter/fibrillation. In the process, he has a peripheral intravenous line inserted and he developed phlebitis. His peripheral intravenous line was discontinued. Blood cultures were intermittently positive (1/2, 0/2, 2/2, 2/2, 2/2, 0/4) during the first week of his hospitalization. He had a history of alcoholism and myxomatous degeneration of his mitral valve years before admission. He had a mitral valve repair and prosthetic ring (not an inserted prosthetic valve). His WBC count was 11 K/mm^3 and his ESR was 37 mm/hr. He had no heart murmur. Cardiac echocardiogram (TEE) after a week and a half of his hospitalization was negative for vegetations.

Commentary on Case # 1 ■ Because the patient had a pre-existing cardiac condition and intermittently positive blood cultures, the possibility of ABE was entertained. Against the diagnosis of ABE was the absence of a continuous/high-grade *S. aureus* bacteremia. Appropriately, 20% of positive blood cultures in hospitals are because of skin contaminants, that is, *S. aureus*- or *S. epidermidis*-introduced during venipuncture. Because his positive blood cultures did not represent a continuous/high-grade bacteremia, they were regarded as nondiagnostic for ABE. *Staphylococcus aureus* bacteremias from peripheral intravenous lines are not associated with endocarditis, but *S. aureus* bacteremias from central intravenous lines have ABE potential. His WBC count and ESR were because of his phlebitis. The ESR in *S. aureus* ABE is usually 50–80 mm/hr. Even though the patient had an abnormal mitral valve, the abnormality was clinically insignificant without a cardiac murmur. Transesophageal echocardiography effectively ruled out *S. aureus* ABE. Peripheral intravenous line infections with positive *S. aureus* blood cultures may mimic ABE but lack the necessary diagnostic requisites as the described case.

Illustrative Case # 2 ■ The patient is a 48-year-old female with a long-standing history of SLE and was admitted to the hospital with fevers and pleuritic chest pain. Her WBC count was 4 K/mm^3 and her ESR was 80 mm/hr. A regurgitant heart murmur was heard at the base. Echocardiography revealed vegetation on the mitral valve. Blood cultures were negative. The patient was thought to have endocarditis on the basis of fever, high ESR, cardiac murmur, and cardiac vegetation on echocardiography.

Commentary on Case # 2 ■ The patient was presented with a flare of her long-standing SLE. Liebman-Sacks endocarditis is a variant of marantic endocarditis that occurs in some patients with SLE. Two of the three criteria for endocarditis were fulfilled, that is, heart murmur and vegetation. However, the third critical factor was absent, that is, a continuous/high-grade bacteremia, which effectively ruled out the diagnosis of endocarditis. It would seem that SLE patients with Liebman-Sacks endocarditis would have a high incidence of infective endocarditis, but this not the case. Infective endocarditis in the presence of Liebman-Sacks vegetations is extremely rare.

Illustrative Case # 3 ■ The patient is a 59-year-old male who was presented with fever, heart murmur, and splinter hemorrhages on the extremities. The patient was admitted with the probable diagnosis of SBE. The patient's WBC count was 12.8 K/mm^3 and his ESR was 120 mm/hr. Blood cultures were drawn. Cardiac echocardiography revealed vegetation on the mitral valve. Serum protein electrophoresis revealed a polyclonal gammopathy. The remainder of his laboratory tests was unremarkable except for a highly elevated serum ferritin level. Blood cultures were incubated for two weeks, but remained negative for growth.

Commentary on Case # 3 ■ The patient was present with possible endocarditis. In favor of the diagnosis of SBE were heart murmur and cardiac vegetation. One of the peripheral manifestations of endocarditis was present, that is, splinter hemorrhages. One key diagnostic requisite is missing which effectively rules the diagnosis of endocarditis, that is, negative blood cultures. The highly elevated ESR (>100 mm/hr) is consistent with collagen-associated diseases, malignancy, drug fevers, abscesses, osteomyelitis, or SBE. Laboratory abnormalities suggest an alternate diagnosis, that is, the SPEP and the highly elevated ferritin suggests a neoplasm. In the absence of an extracardiac malignancy, polyclonal gammopathy on the SPEP and elevated ferritin levels suggests the presence of an atrial myxoma, which was present in this case. Atrial myxoma is a common mimic of infective endocarditis because of the frequent presence of a murmur, highly elevated ESR, and peripheral manifestations, that is, splinter hemorrhages. Patients with SBE do not have a gammopathy polyclonal pattern on SPEP, nor do they have elevated serum ferritin levels, which were the clues to the diagnosis in this case. Once again, negative blood cultures effectively ruled out the diagnosis of IE.

REFERENCES

1. Weinstein L, Brusch JL, eds. Infective Endocarditis. New York: Oxford University Press, 1996.
2. Kaye D, ed. Infective Endocarditis. 2nd ed. New York: Raven Press, 1992.
3. Oram S, ed. Clinical Heart Disease. Philadelphia: F.A. Davis Company, 1971.
4. Cunha BA, Gill MV, Lazar J. Acute infective endocarditis. Infect Dis Clin North Am 1996; 10:811–834.
5. Kim N, Lazar J, Cunha BA. Temperatures ≥102°F as a prognostic feature of acute bacterial endocarditis. Infect Dis Pract 1999; 23:90–92.
6. Braunwald E, Fauci AS, Kasper DL, Hauser SL, Longo DL, Jameson JL, eds. Harrison's Principles of Internal Medicine. 15th ed. New York: McGraw-Hill, 2001.
7. Vlessis AA, Bolling SF, eds. Endocarditis: A Multidisciplinary Approach to Modern Treatment. New York: Futura Publishing Company Inc., 1999.
8. Rosenblum G, Carsons SE. Mimics of endocarditis. In: Cunha BA, ed. Infectious Diseases in Critical Care Medicine. New York: Marcel Dekker Inc., 1998:435–444.
9. Mugge A, Daniel WG, Haverich A, et al. Diagnosis of noninfective cardiac mass lesions by two-dimensional echocardiography. Comparison of the transthoracic and transesophageal approaches. Circulation 1991; 83:70–78.
10. Lutas EM, Roberts RB, Devereux RB, et al. Relation between the presence of echocardiographic vegetations and the complication rate in infective endocarditis. Am Heart J 1986; 112:107–113.

11. Kooiker JC, MacLean JM, Sumi SM. Cerebral embolism, marantic endocarditis, and cancer. Arch Neurol 1976; 33:260–264.
12. Young RS, Zalneraitis EL. Marantic endocarditis in children and young adults: clinical and pathological findings. Stroke 1981; 12:635–639.
13. Cooper LT Jr, ed. Myocarditis: From Bench to Bedside. New Jersey: Humana Press, 2003.
14. Wallace DJ, Hahn BH, eds. Dubois' Lupus Erythematosus. 5th ed. Baltimore: Williams & Wilkins, 1997.
15. Feldman AR, Keeling JH. Cutaneous manifestations of atrial myxoma. J Am Acad Dermatol 1989; 21:1080–1084.
16. Markel ML, Waller BF, Armstrong WF. Cardiac myxoma: a review. Medicine (Baltimore) 1987; 66:114–125.
17. Pinede L, Duhaut P, Loire R. Clinical presentation of left atrial cardiac myxoma: a series of 112 consecutive cases. Medicine 2001; 80:159–172.
18. Reinen K. Cardiac myxomas. N Engl J Med 1995; 333:1610–1617.
19. Sanyay G. Infected cardiac myxoma case report and literature review. Medicine 1998; 77:337–344.
20. Cunha BA. Diagnostic implications of ANCA associated diseases. Infect Dis Pract 2002; 26:158–159.
21. de Corla-Souza A, Cunha BA. Streptococcal viridans bacterial endocarditis associated with anti-neutrophil cytoplasmic autoantibodies (ANCA). Heart Lung 2003; 32:140–143.
22. Cunha BA. Polyclonal gammopathy on SPEP. Infect Dis Pract 1996; 20:39–40.
23. Cunha BA. Diagnostic significance of non-specific laboratory tests in infectious diseases. In: Gorbach SL, Bartlett JB, Blacklow NR, eds. Infectious Diseases in Medicine and Surgery. 3rd ed. Philadelphia: W.B. Saunders Co., 2002:158–165.
24. Bates DW, Goldman L, Lee TH. Contaminant blood cultures and resource utilization: the true consequences of false-positive results. JAMA 1991; 265:365–369.
25. Rubenson DS, Tucker CR, Stinson EG. The use of echocardiography in diagnosing culture-negative endocarditis. Circulation 1981; 64:641–646.
26. Wong D, Chandraratna AN, Wishnow RM, et al. Clinical implications of large vegetations in infectious endocarditis. Arch Intern Med 1983; 143:1874–1877.
27. Mugge A, Daniel WG, Frank G, et al. Echocardiography in infectious endocarditis: reassessment of prognostic implications of vegetation size determined by the transthoracic and transesophageal approach. J Am Coll Cardiol 1989; 14:631–638.
28. Oates E, Sarno RC. Detection of bacterial endocarditis with indium-111 labeled leukocytes. Clin Nucl Med 1988; 13:691–693.
29. McDermott BP, Mohan S, Thermidor M, et al. Acute bacterial endocarditis: the lack of diagnostic value of the indium scan. Am J Med 2004; 117:621–623.
30. Cannaday PB, Sanford JP. Negative blood cultures in infective endocarditis: a review. South Med J 1976; 69:1420–1424.
31. Croney D, Chandraratna PN, Wishnow R, et al. Common implications of large vegetations in infective endocarditis. Arch Intern Med 1983; 143:1874–1877.
32. Pesanti EL, Smith IM. Infective endocarditis with negative blood cultures: an analysis of 52 cases. Am J Med 1979; 66:43–50.
33. Van Scoy RE. Culture-negative endocarditis. Mayo Clin Proc 1982; 57:149–154.

Index

About the Editor

John L. Brusch is associate chief of medicine, Cambridge Health Alliance, Massachusetts, and medical director, Somerville Hospital, Internal Medicine Associates of Somerville, Massachusetts, U.S.A. He is also chief of medicine, Youville Hospital, Cambridge, Massachusetts, and assistant professor of medicine, Harvard Medical School, Cambridge, Massachusetts, U.S.A. A fellow of the American College of Physicians, Dr. Brusch is a member of the American Society of Microbiology and the Infectious Disease Society of America. He serves on the editorial boards of *Infectious Disease Practice* and *e-Medicine*. Dr. Brusch received the M.D. degree from Tufts Medical School, Boston, Massachusetts, U.S.A.